DATE DUE

APR 2 0 2005	
NOV 2 3 2005	
MAR 0 1 2006	

BRODART, CO.   Cat. No. 23-221-003

OPERATIVE ANATOMY

Second Edition

OPERATIVE ANATOMY

Second Edition

Carol E.H. Scott-Conner, M.D., PH.D., M.B.A.
Professor and Head
Department of Surgery
Professor
Anatomy & Cell Biology
University of Iowa
Roy J. and Lucille A. Carver College of Medicine
Iowa City, Iowa

David L. Dawson, PH.D.
Senior Lecturer of Anatomy
Faculty of Life Sciences
University of Dundee
Dundee, Scotland

with illustrations by
Mary K. Shirazi
Gary G. Wind, M.D., F.A.C.S.

LIPPINCOTT WILLIAMS & WILKINS
A **Wolters Kluwer** Company

Philadelphia • Baltimore • New York • London
Buenos Aires • Hong Kong • Sydney • Tokyo

Acquisitions Editor: Lisa McAllister
Developmental Editor: Jenny Kim
Production Editor: Steven P. Martin
Manufacturing Manager: Benjamin Rivera
Cover Designer: Mark Lerner
Compositor: TechBooks
Printer: Maple Press

© 2003 by LIPPINCOTT WILLIAMS & WILKINS
530 Walnut Street
Philadelphia, PA 19106 USA
LWW.com

Printed in the USA

Library of Congress Cataloging-in-Publication Data

Scott-Conner, Carol E. H.
    Operative anatomy / Carol E. H. Scott-Conner, David L. Dawson ; with
illustrations by Mary K. Shirazi, Gary G. Wind.—2nd ed.
        p. ; cm.
Includes bibliographical references and index.
    ISBN 0-7817-3529-7
    1. Anatomy, Surgical and topographical—Atlases.
    [DNLM: 1. Surgical Procedures, Operative—methods. 2. Anatomy,
Regional. WO 500 S425o 2002] I. Dawson, David L. II. Title.
    QM531 .S42 2002b
    611—dc21   2002067541

Care has been taken to confirm the accuracy of the information presented and
to describe generally accepted practices. However, the authors, editors, and
publisher are not responsible for errors or omissions or for any consequences from
application of the information in this book and make no warranty, expressed or
implied, with respect to the currency, completeness, or accuracy of the contents of
the publication. Application of this information in a particular situation remains the
professional responsibility of the practitioner.
    The authors, editors, and publisher have exerted every effort to ensure that
drug selection and dosage set forth in this text are in accordance with current
recommendations and practice at the time of publication. However, in view of
ongoing research, changes in government regulations, and the constant flow of
information relating to drug therapy and drug reactions, the reader is urged to
check the package insert for each drug for any change in indications and dosage
and for added warnings and precautions. This is particularly important when the
recommended agent is a new or infrequently employed drug.
    Some drugs and medical devices presented in this publication have Food and
Drug Administration (FDA) clearance for limited use in restricted research
settings. It is the responsibility of the health care provider to ascertain the FDA
status of each drug or device planned for use in their clinical practice.

10 9 8 7 6 5 4 3 2 1

To the Memory of
Robert L. Bradley, MD PhD, FACS Surgeon,
anatomist, teacher, friend

Contents

Section I. The Head and Neck

THE FACE

HEAD AND NECK ENDOSCOPY

THE MIDLINE AND STRUCTURES APPROACHED THROUGH THE MIDLINE

THE LATERAL NECK AND STRUCTURES APPROACHED FROM THE SIDE

Section IV. The Abdominal Region

BASIC ABDOMINAL PROCEDURES AND THE ABDOMEN IN GENERAL

THE UPPER GASTROINTESTINAL TRACT AND STRUCTURES OF THE LEFT UPPER QUADRANT

THE LIVER, BILIARY TRACT, AND PANCREAS

THE SMALL AND LARGE INTESTINE

THE PELVIS

THE RETROPERITONEUM

THE INGUINAL REGION

Contributors

Beth A. Ballinger, M.D. *Assistant Professor and Staff Physician, Division of Vascular Surgery, Department of Surgery, University of Iowa, Roy J. and Lucille A. Carver College of Medicine, Iowa City, Iowa*

Phillip C. Camp, M.D. *House Staff Fellow, Division of Cardiothoracic Surgery, Department of Surgery, University of Iowa, Roy J. and Lucille A. Carver College of Medicine, Iowa City, Iowa*

Adam J. Dinnewitzer, M.D. *Research Fellow, Department of Colorectal Surgery, Cleveland Clinic Florida, Weston, Florida*

M. Victoria Gerken, M.D. *1821 West Meadow Avenue, Suite A, Visalia, California 93277*

Sean P. Hedican, M.D. *Assistant Professor, Division of Urology, Department of Surgery, University of Wisconsin-Madison, University of Wisconsin Hospitals and Clinics, Madison, Wisconsin*

Jamal J. Hoballah, M.D. *Professor, Division of Vascular Surgery, Department of Surgery, University of Iowa, Roy J. and Lucille A. Carver College of Medicine, Iowa City, Iowa*

James R. Howe, M.D. *Associate Professor, Director, Endocrine Surgery, Department of Surgery, University of Iowa, Roy J. and Lucille A. Carver College of Medicine, Iowa City, Iowa*

Peter R. Jochimsen, M.D. *Professor Emeritus, Section of Surgical Oncology, Department of Surgery, University of Iowa, Roy J. and Lucille A. Carver College of Medicine, Iowa City, Iowa*

G. Patrick Kealey, M.D., F.A.C.S., F.C.C.M. *Professor, Department of Surgery, University of Iowa, Roy J. and Lucille A. Carver College of Medicine, Iowa City, Iowa*

Kemp H. Kernstine, M.D., Ph.D. *Associate Professor, Division of Cardiothoracic Surgery, Department of Surgery, University of Iowa, Roy J. and Lucille A. Carver College of Medicine, Iowa City, Iowa*

Timothy F. Kresowik, M.D. *Professor, Division of Vascular Surgery, Department of Surgery, University of Iowa, Roy J. and Lucille A. Carver College of Medicine, Iowa City, Iowa*

James W. Maher, M.D., F.A.C.S. *Professor, Section of Gastrointestinal Surgery, Department of Surgery, University of Iowa, Roy J. and Lucille A. Carver College of Medicine, Iowa City, Iowa*

Amanda M. Metcalf, M.D. *Professor, Section of Gastrointestinal Surgery, Department of Surgery, University of Iowa, Roy J. and Lucille A. Carver College of Medicine, Iowa City, Iowa*

Stephen C. Rayhill, M.D. *Assistant Professor and Director of Kidney and Pancreas Transplantation, Division of Transplant Surgery, Department of Surgery, University of Iowa, Roy J. and Lucille A. Carver College of Medicine, Iowa City, Iowa*

Isaac Samuel, M.D., F.R.C.S. *Assistant Professor, Section of Gastrointestinal Surgery, Department of Surgery, University of Iowa, Roy J. and Lucille A. Carver College of Medicine, Iowa City, Iowa*

W. John Sharp, M.D. *Associate Professor, Division of Vascular Surgery, Department of Surgery, University of Iowa, Roy J. and Lucille A. Carver College of Medicine, Iowa City, Iowa*

Kenneth B. Simon, M.D., M.B.A. *Medical Officer and Consultant, Centers for Medicare and Medicaid Services, Baltimore, Maryland*

Timothy L. Van Natta, M.D.   *Fellow, Division of Cardiothoracic Surgery, Department of Surgery, University of Iowa, Roy J. and Lucille A. Carver College of Medicine, Iowa City, Iowa*

Steven D. Wexner, M.D., F.A.C.S., F.R.C.S.   *Professor, The Cleveland Clinic Foundation Health Sciences Center of the Ohio State University, Clinical Professor, Department of Surgery, University of South Florida, College of Medicine, Chairman and Residency Program Director and Chief of Staff, Department of Colorectal Surgery, Cleveland Clinic Florida, Weston, Florida*

Richard D. Williams, M.D.   *Professor and Chair, Department of Urology, University of Iowa, Roy J. and Lucille A. Carver College of Medicine, Iowa City, Iowa*

You Min Wu, M.D.   *Associate Professor, Chair and Director, Division of Transplant Surgery, Department of Surgery, University of Iowa, Roy J. and Lucille A. Carver College of Medicine, Iowa City, Iowa*

Foreword

It is a privilege to introduce this fine and literary volume. It comes at a time when the hours of instruction in gross anatomy that medical students receive have been gradually but drastically reduced in many, if not most, medical schools, often by at least one-half that of thirty years ago. Formal instruction in embryology virtually disappeared from some curricula but has recently been partially restored.

To be sure, different medical specialists have different needs for precise anatomical knowledge. Thus, a significant reduction in gross anatomy hours and detail for the majority of medical students was doubtless justified, as the rise in other disciplines such as genetics, molecular biology, psychiatry, and still others laid claim to increased classroom attention. The surgeon's need for precise anatomical knowledge, however, has not decreased. In fact, it has increased, as mini-invasive surgery, in which the first author has special expertise, has exploded worldwide. Incomplete or imprecise knowledge of the regional anatomy involved in a given operation can result in severe injuries and devastating complications. Hence, the need for this operative anatomy atlas by a practicing academic surgeon, Dr. Carol Scott-Conner, and a professional anatomist, Dr. David L. Dawson, is clear. Their intimate collaboration over a period of some years during and after which Dr. Scott-Conner took her second doctorate degree, in anatomy, has culminated in a volume practical not only for medical students and residents but also for practicing surgeons who may need to refresh their knowledge of regional anatomy.

But, while operative anatomy remains the central focus, this book conveys much additional information and guidance and many admonitions—all of great value. Operative techniques for over 101 procedures, involving six regions of the body, are detailed. With each operation, the discussion is divided into "anatomic points" and "technical points." Operative safeguards and potential errors are stressed. Up-to-date references appear at the end of each section. Normal organ function and its preservation or restoration after surgery are emphasized throughout.

The major strength of the work is represented by the line drawings developed with Michael P. Schenk, James Goodman, Myriam E. Kirkman, Steven H. Oh, Charles Boyter, David J. Mascaro, and Mary K. Shirazi, medical illustrators.

This writer is confident that Operative Anatomy will be received enthusiastically and will quickly become a standard source in its field.

James D. Hardy
Professor of Surgery Emeritus
Department of Surgery
University of Mississippi Medical Center
Jackson, Mississippi

Preface

The challenge in revising a text like *Operative Anatomy* lies not in deciding which procedures to add, but rather in choosing those to delete. Can the author assume, for example, that vagotomy is an obsolete operation? Not yet. What about lumbar sympathectomy? Safest to include these procedures and hope for the clemency of the publisher.

Some of the operations in this text are infrequently performed, having been supplanted by other therapies—surgery for peptic ulcer disease, for example, or for bleeding esophageal varices. And yet there is still the occasional patient for whom these operations are appropriate. If a surgeon cannot turn to a reference such as *Operative Anatomy* for the anatomic and technical details of these procedures, where then?

Hence, very little has been deleted. Some material has been condensed, some has been changed, and much has been added. The first edition had 72 chapters; the new edition has 101. Eighteen new authors have enriched this edition with their contributions and 277 new pieces of art have been added.

As with the first edition, the goal has been to provide the surgeon—whether trainee or experienced—with a reference for both the surgical technique and the relevant anatomy. Emphasis has been placed upon proven, mainstream techniques rather than "how I do it", and references are included for alternative or infrequently employed maneuvers.

Carol EH Scott-Conner M.D., Ph.D., M.B.A.
Iowa City, Iowa

Preface to the First Edition

To paraphrase the familiar proverb "necessity is the mother of invention," *frustration is the genesis of books.* As a surgical resident, the first author was often frustrated because the regional gross anatomy studied as a freshman in medical school had too often been forgotten or was inadequate or inappropriate for the procedures to be done the next day. Various surgical atlases and descriptions were of some help with complex procedures, but these often ignored the anatomy relevant to common procedures that all residents must perform.

The second author, trained as a traditional gross anatomist, also became frustrated when attempting to develop surgical anatomy programs based upon procedures which, although commonplace to surgical residents, had not been included in his training. Moreover, he discovered that dissection in the gross anatomy lab was vastly different, both in technique and in concept, from that practiced by surgeons. Also daunting was the realization that the anatomy taught in such anatomy courses was often inappropriate for a single medical discipline, such as surgery. Finally, he, like most traditional anatomists, was only vaguely familiar with the technical aspects of the many procedures required of developing surgeons.

In light of these frustrations, this book was developed to provide a concise reference to the relevant operative anatomy of procedures encountered by most general surgery residents. We also expect that this text will be useful to medical students rotating through surgery. Finally, we hope that this book will be of value to anatomy instructors and to surgeons who would like a quick review of the anatomy germane to common procedures.

The volume is divided into sections based on anatomic regions, permitting the curious user a rapid review of the relevant operative anatomy of a given region. In each section, individual chapters present technical anatomic considerations for specific operative procedures. The illustrations are designed to show both the topographic and regional anatomy, as well as to focus on the anatomy visualized as the procedure progresses. The text is divided into technical and anatomic points, for successful surgery depends on a knowledge of both. At the end of each section, selected references are provided for the reader who is interested in learning more. These carefully selected entries are, in our opion, benchmark articles. Lastly, appreciating the frustrations inherent in learning the technical aspects of general surgery, we have included an appendix that describes common surgical instruments and their use. Because this text is intended for surgeons-in-training and for practicing surgeons, we have used terminology consistent with current surgical usage. In some cases this corresponds to Nomina Anatomica, but in many cases it does not.

This work is not intended to be all-inclusive, either anatomically or surgically. Rather, our aim is to enable the reader to review the anatomy necessary to perform successfully those procedures that form the core of most general surgery residency programs—procedures that comprise the "bread and butter" of a general surgeon's practice.

Carol Scott-Conner, M.D., Ph.D., M.B.A.
David L. Dawson, Ph.D.

Acknowledgments

The authors wish to thank Dr. James D. Hardy and Dr. Robert S. Rhodes for their enthusiasm and advice during the preparation of the first edition.

Katherine Carolan and Jenny Kim provided invaluable editorial assistance during the preparation of this revised edition.

Lisa McAllister, wise and patient editor, has shepherded this book through two editions.

Finally, we thank our students, residents, and co-workers for their patience. The first author gives special thanks to Dr. Harry F. Conner, whose love and support makes all of this possible.

OPERATIVE ANATOMY

Second Edition

SECTION I

The Head and Neck

This anatomically complex region is presented in four sections: the face and parotid region (Chapter 1), endoscopy of the upper respiratory tract (Chapter 2), the midline of the neck and structures approached through the midline (Chapters 3 through 7), and the lateral neck and structures approached from the side (Chapters 8 through 13). Within each section, procedures commonly performed by general surgeons are used to illustrate regional anatomy. For descriptions of more complex procedures, the reader should consult an atlas of plastic surgery or surgery of the head and neck (see the references listed at the end of Part 1).

REFERENCES

1. Lore JM. *An atlas of head and neck surgery.* 3rd ed. Philadelphia: WB Saunders, 1998. (This classic text provides detailed information on specialized surgical techniques.)
2. Smith JW, Aston SJ, eds. *Grabb and Smith's plastic surgery.* 4th ed. Boston: Little, Brown, 1991. (A brief but comprehensive overview of plastic surgery, this book includes information on suturing facial lacerations and local flaps.)

THE FACE

Facial incisions are designed to preserve facial symmetry and motion and to minimize scarring. Elective incisions to remove small skin tumors should lie, whenever possible, in natural skin "wrinkle lines" (Fig. 1). Generally, these lines run perpendicular to the underlying muscles of facial expression, as they are formed by the repetitive pleating of the skin caused by the action of these muscles. Scars that fall in these lines will be less conspicuous than those that cross these lines. Traumatic lacerations that cross these lines can sometimes be debrided or modified by Z-plasty to conform to natural wrinkle lines.

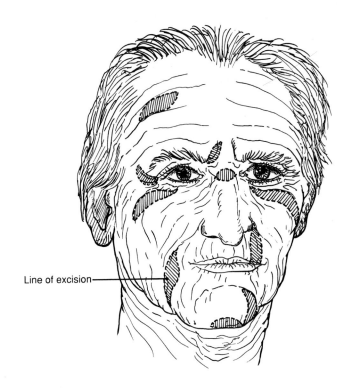

Line of excision

Approximate the eyebrow and vermilion border of the lip with special precision because even a small degree of malalignment will be permanently obvious. Never shave the eyebrow as regrowth of eyebrow hair is unpredictable.

The muscles of facial expression (Fig. 2) are innervated by the seventh cranial nerve, aptly named the facial nerve. The anatomy of the facial nerve and parotid region are illustrated in Chapter 1.

Deep lacerations of the cheek may divide branches of the facial nerve or the parotid (Stensen's) duct. Evaluate nerve function by asking the patient to raise and lower the eyebrows (temporal branches of the facial nerve), close the eyes tightly (zygomatic branches),

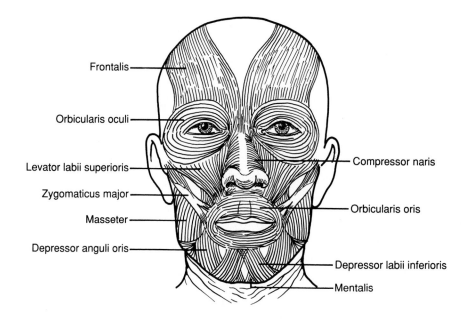

and smile (zygomatic and buccal branches). If a nerve injury is diagnosed, attempt primary repair.

Look inside the mouth, gently retracting the cheek with a tongue blade, and identify the internal opening of the parotid duct as a small punctum opposite the maxillary second molar. Cannulate this with a fine Silastic tube. The appearance of the tube within the wound confirms injury to the duct. Identify both ends of the duct, repairing it with fine, interrupted sutures of an absorbable material. Use the Silastic tube to stent the repair.

Close deep lacerations in layers, carefully approximating muscle, fascia, and skin. Complex injuries involving muscle, nerve, or the parotid duct are best repaired in the operating room.

REFERENCES

1. Kreissl CJ. The selection of appropriate lines for elective surgical incisions. *Plast Reconstr Surg* 1951;8:1. (This brief paper discusses the rationale for choosing various incisions to minimize scarring.)
2. Schultz RC. Soft tissue injuries of the face. In: Smith JW, Aston SJ, eds. *Grabb and Smith's plastic surgery*. 4th ed. Boston: Little, Brown, 1991:325–345.

CHAPTER 1

Parotidectomy

The parotid gland is divided into a superficial lobe and a deep lobe for purposes of surgical dissection. Because 70% to 80% of the parotid tissue lies in the superficial lobe, most tumors, whether benign or malignant, arise in this lobe. Superficial lobectomy is the standard treatment for small benign tumors. Simple enucleation is unwise, even when technically feasible, because even histologically benign tumors are likely to recur. A recurrent tumor is much more difficult to resect with preservation of the facial nerve and is more likely to be malignant.

The safe performance of superficial parotidectomy involves careful identification and preservation of the facial nerve and its branches (see Fig. 1.1A). Total parotidectomy is sometimes required when the deep lobe is involved. This procedure is briefly described in Fig. 1.5. More complex problems, including reconstruction of branches of the facial nerve, are covered in the references at the end of this chapter. In this chapter, the anatomy of the parotid region is illustrated as it is demonstrated during the performance of parotidectomy.

Positioning the Patient (Fig. 1.1)

Technical Points

Position the patient supine on the operating table. General anesthesia is preferred; however, avoid muscle relaxants, so that, if necessary, nerve function can be assessed intraoperatively. Place the operating table in a head-up position to improve exposure and minimize bleeding. Turn the head to the contralateral side and slightly hyperextend the neck to enhance exposure of the preauricular region. Place a cotton plug in the external ear to prevent blood accumulation within the external auditory meatus and on the eardrum. Drape an operative field that includes the external ear and mastoid process, the neck, and the angle of the mouth and the lateral palpebral commissure of the eye. Motion of the angle of the mouth or eyelid in response to stimulation of facial nerve branches may assist in the dissection.

Plan the preauricular skin incision so that it lies in a skin fold (Fig. 1.1B). Draw an incision in the skin fold anterior to the ear and extend the line of incision along the inferior margin of the mandible anteriorly. This incision provides adequate exposure to the area, can be extended if necessary, and lies in an inconspicuous position behind the mandible. Extend the incision posteriorly in an inverted T to provide additional exposure in difficult cases. Deepen the incision through the platysma muscle and achieve hemostasis with electrocautery.

LIST OF STRUCTURES

Parotid gland and associated structures
  Parotid gland
    Superficial lobe
    Deep lobe
    Parotid duct
  Superficial parotid lymph nodes
  Parotid fascia
  Deep cervical fascia
Nerves
  Facial nerve
    Temporofacial division
      Temporal branches
      Zygomatic branches
      Buccal branches
    Cervicofacial division
      Marginal mandibular branch

Cervical branch
Great auricular nerve
Auriculotemporal nerve
Muscles
  Masseter muscle
  Sternocleidomastoid muscle
  Digastric muscle
    Posterior belly of digastric muscle
  Platysma muscle
Vessels
  External carotid artery
    Superficial temporal artery
      Transverse facial artery
    Maxillary artery
  External jugular vein
    Superficial temporal vein
    Maxillary vein

Retromandibular vein
Facial vein
Landmarks
  Lateral palpebral commissure
    (canthus)
  External auditory meatus
  Mandible
    Ramus of mandible
  Zygomatic arch
  Temporal bone
    Tympanic portion
    Mastoid process
    Styloid process
    Styloid vaginal process
    Stylomastoid foramen
  Atlas
    Transverse process

FIGURE 1.1
POSITIONING THE PATIENT

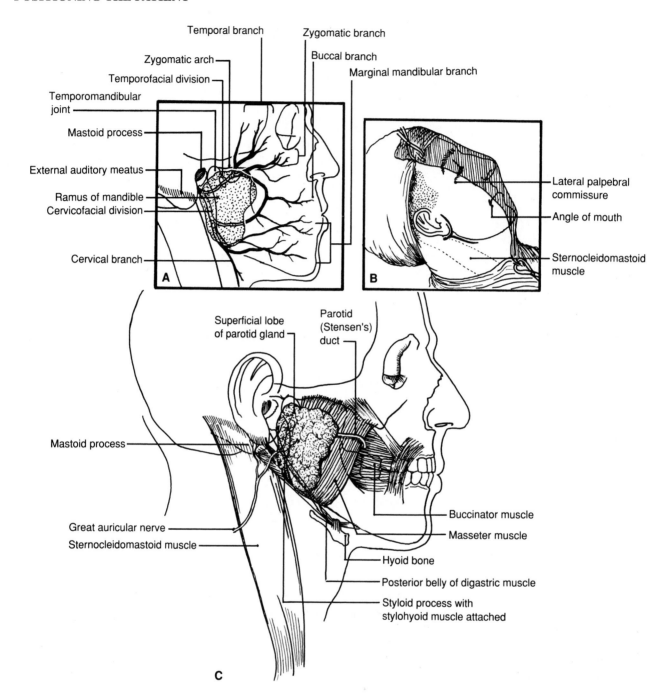

Anatomic Points

The parotid region is bounded anteriorly by the mandibular ramus, posteriorly by the tympanic part of the temporal bone and the mastoid process, and superiorly by the external acoustic meatus, zygomatic arch, and temporomandibular joint (Fig. 1.1C). The deep structures in this region include the styloid process and, more inferiorly, the transverse process of the atlas. The gland overlies portions of the surrounding masseter muscle, the sternocleidomastoid muscle, and the posterior belly of the digastric muscle.

The parotid is enclosed in a sheath derived from the superficial (investing) lamina of deep cervical fascia. Branches of the great auricular nerve (the largest sensory branch of the cervical plexus, with fibers derived from C2 and C3), part of the platysma muscle, and a variable number of superficial

CHAPTER 1

Parotidectomy

The parotid gland is divided into a superficial lobe and a deep lobe for purposes of surgical dissection. Because 70% to 80% of the parotid tissue lies in the superficial lobe, most tumors, whether benign or malignant, arise in this lobe. Superficial lobectomy is the standard treatment for small benign tumors. Simple enucleation is unwise, even when technically feasible, because even histologically benign tumors are likely to recur. A recurrent tumor is much more difficult to resect with preservation of the facial nerve and is more likely to be malignant.

The safe performance of superficial parotidectomy involves careful identification and preservation of the facial nerve and its branches (see Fig. 1.1A). Total parotidectomy is sometimes required when the deep lobe is involved. This procedure is briefly described in Fig. 1.5. More complex problems, including reconstruction of branches of the facial nerve, are covered in the references at the end of this chapter. In this chapter, the anatomy of the parotid region is illustrated as it is demonstrated during the performance of parotidectomy.

Positioning the Patient (Fig. 1.1)

Technical Points

Position the patient supine on the operating table. General anesthesia is preferred; however, avoid muscle relaxants, so that, if necessary, nerve function can be assessed intraoperatively. Place the operating table in a head-up position to improve exposure and minimize bleeding. Turn the head to the contralateral side and slightly hyperextend the neck to enhance exposure of the preauricular region. Place a cotton plug in the external ear to prevent blood accumulation within the external auditory meatus and on the eardrum. Drape an operative field that includes the external ear and mastoid process, the neck, and the angle of the mouth and the lateral palpebral commissure of the eye. Motion of the angle of the mouth or eyelid in response to stimulation of facial nerve branches may assist in the dissection.

Plan the preauricular skin incision so that it lies in a skin fold (Fig. 1.1B). Draw an incision in the skin fold anterior to the ear and extend the line of incision along the inferior margin of the mandible anteriorly. This incision provides adequate exposure to the area, can be extended if necessary, and lies in an inconspicuous position behind the mandible. Extend the incision posteriorly in an inverted T to provide additional exposure in difficult cases. Deepen the incision through the platysma muscle and achieve hemostasis with electrocautery.

LIST OF STRUCTURES

Parotid gland and associated structures
  Parotid gland
    Superficial lobe
    Deep lobe
    Parotid duct
  Superficial parotid lymph nodes
  Parotid fascia
  Deep cervical fascia
Nerves
  Facial nerve
    Temporofacial division
      Temporal branches
      Zygomatic branches
      Buccal branches
    Cervicofacial division
      Marginal mandibular branch

    Cervical branch
  Great auricular nerve
  Auriculotemporal nerve
Muscles
  Masseter muscle
  Sternocleidomastoid muscle
  Digastric muscle
    Posterior belly of digastric muscle
  Platysma muscle
Vessels
  External carotid artery
    Superficial temporal artery
      Transverse facial artery
    Maxillary artery
  External jugular vein
    Superficial temporal vein
    Maxillary vein

  Retromandibular vein
  Facial vein
Landmarks
  Lateral palpebral commissure
    (canthus)
  External auditory meatus
  Mandible
    Ramus of mandible
  Zygomatic arch
  Temporal bone
    Tympanic portion
    Mastoid process
    Styloid process
    Styloid vaginal process
    Stylomastoid foramen
  Atlas
    Transverse process

FIGURE 1.1
POSITIONING THE PATIENT

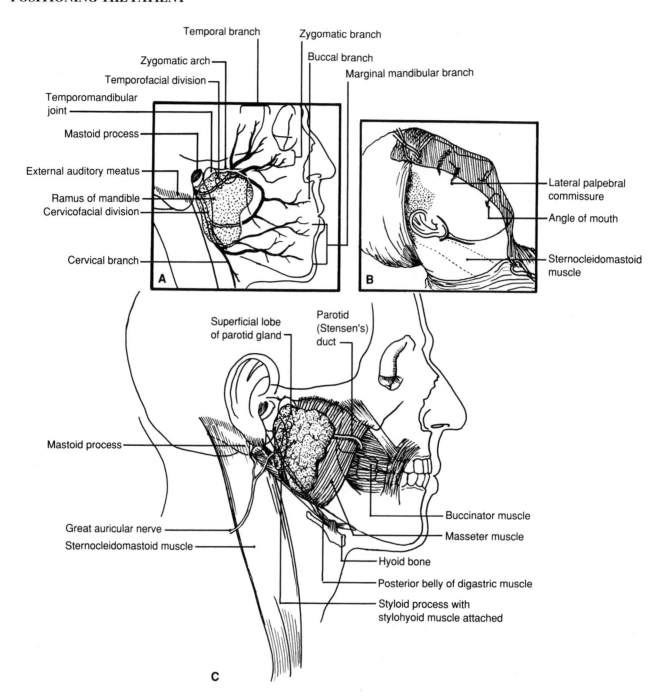

Temporal branch

Zygomatic branch

Buccal branch

Marginal mandibular branch

Zygomatic arch

Temporofacial division

Temporomandibular joint

Mastoid process

External auditory meatus

Ramus of mandible

Cervicofacial division

Cervical branch

A

Lateral palpebral commissure

Angle of mouth

Sternocleidomastoid muscle

B

Superficial lobe of parotid gland

Parotid (Stensen's) duct

Mastoid process

Great auricular nerve

Sternocleidomastoid muscle

Buccinator muscle

Masseter muscle

Hyoid bone

Posterior belly of digastric muscle

Styloid process with stylohyoid muscle attached

C

Anatomic Points

The parotid region is bounded anteriorly by the mandibular ramus, posteriorly by the tympanic part of the temporal bone and the mastoid process, and superiorly by the external acoustic meatus, zygomatic arch, and temporomandibular joint (Fig. 1.1C). The deep structures in this region include the styloid process and, more inferiorly, the transverse process of the atlas. The gland overlies portions of the surrounding masseter muscle, the sternocleidomastoid muscle, and the posterior belly of the digastric muscle.

The parotid is enclosed in a sheath derived from the superficial (investing) lamina of deep cervical fascia. Branches of the great auricular nerve (the largest sensory branch of the cervical plexus, with fibers derived from C2 and C3), part of the platysma muscle, and a variable number of superficial

FIGURE 1.2
ELEVATION OF FLAPS TO EXPOSE THE PAROTID GLAND

Temporal branch of VII

Great auricular nerve
Sternocleidomastoid muscle
Cervical branch
Marginal mandibular branch of VII

Zygomatic branch of VII
Masseter muscle
Parotid fascia (capsule)
Parotid (Stensen's) duct
Buccal branch of VII

parotid lymph nodes (draining the auricle, external acoustic meatus, eyelids, and frontotemporal region of the scalp) are superficial to the gland.

Elevation of Flaps to Expose the Parotid Gland (Fig. 1.2)

Technical Points

Elevate flaps in the plane just superficial to the dense superficial parotid fascia. Use skin hooks or fine-pointed rake retractors to exert upward traction on the skin flap as the plane is developed between subcutaneous tissue and superficial parotid fascia by sharp dissection. Identify the main trunk of the great auricular nerve and preserve it. Branches from the great auricular nerve will enter the substance of the parotid gland and must be divided. Divide the posterior facial vein, but preserve the retromandibular vein to avoid venous engorgement.

As the dissection progresses anteriorly, peripheral branches of the facial nerve will emerge from the parotid to innervate facial muscles. Look for them, and take care to preserve them by dissecting in a plane superficial to these terminal branches. Terminate the dissection at the anterior and inferior margins of the parotid gland to avoid injuring these tiny terminal branches.

Anatomic Points

The flap to be elevated includes the skin, superficial fascia, and platysma muscle. The anterior branches of the great auricular nerve, which lie deep to the platysma but superficial to the parotid fascia, give the surgeon a guide for attaining the proper plane of dissection. As the anterior margin of the parotid gland is reached, however, motor branches of the facial nerve (VII) that innervate the very superficial muscles

of facial expression will begin to emerge into the operating field. Although branches of the great auricular nerve must necessarily be sacrificed, branches of the facial nerve must be preserved.

Identification of the Main Trunk of the Facial Nerve (Fig. 1.3)

Technical Points

Locate the anterior border of the sternocleidomastoid muscle and mobilize it from the posterior aspect of the parotid gland by incising the fascia. The alternative approach of following the tail of the parotid gland to define the inferior border risks injury to the mandibular branch of the facial nerve. Incise the connective tissue between the external auditory meatus and the parotid. Visualize the posterior belly of the digastric muscle. Careful sharp and blunt dissection in the plane along the periosteum of the mastoid process provides a safe route to deeper structures. Spread the tissues gently, using the tips of a fine-pointed hemostat, in a direction parallel to the anticipated path of the nerve.

Expose the main trunk of the facial nerve about one fingerbreadth inferior to the membranous portion of the external auditory canal and the same distance anterior to the mastoid process (Fig. 1.3A). Identify the nerve by its position and the characteristic appearance of a nerve trunk (white, glistening, with a faintly discernible linear structure, and often with one or two minute longitudinal blood vessels visible on the surface). The nerve will be a sizeable structure, commonly about 2 to 3 mm in diameter. Trace the trunk of the facial nerve into the parotid gland and commence dissection, progressing from proximal to distal, by spreading a fine hemostat parallel and superficial to the nerve. Some surgeons prefer to use a blunt Freer elevator to develop the plane.

FIGURE 1.3
IDENTIFICATION OF THE MAIN TRUNK OF THE FACIAL NERVE

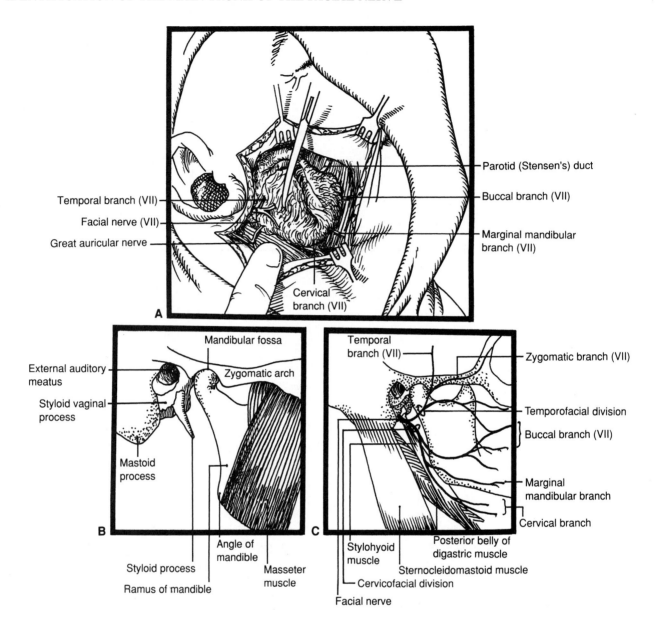

A

Parotid (Stensen's) duct
Buccal branch (VII)
Marginal mandibular branch (VII)
Temporal branch (VII)
Facial nerve (VII)
Great auricular nerve
Cervical branch (VII)

B

External auditory meatus
Styloid vaginal process
Mastoid process
Styloid process
Ramus of mandible
Mandibular fossa
Zygomatic arch
Angle of mandible
Masseter muscle

C

Temporal branch (VII)
Zygomatic branch (VII)
Temporofacial division
Buccal branch (VII)
Marginal mandibular branch
Cervical branch
Stylohyoid muscle
Cervicofacial division
Facial nerve
Posterior belly of digastric muscle
Sternocleidomastoid muscle

Anatomic Points

Bony landmarks of this region include the zygomatic arch (superior), the ramus of the mandible (deep), and the styloid process (posterior) (Fig. 1.3B). Although it would seem reasonable to locate the stylomastoid foramen, and thus the main trunk of the facial nerve, by locating the interval between the mastoid process and the styloid process, this cannot be accomplished reliably. The superficial lamina of the deep cervical fascia, here investing the sternocleidomastoid muscle and the parotid gland and fusing with the perichondrium and periosteum with which it comes into contact, effectively prevents palpation of deeper structures. In addition, the styloid

process is quite variable in that it may be shielded by the variably developed styloid vaginal process, is frequently absent, and can vary in length from 0.1 to 4.2 cm.

By cutting the fascia and retracting the sternocleidomastoid muscle posteriorly and the parotid gland anteriorly, one can visualize the posterior belly of the digastric muscle and the anterior border of the mastoid process (Fig. 1.3C). At this point, the main trunk of the facial nerve (VII) is directed almost in a coronal plane, running from the stylomastoid foramen to the "plane" between the superficial and deep lobes of the parotid gland, where it makes an approximate right-angle turn to run anteriorly in the sagittal plane. If the trunk of the nerve cannot be located easily, bluntly dissect slightly

FIGURE 1.4
REMOVAL OF THE SUPERFICIAL LOBE

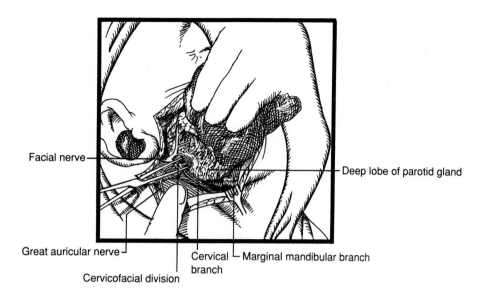

Facial nerve — Deep lobe of parotid gland

Great auricular nerve — Cervicofacial division — Cervical branch — Marginal mandibular branch

anteriorly rather than posteriorly, restricting the vertical extent of the dissection to the region from the tip of the mastoid craniad to about 1 to 2 cm. This will prevent trauma to the only other sizeable nerve in this region, the auriculotemporal nerve. The auriculotemporal nerve is a sensory branch of the mandibular division of the trigeminal nerve, which innervates the temporomandibular joint, external auditory meatus, tympanic membrane, most of the anterior part of the external ear, and most of the temporal region. It enters the region at the level of the external auditory meatus.

Removal of the Superficial Lobe (Fig. 1.4)

Technical Points

Remove the superficial lobe by dissection in the plane of the branches of the facial nerve. Elevate the parotid by traction with a gauze sponge, by grasping it with forceps, or by placing traction sutures. Identify the two major divisions of the facial nerve and trace each by spreading in the plane immediately superficial to the nerve trunks. Gently stimulate any structure in doubt before division. This may be done by very gentle mechanical stimulation (gentle squeezing with forceps or hemostat) or by the use of a disposable nerve stimulator. Stimulation of a motor nerve, such as a branch of the facial nerve, will cause a twitch of the innervated muscle in a nonparalyzed patient. Motion of the eyelids or the corner of the mouth, which were purposefully left exposed when the operative field was draped, can easily be observed. Do not stimulate branches of the facial nerve unless truly uncertain of the anatomy because paresis may result from mechanical or electrical stimulation. Attain hemostasis using fine suture ties. Use cautery judiciously, taking care not to contact nerve fibers.

Anatomic Points

The facial nerve usually separates into two major divisions at a point posterior and slightly medial to the mandibular ramus, about one third of the distance from the temporomandibular joint to the angle of the mandible. The more superior temporofacial division is usually smaller than the more inferior cervicofacial division.

Anatomists still debate the existence of distinct superficial and deep parotid lobes, separated by the plane through which the facial nerve passes. The anatomy is variable, and one or more isthmi of parotid tissue connect the superficial and deep lobes. However, by careful dissection immediately superficial to the facial nerve, an apparent superficial lobe can be removed with a minimum of trauma to other important structures traversing the substance of the parotid gland. Isthmi of parotid tissue are divided sharply as encountered.

The facial nerve is immediately superficial to the external jugular vein and its tributaries, which are themselves superficial to the external carotid artery and its regional branches (superficial temporal and maxillary arteries).

Dissection of the Deep Lobe, Ligation of the Parotid Duct, and Closure of the Wound (Fig. 1.5)

Technical Points

If the tumor involves the deep lobe, dissection of parotid tissue from underneath and around the facial nerve branches is necessary. Elevate the branches of the facial nerve gently with a nerve hook and dissect parotid tissue from around and beneath them (Fig. 1.5A). Do not hesitate to sacrifice nerve branches that are involved by tumor. Perform an immediate reconstruction using a nerve graft (see references).

FIGURE 1.5
DISSECTION OF THE DEEP LOBE, LIGATION OF THE PAROTID DUCT, AND CLOSURE OF THE WOUND

Ligate the parotid duct. Check the field for hemostasis and close with fine interrupted sutures. Leave a small drain under the flap (Fig. 1.5B).

Anatomic Points

Removal of the deep lobe presents many technical difficulties, which may ultimately result in picking out parotid tissue piecemeal. Care must be taken to avoid trauma to the terminal branches of the facial nerve.

The number of branches of the facial nerve within the parotid gland is variable, and there are fine anastomoses between the terminal points of some branches. It is convenient to consider five major branches, which correspond to the common anatomic pattern and the typical pattern of innervation. The first branch after the facial nerve exits the stylomastoid foramen is the posterior auricular, which passes posterosuperiorly between the parotid gland and anterior border of the sternocleidomastoid to supply the muscles of facial expression posterior to the external acoustic meatus. The main trunk of the facial nerve then supplies the muscles originating from the styloid process and the posterior belly of the digastric muscle. Upon entering the parotid gland proper, the nerve divides into its temporofacial and cervicofacial divisions.

The temporofacial division subsequently divides into several branches. The temporal branches supply the auricular muscles, muscles of the forehead, and most of the orbicularis oculi. The zygomatic branches innervate part of the orbicularis oculi, muscles of the nose, and most elevators of the upper lip. The buccal branches innervate the muscles of both lips and the buccinator muscle.

The cervicofacial branches typically include a single marginal mandibular branch and a single cervical branch. The marginal mandibular branch supplies the muscles of the lower lip. Damage to this branch causes a severe deformity, which is especially pronounced during phonation. There are frequently multiple anastomoses between branches, resulting in the formation of a parotid plexus (pes anserinus of the face). This is especially true with the temporofacial branches.

The external jugular vein and its regional tributaries, the superficial temporal vein, maxillary vein, and facial vein, can all be ligated with impunity. The still deeper external carotid artery and its regional ramifications, the superficial temporal artery (and its sole major branch, the transverse facial artery), and the (internal) maxillary artery can also be ligated. The deepest parotid tissue should be approached very cautiously because of the relationship of the gland to deeper structures, notably, the lateral pharyngeal wall.

The buccal branches of the facial nerve typically lie just inferior to the duct. When ligating the parotid duct, be careful not to injure this structure. The transverse facial artery lies just superior to the duct and will generally need to be ligated.

SURGICAL REFERENCES

1. Attie JN, Sciubba J. Operations on the submandibular and sublingual glands. In: Nyhus, Baker, Fischer, eds. *Mastery of surgery.* 3rd ed. Philadelphia: Lippincott-Raven, 1996:310–318. (Describes the anatomy of the submandibular region in detail and gives surgical technique.)
2. Beahrs OH. The surgical anatomy and technique of parotidectomy. *Surg Clin North Am* 1977;57:477. (An excellent description of anatomy and safe technique backed by vast experience.)
3. Beahrs OH, Adson MA. The surgical anatomy and technique of parotidectomy. *Am J Surg* 1958;95:885. (Detailed analysis of the anatomy of the region as it relates to surgical technique.)
4. Christensen NR, Jacobsen SD. Parotidectomy: preserving the posterior branch of the great auricular nerve. *J Laryngol Otol* 1997;111:556.
5. Gaisford JC, Hanna DC. Parotid tumor surgery. In: Goldwyn RM, ed. *The unfavorable result in plastic surgery.* Boston: Little, Brown, 1984:419. (Techniques for avoiding and repairing nerve injuries.)
6. Hanna DC. Salivary gland tumors. In: Gaisford JC, ed. *Symposium on cancer of the head and neck.* Vol 2. St. Louis: CV Mosby, 1968:352.
7. Ollilia DW, Foshag LJ, Essner R, et al. Parotid region lymphatic mapping and sentinel lymphadenectomy for cutaneous melanoma. (Discusses the rationale for including parotidectomy when radical neck dissection is performed for malignant melanoma of the head and neck and provides an alternative technique.)
8. Terrell JE, Kileny PR, Yian C, et al. Clinical outcome of continuous facial nerve monitoring during primary parotidectomy. *Arch Otolaryngol Head Neck Surg* 1997;123:1081.
9. Woods JE. Parotidectomy: points of technique for brief and safe operations. *Am J Surg* 1983;145:678. (Presents surgical shortcuts, emphasizing safety.)
10. Woods JE, Beahrs OH. A technique for the rapid performance of parotidectomy with minimal risk. *Surg Gynecol Obstet* 1976;142:87. (Summarizes the Mayo Clinic technique; an excellent brief description.)

ANATOMIC REFERENCES

1. Bernstein L, Nelson RH. Surgical anatomy of the extraparotid distribution of the facial nerve. *Arch Otolaryngol Head Neck Surg* 1984;110:177. (Reviews the common variants in facial nerve anatomy.)
2. Davis RA, Anson BJ, Budinger JM, et al. Surgical anatomy of the facial nerve and parotid gland based upon a study of 350 cervicofacial halves. *Surg Gynecol Obstet* 1956;102:385. (Offers a detailed description of the anatomy of the region, including variations in facial nerve distribution, parotid gland and duct anatomy, and bony structures.)
3. McCormack LJ, Cauldwell EW, Anson BJ. The surgical anatomy of the facial nerve with special reference to the parotid gland. *Surg Gynecol Obstet* 1945;80:620. (Gives particular attention to the relationship between deep and superficial lobes of the parotid gland and the facial nerve.)
4. McKenzie J. The parotid gland in relation to the facial nerve. *J Anat* 1948;82:183. (Clearly demonstrates the lobulated nature of the parotid gland enfolding the facial nerve.)
5. McWhorter GL. The relations of the superficial and deep lobes of the parotid gland to the ducts and to the facial nerve. *Anat Rec* 1917;12:149. (Provides an original description of the isthmus of parotid tissue connecting the superficial and deep lobes.)
6. Saunders JR, Hirata RM, Jaques DA. Salivary glands. *Surg Clin North Am* 1986;66:59. (Discusses anatomy and surgical techniques for excision of submandibular gland tumors as well as parotid gland tumors.)

HEAD AND NECK ENDOSCOPY

Although not strictly operative procedures, laryngoscopy and endotracheal intubation are frequently performed by surgeons. Accurate diagnosis and management of upper airway problems demand a thorough understanding of the anatomy of this region.

CHAPTER 2

Laryngoscopy and Endotracheal Intubation

Laryngoscopy, or visualization of the larynx, is performed for both diagnostic and therapeutic purposes. In this chapter, indirect (or mirror) laryngoscopy and the visualization of the larynx for the purpose of endotracheal intubation are discussed. The use of the fiberoptic laryngoscope is not presented here because visualization of the upper airway using this instrument is similar to that described for fiberoptic bronchoscopy (see Chapter 21).

Indirect Laryngoscopy

Mirror Laryngoscopy (Fig. 2.1)

Technical Points

The patient should be seated facing the examiner for this procedure. Adequate topical anesthesia of the posterior pharynx is essential. Ask the patient to open the mouth and stick out the tongue. Spray a topical anesthetic over the tongue, soft palate, uvula, and posterior pharynx. Gently grasp the tongue with a dry sponge, or deflect it down with a tongue blade to improve visibility. Use a headlamp to provide illumination. Warm a dental mirror by holding it under hot running water so that it does not fog when placed in the warm, moist environment of the posterior pharynx.

Place the mirror in the oropharynx, just anterior to the uvula. Push back gently on the uvula and visualize the larynx by adjusting the angle of the mirror slightly (Fig. 2.1). Observe the vocal cords for color, symmetry, abnormal growths, and mobility during phonation. The mirror can also be used to inspect the lateral pharyngeal wall and can be reversed to view the posterior nasopharynx.

Recognize that the mirror produces an apparent reversal of anterior and posterior regions. Visualization of the anterior commissure and base of the epiglottis, the ventricles, and the subglottic regions is limited by overhanging structures.

Anatomic Points

The upper aerodigestive tract is divided into the oral cavity proper and the pharynx on the basis of embryologic origin. The oral cavity is lined by epithelium of ectodermal origin. It ends at about the level of the palatoglossal arch. The pharynx is lined with epithelium that is endodermally derived. It is divided into the nasopharynx, the oropharynx, and the laryngopharynx. The nasopharynx is posterior to the nose and superior to the soft palate. The oropharynx extends from the soft palate to the hyoid bone. The laryngopharynx extends from the hyoid bone to the cricoid cartilage.

Endotracheal Intubation

Positioning the Patient to Straighten and Shorten the Airway Before Intubation (Fig. 2.2)

Technical Points

Position the patient supine with the neck slightly flexed and a small roll under the head. Stand at the head of the operating table or bed. If you are intubating a patient in bed, remove the headboard whenever possible to gain better access to the patient.

The "sniffing position" (Fig. 2.2A) decreases the distance from the teeth to the larynx and facilitates visualization of the larynx. Hyperextension of the neck (Fig. 2.2B) increases the

LIST OF STRUCTURES

Larynx
  Laryngeal aditus
  Rima glottidis
  Thyroid cartilage
  Ventricular folds
Tongue
Uvula

Epiglottis
Hyoid bone
Hyoglossus muscle
Hyoepiglottic ligament
Trachea
  Cricoid cartilage
  Carina

Pharynx
  Nasopharynx
  Oropharynx
  Laryngopharynx
  Palatine tonsil
  Palatoglossal arch

FIGURE 2.1
MIRROR LARYNGOSCOPY

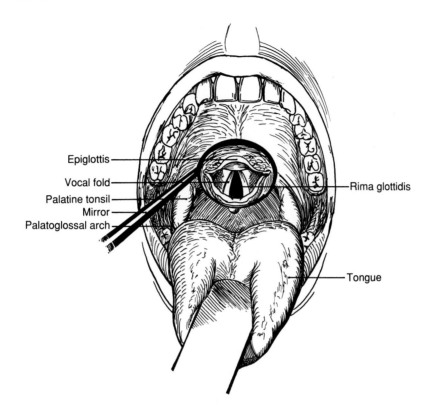

Epiglottis

Vocal fold

Palatine tonsil

Mirror

Palatoglossal arch

Rima glottidis

Tongue

distance from the teeth to the larynx and makes intubation more difficult. Flexion of the head on the neck compresses the airway, again making intubation more difficult. Achieve the correct position by placing a small pillow or folded sheet under the head.

Do not manipulate the head and neck in a patient with a known or possible cervical spine injury. Displacement of vertebrae can cause irreversible damage to the spinal cord. In the situation of known or suspected injury to the cervical spine, fiberoptic laryngoscopy, blind nasotracheal intubation (generally only successful in breathing patients), or cricothyroidotomy is safer than orotracheal intubation. These difficult airway problems are discussed in the references.

Anatomic Points

Note the relative orientation of the structures involved in endotracheal intubation. In the anatomic position, the orientation of the horizontally displaced oral cavity is about 90 degrees with respect to the vertical laryngeal pharynx. The laryngeal aditus (entrance) forms the anterior wall of the cranial portion of the laryngeal pharynx. The rima glottidis is again approximately horizontal, but the infraglottic cavity and trachea are oblique, coursing from superoanterior to inferoposterior. With the neck gently flexed and the atlantooccipital joint extended, the involved pathway has gentle curves

rather than acute angles. Straightening the airway in this manner also shortens the distance from the teeth to the trachea. Allow for this when tube length is estimated before intubation.

Using Straight and Curved Laryngoscope Blades (Fig. 2.3)

Technical Points

Preoxygenate the patient by bag-and-mask ventilation with 100% oxygen before attempting intubation. This allows intubation to progress in an orderly, unhurried fashion. Check all equipment carefully. Verify that the laryngoscope light works and that the proper size of endotracheal tube is available, and check the cuff on the endotracheal tube. Have suction available and working, and have at hand an assortment of laryngoscope blades, endotracheal tubes, and a stylet.

Use the fingers of your gloved dominant hand to open the jaws by spreading apart the upper and lower incisors. Hold the laryngoscope by its handle in your nondominant hand and gently introduce the blade, sliding it over the tongue toward the oropharynx.

When opening the jaws and inserting the laryngoscope, be very careful to avoid chipping the teeth or using them as a fulcrum to lever the laryngoscope blade. Think of the laryngoscope as a lighted tongue blade with a handle that is used to elevate the tongue, mandible, and epiglottis to expose the larynx.

FIGURE 2.2
POSITIONING THE PATIENT TO STRAIGHTEN AND SHORTEN THE AIRWAY BEFORE INTUBATION

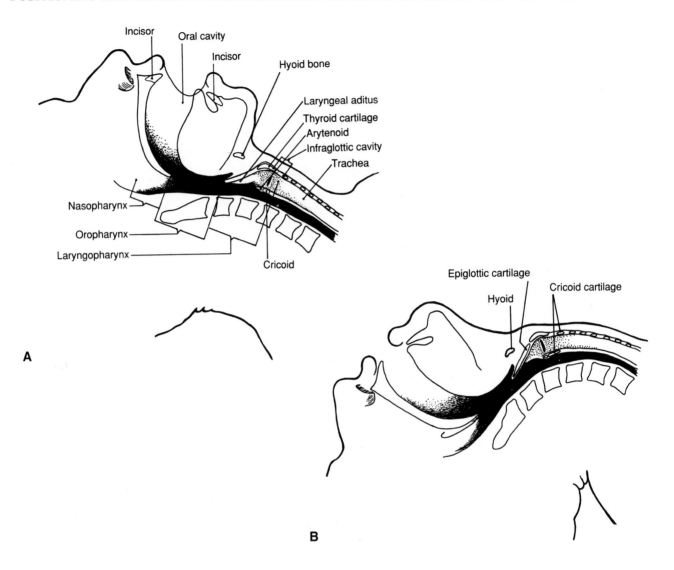

Two types of laryngoscope blades (straight and curved) are commonly used. To some extent, personal preference dictates which blade is used. Many people prefer the curved blade for routine intubation, using the straight blade only when exposure is difficult.

Insert the curved (MacIntosh) blade to a point just in front of the epiglottis (Fig. 2.3A). The curve of the blade tends to follow the curve of the tongue and is advanced downward until the tip of the blade rests against the hyoepiglottic ligament. Gentle upward and forward pressure elevates the epiglottis and reveals the larynx. Be careful not to injure the teeth.

Insert the straight (Miller) blade past the epiglottis (Fig. 2.3B). Elevate the epiglottis by direct pressure to expose the vocal cords. Careful positioning of the patient to align the airway before insertion of the blade will help to ensure success. Note that the view obtained is slightly different because the straight blade covers and obscures the view of the epiglottis.

Anatomic Points

Note that the base of the tongue and the anterior surface of the epiglottis are apposed. Both have attachments to the hyoid bone (the tongue via the hyoglossus muscle, the epiglottis via the hyoepiglottic ligament). Elevating the tongue and mandible will reduce tension on the hyoid bone and epiglottis and will allow increased mobility of the epiglottis. Moving the epiglottis anteriorly is accomplished with a straight blade by applying gentle pressure on the epiglottic cartilage itself. The curved blade presses on the hyoepiglottic ligament to pull the epiglottis anteriorly.

Visualization of the Vocal Cords (Fig. 2.4)

Technical Points

The larynx and vocal cords should be easily visible (Fig. 2.4). The view of the larynx obtained is similar to that seen in

FIGURE 2.3
USING STRAIGHT AND CURVED LARYNGOSCOPE BLADES

Fig. 2.1. Although one is now looking at the larynx directly, rather than using a mirror, the examiner's position relative to the airway has changed, and thus the view obtained has the same orientation. If the cords cannot be visualized, press down on the thyroid cartilage to bring an anterior larynx into view.

Anatomic Points

The true vocal cords appear whitish. The more cephalad ventricular folds (false vocal cords) are pink and are not as prominent. Gentle downward pressure on the thyroid cartilage will compress the esophagus and other soft tissues posterior to the larynx, thus enhancing the alignment of the laryngeal cavity with the passageway from mouth to vocal cords.

Passage of the Endotracheal Tube Through the Cords (Fig. 2.5)

Technical Points

If the patient is awake, anesthetize the throat with topical anesthetic. Introduce the tube at the angle of the mouth and pass it along the side of the laryngoscope, usually on the right (for a right-handed operator). It can thus be introduced without blocking the view of the cords. Pass the tube under direct vision through the vocal cords (Fig. 2.5A).

The endotracheal tube is constructed with a gentle curve, which aids in passage through the cords (Fig. 2.5B). If a greater curvature is needed because of a very anterior larynx,

use a stylet. This stiffens the tube but increases the risk for laryngeal damage if the tube is forced. The tube should pass easily. The patient may react to passage of the tube into the trachea by coughing.

Anatomic Points

Observe the epiglottis, aryepiglottic folds, ventricular folds, and vocal cords, along with the intervening rima glottidis, during the preceding steps (Fig. 2.5A, *inset*). In inserting the tube, guide it through the rima glottidis to inflict as little trauma as possible to the laryngeal mucosa. Such trauma can denude regions of the larynx and elicit involuntary reflexes carried by sensory fibers of the internal branch of the superior laryngeal nerve cephalad to the vocal cords and fibers of the recurrent laryngeal nerve inferior to the vocal cords.

Positioning the Tube (Fig. 2.6)

Technical Points

Inflate the cuff of the tube and confirm its placement within the trachea. The cuff should be inflated until no air leak is detected around it while maintaining the cuff pressure below 25 mm Hg. This ensures that the cuff pressure is less than the tracheal capillary perfusion pressure, thereby minimizing pressure necrosis of the trachea. The esophagus lies directly posterior to the trachea; blind passage of the tube, particularly when the larynx is more anterior than usual, may result in esophageal intubation. Guard against this by always passing

FIGURE 2.4
VISUALIZATION OF THE VOCAL CORDS

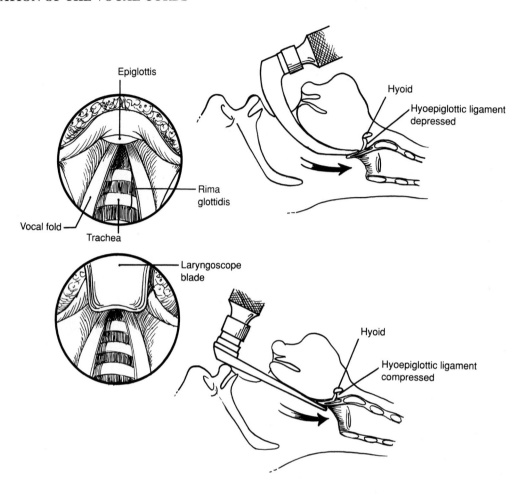

the tube under direct vision and ascertaining the position of the tube by confirming that there is easy exchange of air during respiration as well as the presence of bilateral breath sounds. In the operating room or intensive care unit, pulse oximetry or end-tidal CO_2 measurement can help to confirm adequacy of ventilatory exchange.

Inflate the cuff using the recommended volume of air for the tube. Overinflation may rupture the cuff or cause pressure and ischemic damage to the trachea.

The tip of the tube should lie 2.5 cm above the carina to allow downward migration with increasing neck flexion (Fig. 2.6B). Confirm the position of the tube by auscultation. Breath sounds should be heard clearly over both lung fields. If the tube is inserted too far, it will enter one of the principal bronchi, usually the right. Overinflation of one lung and collapse of the contralateral lung will result. When this occurs, deflate the cuff and reposition the tube. Confirm the position of the tube by obtaining a chest radiograph.

Anatomic Points

The blood supply to the trachea, derived from branches of the inferior thyroid arteries, is not particularly rich. In addition, the tracheal cartilages provide a relatively rigid framework. Thus, overinflation of the cuff can easily compromise the blood supply to the mucosa—in particular, that covering the cartilages.

Estimate the distance from the incisor teeth to the carina in order to ensure that the tip of the tube is properly placed. The distance from incisors to vocal cords and then to the carina increases with age. Further, there is a disproportionate increase in the length of the trachea. The length of the trachea (cords to carina) essentially triples from birth to the age of 65 years, whereas the length of the oropharyngeal cavity (incisors to vocal cords) essentially doubles. The approximate length of tube needed can be determined before intubation by placing the tube alongside the face and neck and extending it to the sternal angle (of Louis), which approximates the level of the carina. The tube should be 2 to 3 cm shorter than this distance.

At the carina, the trachea divides into left and right principal bronchi. The left principal bronchus is smaller in diameter than the right and takes off at a more acute angle. This explains why endotracheal tubes, if inserted too far, typically enter the right principal bronchus.

FIGURE 2.5
PASSAGE OF THE ENDOTRACHEAL TUBE THROUGH THE CORDS

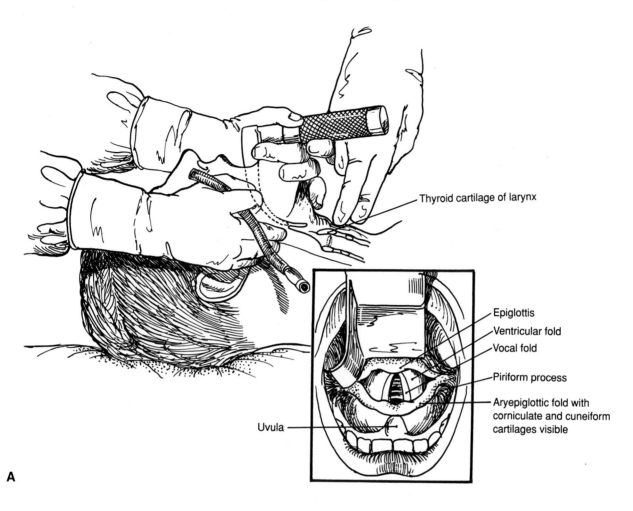

Thyroid cartilage of larynx

Epiglottis
Ventricular fold
Vocal fold
Piriform process
Aryepiglottic fold with corniculate and cuneiform cartilages visible

Uvula

A

Larynx

B

FIGURE 2.6
POSITIONING THE TUBE

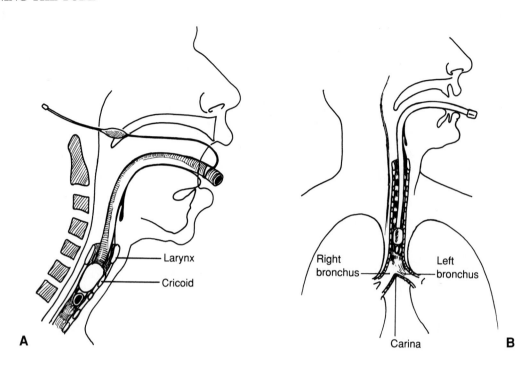

Larynx

Cricoid

Right bronchus — Left bronchus

Carina

A   B

REFERENCES

1. Applebaum EL, Bruce DL. *Tracheal intubation.* Philadelphia: WB Saunders, 1976. (This monograph describes basic intubation techniques, including tracheostomy.)
2. Blanc VF, Tremblay NAG. The complications of tracheal intubation. *Anesth Analg* 1974;53:202.
3. Dripps RD, Eckenhoff JE, Van Dam LD. Intubation of the trachea. In: Dripps RD, Eckenhoff JE, Van Dam LD, eds. *Anesthesia: the principles of safe practice.* 6th ed. Philadelphia: WB Saunders, 1982.
4. McGovern FH, Fitz-Hugh GS, Edgeman LJ. The hazards of endotracheal intubation. *Ann Otolaryngol* 1971;80:556.
5. Orringer MB. Endotracheal intubation and tracheostomy: Indications, techniques, and complications. *Surg Clin North Am* 1980;60:1447. (Provides a clear description of blind nasotracheal intubation, as well as of other techniques; also discusses what to do if intubation is not possible after induction of anesthesia.)
6. Thierbach AR, Lipp MD. Airway management in trauma patients. *Anesth Clin North Am* 1999;17:63–81. (Discusses options when possible cervical spine injury complicates management.)
7. Wilson WC, Benumof JL. Pathophysiology, evaluation, and treatment of the difficult airway. *Anesth Clin North Am* 1998;16:29–75.

THE MIDLINE AND STRUCTURES APPROACHED THROUGH THE MIDLINE

The fascial spaces and anatomic triangles of the neck provide a good orientation to the complex anatomy of the neck. An understanding of the infrahyoid deep (or investing) cervical fascia is essential to good surgical technique in the neck. For simplicity, visualize the cervical fascia as a set of "tubes within tubes" (Fig. 1).

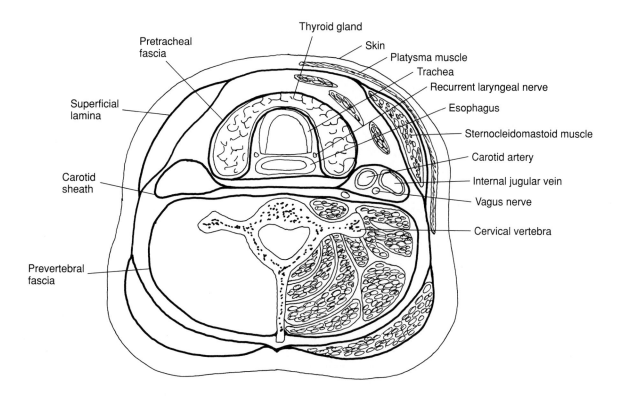

The outermost tube, or superficial lamina, which invests all cervical structures, splits to encompass the sternocleidomastoid muscle, trapezius muscle, the corresponding motor nerve (cranial nerve XI), and the strap muscles. This fascial layer attaches posteriorly to the ligamentum nuchae. In the root of the neck, the fascia is attached to both the anterior and posterior surfaces of the manubrium. The intervening suprasternal space (of Burns) contains the lower portion of the anterior jugular veins and their connecting branch, the jugular venous arch.

Four tubes are located within this superficial tube. Two of these tubes—the carotid sheaths—are paired. The carotid sheaths contain the vagus nerve, carotid artery complex, and internal jugular vein and compose the major neurovascular bundles of the neck. One of the four tubes—the prevertebral fascia—encompasses the cervical vertebrae and their associated muscles, the emerging cervical spinal nerve roots and branches thereof (including the phrenic nerve), the cervical portion of the sympathetic chain, and the cervical part of the subclavian artery. Pretracheal fascia forms the fourth tube. This fascial tube surrounds the larynx, esophagus, thyroid and parathyroid glands, and recurrent laryngeal nerve. In the vicinity of the thyroid gland, the tube splits to invest entirely the thyroid and parathyroid glands, forming the false capsule of the thyroid gland. Between the deep surface of the thyroid gland and the upper two or three tracheal rings, this fascia is strongly adherent to the gland and trachea, forming the so-called adherent zone or lateral suspensory ligament (of Berry). The recurrent laryngeal nerve can pass anterior to, posterior to, or through (about 25% of cases) this ligament. Parathyroid glands are typically located within the capsule derived from pretracheal fascia, but outside the true capsule of the thyroid gland.

The superficial neck is divided into triangles (Fig. 2) for convenience. These triangles are bounded by bony or muscular fixed landmarks and provide important guides to the location of nerves and other critical structures.

Triangles of the Neck

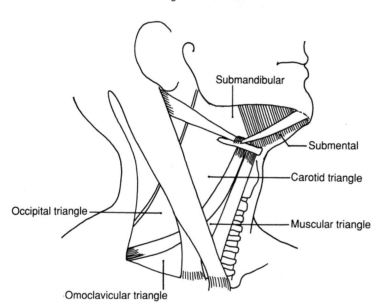

Two major triangles, both of which are roofed by deep (investing) cervical fascia on each side of the neck, are based on the location of the sternocleidomastoid muscle (Fig. 3). Each triangle can be further subdivided. The *anterior triangle* is bounded posteriorly by the sternocleidomastoid muscle, superiorly by the body of the mandible, and anteriorly by the midline. The *posterior triangle* is bounded anteriorly by the sternocleidomastoid muscle, inferiorly by the clavicle, and posteriorly by the trapezius muscle.

The *anterior triangle* can be divided into four lesser triangles. The *submandibular triangle* lies between the body of the mandible and the two bellies of the digastric muscle. The *carotid triangle* is delimited by the sternocleidomastoid muscle, the superior belly of the omohyoid muscle, and the posterior belly of the digastric muscle. The *muscular triangle* is bounded by the sternocleidomastoid muscle, the superior belly of the omohyoid muscle, and the midline. The *submental triangle* is bounded by the hyoid bone, the midline of the neck, and the anterior belly of the digastric muscle.

The *posterior triangle* is subdivided into two triangles. The larger of these is the *occipital triangle,* which is bounded by the trapezius muscle, the sternocleidomastoid muscle, and

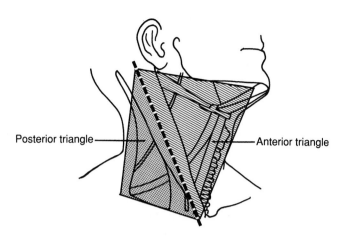

Posterior triangle ——————————— Anterior triangle

the inferior belly of the omohyoid muscle. The much smaller *omoclavicular triangle* is delimited by the inferior belly of the omohyoid muscle, the clavicle, and the sternocleidomastoid muscle. It is quite important to realize that several important structures of the neck are not, in the strictest sense, located in either the anterior or posterior triangle or their subdivisions, but rather are located deep to the sternocleidomastoid muscle itself. These structures are typically rendered accessible either by lateral retraction of the sternocleidomastoid muscle or, immediately superior to the clavicle, by dissecting in the interval between the sternal and clavicular heads of the sternocleidomastoid muscle, a space known as the minor supraclavicular fossa or *scalene triangle*.

General surgical procedures involving the neck can be divided into those that are performed through a midline approach and those that are performed through a lateral incision. Accordingly, the anatomy of the neck is explored in this section first through structures approached through the midline (trachea, thyroid, parathyroid), and then through structures approached laterally (lymph nodes, major vessels, cervical esophagus).

Important structures of the midline of the neck include the thyroid and parathyroid glands, the trachea, and the esophagus. In this section, the anatomy of the trachea (Chapters 3 and 4), thyroid (Chapters 5 and 6), and parathyroids (Chapter 7) will be developed.

Although the esophagus is a midline structure, it is approached laterally because it lies deep to the trachea. Surgical anatomy of the cervical esophagus (Chapters 12 and 13), therefore, is included with other structures approached from the side.

CHAPTER 3

Tracheostomy and Cricothyroidotomy

Tracheostomy is necessary when long-term access to the airway for ventilatory support or respiratory toilet is required. This chapter describes formal tracheostomy; percutaneous tracheostomy (Chapter 4) is an alternative in selected patients. Formal tracheostomy is best performed over a previously placed endotracheal tube in a fully equipped operating room where adequate lighting, electrocautery, and suction are available.

Tracheostomy may also be required in an emergency when the patient cannot be intubated in the normal fashion (e.g., when massive facial trauma or edema precludes safe intubation). In this situation, cricothyroidotomy (see Fig. 3.8) can be performed more quickly and more safely than formal tracheostomy.

Positioning the Patient (Fig. 3.1)

Technical Points

Slightly hyperextend the neck by placing a small roll under the patient's shoulders (Fig. 3.1A). If the roll is placed under the neck instead of the shoulders, a larger roll will be needed and the head may be elevated as well, thereby preventing the desired hyperextension. Do not hyperextend the neck in a patient with a known or suspected cervical spine injury because the resulting vertebral motion may cause irreversible damage to the spinal cord.

Select a tracheostomy tube appropriate to the size of the patient; for an average-sized adult, a number 7 or 8 tube will work well. Test the balloon and then deflate and lubricate it with sterile lubricant. Place the obturator inside the tube. Be sure that a soft rubber suction catheter is available on the sterile field for suctioning the tracheostomy after the tube is inserted.

Anatomic Points

The phrenic nerve arises from spinal cord levels C3 to C5, and the brachial plexus is derived from C5 to T1. Spinal cord damage at or above C3 will result in death secondary to paralysis of all respiratory muscles. Damage of the cord at levels involving the brachial plexus can result in quadriplegia. Hyperextension of the neck stretches the cord and may compress the cord against a damaged cervical vertebra; such a maneuver may also result in complete transection as the cord is caught between broken fragments of cervical vertebrae.

Landmark structures of this region are shown in Fig. 3.1B. The thyroid gland, often with a pyramidal lobe, overlies the trachea. The paired sternocleidomastoid muscles are located well lateral to it. The thyroid cartilage and cricoid cartilage are easily palpable above the thyroid gland. The hyoid bone can be palpated above the thyroid cartilage.

Identification of Landmarks (Fig. 3.2)

Technical and Anatomic Points

Palpate five midline landmarks, including the mental protuberance, or tip of the chin; the body of the hyoid bone; the laryngeal prominence of the thyroid cartilage (Adam's apple); the cricoid cartilage; and the suprasternal or jugular notch of the manubrium sterni. All of these constant bony or cartilaginous landmarks should be identified with certainty to avoid inadvertent supraglottic incision. Repeated palpation of these readily identifiable midline structures will help to ensure that the dissection remains in the midline.

Skin Incision (Fig. 3.3)

Technical Points

A vertical incision about midway between the cricoid

LIST OF STRUCTURES

Larynx	Hyoid bone	Anterior jugular vein
Thyroid cartilage	Laryngeal prominence	External jugular vein
Cricoid cartilage	Manubrium sterni	Platysma muscle
Cricothyroid membrane	Jugular (suprasternal) notch	Brachiocephalic (innominate) artery
Cricothyroid artery	**Associated structures**	Brachiocephalic (innominate) vein
Trachea	Thyroid gland	Jugular venous arch
Landmarks	Isthmus	Brachial plexus
Mental protuberance	Pyramidal lobe	

FIGURE 3.1
POSITIONING THE PATIENT

Cricothyroid membrane

Thyroid gland

Sternocleidomastoid muscle

Cricoid cartilage

Pyramidal lobe of thyroid

FIGURE 3.2
IDENTIFICATION OF LANDMARKS

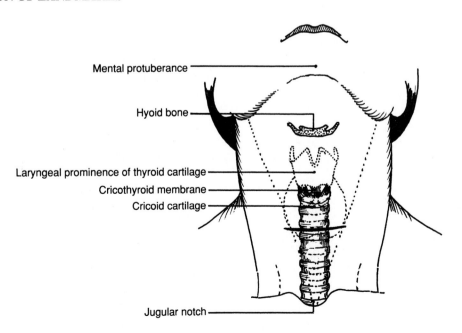

Mental protuberance

Hyoid bone

Laryngeal prominence of thyroid cartilage

Cricothyroid membrane

Cricoid cartilage

Jugular notch

FIGURE 3.3
SKIN INCISION

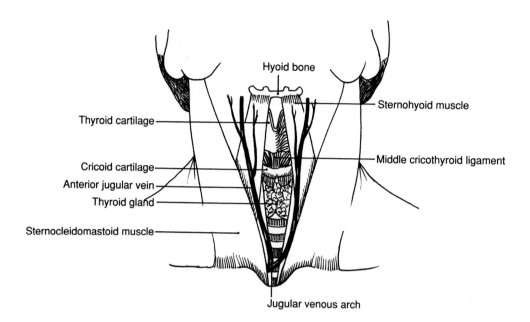

cartilage and the jugular notch provides the best exposure and is preferred in emergency situations. With this incision, there is less bleeding and less risk for damage to nerves and vessels. The incision shown is slightly larger than usually required. Do not hesitate to make a generous incision if exposure is difficult.

A transverse incision, made at the same level, yields a somewhat better cosmetic result; however, the advantage is marginal because scarring occurs around the tracheal stoma. Formal tracheostomy is performed between the second and third tracheal rings. Cricothyroidotomy is done through the cricothyroid membrane. If a transverse incision is used, it should be planned to lie directly over the appropriate level, confirmed by palpation of the anatomic landmarks.

Anatomic Points

The theoretic cosmetic advantage of a transverse incision is that it follows the direction of Langer's lines (resulting from the predominant orientation of dermal collagen bundles and elastic fibers in the skin) and also parallels the natural wrinkle lines of the area.

Dissection Down to the Trachea (Fig. 3.4)

Technical Points

Proceed with sharp and blunt dissection in the midline, confirming correct placement by repeated palpation of anatomic landmarks.

Anatomic Points

The paired platysma muscles, which should be identified and retracted, are deficient in the median plane. The superficial

veins in this region (anterior and external jugulars and their tributaries) run in a predominantly vertical direction deep to the platysma. With the exception of the jugular venous arch, these superficial veins do not cross or occupy the median plane. No motor nerves, and only the terminal branches of sensory nerves, cross or occupy the median plane.

Isthmus of Thyroid Gland (Fig. 3.5)

Technical Points

The next important structure to identify is the isthmus of the thyroid gland. The isthmus may be retracted cephalad or caudad, or divided, to obtain access to the appropriate segment of the trachea. To facilitate retraction of the isthmus, spread the tissues with a blunt-tipped hemostat (such as a small Kelly clamp) in the plane between the thyroid and the trachea. Then place a vein retractor on the isthmus to retract it away from the second and third tracheal rings. Decide whether to divide the isthmus according to the amount of dissection necessary to expose the second and third tracheal rings and the space between. Generally, it is possible to achieve this exposure by retraction.

If it is necessary to divide the isthmus of the thyroid partially or completely, first confirm that the plane between the thyroid and trachea has been developed adequately. Then double-clamp and oversew or suture-ligate the highly vascular thyroid tissue before proceeding.

Anatomic Points

The thyroid begins its development as a diverticulum in the region of the incipient tongue and migrates from its site of origin (marked by the foramen cecum) to its definitive

FIGURE 3.4
DISSECTION DOWN TO THE TRACHEA

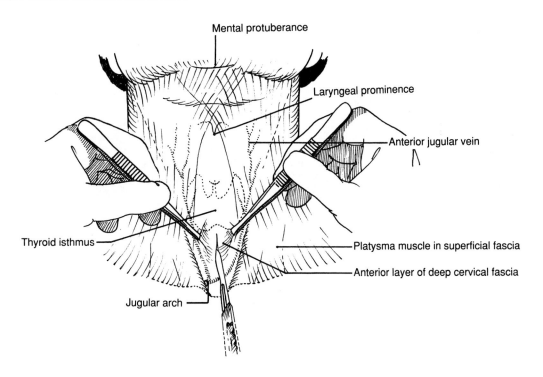

Mental protuberance

Laryngeal prominence

Anterior jugular vein

Thyroid isthmus

Platysma muscle in superficial fascia

Anterior layer of deep cervical fascia

Jugular arch

FIGURE 3.5
ISTHMUS OF THYROID GLAND

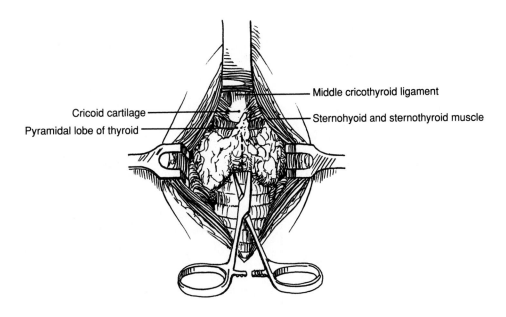

Middle cricothyroid ligament

Cricoid cartilage

Sternohyoid and sternothyroid muscle

Pyramidal lobe of thyroid

FIGURE 3.6
EXPOSURE OF PRETRACHEAL FASCIA

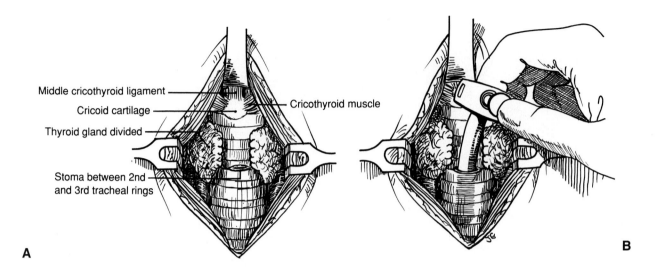

FIGURE 3.7
TRACHEOBRACHIOCEPHALIC ARTERY FISTULA

FIGURE 3.8
CRICOTHYROIDOTOMY

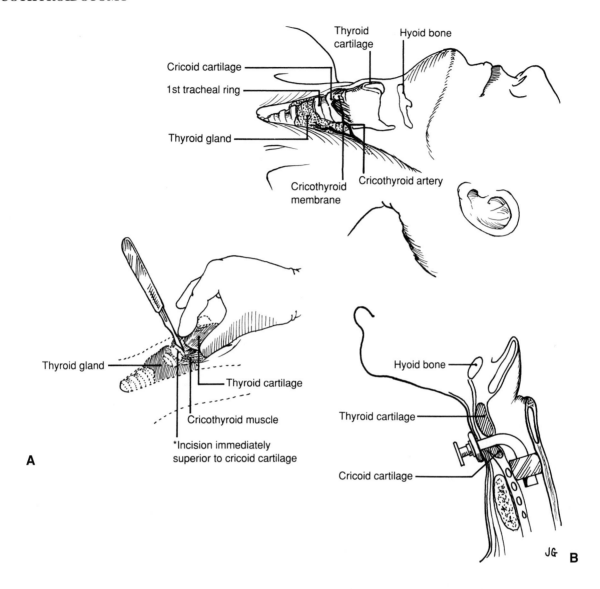

location. Although the large lobes are paratracheal, the isthmus is in the median plane and typically covers the second and third tracheal rings. Further, its developmental route is frequently indicated by the presence of a pyramidal lobe, the result of "residual" thyroid tissue being deposited along the path of descent. This lobe is usually slightly to the left of the midline, but it may be in the midline or on the right.

Exposure of Pretracheal Fascia (Fig. 3.6)

Technical Points

Dissect the pretracheal fascia (which invests the thyroid gland) from the trachea to provide a clear view of the trachea. To perform a formal tracheostomy, count the rings down from the cricoid cartilage. Incise and spread the tissue between the second and third rings (Fig. 3.6A). A simple transverse incision is generally all that is required; however, some prefer to make an H-shaped or T-shaped cut. It is rarely necessary to excise any cartilage.

Have an assistant at the head of the table deflate the cuff of the endotracheal tube and withdraw it slowly until it is just below the vocal cords but above the tracheal stoma. With the stoma spread, insert the pretested tracheostomy tube, with the obturator in place, by pushing it straight in and then downward (Fig. 3.6B). Push downward only after feeling the tube pop into the tracheal lumen; otherwise, it is possible to place the tube in the pretracheal space. Inflate the cuff, have the endotracheal tube removed, and connect the tracheostomy to the ventilator or to oxygen. Pass a soft suction catheter down the tracheostomy tube to remove blood and mucus from the airway. Free passage of the catheter into the bronchial tree confirms position of the tracheostomy tube within the airway.

A tracheostomy hook—a small, sharp, hooked device—may be used to pull the trachea up into the field and maintain visibility when the incision is deep. However, care must be taken to avoid puncture of the cuff of the tracheostomy tube when using the hook. A better method is to place a 2-0 monofilament suture through the third tracheal cartilage and use that for retraction. The suture can be left long and brought out through the skin incision to aid in replacing the tube if it becomes dislodged.

Anatomic Points

It is critical that the incision *not* be made through the cricoid. This is the only totally circumferential cartilage in the airway and provides important stability. Repeated identification of anatomic landmarks and careful dissection in a bloodless field will prevent such an error as well as the equally unfortunate circumstance of entering the airway above the glottis.

Tracheobrachiocephalic Artery Fistula (Fig. 3.7)

Technical and Anatomic Points

If a tracheostomy is performed below the level of the fourth ring, the tip of the tracheostomy tube may erode into the brachiocephalic (innominate) artery, which runs obliquely across the thoracic outlet immediately anterior to the trachea (Fig. 3.7A). This will result in delayed massive bleeding into the airway. The left brachiocephalic (innominate) vein often lies in the jugular notch in its passage from the root of the neck to the superior vena cava (Fig. 3.7B). A very low incision could injure this vessel.

Should bleeding from either of these vessels occur, obtain temporary control by placing a finger in the stoma and pressing anteriorly. This will compress the vessel against the undersurface of the manubrium, allowing time to transport the patient to the operating room. Definitive management of this difficult problem is detailed in the surgical references at the end of this chapter.

Cricothyroidotomy (Fig. 3.8)

Technical Points

Cricothyroidotomy is performed through the cricothyroid membrane, which is the most superficial part of the airway (closest to the skin) and hence affords the easiest approach during emergency situations. In a dire emergency, percutaneous needle cannulation of the cricothyroid membrane may be lifesaving, allowing time for subsequent, more orderly control of the airway. The landmarks for this procedure are the thyroid cartilage, the cricoid cartilage, and the hyoid bone (Fig. 3.8A).

To perform an emergency cricothyroidotomy, first stabilize the larynx with the fingers of the nondominant hand and palpate the cricothyroid membrane (Fig. 3.8B). Stab into the cricothyroid membrane transversely with a scalpel. Spread the hole with a Kelly clamp and insert a tracheostomy tube. Be careful to avoid injury to the cricoid cartilage! Most bleeding will be venous; control it by direct pressure with the fingers of your nondominant hand until the tube is in and the patient is successfully ventilated. Then expose and ligate individual bleeders.

If time permits, cricothyroidotomy may be performed by dissection in a manner similar to that described for tracheostomy. Visualize the cricothyroid membrane and incise it transversely, then spread the tissues and insert the tracheostomy tube as discussed previously (Fig. 3.8C).

Anatomic Points

The cricoid cartilage is the narrowest part of the airway. Concern about subglottic stenosis limits the application of this approach.

A branch of the superior thyroid artery—the cricothyroid artery (and its accompanying vein)—runs transversely across the cricothyroid membrane. This artery occasionally has a branch that penetrates the cricothyroid membrane to anastomose with the laryngeal arteries. It is typically closer to the thyroid cartilage than to the cricoid cartilage. Thus, to avoid injury to these vessels, as well as to avoid damage to the closely situated vocal cords, cricothyroidotomy should be performed by making a transverse incision along the superior border of the cricoid cartilage, rather than along the inferior border of the thyroid cartilage.

SURGICAL REFERENCES

1. Chew JW, Cantrell RW. Tracheostomy: complications and their management. *Arch Otolaryngol* 1972;96:538. (Provides an excellent review of complications, including tracheoinnominate artery fistula.)
2. Dulguerov P, Gysin C, Perneger TV, et al. Percutaneous or surgical tracheostomy: a meta-analysis. *Crit Care Med* 1999;27:1617. (Compares complications as reported in literature.)
3. Eliachar I, Zohar S, Golz A, et al. Permanent tracheostomy. *Head Neck Surg* 1984;7:99. (Describes construction of a permanent stoma.)
4. Gysin C, Dulguerov P, Guyot JP, et al. Percutaneous versus surgical tracheostomy: a double-blind randomized trial. *Ann Surg* 1999;230:708. (Details complications associated with both techniques.)
5. Heffner JE, Miller KS. Tracheostomy in the intensive care unit. I. Indications, techniques, management. *Chest* 1986;90:269. (Offers a good description of the management of a patient with a tracheostomy.)
6. Orringer MB. Endotracheal intubation and tracheostomy: indications, techniques, and complications. *Surg Clin North Am* 1980;60:1447.
7. Van-Hasselt EJ, Bruining HA. Elective cricothyroidotomy. *Intensive Care Med* 1985;11:207. (Provides reviews of clinical experience.)

ANATOMIC REFERENCES

1. American Association of Clinical Anatomists, Educational Affairs Committee. The clinical anatomy of several invasive procedures. *Clin Anat* 1999;12:43.

2. Ger R, Evans JT. Tracheostomy: an anatomico-clinical review. *Clin Anat* 1993;6:337.
3. Salassa JR, Pearson BW, Payne WS. Gross and microscopical blood supply of the trachea. *Ann Thorac Surg* 1977;24:100.

TECHNICAL COMPLICATIONS: MANAGEMENT OF TRACHEOINNOMINATE ARTERY FISTULA REFERENCES

1. Courcy PA, Rodriguez A, Garrett HE. Operative technique for repair of tracheo-innominate artery fistula. *J Vasc Surg* 1985;2:332.

2. Hafez A, Couraud L, Velly JF, et al. Late cataclysmic hemorrhage from the innominate artery after tracheostomy. *Thorac Cardiovasc Surg* 1984;32:315.

CHAPTER 4

Percutaneous Dilatational Tracheostomy

Timothy Van Natta and G. Patrick Kealey

Percutaneous dilatational tracheostomy is now an accepted operative technique. There are two slightly different technical approaches to this procedure, which differ primarily in the use or omission of bronchoscopic guidance. Both are discussed in this chapter.

Percutaneous dilatational tracheostomy is not recommended for achieving emergency airway control or access. Endotracheal intubation or cricothyrotomy is the most appropriate emergency technique to achieve adequate airway control and ventilation. Percutaneous dilatational tracheostomy is a safe and appropriate technique for use in the intubated patient who requires elective tracheostomy. It may be done at the bedside in the intensive care unit.

Contraindications to percutaneous dilatational tracheostomy include the following:

1. Inability to extend the cervical spine
2. Unstable cervical spine
3. Inability to palpate anatomic landmarks due to edema, obesity, or anatomic abnormalities
4. Patients who are not intubated
5. Calcification of the tracheal rings on chest radiograph
6. Pediatric patients (younger than 16 years of age) and adults with small airways
7. Need for emergency airway management

Appropriate positioning and preparation of the patient are essential to achieving good operative results. Therefore, in both techniques, the following preparations must be made. Place the intubated patient in a supine position. Continuous monitoring should include electrocardiographic monitoring of heart rate, blood pressure, pulse oximetry, inspired title volume, and ventilator pressures. Increase the inspired oxygen fraction to 100% percent and ensure adequate ventilation. Because a firm operating surface is necessary, place a cardiopulmonary resuscitation board under the patient's upper torso. Extend the cervical spine by placing a rolled towel between the shoulder blades (see Fig. 3-1A in Chapter 3). Prep and drape the anterior neck with sterile towels.

Percutaneous Dilatational Tracheostomy Without Bronchoscopic Guidance (Fig. 4.1)

Technical and Anatomic Points

Palpate the anterior neck and identify the landmarks, including the cricoid cartilage (see also Fig. 3.1B in Chapter 3). Infiltrate the skin and subcutaneous tissues with 1% lidocaine solution with epinephrine before making the skin incision. Make the skin incision starting at the inferior edge of the cricoid cartilage and extending inferiorly 2 cm. Divide the subcutaneous tissues bluntly with hemostats until the trachea is visualized and its cartilage rings are palpable. This allows for a clear visual delineation of tracheal anatomy, including the location of the tracheal midline, and obviates the need for concomitant bronchoscopy.

Achieve hemostasis with absorbable suture or electrocautery as necessary. Partially deflate the cuff of the endotracheal tube and slowly withdraw it until the cuff is palpable at the level of the cricoid cartilage. Attach a 17-gauge needle with an overlying plastic catheter to a syringe partially filled with 1% lidocaine solution with epinephrine. Insert this into the trachea between the first and third cartilage rings under direct vision. Confirm entry into the trachea by free aspiration of air. Advance the overlying plastic catheter into the trachea and withdraw the needle. Again confirm the position of the plastic catheter within the trachea by aspirating air, and inject 1 mL of 1% lidocaine with epinephrine into the trachea for local anesthesia and hemostasis.

Advance a 1.32 J-tipped guidewire through the catheter into the trachea (Fig. 4.1A) and remove the overlying plastic catheter. Next, place a dilator guide over the guidewire, followed by a lubricated, flexible, tapered dilator up to its external 38 French mark (Fig. 4.1B,C). Perform this dilation carefully and without excessive force. Remove the

LIST OF STRUCTURES

Trachea
    Cricoid cartilage

FIGURE 4.1
PERCUTANEOUS DILATATIONAL TRACHEO-STOMY WITHOUT BRONCHOSCOPIC GUIDANCE
(From Singh RK. Timing and type of tracheostomy. *Probl Gen Surg* 2000;17:101–109, with permission.)

A

B

C

D

dilator, leaving the dilator guide and guidewire in place. Pass a size 6 or 8 Shiley tracheostomy tube over the appropriate dilator, which will function as an obturator. Lubricate the tracheostomy tube and dilator and pass these into the trachea (Fig. 4.1D).

When the tracheostomy tube is seated in its final position, remove the dilator, dilator guide, and guidewire as a unit. Inflate the tracheostomy balloon. Leave the endotracheal tube in place, but disconnect it from the ventilator. Connect the tracheostomy tube to the ventilator tubing with a flexible adaptor. Initiate ventilation. Confirm satisfactory oxygenation and minute ventilation before withdrawing the endotracheal tube. Secure the tracheostomy tube by four-point fixation using sutures and a tracheostomy tape. Obtain a portable upright chest radiograph to determine proper positioning of the tracheostomy tube and to evaluate for pneumothorax or hemothorax.

Percutaneous Dilatational Tracheostomy with Bronchoscopic Guidance (Fig. 4.2)

Technical and Anatomic Points

After preparing the patient as described previously, attach a bronchoscopy adapter between the endotracheal tube and the ventilator tubes. Perform a bronchoscopic inspection of the airway. Withdraw the endotracheal tube to immediately below the vocal folds. Reinflate the cuff of the endotracheal tube to ensure adequate ventilation.

Bronchoscopic transillumination of the anterior trachea is a useful guide but does not absolutely guarantee an initial midline tracheal puncture. Palpate and define the cricoid and tracheal rings. Infiltrate the skin and subcutaneous tissue over the second and third tracheal rings with 1% lidocaine solution with epinephrine. Insert a 17-gauge needle with an overlying plastic catheter percutaneously between the first and third tracheal rings into the trachea. Attach the needle to a syringe partially filled with the lidocaine solution. Confirm the presence of air by aspirating with a syringe. Use the bronchoscope to confirm that the needle entry is midline (Fig. 4.2A). Withdraw the needle, leaving the plastic catheter in place as previously described. Pass the J wire until bronchoscopic observation, confirming that the J wire passes toward the carina (Fig. 4.2B).

Make a 2-cm transverse skin incision 1 cm on either side of the guidewire. Insert the dilator guide over the guidewire into the trachea. Dilate the trachea using the tapered flexible dilator up to its external 38 French mark. In both techniques, perform the dilatation carefully and without excessive force. Remove the tapered dilator. Place a size 6 or 8 Shiley tracheostomy tube snugly over the appropriate dilator. Lubricate the tracheostomy tube and dilator and pass them over the guidewire and into the trachea. Use bronchoscopic visualization to confirm that the tracheostomy tube is within the trachea (Fig. 4.2C). Withdraw the dilator, dilator guide, and guidewire as a single unit. Insert the inner cannula of

FIGURE 4.2
PERCUTANEOUS DILATATIONAL TRACHEOSTOMY WITH BRONCHOSCOPIC GUIDANCE

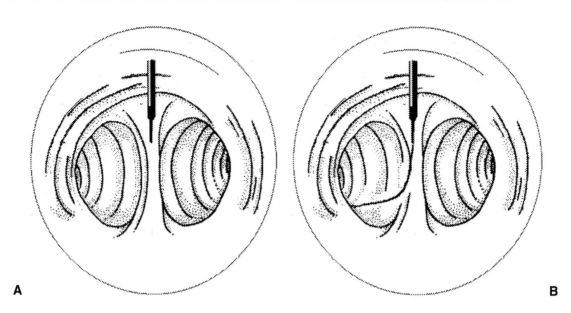

A

B

the tracheostomy tube, inflate the cuff of the tube, and attach the ventilator.

Insert the bronchoscope into the tracheostomy tube to confirm the intratracheal position of the tracheostomy tube and to inspect for bleeding. Withdraw the oral endotracheal tube only after confirmation of appropriate positioning of the tracheostomy tube. Secure the tracheostomy tube using four-point fixation sutures and the tracheostomy tape. Obtain a portable upright chest radiograph to evaluate

the tracheostomy position and for the presence of either hemothorax or pneumothorax.

The key to successful percutaneous dilatation tracheostomy is careful surgical technique preceded by appropriate positioning of an intubated patient. Bronchoscopically directed guidewire insertion into the trachea ensures anterior midline placement of the tracheostomy tube and eliminates the anterior dissection of the neck structures and paratracheal tissues.

REFERENCES

1. Ciaglia P, Graniero K. Percutaneous dilatational tracheostomy: results and long-term follow-up. *Chest* 1992;101:464–467.
2. Ciaglia P, Firsching R, Syniec C. Elective percutaneous dilatational tracheostomy: a new simple bedside procedure, preliminary report. *Chest* 1985;87:715–719.
3. Moe KS, Schmid S, Stoeckli SJ, et al. Percutaneous tracheostomy: a comprehensive evaluation. *Ann Otol Rhinol Laryngol* 1999;108:384–391.
4. Fernadez L, Norwood S, Roettger R, et al. Bedside percutaneous tracheostomy with bronchoscopic guidance in critically ill patients. *Arch Surg* 1996;131:129–132.
5. Rosenbower TJ, Morris JA Jr, Eddy VA, et al. The long-term complications of percutaneous dilatational tracheostomy. *Am Surg* 1998;64:82–87.
6. Van Natta TL, Morris JA Jr, Eddy VA, et al. Elective bedside surgery in critically injured patients is safe and cost-effective. *Ann Surg* 1998;227:618–626.
7. Hinerman R, Alvarez F, Keller CA. Outcome of bedside percutaneous tracheostomy with bronchoscopic guidance. *Intensive Care Med* 2000;26:1850–1856.
8. Byhahn C, Wilke HJ, Halbig S, et al. Percutaneous tracheostomy: Ciaglia blue rhino versus the basic Ciaglia technique of percutaneous dilatational tracheostomy. *Anesth Analg* 2000;91:882–886.
9. Cheng E, Fee Jr WE. Dilatational versus standard tracheostomy: a meta-analysis. *Ann Otol Rhinol Laryngol* 2000;109:803–807.
10. Norwood S, Valina VL, Short K, et al. Incidence of tracheal stenosis and other late complications after percutaneous tracheostomy. *Ann Surg* 2000;232:233–241.

CHAPTER 5

Thyroglossal Duct Cyst

Thyroglossal duct cysts form along the path of descent of the thyroid gland. They present as upper midline neck masses. Often, these cysts become infected and present as abscesses. Incision and drainage or simple excision of the cyst results in a high recurrence rate. Complete removal of the cyst and its associated tract is necessary for cure.

In this section, the anatomy of the upper midline of the neck is explored, and the embryology of the thyroid gland and associated anomalies is discussed.

Positioning the Patient and Incising the Skin (Fig. 5.1)

Technical Points

Position the patient supine, with the neck hyperextended and the chin directly anterior. Include the lower face and lips in the surgical field. (Access to the mouth may facilitate subsequent dissection.)

Make a transverse skin incision over the cyst (Fig. 5.1A). If previous drainage of the cyst has resulted in an external sinus tract or scar, excise this in transverse elliptical fashion with the skin incision. Plan the incision to lie parallel to, or within, the natural skin lines. Elevate flaps in the plane deep to the platysma muscle to expose the deep cervical fascia and paired sternohyoid muscles overlying the cyst. Incise this fascia in the midline.

Anatomic Points

Thyroid anlagen begin as an epithelial thickening of endodermal origin during the fourth intrauterine week. This thickening is located in the floor of pharyngeal arch II, between the tuberculum impar (pharyngeal arch I) and copula (arches II through IV) that participate in the formation of the tongue. The anlage rapidly evaginates, coming into contact with the aortic sac of the developing heart. Owing to differential growth, the thyroid migrates from its point of origin, marked by the foramen cecum of the mature tongue (at the junction of the anterior two thirds and posterior one third), to its definitive location. During this migration, the gland is connected to the tongue by the thyroglossal duct (Fig. 5.1B). The path of migration passes anterior to the developing hyoid bone, whose paired anlagen, from pharyngeal arch II, fuse in the ventral midline and also undergo some rotation. Because of the relationship of the thyroglossal duct to the developing hyoid bone, the duct can (a) be drawn posterocranially with respect to the hyoid, (b) be enveloped in hyoid periosteum or hyoid bone proper, or (c) pass posterior to the hyoid. Typically, the duct degenerates, leaving a short diverticulum at the foramen cecum proximally, a longer cord distally that develops into the pyramidal lobe of the thyroid gland (typically displaced slightly to the left of the median plane), and an intervening fibrous cord. If the discontinuous epithelial cells present in the fibrous remnant differentiate and subsequently assume a secretory function, a thyroglossal duct cyst results.

A thyroglossal duct cyst should be suspected in any person presenting with a median or paramedian lump in the neck, especially if the lump is superior to the level of the cricoid cartilage and if it moves with the excursion of the hyoid bone during swallowing or tongue protrusion (Fig. 5.1C). A lingual thyroid, usually the result of maldescent of the thyroid, has to be considered if the lump is located intralingually. In this case, preoperative evaluation with a radioisotope scan is essential because 65% to 75% of patients with this condition lack other thyroid tissue.

LIST OF STRUCTURES

Embryologic structures and terms
  Thyroid anlagen
  Pharyngeal arches
  Tuberculum impar (pharyngeal arch I)
  Copula (pharyngeal arches II through IV)
  Thyroglossal duct

Adult structures
  Tongue
    Foramen cecum
  Hyoid bone
  Suprahyoid muscles
    Mylohyoid muscle
    Geniohyoid muscle
  Sternohyoid muscle
  Genioglossus muscle

  Hypoglossal nerve (XII)
  Mandibular division of trigeminal nerve (V)
    Mylohyoid branch
    Lingual branch
  Thyroid gland
    Pyramidal lobe
  Thyroid cartilage

FIGURE 5.1
POSITIONING THE PATIENT AND INCISING THE SKIN

Hyoid
Line of incision
Sinus
Thyroid cartilage

Thyroid gland

Trachea

A

Hyoid
Tract
Cyst
Cricoid cartilage

Thyroid gland

B

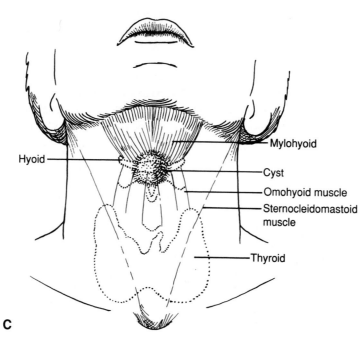

Hyoid

Mylohyoid
Cyst
Omohyoid muscle
Sternocleidomastoid muscle

Thyroid

C

FIGURE 5.2
DISSECTION OF THE CYST

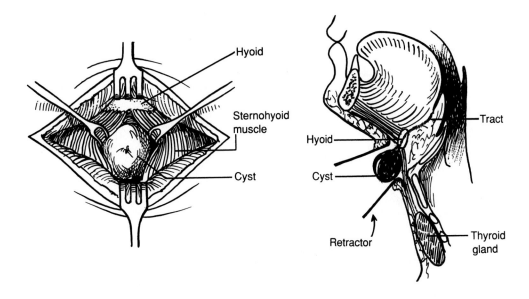

Dissection of the Cyst (Fig. 5.2)

Technical Points

Retract the paired sternohyoid muscles laterally to expose the cyst. Carefully dissect the cyst from the surrounding soft tissues on all sides. Often, the inferior border can be delineated most easily. Start the dissection here, and divide any attachments to the pyramidal lobe of the thyroid that may be present (Fig. 5.2A). Search for and identify the tract leading up to the hyoid bone. This will be palpable as a firm, cordlike structure passing superiorly and deep in a relatively straight path to the midportion of the hyoid (Fig. 5.2B). If the cyst is densely adherent to the hyoid and the tract cannot be identified, simply proceed to excise the cyst and midportion of the hyoid *en bloc.*

Anatomic Points

The tract typically is to the left of midline, juxtaposed to the thyroid cartilage. If a pyramidal lobe is present, the dissection should start at its apex and proceed superiorly to the body of the hyoid bone. Although the tract typically ascends posterior to the body of the hyoid and then is recurved to pass superficial to the anterior surface of the hyoid, it must be emphasized

FIGURE 5.3
DISSECTION THROUGH THE HYOID TO THE BASE OF THE TONGUE

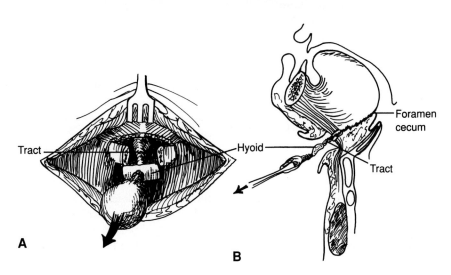

FIGURE 5.4
TRACT FOLLOWED TO THE FORAMEN CECUM

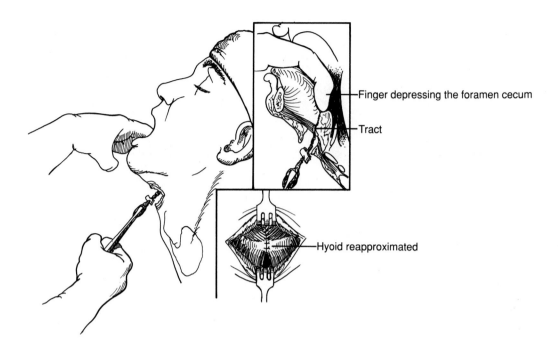

Finger depressing the foramen cecum

Tract

Hyoid reapproximated

that the tract can lie within the hyoid periosteum or within the bone, or it can continue its ascent to the foramen cecum posterior to the hyoid.

Dissection Through the Hyoid to the Base of the Tongue (Fig. 5.3)

Technical Points

Detach the mylohyoid and deeper geniohyoid muscles from the hyoid superiorly and the sternohyoid muscles inferiorly. Divide the hyoid laterally with a small, heavy scissor. Excise a block of the midportion of the hyoid bone in continuity with the cyst and its tract (Fig. 5.3A). Continue the dissection proximally. Excise a core of tissue surrounding the fibrous tract (Fig. 5.3B).

Anatomic Points

Because of the variability of the path of the thyroglossal duct with respect to the hyoid, resect a portion of the body of the hyoid bone in continuity with soft tissues to ensure that no part of the duct remains.

Tract Followed to the Foramen Cecum (Fig. 5.4)

Technical Points

Place a second surgical glove (one-half size larger than the size normally worn) over the glove of your nondominant hand or have an assistant do this. Insert the index and second finger

of this hand into the mouth and press downward in the vicinity of the foramen cecum. Then continue the dissection up toward the foramen cecum, using the hand within the mouth as a guide. Excise the tract. Do not excise the foramen cecum through the cervical incision. Suture-ligate the base of the tract just below the foramen cecum.

Check hemostasis in the operated field. If only a small portion of the hyoid bone has been resected, reapproximate it with a monofilament nonabsorbable suture. When a large cyst necessitates removal of a large portion of the hyoid bone, close the defect by suturing the sternohyoid muscle inferiorly to the mylohyoid muscle superiorly. Then close the cervical fascia and skin.

Anatomic Points

As the tract is followed to the foramen cecum, the surrounding soft tissues are "cored out" along with the tract. This includes the median portions of the mylohyoid muscle and its raphe, the geniohyoid muscle, and the genioglossus muscles. Removing this median core should not endanger the nerves of this region, the hypoglossal nerve (cranial nerve XII) or the mylohyoid and lingual branches of the mandibular division of the trigeminal nerve (cranial nerve V), because these arise posterolaterally, course anterolaterally, and remain lateral to the anterior midline.

Because the foramen cecum lies posterosuperior to the hyoid, digital pressure in the vicinity of the foramen cecum not only stabilizes the soft tissues but also forces these tissues anteriorly, enhancing their excision.

SURGICAL REFERENCES

1. Bennett KG, Organ CH, Williams GR. Is the treatment for thyroglossal duct cysts too extensive? *Am J Surg* 1986;152:602. (This clinical review confirms the need for excision of the midportion of the hyoid.)
2. Gupta P, Maddalozzo J. Preoperative sonography in presumed thyroglossal duct cysts. *Arch Otolaryngol Head Neck Surg* 2001;127:200–202. (Discusses the use of preoperative ultrasound to confirm the existence of normally placed thyroid.)
3. Maddalozzo J, Venkatesan TK, Gupta P. Complications associated with the Sistrunk procedure. *Laryngoscope* 2001;111:119–123. (Wound complications dominate.)
4. Organ GM, Organ CH Jr. Thyroid gland and surgery of the thyroglossal duct: exercise in applied embryology. *World J Surg* 2000;24:886–890. (Reviews surgery and associated embryology.)
5. Sistrunk WE. The surgical treatment of cysts of the thyroglossal tract. *Ann Surg* 1920;71:121. (Provides an original description of the classic procedure.)
6. Sistrunk WE. Technique of removal of cysts and sinuses of the thyroglossal duct. *Surg Gynecol Obstet* 1928;46:109.

GENERAL REFERENCES

1. Brown RL, Azizkhan RG. Pediatric head and neck lesions. *Pediatr Clin North Am* 1998;45:889–905. (Discusses this and other common lesions.)
2. Marshall SF. Thyroglossal cysts and sinuses. *Surg Clin North Am* 1953;33:633. (Reviews the results of extensive experience with the Sistrunk technique.)
3. McClintock JC, Mahaffey DE. Thyroglossal tract lesions. *J Clin Endocrinol* 1950;10:1108. (Discusses embryology with particular reference to development of the hyoid bone.)
4. Nichollas R, Girelfucci B, Roman S, et al. Congenital cysts and fistulas of the neck. *Int J Pediatr Otorhinolaryngol* 2000;55:117–124. (Good review of branchial cleft and thyroglossal duct cysts.)
5. Sprinzl GM, Koebke J, Wimmers-Klick J, et al. Morphology of the human thyroglossal tract: a histologic and macroscopic study in infants and children. *Ann Otol Rhinol Laryngol* 2000;109:1135–1139. (Reaffirms the need to excise part of the hyoid bone.)

EMBRYOLOGY REFERENCES

1. Albers GD. Branchial anomalies. *JAMA* 1963;183:399.
2. Boyd JD. Development of the thyroid and parathyroid glands and the thymus. *Ann R Coll Surg Engl* 1950;7:455.
3. Gilmour JR. The embryology of the parathyroid glands, the thymus and certain associated rudiments. *J Pathol Bacteriol* 1937;45:507.
4. Sgalitzer KE. Contribution to the study of the morphogenesis of the thyroid gland. *J Anat* 1941;75:389.
5. Weller GL. Development of the thyroid, parathyroid and thymus glands in man. *Contrib Embryol* 1933;24:93.
6. Wilson CP. Lateral cysts and fistulas of the neck of developmental origin. *Ann R Coll Surg Engl* 1955;17:1.

CHAPTER 6

Thyroid Lobectomy

The thyroid gland is composed of left and right lobes, a connecting isthmus, and a variable pyramidal lobe. Both total and subtotal lobectomies are described in this chapter. Modified neck dissection (see Chapter 11) is sometimes added to these procedures to remove lymph nodes involved by thyroid cancer.

In this chapter, the anatomy of the thyroid gland, parathyroid glands, and recurrent laryngeal nerve is discussed.

Position of Patient and Choice of Skin Incision (Fig. 6.1)

Technical Points

Position the patient supine with the neck in slight hyperextension (Fig. 6.1A). A moderate reverse Trendelenburg position of 20 to 30 degrees helps to minimize bleeding by decreasing venous pressure. Stabilize the head in the midline. Plan an incision two fingerbreadths above the sternal notch (Fig. 6.1B). Mark the incision by pressing down firmly with a heavy silk suture. Measure the distance on each side of the midline to ensure symmetry. If the thyroid is asymmetrically enlarged, make the incision very slightly higher on the side of the enlarged lobe. Because the skin tends to fall down (droop) after resection of the underlying mass, an asymmetric scar will result if one does not anticipate this and compensate for it.

Carry the incision through the skin, superficial fat, and platysma (Fig. 6.1C). Identify the platysma laterally and cut through it. Identification of the platysma at this stage makes elevation of skin flaps in the proper plane easier. Careful and meticulous hemostasis is essential throughout the operation because critical structures are much easier to identify if the tissues do not become stained with blood.

Anatomic Points

A horizontal skin incision about 5 cm superior to the jugular notch will be located almost directly over the isthmus of the thyroid gland. Superficial to the plane of the platysma muscle, only very small tributaries of the jugular veins and the terminal branches of the transverse cervical nerve (C2 and C3), which is oriented horizontally, are present. Be especially careful incising the area between the paired platysma muscles.

The platysma arises in the superficial fascia covering the pectoralis major and deltoid muscles. It is located in the superficial fascia of the neck and is innervated by the cervical branch of the facial nerve (cranial nerve VII). Anterior fibers of the left and right platysma muscles decussate inferior to the mental symphysis. The more posterior fibers either attach to the body of the mandible or ascend to insert on the skin and subcutaneous tissue of the lower face. The course of these muscles is such that the gap between left and right is wider inferiorly than superiorly. The anterior jugular vein frequently lies just deep to or medial to the anterior borders of these muscles.

LIST OF STRUCTURES

Thyroid gland and associated structures
  Thyroid gland
    Left and right lobes
    Isthmus
    Pyramidal lobe
  Parathyroid glands
    Superior parathyroid glands
    Inferior parathyroid glands
Nerves
  Vagus (X) nerve
  Recurrent laryngeal nerve
  Superior laryngeal nerve
  Ansa cervicalis

Muscles
  Platysma
  Infrahyoid (strap) muscles
    Sternohyoid muscle
    Sternothyroid muscle
    Thyrohyoid muscle
    Omohyoid muscle
  Sternocleidomastoid muscle
Vessels
  Middle thyroid vein
  External jugular vein
  Internal jugular vein
  Anterior jugular vein
  Thyrocervical trunk

  Inferior thyroid artery
  Thyroidea ima artery
  Superior thyroid artery
Landmarks
  Trachea
  Thyroid cartilage
  Cricoid cartilage
  Esophagus
  Pretracheal fascia
    Ligaments of Berry
  Hyoid bone

FIGURE 6.1
POSITION OF PATIENT AND CHOICE OF SKIN INCISION

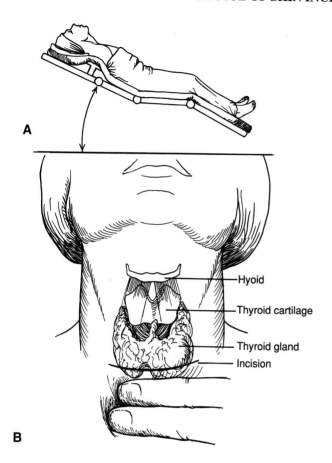

A

B

Hyoid
Thyroid cartilage
Thyroid gland
Incision

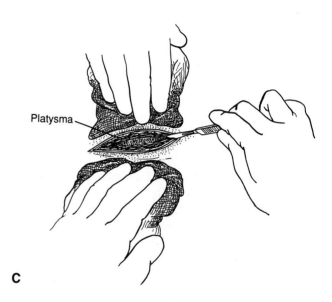

Platysma

C

Raising Skin Flaps (Fig. 6.2)

Technical Points

Identify the platysma in the lateral part of the incision, off the midline. Raise flaps beneath the platysma, using traction and countertraction to aid in dissection. Fine skin hooks or Lahey clamps may be used to put traction on the flap. Supply countertraction by pulling downward with a gauze sponge. Proceed with sharp dissection using a knife or Metzenbaum scissors to develop the plane. Raise the flaps to just above the thyroid cartilage superiorly and the sternal notch inferiorly, and laterally to the sternocleidomastoid muscle. Very few vessels should be encountered.

Anatomic Points

Elevation of the platysma will expose the four infrahyoid strap muscles: thyrohyoid, sternohyoid, sternothyroid, and omohyoid muscles. These muscles are named according to their origins and insertions (*omo* is Greek for shoulder). The sternohyoid and more lateral omohyoid muscles are superficial to the sternothyroid and thyrohyoid.

The thyrohyoid muscle receives its nerve supply from an independent branch of the cervical nerve fibers (C1) that ac-

company the hypoglossal nerve. The other three strap muscles are innervated by branches of the ansa cervicalis (C1 to C3).

The paired sternohyoid muscles lie immediately beneath the platysma. These are the strap muscles closest to the midline. Their nerve supply—typically, an upper and a lower branch from the ansa cervicalis—enters from a posterior and lateral aspect to course in the space between the platysma and sternohyoid. Exercise care in retraction of the platysma to avoid injuring these nerves.

Keep in mind that the external jugular vein and its tributaries are located immediately deep to the platysma but superficial to the strap muscles. Although these veins can be ligated and divided, it is always wise to appreciate them before division rather than after division.

Division or Mobilization of Strap Muscles (Fig. 6.3)

Technical Points

Incise the fascia in the midline and dissect in the midline until the thyroid gland (recognized as a purple-pink organ covered by a network of vessels) is encountered. Identify the midline by palpation, by the symmetric jugular venous arch, and by the division between the strap muscles. There will generally be a large superficial branch of the external

FIGURE 6.2
RAISING SKIN FLAPS

jugular vein on each side of the midline; stay between these. Identify the strap muscles through the surrounding fascia by noting a slight change in color. The midline, with no strap muscle directly under the fascia, will appear somewhat whiter than the fascia overlying the lateral strap muscles.

Develop the plane between the strap muscles and the thyroid gland by sharp and blunt dissection. Place Kocher clamps on the strap muscles to provide traction and exposure. When the thyroid is only minimally or moderately enlarged, excellent exposure may be obtained by retracting the strap muscles without dividing them. Use a small Richardson or Greene retractor to do this.

Do not hesitate to divide the strap muscles between Kocher clamps when necessary to improve exposure for large goiters.

Divide the strap muscles as high as possible to avoid denervating the main portion of the muscle. Suture the strap muscles together at the conclusion of the operation.

Anatomic Points

During the dissection necessary to expose the investing fascia of the neck, tributaries of the external jugular vein will be encountered. As with all veins in superficial fascia, these veins are quite variable, but they tend to follow a pattern. The anterior jugular veins typically lie just medial to, or slightly covered by, the medial border of the platysma muscle. Occasionally, there is a small tributary from the thyroid gland. The jugular venous arch is encountered in the lower part of the

FIGURE 6.3
DIVISION OR MOBILIZATION OF STRAP MUSCLES

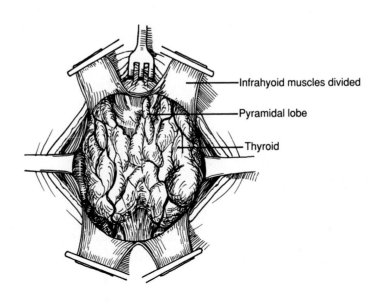

neck, at a variable distance superior to the manubrium. This is a communication between right and left anterior jugular veins. It may have to be ligated and divided to provide adequate exposure of deeper structures. Other communications of the anterior jugular veins with other veins, such as with the external jugular or internal jugular vein, may occur, and these can be safely ligated and divided. In about 6% of individuals, a median, unpaired cervical vein is present; this usually occurs when one of the anterior jugular veins is missing.

Generally, only the sternohyoid, sternothyroid, and omohyoid muscles are encountered and must be retracted or divided. If it is necessary to cut the strap muscles to improve exposure of the thyroid gland, they should be divided relatively high in the surgical field. Motor nerves (branches of the ansa cervicalis) usually enter the muscles at two points, one close to the level of the thyroid cartilage and one just superior to the jugular notch (sternohyoid and sternothyroid) or clavicle (omohyoid). Although no major morbidity results from denervating or otherwise impairing the functions of these muscles, they all are involved in deglutition. Because they depress the elevated hyoid and larynx, impairment of their function thus adversely affects swallowing and may be cosmetically undesirable as well.

Ligation of Middle Thyroid Vein (Fig. 6.4)

Technical Points

Retract the thyroid medially into the field by traction with a gauze sponge or traction suture. Identify, double-ligate, and divide the middle thyroid vein. This fragile vessel is easily torn and may be the source of troublesome bleeding if not divided early. Sometimes, several venous branches are identified and must be ligated.

Be aware that, in the case of large goiters, the external jugular vein may become "tented up" and splayed over the gland. In such situations, it may be injured or inadvertently ligated.

If the middle thyroid vein cannot be identified, proceed to the next step.

Anatomic Points

The venous drainage of the thyroid gland does not exactly parallel the arterial supply. The superior thyroid veins accompany the superior thyroid arteries, the inferior thyroid veins lie on the trachea and empty into the brachiocephalic veins, and typically, there are also one or more middle thyroid veins. The latter vein arises from the lateral surface of the gland somewhat inferior to its midpoint, typically at about the junction of the lower and middle third of the gland. They then passes laterally superficial to the common carotid artery to empty into the internal jugular vein about at the level of the lower pole of the thyroid gland. Although the middle thyroid vein must always be sought, in actuality, its presence is quite variable. It has been reported to be present in only slightly more than half of patients. Often, several veins are encountered in the region of the middle thyroid vein.

Ligation of Superior Pole Vessels (Fig. 6.5)

Technical Points

Use downward and medial traction on the thyroid to gain exposure of the superior pole. Place a small retractor in the upper part of the incision. Slide a right-angle clamp under the upper pole vessels and double-ligate and divide them right on the thyroid under direct visual control. Use a suture-ligature on the "up" side because the vessels are difficult to control if the tie does not hold and tend to retract up into the neck. Place a gauze sponge in the region of the upper pole, remove the retractor, and proceed to free the lower pole of the lobe.

Some surgeons prefer to mobilize and divide the superior pole vessels after identification of the recurrent laryngeal nerve. To mobilize the lobe in this manner, perform the maneuvers described in Figs. 6.6 and 6.7 first, delivering the lower pole of the thyroid into the incision in order to visualize

FIGURE 6.4
LIGATION OF MIDDLE THYROID VEIN

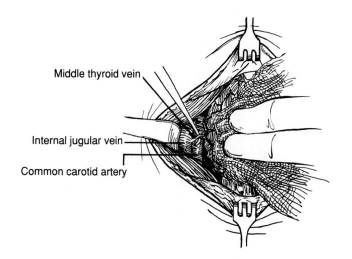

Middle thyroid vein

Internal jugular vein

Common carotid artery

FIGURE 6.5
LIGATION OF SUPERIOR POLE VESSELS

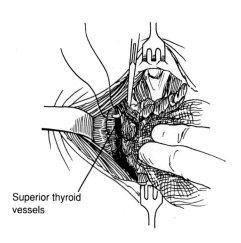

Superior thyroid vessels

FIGURE 6.6
MOBILIZATION OF THE INFERIOR POLE

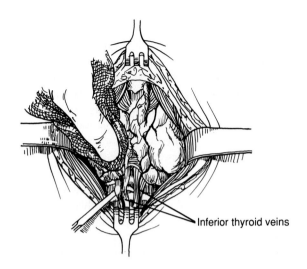

Inferior thyroid veins

the recurrent nerve; then, ligate the vessels of the superior pole.

Anatomic Points

Carefully identify the superior thyroid artery and vein as close to the upper pole of the thyroid gland as possible. Skeletonize these vessels before ligation to avoid including the delicate external branch of the superior laryngeal nerve. This delicate branch innervates the cricothyroid muscle. Denervation of this muscle will result in subtle voice changes because the cricothyroid muscle tenses and elongates the true vocal cords. This nerve typically is slightly superior to the superior

thyroid artery, but is located in a deeper plane (actually deep to the investing fascia of the inferior pharyngeal constrictor and cricothyroid muscles), which helps to protect it when the superior thyroid vessels are meticulously skeletonized as close to thyroid tissue as possible.

Mobilization of the Inferior Pole (Fig. 6.6)

Technical Points

The vessels at the inferior pole of the thyroid are divided next. Place a retractor in the inferior pole of the incision. Slide a right-angle clamp from the midline laterally, sweeping under the vessels, and then pass it from lateral to medial and double-ligate and divide the vessels. Do not try to divide too much because the recurrent laryngeal nerve, which generally runs laterally and deep in the tracheoesophageal groove but which can be variable in location, has not yet been identified. Place a gauze sponge in this area and remove the retractor. Some surgeons identify the recurrent laryngeal nerve before performing this step.

Anatomic Points

Vessels ligated in this stage of the operation are mainly inferior thyroid veins and occasionally are thyroidea ima arteries.

The inferior thyroid vein takes a different course than the inferior thyroid artery. The inferior thyroid arteries are related to the posterolateral aspect of the gland. By contrast, the inferior thyroid veins are related to the inferior and medial aspect of the gland. They usually arise as two trunks on the medial aspect of the lateral lobes, close to the midline. From here, they pass inferiorly, emptying into their corresponding brachiocephalic veins. Sometimes, the right and left veins

FIGURE 6.7
IDENTIFICATION OF THE RECURRENT LARYNGEAL NERVE AND LIGATION OF THE INFERIOR THYROID ARTERY

Recurrent laryngeal nerve

A Inferior thyroid artery **B**

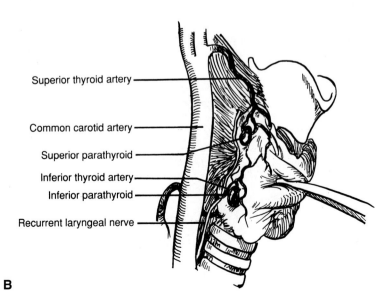

Superior thyroid artery
Common carotid artery
Superior parathyroid
Inferior thyroid artery
Inferior parathyroid
Recurrent laryngeal nerve

join, forming a thyroidea ima vein that empties into the left brachiocephalic vein.

Identification of the Recurrent Laryngeal Nerve and Ligation of the Inferior Thyroid Artery (Fig. 6.7)

Technical Points

Retract the lobe medially. The additional mobility gained by ligating the upper and lower poles should help in mobilization. It should be possible to "dislocate" the lobe of the thyroid up into the operative field, thereby exposing important structures (inferior thyroid artery, recurrent laryngeal nerve, and parathyroids) that lie posterior. If the middle thyroid vein was not previously identified, look for it again and ligate and divide it. Recheck hemostasis and ensure a dry operative field. If bleeding has occurred, irrigate the field with warm saline solution and reassess hemostasis. The inferior thyroid artery, recurrent laryngeal nerve, and parathyroids are much easier to identify in a dry field. Place a small retractor on the carotid sheath and its contents, and have an assistant apply gentle traction to open the space between the carotid artery and thyroid gland.

Identify the inferior thyroid artery, which enters the thyroid laterally (not from below). With the tips of a fine hemostat, gently spread the areolar tissue between the inferior thyroid artery and the thyroid gland. The recurrent laryngeal nerve is most commonly found in close proximity to, and deep to, the inferior thyroid artery (Fig. 6.7B). It has the characteristic glistening white appearance of a peripheral nerve; one or more fine branching vessels may be seen running longitudinally, and faint linear striations are apparent on close inspection. The recurrent laryngeal nerve generally lies deep, in the vicinity of the tracheoesophageal groove. Locate this nerve and trace it for a sufficient distance to verify its identity, its relation to the thyroid, and its course. Ligate the inferior thyroid artery close to the thyroid gland.

Next, identify the superior and inferior parathyroid glands. These are most commonly located within the capsule of the thyroid gland and are identified by their slightly brownish color and the fine blood vessels that can frequently be seen to supply them. Variations in the pattern of location of the parathyroid glands are discussed in detail in Chapter 7.

Subtotal lobectomy preserves a rim of thyroid tissue posteriorly, including the thyroid adjacent to the parathyroids. Risk for damage to the parathyroids and to the recurrent laryngeal nerve is thereby minimized. Total lobectomy requires removal of the entire lobe. In either case, the parathyroids and the recurrent laryngeal nerve should be identified and preserved. If a parathyroid gland is inadvertently removed, it may be autotransplanted.

Anatomic Points

The inferior thyroid artery enters the posterolateral margin of the thyroid gland at about the level of the thyroid isthmus. If the artery cannot be located at that level, look inferiorly first, then explore more superiorly. The inferior thyroid artery arises from the thyrocervical trunk, ascends to the level of the cricoid cartilage deep to prevertebral fascia on the anterior scalene muscle, and then loops medially and inferiorly deep to the prevertebral fascia. Here, it is anterior to the vertebral artery, is posterior to the carotid sheath, and has a variable relationship to the cervical sympathetic trunk (although the middle cervical ganglion is typically in contact with the anterior surface of the inferior thyroid artery). It then pierces the prevertebral fascia at about the level of the middle of the thyroid gland, and divides into an upper and a lower branch. These branches are usually in close proximity to the inferior (recurrent) laryngeal nerve, being either anterior to, posterior to, or on both sides of this nerve. The inferior thyroid artery is intimately associated with the inferior (recurrent) laryngeal nerve and usually is not located at the inferior pole of the gland (as the name might suggest), but rather is higher. It is about at the level of the middle thyroid vein, when that is present.

The relationship of the inferior thyroid artery and the inferior (recurrent) laryngeal nerve is quite variable. Typically, the artery branches immediately posterior to thyroid tissue. The inferior (recurrent) laryngeal nerve is most often found posterior to the inferior thyroid artery and its branches (70%), but it may pass between the branches of the inferior thyroid artery, or it may lie completely anterior to the artery. The recurrent laryngeal nerve lies in the tracheoesophageal groove in almost half of cases; in most of the remaining cases, it lies anterior to the groove, between the trachea and thyroid gland. Occasionally, the nerve is located more posteriorly, between the esophagus and thyroid gland (6%). Even less often, it is anterior to the tracheoesophageal groove, in the substance of the thyroid gland itself (2%). Obviously, the nerve can lie anterior to, in, or posterior to the suspensory ligament (of Berry).

In about 1% of cases, the right inferior laryngeal nerve is nonrecurrent. It then arises normally from the vagus nerve but passes medially without looping under the subclavian artery. In these cases, the right subclavian artery arises from the aorta distal to the left subclavian artery and then courses to the right, posterior to the esophagus. Similarly, the left recurrent nerve can pass directly to the larynx if there is a persistent right aortic arch and a retroesophageal left subclavian artery. This situation is extremely rare.

Be careful to identify the parathyroid glands. These are usually located on the posterior surface of the thyroid gland, each in its own capsule. Usually, the superior glands are located near where the inferior thyroid artery bifurcates and enters the gland (middle third), whereas the inferior parathyroids are located inferior to this and are frequently inferior to the inferior pole of the thyroid glands. The blood supply to both superior and inferior parathyroids derives from the inferior thyroid artery.

Occasionally (1% to 13% of cases), there is an unpaired thyroidea ima artery, which either replaces or supplements the inferior thyroid artery. This artery, when present, can arise from a variety of sources, such as the brachiocephalic, right common carotid, internal thoracic, or subclavian arteries, or from the arch of the aorta.

FIGURE 6.8
DIVISION OF THE ISTHMUS AND COMPLETION OF LOBECTOMY (TOTAL VERSUS SUBTOTAL)

Division of the Isthmus and Completion of Lobectomy (Total versus Subtotal) (Fig. 6.8)

Technical Points

The isthmus should have been well-delineated by the superior and inferior pole ligation. Pass a blunt-tipped hemostat, such as a Kelly clamp, between the thyroid and the trachea to develop this plane (Fig. 6.8A). Divide the isthmus either at its narrowest point or (if resection of the isthmus is to be done with lobectomy) on the far side (Fig. 6.8B). Generally, the isthmus can be divided between one or two pairs of hemostats.

Rotate laterally the lobe that is being removed and sharply incise the attachments of the thyroid to the trachea

FIGURE 6.9
CONCLUSION OF DISSECTION

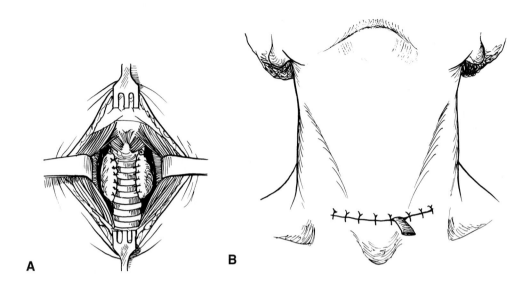

A   B

(Fig. 6.8C,D), taking care not to injure the trachea. The surface of the tracheal rings should be easily visualized. Hold the lobe of the thyroid, now attached only laterally and by a small thyroid remnant, in your nondominant hand as dissection progresses.

For a subtotal lobectomy, divide the lobe with Kelly clamps, leaving a remnant that is less than 5 g, sufficient only to preserve the parathyroids. Place the Kelly clamps at such an angle that the posterior capsule is preserved; this helps to protect the posterior-lying parathyroid glands and simplifies closure of the thyroid remnant.

Total lobectomy requires meticulous dissection of the entire lobe from both parathyroid glands. Often, this is best accomplished before division of the isthmus, unless the lobe is very large. Carefully dissect each parathyroid gland, preserving its blood supply, from the capsule of the thyroid.

Anatomic Points

If the isthmus is to be divided, division along or adjacent to the median sagittal plane is safest. Be sure that instruments passed deep to the isthmus of the thyroid gland are in the proper plane (between the trachea and the true capsule of the thyroid gland). This plane should be able to be easily developed by blunt dissection with a Kelly clamp.

Removal of a lobe requires that the lateral lobes be dissected from the trachea, to which they are attached by the suspensory ligament (of Berry). This so-called ligament is really connective tissue derived from pretracheal fascia. It attaches the medial surface of the thyroid gland to the cricoid cartilage. Remember that recurrent laryngeal nerves can lie anterior or posterior to or in the substance of this ligament.

Identify the nerve before freeing and removing the thyroid, not after.

Conclusion of Dissection (Fig. 6.9)

Technical and Anatomic Points

Oversew the isthmus with a running lock stitch to achieve hemostasis. Check the thyroid remnant for hemostasis, placing suture ligatures if needed. Then tack the thyroid remnant (in a subtotal lobectomy) to the trachea with a running suture. Take care in placing this suture not to injure the parathyroid glands or recurrent laryngeal nerve. Place the sutures through the strong pretracheal fascia and try to avoid entering the lumen of the trachea. Some surgeons prefer not to tack the remnant to the trachea.

If a bilateral lobectomy is planned, place a pack in the operated field and proceed with lobectomy on the contralateral side. The appearance of the field at the completion of bilateral subtotal lobectomy is shown in Fig. 6.9A.

At the conclusion of the operation, recheck hemostasis and remove all packs. A drain is optional. If one is used, place it through a gap in the midline fascial closure and bring it out through the middle of the incision. Close the strap muscles with horizontal mattress sutures if they were divided. Close the midline with interrupted sutures, but do not close it completely. Rather, bring the drain out through the midline, leaving a 2- to 3-cm opening at the inferior pole to allow leakage of blood into the subcutaneous tissues if postoperative hemorrhage occurs. Approximate the platysma with fine interrupted absorbable sutures and then close the skin incision with fine interrupted sutures (Fig. 6.9B).

TECHNICAL REFERENCES

1. Agarwal A, Agarwal G, Mishra SK. Thyroid surgery and the recurrent laryngeal nerve. *Br J Surg* 1999;86:291–292.
2. Allo MD, Thompson NW. Rationale for the operative management of substernal goiters. *Surgery* 1983;94:969. (Discusses modifications of the technique for dealing with a large substernal component.)
3. Harness JK, Gung L, Thompson NW, et al. Total thyroidectomy: complications and technique. *World J Surg* 1986;10:781. (Reviews a large series of total thyroidectomies, including a discussion of the incidence of various complications.)
4. Levin KE, Clark OH. Reoperative thyroid and parathyroid surgery. In: Thompkins RK, ed. *Reoperative surgery.* Philadelphia: JB Lippincott, 1988:509. (Provides an excellent discussion of strategy for preoperative evaluation and reoperation.)
5. Moley JF, Lairmore TC, Doherty GM, et al. Preservation of the recurrent laryngeal nerves in thyroid and parathyroid reoperations. *Surgery* 1999;126:677–679. (Emphasizes working, wherever possible, in a previously undissected area.)
6. Schwartz AE, Griedman EW. Preservation of the parathyroid glands in total thyroidectomy. *Surg Gynecol Obstet* 1987;165:327. (Emphasizes identification and preservation of the blood supply to the parathyroids.)
7. Shahian DM. Surgical treatment of intrathoracic goiter. In: Cady B, Rossi RL, eds. *Surgery of the thyroid and parathyroid glands.* 3rd ed. Philadelphia: WB Saunders, 1991:215. (Provides additional information on substernal goiter.)
8. Thompson NW, Olsen WR, Hoffman GL. The continuing development of the technique of thyroidectomy. *Surgery* 1973;73:913. (Includes good illustrations of points of danger to the superior and recurrent laryngeal nerves as well as a discussion of strategy to avoid nerve damage.)

ANATOMIC REFERENCES

1. Bachhuber CA. Complications of thyroid surgery: anatomy of the recurrent laryngeal nerve, middle thyroid vein and inferior thyroid artery. *Am J Surg* 1943;60:96.
2. Dozois RR, Beahrs OH. Surgical anatomy and technique of thyroid and parathyroid surgery. *Surg Clin North Am* 1977;57:647.
3. Harlaftis N, Tzinas S, Droulias C, et al. Rare complications of thyroid surgery. *Am J Surg* 1976;42:645. (Discusses rare injuries to the sympathetic ganglia, pleura, trachea, esophagus, and thoracic duct.)
4. Henry JF, Audiffret J, Cenizot A, et al. The nonrecurrent inferior laryngeal nerve: review of 33 cases, including two on the left side. *Surgery* 1988;104:977.
5. Katz AD. Extralaryngeal division of the recurrent laryngeal nerve: report on 400 patients and the 721 nerves measured. *Am J Surg* 1986;152:407.
6. Lendquist S, Cahlin C, Smeds S. Superior laryngeal nerve in thyroid surgery. *Surgery* 1987;102:999. (Provides a clear description, with excellent drawings, of variant anatomy of superior laryngeal nerve.)
7. Moosman DA, DeWeese MS. The external laryngeal nerve as related to thyroidectomy. *Surg Gynecol Obstet* 1968;127:1011. (Offers an excellent review of the anatomy of the external laryngeal nerve.)
8. Nemiroff P, Katz AD. Extralaryngeal divisions of the recurrent laryngeal nerve: surgical and clinical significance. *Am J Surg* 1982;144:466–469.
9. Pelizzo MR, Toniato A, Gemo G. Zuckerkandl's tuberculum: an arrow pointing to the recurrent laryngeal nerve (constant anatomical landmark). *J Am Coll Surg* 1998;187:333–336. (A variable—despite the title of the article—landmark that may be of assistance.)
10. Rossi RL, Cady B. Surgical anatomy. In: Cady B, Rossi RL, eds. *Surgery of the thyroid and parathyroid glands.* 3rd ed. Philadelphia: WB Saunders, 1991:13. (Provides an excellent review of anatomy and surgical technique.)
11. Wang C. The use of the inferior cornu of the thyroid cartilage in identifying the recurrent laryngeal nerve. *Surg Gynecol Obstet* 1975;140:91. (Discusses an alternate technique for identification of the recurrent nerve.)

CHAPTER 7

Parathyroidectomy

Parathyroidectomy is performed for hyperparathyroidism; this condition may be caused by overactivity of one gland (secondary to parathyroid adenoma or, rarely, carcinoma) or of several glands (secondary to multiple adenomas or diffuse hyperplasia). Often, it is difficult to be certain preoperatively how many glands are involved. Newer imaging modalities such as radionuclide scans have increased the precision but not eliminated the need for careful exploration.

The goal of surgery for hyperparathyroidism is to remove any or all abnormal glands, leaving only normal parathyroids or, if all glands are involved, a small remnant of parathyroid tissue to prevent hypoparathyroidism. The best chance for a good result is at the time of the first operation because reoperation for hyperparathyroidism is difficult, even though improved preoperative localization techniques have made it somewhat easier. Every attempt must be made to locate and identify all parathyroids and to document carefully the exact findings. Use a standard diagram, such as that shown here, to record the operation.

This chapter describes the standard formal exploration. A more focused technique, such as the lateral approach described in Fig. 7.4, is used by some surgeons when preoperative imaging studies are highly suggestive of single-gland disease.

Positioning and Skin Incision (Fig. 7.1)

Technical Points

Most abnormal parathyroids are found in the neck. Neck exploration is the first (and often the only) maneuver to perform when operating for hyperparathyroidism. If no abnormal glands are found in the neck, mediastinal exploration is the next step. This is generally performed at a second operation.

Because the parathyroids are in close proximity to the thyroid gland, the surgical exposure is the same as that used for thyroidectomy. Position the patient as for thyroidectomy and raise flaps under the platysma. Meticulous hemostasis is critical; a bloodless field and tissues that have not become bloodstained are important for accurate identification. Expose the posterior surface of the thyroid gland as described in Figs. 6.1 through 6.7 in Chapter 6.

Anatomic Points

The surgical strategy for parathyroidectomy is based on an understanding of the embryology of these glands and other pharyngeal derivatives. The inferior parathyroid glands (parathyroids III) develop from the epithelium of the dorsal wing of pharyngeal pouch III. The ventral wing of this pouch gives rise to the thymus. The superior parathyroid glands (parathyroids IV) are derived from the dorsal wing of pharyngeal pouch IV. The ventral wing is thought to give rise either to transitory thymic tissue or to a component of the definitive thyroid gland.

Differential migration of the developing ventral wing derivatives of both pouches also involves the dorsal wing derivatives (parathyroids), resulting in glands derived from pharyngeal pouch III being typically located inferior and caudal to glands derived from pharyngeal pouch IV. Although such migration increases the possibility of ectopic parathyroids and supernumerary glands, a definite pattern exists with respect to location and number.

Typically (80% to 98% of cases), there are four glands, which are oval, spherical, or bean shaped. Each is encapsulated in a well-circumscribed fat lobule. The superior parathyroid glands are usually (75% to 80% of cases) located in connective tissue associated with the posterior edge of the thyroid

LIST OF STRUCTURES

Adult structures		Embryologic structures
Parathyroid glands	Recurrent laryngeal nerve	Pharyngeal pouch III
Superior parathyroid glands	Thymus	Ventral wing
Inferior parathyroid glands	Mediastinum	Dorsal wing
Thyroid gland	Cricoid cartilage	Pharyngeal pouch IV
Middle thyroid vein	Thyroid cartilage of larynx	Ventral wing
Inferior thyroid artery	Esophagus	Dorsal wing
	Tracheoesophageal groove	

ORIENTATION

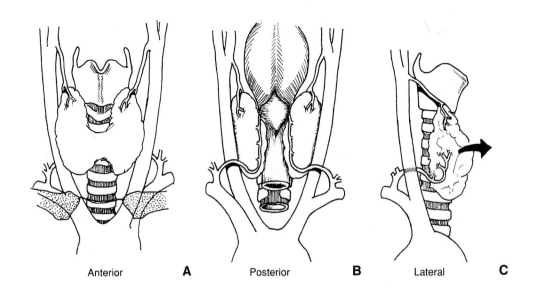

Anterior   **A**   Posterior   **B**   Lateral   **C**

FIGURE 7.1
POSITIONING AND SKIN INCISION

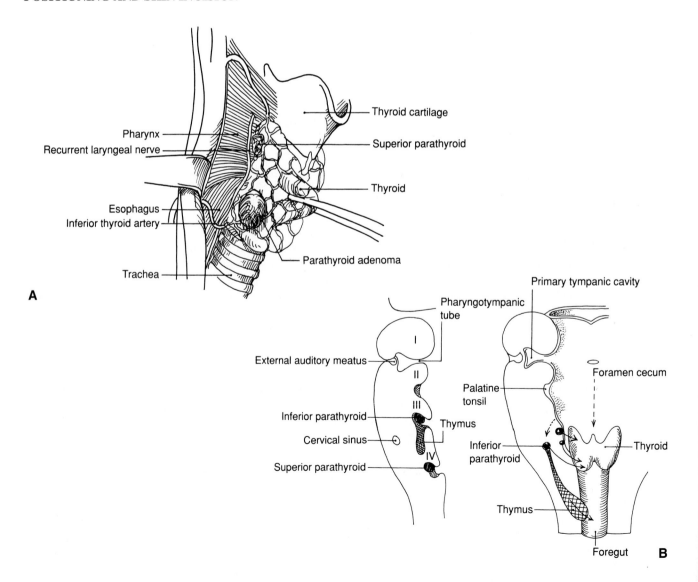

A

Thyroid cartilage
Pharynx
Recurrent laryngeal nerve
Superior parathyroid
Thyroid
Esophagus
Inferior thyroid artery
Parathyroid adenoma
Trachea

Primary tympanic cavity
Pharyngotympanic tube
External auditory meatus
Foramen cecum
Palatine tonsil
Inferior parathyroid
Thymus
Cervical sinus
Inferior parathyroid
Thyroid
Superior parathyroid
Thymus
Foregut   **B**

FIGURE 7.2
IDENTIFICATION OF THE UPPER PARATHYROID GLAND ON THE RIGHT SIDE

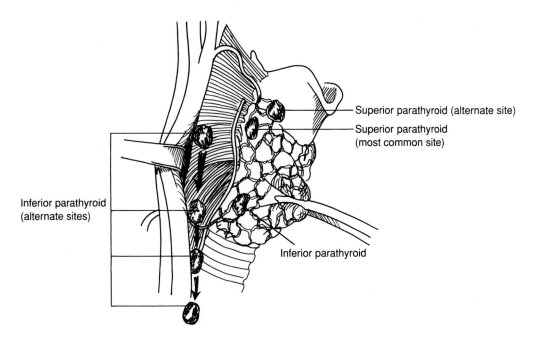

Superior parathyroid (alternate site)
Superior parathyroid (most common site)
Inferior parathyroid (alternate sites)
Inferior parathyroid

gland superior to the inferior thyroid artery–recurrent laryngeal nerve junction.

Although the location of the inferior parathyroids is more variable, they are most frequently (40% to 60% of cases) found along the superficial surface of the lower pole of the thyroid (inferior to the inferior thyroid artery–recurrent laryngeal nerve junction). With almost equal frequency (30% to 40% of cases), the inferior parathyroids are located inferior to the thyroid gland, either in the connective tissue connecting the thyroid gland and thymus gland or within the substance of the thymus gland proper.

When glands on one side are located in their normal position, there is typically contralateral symmetry (in about 80% of cases with respect to superior parathyroids and in about 70% of cases with respect to inferior parathyroids).

Identification of the Upper Parathyroid Gland on the Right Side (Fig. 7.2)

Technical Points

Mobilize the right lobe of the thyroid by placing traction sutures in the midportion and superior pole of the gland. Identify, ligate, and divide the middle thyroid vein. Rotate the right lobe of the thyroid medially and up into the wound. Divide the superior pole vessels, if necessary, to improve exposure.

Search for the upper parathyroid gland in the following locations:

1. At the posterior cricothyroid juncture
2. Behind the upper pole of the thyroid
3. In the retroesophageal or retropharyngeal space

If you are having difficulty locating a superior parathyroid gland, remember that a common error is failure to explore the retroesophageal space adequately. Develop the plane between the esophagus and the vertebral column bluntly and visually explore it for the entire length of the operative field. Gently pass your index finger into this plane and palpate well down into the mediastinum (as far as you can reach).

The blood supply of the superior parathyroid gland generally derives from the inferior thyroid artery. Tracing the branches of this artery may help to locate the parathyroid.

Anatomic Points

Because of the short migratory route, the frequency of ectopic superior parathyroids is less than that of inferior parathyroids. An excellent recent study of 503 autopsies (anatomic reference 1) revealed that 80% of superior parathyroids were located in an area 2 cm in diameter and about 1 cm superior to the intersection of the recurrent laryngeal nerve and the inferior thyroid artery–within the so-called surgical capsule of the thyroid in the connective tissue binding the posterior edge of the thyroid to the pharynx. The next most frequent locations reported were more superior but in the same tissue plane, although typically the glands were inferior to the superior thyroid artery. Rarely, the superior parathyroids were located more inferiorly. They have also been reported to occur posterior or inferior to the junction of the inferior thyroid artery and recurrent laryngeal nerve, posterior to the inferior pole of the thyroid, in the retropharyngeal or retroesophageal space, posterior to the carotid sheath, in the posterior part of the superior mediastinum, and very rarely, within the true capsule of the thyroid gland.

FIGURE 7.3
IDENTIFICATION OF THE LOWER
PARATHYROID GLAND

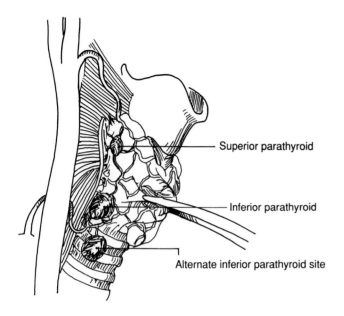

Superior parathyroid

Inferior parathyroid

Alternate inferior parathyroid site

Identification of the Lower Parathyroid Gland (Fig. 7.3)

Technical Points

Search for the lower parathyroid gland in the following locations:

1. Adherent to the lower pole of the thyroid
2. Within a cervical tongue of thymus
3. In close proximity to the lower pole of the thyroid

The lower parathyroid glands are more variable in location than are the upper parathyroid glands.

After identifying two glands on the first side, explore the second side in a similar manner. Identify and examine all four parathyroids before excision or biopsy. If you cannot locate all four parathyroid glands, remove all fatty and areolar tissue within reach from the superior mediastinum. Check the tracheoesophageal groove carefully and probe down into the mediastinum in this space, being careful to avoid injury to the recurrent laryngeal nerve. Clean fatty tissue from the region of the carotid sheath. Open the carotid sheath. Remember that the blood supply of the parathyroid usually derives from the inferior thyroid artery; tracing branches of this artery may help to locate an elusive gland. Finally, look within the substance of the thyroid gland by incising the lobe on the side of the missing parathyroid (thyroidotomy) or removing it.

Normal parathyroid glands are oval or bean-shaped, measure about 2 to 4 mm × 4 to 6 mm, and weigh 40 to 60 mg. They are commonly yellow-brown and tend to become darker when manipulated ("parathyroid blush"). Although adherent to the thyroid, a parathyroid gland will move slightly when

touched with the tip of a hemostat, whereas a follicle of thyroid tissue generally will not.

If you find a single enlarged gland, excise it in its entirety, ligating the small vascular pedicle. Perform a biopsy on at least one of the normal-appearing glands to exclude hyperplasia.

If several glands are enlarged, remove them. When all four glands are enlarged, remove three and leave only a small remnant of the fourth gland. Alternatively, all four may be removed. In such cases, save a remnant of one, mince it into fine fragments, and implant it within the muscles of the forearm. Mark the location of the implant with Fine clips or permanent sutures.

To obtain a biopsy specimen of a normal-appearing parathyroid gland, gently tease it free of the surrounding tissue, carefully preserving the blood supply. Then place a fine suture-ligature through the tip of it (for traction) and shave off a piece with Fine iris scissors. The cut surface of a parathyroid gland will bleed in a fine, diffuse pattern. By contrast, fat or lymph node (commonly mistaken for parathyroid tissue) will bleed unevenly.

Anatomic Points

The inferior parathyroid glands develop from the dorsal wing of pharyngeal pouch III, whereas the ventral wing of this pouch develops into the definitive thymus gland. As the thymus migrates from its site of origin to its definitive location, it drags the inferior parathyroids with it until the parathyroids adhere to the true capsule of the developing thyroid gland. Because of the rather long migratory path of the pharyngeal pouch III derivatives, inferior parathyroid tissue is most likely to be found in ectopic locations. In about half of cases, the inferior parathyroids are located on the superficial surface (either anterior or posterior) of the inferior pole of the thyroid gland. Also in about half of the cases, the parathyroids are located in the thyrothymic ligament, or in the cervical part of the thymus. Other locations reported include within the mediastinal part of the thymus, at the carotid bifurcation, in the carotid sheath, in the anterior part of the superior mediastinum not associated with thymus, in the pericardium, and superior to the superior thyroid artery.

Supernumerary glands may occur as a result of "seeding" of parathyroid cells along this lengthy path of embryologic descent. As many as five supernumerary glands have been reported, with about two thirds being located in the thyrothymic ligament or thymus gland, suggesting an origin from pharyngeal pouch III. About one third of supernumerary glands are located in the vicinity of the thyroid, between the superior and inferior parathyroids.

Recurrent Hyperparathyroidism: Lateral Approach, Mediastinal Exploration (Fig. 7.4)

Technical and Anatomic Points

When hyperparathyroidism persists or recurs after surgery, reexploration is necessary. Most missed parathyroid glands

FIGURE 7.4
RECURRENT HYPERPARATHYROIDISM: LATERAL APPROACH, MEDIASTINAL EXPLORATION

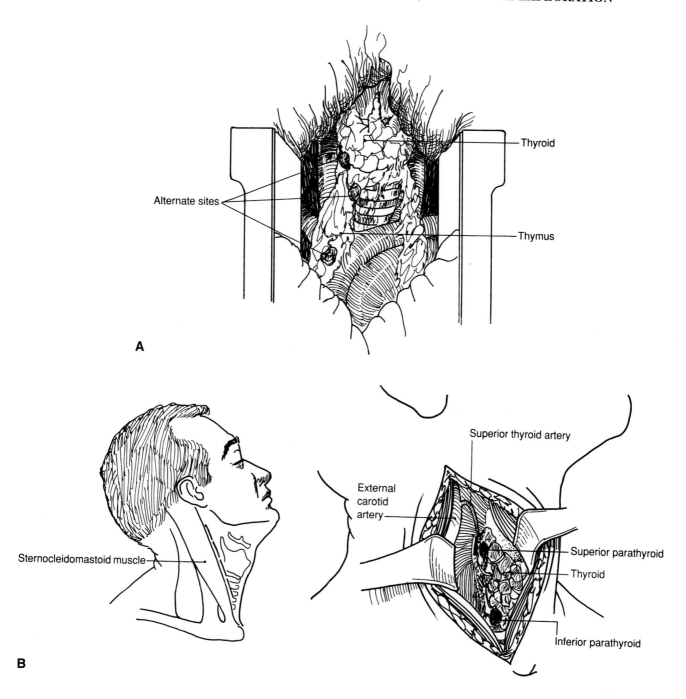

are in the neck. Hence, unless excellent localization studies or a thorough prior neck exploration by an experienced surgeon mandates otherwise, repeat the neck exploration. Before proceeding, carefully review operative notes and pathology reports. A standard diagram, such as that shown in the orientation figure at the beginning of this chapter, facilitates the recording of information and is invaluable when reexploration is needed.

Reopen the old cervical incision and develop flaps under the platysma. If only one gland was found on one side at initial exploration, recheck that side first. If the plane between the strap muscles and thyroid is densely scarred, make a lateral incision between the anterior border of the sternocleidomastoid muscle and the strap muscles (Fig. 7.4A). Gentle dissection through this lateral approach will lead to the inferior thyroid artery and recurrent laryngeal nerve. Often, this area is relatively "virgin" and free of scar tissue. This approach is also sometimes used for initial exploration when there is high confidence in preoperative imaging techniques.

Missed cervical parathyroids are commonly found in the tracheoesophageal groove, in the thymic fat pad, within the substance of the thyroid gland, in the fatty areolar tissue adjacent to the thyroid, or in the carotid sheath.

Mediastinal exploration is performed when thorough neck exploration has failed to cure hyperparathyroidism (Fig. 7.4B). An upper median sternotomy is performed and the fatty and areolar tissue, including the entire thymic fat pad, is removed (see Chapter 20). Most mediastinal parathyroids lie in the anterior mediastinum. Occasionally, an ectopic superior parathyroid gland lies deep in the posterior mediastinum in the vicinity of the esophagus.

SURGICAL REFERENCES

1. Akerstrom G, Rudberg C, Grimelius L, et al. Causes of failed primary exploration and technical aspects of reoperation in primary hyperparathyroidism. *World J Surg* 1992;16:562. (Analyzes patterns of failure and emphasizes corrective strategies.)
2. Edis AJ. Surgical anatomy and technique of neck exploration for primary hyperparathyroidism. *Surg Clin North Am* 1977;57:495. (Provides a general review.)
3. Esselstyn CB, Levin H. A technique for parathyroid surgery. *Surg Clin North Am* 1975;55:1047. (Clearly describes the technique, including transcervical thymectomy.)
4. Kaplan EL, Yashiro T, Salti G. Primary hyperparathyroidism in the 1990's: choice of surgical procedure for this disease. *Ann Surg* 1992;215:300–317.
5. Kilgo MS, Pirsch JD, Warner TF, et al. Tertiary hyperparathyroidism after renal transplantation: surgical strategy. *Surgery* 1998;124:677–684.
6. Levin K, Clark OH. The reasons for failure in parathyroid operations. *Arch Surg* 1989;124:911.
7. Moley JF, Lairmore TC, Doherty GM, et al. Preservation of the recurrent laryngeal nerves in thyroid and parathyroid reoperations. *Surgery* 1999;125:673–679. (Describes lateral approach and other strategies for working through undissected territory.)
8. Monchik JM, Bendinelli C, Passero MA Jr, et al. Subcutaneous forearm transplantation of autologous parathyroid tissue in patients with renal hyperparathyroidism. *Surgery* 1999;126:1152–1159. (Clearly explains technique of autotransplantation)
9. Pollock WF. Surgical anatomy of the thyroid and parathyroid glands. *Surg Clin North Am* 1964;44:1161.
10. Pyrtek LJ, Painter RL. An anatomic study of the relationship of the parathyroid glands to the recurrent laryngeal nerve. *Surg Gynecol Obstet* 1964;119:509.
11. Scholz DA, Purnell DC, Woolner LB, et al. Mediastinal hyperfunctioning parathyroid tumors: review of 14 cases. *Ann Surg* 1973;178:173. (Discusses mediastinal locations.).
12. Sitges-Serra A, Caralps-Riera A. Hyperparathyroidism associated with renal disease: pathogenesis, natural history, and surgical treatment. *Surg Clin North Am* 1987;67:359.
13. Wang C. Surgical management of primary hyperparathyroidism. *Curr Probl Surg* 1985;22:1. (Provides an excellent review of anatomy, pathology, and surgical management.)
14. Wells SA, Leight GS, Hensley M, et al. Hyperparathyroidism associated with the enlargement of two or three parathyroid glands. *Ann Surg* 1985;202:533. (Emphasizes the prevalence of two- or three-gland enlargement and stresses the need to visualize all parathyroids.)

DIFFICULT SURGICAL PROBLEM REFERENCES

1. Beahrs OH, Edis AJ, Purnell DC. Unusual problems in parathyroid surgery. *Am J Surg* 1977;134:502. (Reviews the anomalous locations encountered during 122 explorations.)
2. Cheung PS, Borgstrom A, Thompson NW. Strategy in reoperative surgery for hyperparathyroidism. *Arch Surg* 1989;124:676. (Discusses the locations of missed adenomas.)
3. Freeman JB, Sherman BM, Mason EE. Transcervical thymectomy: an integral part of neck exploration for hyperparathyroidism. *Arch Surg* 1976;111:369.
4. Patow CA, Norton JA, Brennan MF. Vocal cord paralysis and reoperative parathyroidectomy: a prospective study. *Ann Surg* 1986;203:282.
5. Saxe AW, Brennan MF. Reoperative parathyroid surgery for primary hyperparathyroidism caused by multiple gland disease: total parathyroid autotransplantation with cryopreserved tissue. *Surgery* 1982;91:616. (Describes cryopreservation and autotransplantation.)
6. Speigel AM, Marx J, Doppman JL, et al. Intrathyroidal parathyroid adenoma or hyperplasia: an occasionally overlooked cause of surgical failure in primary hyperparathyroidism. *JAMA* 1975;234:1029. (Describes six cases, emphasizing the normal appearance of the thyroid and characteristics of a normal thyroid scan.)
7. Turner WW, Snyder WH. Parathyroid map. *Surgery* 1981;89:770. (Offers an excellent diagram that can be used to record operative findings.)
8. Wells SA, Ross AJ, Dale JK, et al. Transplantation of the parathyroid glands: current status. *Surg Clin North Am* 1979;59:167.

ANATOMIC REFERENCES

1. Akerstrom G, Malmaeus J, Bergstrom R. Surgical anatomy of human parathyroid glands. *Surgery* 1984;95:14.
2. Fraker DL, Doppman JL, Shawker TH, et al. Undescended parathyroid adenoma: an important etiology for failed operations for primary hyperparathyroidism. *World J Surg* 1990;14:342–348.
3. Gilmour JR. The gross anatomy of the parathyroid glands. *J Pathol* 1938;46:133. (Reviews the size, number, and location of parathyroid glands based on data from an autopsy series.)
4. Liechty RD, Weil R. Parathyroid anatomy in hyperplasia. *Arch Surg* 1992;127:813. (Reviews anomalous locations encountered in surgery for hyperplasia.)
5. Nathaniels EK, Nathaniels AM, Chiu-an W. Mediastinal parathyroid tumors: a clinical and pathological study of 84 cases. *Ann Surg* 1970; 171:165. (Provides an excellent summary of the location of mediastinal glands, emphasizing that most are accessible via a cervical incision.)
6. Pyrtek LJ, Painter RL. An anatomic study of the relationship of the parathyroid glands to the recurrent laryngeal nerve. *Surg Gynecol Obstet* 1964;119:509. (Describes the rectangular area traversed by the recurrent nerve, which, in this autopsy series, was the location of 93% of the parathyroids studied.)
7. Wang C. The anatomic basis of parathyroid surgery. *Ann Surg* 1976;183:271. (Offers an excellent review of a large series of parathyroid glands examined at autopsy; discusses variations in size and shape, as well as location.)

THE LATERAL NECK AND STRUCTURES APPROACHED FROM THE SIDE

Structures of significance in the lateral neck are primarily vascular. The internal and external jugular veins and the common, internal, and external carotid arteries are all approached from the side. The internal and external jugular veins are primarily used for vascular access (Chapter 8), either by percutaneous puncture or by cutdown. Surgery for stroke prevention is performed on the carotid artery in the region of its bifurcation (Chapter 9).

As are all major vessels, the carotid arteries and jugular veins are accompanied by lymph nodes. Lymph node biopsy (Chapter 10) introduces the anatomy of the cervical lymph node groups. The anatomy of the major lymph node groups is related to major vascular structures and nerves by the meticulous operation undertaken for cancer (termed *radical neck dissection*) (Chapter 11).

Although the esophagus is a midline structure, it lies so deep in the neck that it is easier to approach from the side. Therefore, exposure of the cervical esophagus and the anatomic relationships of this portion of the gastrointestinal tract are included in this section (Chapter 12).

Neck exploration for trauma (Chapter 13)—a systematic inspection of major vascular and visceral compartments of the neck—completes the procedures commonly performed in this area.

CHAPTER 8

Venous Access: External and Internal Jugular Veins

The external and internal jugular veins are frequently used for access to the central venous circulation. In this chapter, external jugular venous cutdown, internal jugular venous cutdown, and percutaneous internal jugular venous cannulation are presented. The anatomy of the carotid sheath is introduced. The carotid artery and the anatomy of the carotid region are discussed in greater detail in Chapter 9.

External Jugular Venous Cutdown

The external jugular vein, because of its superficial location, is an easy site for venous cutdown or percutaneous cannulation. Difficulty is often encountered in passing a catheter centrally from this location. In addition, the vein is often thrombosed in patients in whom the procedure has been attempted before. For these reasons, the more difficult internal jugular approaches may be required.

Venous Anatomy of the Neck and External Jugular Venous Cutdown (Fig. 8.1)

Technical Points

Position the patient with the head turned to one side. A slight Trendelenburg position will increase venous pressure in the neck, facilitating identification of the vein and decreasing the chance of venous air embolism. Apply pressure to the platysma muscle just above the clavicle and identify the external jugular vein as it distends with blood. Infiltrate the area overlying the vein with local anesthetic and make a small transverse skin incision over the vein in the midneck. Make the incision with care to avoid injury to the vein, which lies very superficially. Identify the vein and dissect parallel to the

LIST OF STRUCTURES

External jugular vein
Internal jugular vein
Common facial vein
Common carotid artery
Platysma muscle
Sternocleidomastoid muscle

vein proximally and distally for a length of about 1 cm. Elevate the vein into the wound with a hemostat. Ligate the vein proximally (cephalad) and place a ligature around the distal vein.

The catheter should enter the skin at a separate site, rather than through the cutdown incision. Make a small incision about 2 cm above the skin incision and tunnel the catheter under the skin to the incision. A Broviac or Hickman-type catheter is tunneled under the skin of the chest wall to an exit site located at a flat, stable location. Generally, the parasternal region, about 10 cm below the clavicle, is selected as the exit site.

Use a number 11 blade for performing a small anterior venotomy, then introduce the catheter. Because of angulation at the juncture of the external jugular vein and the subclavian vein, there may be a tendency for the catheter to "hang up" or to pass out toward the arm rather than centrally. If this occurs, turn the patient's head back toward the side of cannulation and reattempt to pass the catheter centrally. If necessary, use a floppy-tipped guidewire, under fluoroscopic control, to guide the catheter into the superior vena cava. Tie the catheter in place distally.

Secure the catheter in position and close the incision with interrupted absorbable sutures.

If the external jugular vein cannot be cannulated or the central venous circulation cannot be accessed using this approach, extend the incision medially and proceed to the internal jugular vein (Fig. 8.2).

Anatomic Points

The external jugular vein begins in the vicinity of the angle of the mandible, within or just inferior to the parotid gland. It runs just deep to the platysma muscle. Its course is approximated by a line connecting the mandibular angle and the middle of the clavicle. It crosses the sternocleidomastoid muscle and pierces the superficial lamina of the deep cervical fascia roofing the omoclavicular triangle. It continues its vertical course to end in either the subclavian or, about one third of the time, the internal jugular vein. When it pierces the superficial lamina, its wall adheres to the fascia. This tends to hold a laceration of the vein open and predisposes the patient to air entrance if the vein is severed at this site. The vein can be occluded by pressure just superior to the middle of

FIGURE 8.1
VENOUS ANATOMY OF THE NECK AND EXTERNAL JUGULAR VENOUS CUTDOWN

the clavicle, a point slightly posterior to the clavicular origin of the sternocleidomastoid muscle. The diameter of the external jugular vein is quite variable and appears to have an inverse relation to the diameter of the internal jugular veins. The right external jugular vein is typically larger in diameter than the left, partly because it is more closely aligned with the superior vena cava and thus the right atrium.

At midneck, the external jugular vein is covered only by the platysma muscle and minor branches of the transverse cervical nerve. This branch of the cervical plexus, carrying sensory fibers of C2 and C3, pierces the superficial lamina of the cervical fascia at the posterior edge of the middle of

the sternocleidomastoid, then crosses the sternocleidomastoid muscle, passing deep to the external jugular vein, to innervate the skin of the anterior triangle of the neck.

Internal Jugular Venous Cutdown

Dissection to the Internal Jugular Vein (Fig. 8.2)

Technical Points

Choose the right internal jugular vein whenever possible. Position the patient supine with the head turned to the contralateral side. The table should be flat or in a slight Trendelenburg

FIGURE 8.2
DISSECTION TO THE INTERNAL JUGULAR VEIN

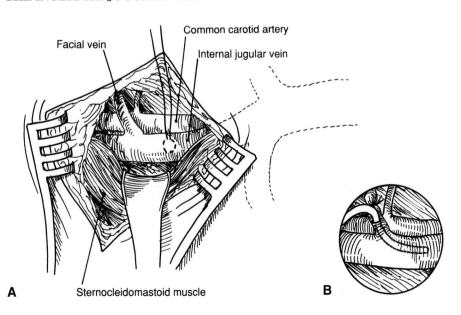

position to distend the veins of the neck and minimize the chances of venous air embolism. Infiltrate the skin of a planned transverse skin incision about 2 cm above the clavicle. Make an incision about 3 cm in length, centered over the triangle formed by the division of the sternocleidomastoid muscle into its medial and lateral heads.

Deepen the incision through the platysma until the sternocleidomastoid muscle is encountered, then spread the tissue between the two heads of the muscle to expose the underlying internal jugular vein.

If approaching the internal jugular vein after a failed external jugular vein cutdown, the incision may be high enough to access the common facial vein as it empties into the internal jugular vein. Extend the incision medially across the medial border of the sternocleidomastoid muscle. Retract the sternocleidomastoid muscle and identify the internal jugular vein just deep to the muscle and lying within the carotid sheath. Search along the anterior and upper aspect of the vein for a large common facial vein. If this can be identified, it can often be cannulated and ligated. This is a simpler way to access the internal jugular vein than is the pursestring suture method (Fig. 8.3).

Anatomic Points

The right internal jugular vein takes a relatively straight course to the central venous circulation, unlike the left, which first enters the brachiocephalic vein. For this reason, it is the preferred site of cannulation.

The minor supraclavicular fossa is the triangle bounded by the clavicle and the sternal and clavicular heads of the sternocleidomastoid muscle. This fossa is covered by skin, superficial fascia (in which there may be branches of the medial supraclavicular nerve), fibers of the platysma muscle, and the superficial lamina of the cervical fascia.

The internal jugular vein is the dominant structure within the fossa itself. Its exposure may be somewhat tedious owing to the presence of deep cervical lymph nodes. It is located in its own compartment in the carotid sheath and tends to diverge anteriorly from the common carotid artery. This facilitates circumferential dissection of the vein. Because the vein is completely surrounded by the connective tissue elements of the carotid sheath, it does not collapse completely. This can lead to the complication of air embolus. Remember that the common carotid artery is posterior to the internal jugular vein at this level and that the apex of the lung is posterior to the common carotid artery. Slightly more inferior, the termination of the internal jugular vein and the beginning of the brachiocephalic vein are in contact with parietal pleura and the apex of the lung.

Placement of Pursestring Suture and Cannulation of the Internal Jugular Vein (Fig. 8.3)

Technical and Anatomic Points

Carefully dissect in the anterior adventitial plane of the vein to free several centimeters of vein proximally and distally. Pass

FIGURE 8.3
PLACEMENT OF PURSESTRING SUTURE AND CANNULATION OF THE INTERNAL JUGULAR VEIN

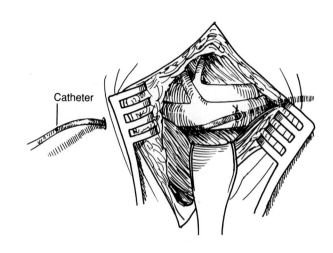

a right-angle clamp under the vein and place Silastic loops proximal and distal to the vein. Lift up on the vein gently with DeBakey pickups, if necessary, to facilitate passage of the right-angle clamp. The internal jugular vein can be ligated if necessary. If injury to the vein occurs, ligation and division of the vein is the safest course.

Place a 4-0 Prolene pursestring suture on the anterior surface of the vein. Place this suture in four bites, drawing a small square on the vein. Make a small incision, using a number 11 blade, in the center of the pursestring and insert the catheter. Confirm passage into the central circulation and good position of the catheter tip. Tie the pursestring suture and close the incision in layers with interrupted absorbable suture.

Percutaneous Cannulation of the Internal Jugular Vein

Posterior Approach to the Internal Jugular Vein (Fig. 8.4)

Technical Points

Position the patient supine, in a moderate Trendelenburg position, with the head turned to the contralateral side. Palpate the lateral border of the sternocleidomastoid muscle about two fingerbreadths above the clavicle. Use the thumb of the nondominant hand to stabilize and elevate the sternocleidomastoid muscle by hooking the tip of the thumb under the edge of the muscle and lifting slightly. Place the index finger of the same hand in the sternal notch for orientation. Visualize an imaginary line passing just deep to the thumb of that hand and aiming at the index finger. Infiltrate the skin with local anesthetic, then infiltrate the deeper tissues, aspirating carefully as the needle is advanced. Use this small-gauge needle to identify the internal jugular vein by aspirating venous blood about 1 to 2 cm deep to the skin. If no blood is obtained, vary the depth below the sternocleidomastoid muscle, but not the angle of the needle, until blood is obtained.

FIGURE 8.4
POSTERIOR APPROACH TO THE INTERNAL JUGULAR VEIN

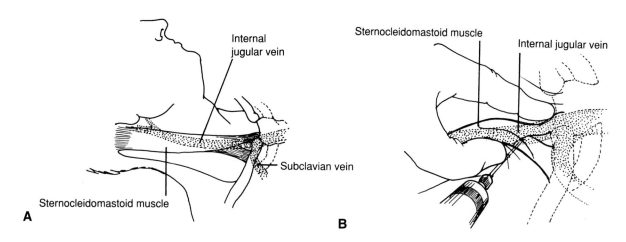

After identifying the vein with a small-caliber needle, use a slightly larger needle to cannulate the vein, then introduce the floppy end of a guidewire into the vein. It should pass easily. A vessel dilator and introducer of the desired size can then be passed over the guidewire and the catheter placed. If bright-red blood is obtained when the vessel is cannulated, the carotid artery may have been entered. Before making another attempt, withdraw the needle and apply firm but gentle pressure to the site for 10 minutes. If attempting a new venipuncture on the opposite internal jugular vein, it is always safest to obtain a chest radiograph before proceeding any further. Although rare, a bilateral pneumothorax can occur and is a potentially serious, if not lethal, complication if it is not recognized.

After the catheter is successfully positioned, confirm its location by chest radiography and check carefully for the presence of a pneumothorax.

Anatomic Points

At the entrance site of the needle, no major anatomic structures should be located. Remember that the internal jugular vein is immediately deep to the sternocleidomastoid muscle and anterolateral to the common carotid artery. The apex of the lung is protected by the anterior scalene muscle and its fascia, but it can be entered if the needle is directed too deeply. An improperly placed needle can enter the common carotid artery medial to the vein or damage the vagus nerve posteromedial to the vein.

REFERENCES

1. Albarran-Sotelo R, Atkins JM, Bloom RS, et al. Intravenous techniques. In: *Textbook of advanced cardiac life support.* 2nd ed. New York: American Heart Association, 1987:147. (Offers an excellent review of currently recommended techniques for central venous access.)
2. American Association of Clinical Anatomists, Educational Affairs Committee. The clinical anatomy of invasive procedures. *Clin Anat* 1999;12:43.
3. Benotti PN, Bothe A Jr, Miller JD, et al. Safe cannulation of the internal jugular vein for long-term hyperalimentation. *Surg Gynecol Obstet* 1977;144:574.
4. Caridi JG, Hawkins IF Jr, Wiechmann BN, et al. Sonographic guidance when using the right internal jugular vein for central vein access. *AJR Am J Roentgenol* 1998;171:1259–1263. (Describes use of ultrasound to facilitate percutaneous cannulation.)
5. Kaushik S, Dubey PK, Ambesh SP. Internal jugular vein cannulation in neurosurgical patients: a new approach. *J Neurosurg Anesthesiol* 1999;11:185–187. (Describes a modified technique that is useful when head and neck must be maintained in neutral position.)
6. Krausz MM, Berlarzky Y, Ayalon A, et al. Percutaneous cannulation of the internal jugular vein in infants and children. *Surg Gynecol Obstet* 1979;148:591. (Describes variations in anatomy in young children.)
7. Lowell JA, Bothe A Jr. Venous access: preoperative, operative, and postoperative dilemmas. *Surg Clin North Am* 1991;71:1231.
8. Recht MP, Burke DR, Meranze SG, et al. Simple technique for redirecting malpositioned central venous catheters. *AJR Am J Roentgenol* 1990;154:183. (Describes a useful technique when the catheter is misdirected.)
9. Silberzweig JE, Mitty HA. Central venous access: low internal jugular vein approach using imaging guidance. *AJR Am J Roentgenol* 1998;170:1617–1620. (Explains rationale for low approach; advocates adjunctive use of ultrasound.)
10. Teichgraber UKM, Benter TM, Gebel M, et al. A sonographically guided technique for central venous access. *AJR Am J Roentgenol* 1997;169:731–733. (Describes use of ultrasound to facilitate cannulation.)

CHAPTER 9

Carotid Endarterectomy

Timothy F. Kresowik

The carotid bifurcation in the neck is a frequent site of atherosclerosis. Thromboembolic events originating from atherosclerotic plaque at this location are a common cause of ischemic stroke. Fortunately, the disease is almost always limited to the region of the bifurcation and is surgically accessible. Randomized clinical trials have established the efficacy of carotid endarterectomy (surgical plaque removal) for stroke prevention in patients who have high-grade stenosis of the internal carotid artery in the neck.

Regional Anatomy and Skin Incision (Fig. 9.1)

Technical Points

Preoperative determination of extent of disease and location of the carotid bifurcation, through either duplex ultrasound imaging or angiography, allows the skin incision to be planned for optimal access. The description that follows would apply to patients whose carotid bifurcation is in the typical position in the midneck, and in whom the disease does not extend unusually far distally or proximally.

Position the patient with the neck extended and the head rotated to the side opposite the procedure. It is also helpful to have the head of the bed elevated about 30 degrees to decrease venous pressure and bleeding. The most important landmark for planning the incision is the anterior border of the sternocleidomastoid muscle, which can be visualized or palpated. Initiate the distal end of the incision along this border at the level of the angle of the mandible or 2 to 3 cm from the mastoid process. The upper portion of the incision should follow the border of the sternocleidomastoid muscle. At a point two thirds of the distance between the mastoid process and the head of the clavicle, curve the incision into a more transverse direction to produce a better cosmetic result than the traditional straight incision.

Anatomic Points

The incision described previously allows the best balance between exposure and cosmesis. Langer's lines in the neck are predominately horizontal, and making the inferior portion of the incision more transverse results in a better scar that follows the normal skin creases.

Exposure of the Sternocleidomastoid Muscle (Fig. 9.2)

Technical Points

Deepen the skin incision through the subcutaneous tissue and platysmal layer. Mobilize the medial border of the sternocleidomastoid muscle along the entire length of the incision. If the incision is extended superiorly, the tail of the parotid gland is encountered. If necessary for exposure, this portion of the parotid can be mobilized along the inferior and posterior aspects of the gland. The external jugular vein and great auricular nerve may be encountered at this level. The external jugular vein may be ligated. Preserve the greater auricular nerve if possible. The dissection plane should remain over the medial border of the sternocleidomastoid muscle and not drift anteriorly toward the mandible because injury

LIST OF STRUCTURES

Sternocleidomastoid muscle	Marginal mandibular branch of facial nerve	Ansa cervicalis
Mandible	Internal jugular vein	Vagus nerve
Mastoid process	Facial vein	Glossopharyngeal nerve
Clavicular head	Spinal accessory nerve	Omohyoid muscle
Langer's lines	Digastric muscle	Common carotid artery
Platysma muscle	Hypoglossal nerve	Internal carotid artery
Parotid gland	Sternocleidomastoid branch of occipital artery	External carotid artery
External jugular vein		Superior thyroid artery
Great auricular nerve		Superior laryngeal nerve

FIGURE 9.1
REGIONAL ANATOMY AND SKIN INCISION

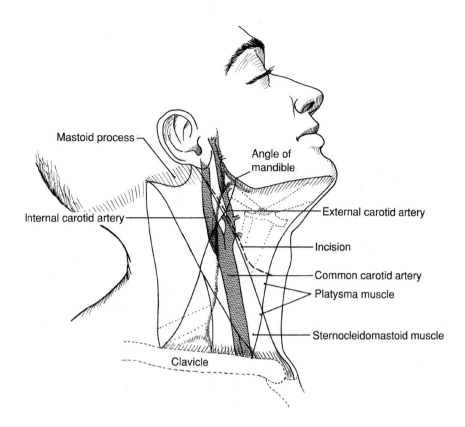

Mastoid process

Angle of mandible

Internal carotid artery

External carotid artery

Incision

Common carotid artery

Platysma muscle

Sternocleidomastoid muscle

Clavicle

to the marginal mandibular branch of the facial nerve could result. Near the upper end of the incision, an arterial branch from the occipital artery going to the sternocleidomastoid muscle may be encountered and should be divided. This arterial branch usually loops over the hypoglossal nerve in its course from the occipital artery, and division allows the hypoglossal nerve to retract medially away from the dissection plane.

If more proximal exposure of the common carotid is necessary, develop a subplatysmal flap at the inferior end of the incision to allow continued mobilization of the medial border of the sternocleidomastoid muscle to its clavicular insertion despite the transverse course of the skin incision.

Anatomic Points

The platysmal muscle has little functional importance but is the division between a plane superficial to the muscle, which is devoid of significant neurovascular structures, and the plane deep to the muscle that contains nerves that should be preserved if possible. The great auricular nerve is a sensory branch of C2 and C3 that parallels the external jugular vein. Sacrifice or injury to the greater auricular nerve leads to numbness or paresthesia of the ear. The marginal mandibular branch of the facial nerve normally parallels the ramus of the mandible but can extend as much as 2.5 cm inferior to the

mandible. The nerve is a motor branch to the muscles of the corner of the mouth. Injury to this nerve can lead to a significant cosmetic and functional impairment, with drooping of the corner of the mouth and drooling. Keeping the dissection plane along or posterior to the border of the sternocleidomastoid muscle will usually avoid direct injury to this nerve. This nerve can also be injured by injudicious placement of mechanical retractors against the mandible.

Exposure of the Carotid Sheath and Internal Jugular Vein (Fig. 9.3)

Technical Points

The next portion of the dissection involves mobilizing the medial border of the internal jugular vein. It is important to perform the dissection using this anatomic landmark rather than proceeding directly to dissecting out the carotid artery. Take care to stay along the border of the vein to minimize the chance of cranial nerve injury. As the medial border of the vein is mobilized, the common facial vein is encountered. Ligate and divide it. As the dissection progresses superiorly, additional small draining veins may be encountered and may need to be ligated. If very distal exposure of the internal carotid is necessary, the posterior belly of the digastric muscle can be divided, but dissection at

FIGURE 9.2
EXPOSURE OF THE STERNOCLEIDOMASTOID MUSCLE

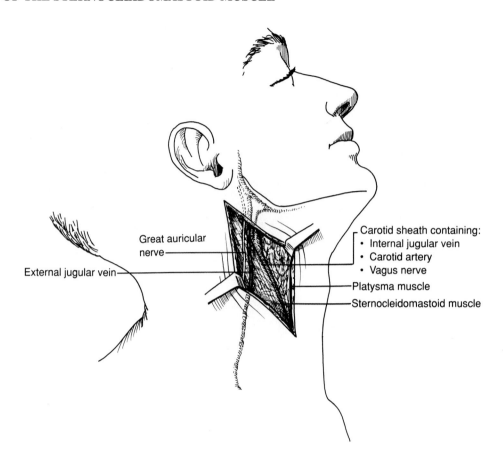

Great auricular nerve

External jugular vein

Carotid sheath containing:
• Internal jugular vein
• Carotid artery
• Vagus nerve
Platysma muscle
Sternocleidomastoid muscle

this level is not necessary in most carotid endarterectomy procedures.

In performing the superior portion of the dissection, avoid drifting laterally in the plane between the posterior aspect of the sternocleidomastoid muscle and the internal jugular vein. The eleventh cranial nerve (spinal accessory) may be encountered in this area.

At the inferior end of the dissection, the omohyoid muscle is encountered looping across the field. The muscle may be divided, but adequate exposure is often obtained by mobilizing and retracting the muscle inferiorly.

Anatomic Points

The common facial vein is the largest vein draining into the internal jugular. It is formed from the confluence of the retro-mandibular vein and facial vein. The junction of the common facial and internal jugular veins is usually a good marker of the level of the carotid bifurcation. The spinal accessory nerve is found deep to the sternocleidomastoid muscle lateral to the internal jugular vein. Injury to this nerve, which supplies the trapezius muscle, can lead to a shoulder drop and difficulty in arm abduction.

Exposure of the Carotid Bifurcation (Fig. 9.4)

Technical Points

Exposure and mobilization of the carotid is normally begun along the lateral aspect of the common carotid artery and then extended distally. Gently mobilize the vagus nerve from the lateral aspect of the carotid. Take care not to create inadvertently a crush injury of the nerve by injudicious use of the forceps during dissection. Continue the dissection distally along the lateral aspect of the internal carotid. Locate the hypoglossal nerve as it runs between the internal carotid and external carotid and then courses anteriorly. If the previously mentioned arterial branch looping over the nerve from the occipital artery to the sternocleidomastoid muscle has been divided, mobilizing the nerve along the posterior and inferior aspects will generally cause it to fall medially and out of danger.

The superior (descending) branch of the ansa cervicalis will also usually retract medially, but it may be occasionally necessary to divide this branch or the inferior branch arising from the cervical plexus to obtain adequate exposure.

Completely mobilize the internal carotid artery to allow clamping well distal to the most distal aspect of the carotid

FIGURE 9.3
EXPOSURE OF THE CAROTID SHEATH AND INTERNAL JUGULAR VEIN

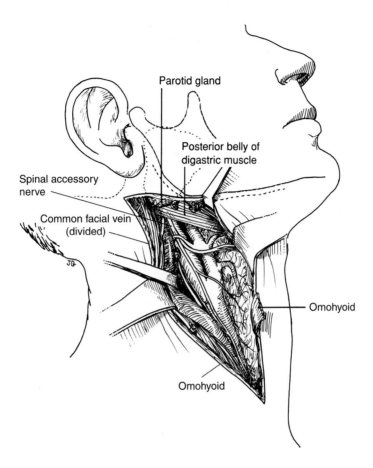

Parotid gland

Posterior belly of
digastric muscle

Spinal accessory
nerve

Common facial vein
(divided)

Omohyoid

Omohyoid

plaque. Minimize manipulation of the bifurcation to decrease the likelihood of dislodging atherothrombotic debris by gently dissecting the tissues away from the artery. In addition, avoid dissecting the internal carotid on its medial aspect (i.e., in the crotch between the internal and external carotid) in order to minimize trauma to the carotid baroreceptors and carotid sinus nerve.

Mobilize the proximal portion of the external carotid and its first branch, the superior thyroid artery, for clamping. In a similar fashion, completely mobilize the common carotid artery proximally and identify a minimally diseased section for clamping.

Anatomic Points

The vagus nerve is within the carotid sheath and, in the superior portion of the dissection, is posterior to the internal carotid and then courses lateral to the common carotid. The nerve may course anterior to the carotid, especially proximally in the neck. The major disability associated with injury to the vagus in the neck is vocal cord paresis because of the recurrent laryngeal nerve fibers that are traveling with the

vagus in the neck. The hypoglossal nerve emerges between the internal jugular vein and internal carotid. The nerve loops anterior to the branches of the external carotid artery superficial to the carotid sheath, usually just superior to the carotid bifurcation. The hypoglossal nerve is a motor nerve to the intrinsic muscles of the tongue, and injury to this nerve can cause significant disability owing to speech and eating difficulties. Traveling with the hypoglossal nerve are fibers from C1 that form the superior root of the ansa cervicalis. The ansa fibers normally diverge from the hypoglossal nerve as it crosses the internal carotid and descend superficial to the internal and common carotid arteries. The superior root is joined by the inferior root, which comprises fibers originating from C2 and C3 and emerges from between the internal jugular and common carotid. The ansa cervicalis innervates the strap muscles. Although the nerve is spared if possible, division of the inferior or superior root is sometimes necessary to obtain adequate mobilization of the hypoglossal nerve or exposure of the carotid and does not result in significant disability.

There are other nerves in the vicinity that are not encountered in the usual carotid endarterectomy procedure.

FIGURE 9.4
EXPOSURE OF THE CAROTID BIFURCATION

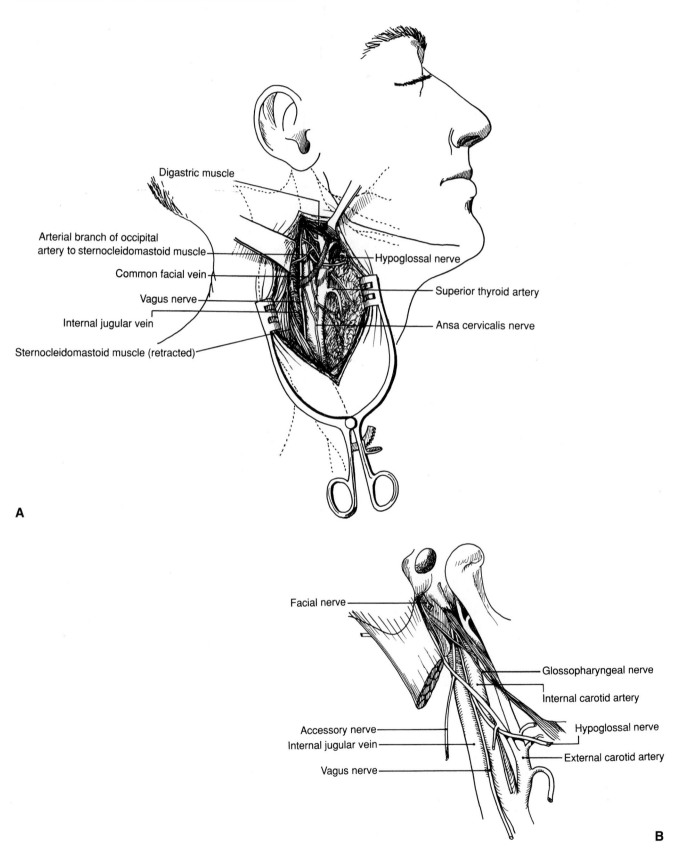

The glossopharyngeal nerve parallels the course of the hypoglossal but is much more superior; its inferior extent is rarely below the angle of the mandible. It may, however, be encountered in very high dissections of the internal carotid. The nerve superiorly is located between the internal jugular vein and internal carotid artery. It then passes superficial to the internal carotid and courses between the internal and external carotid arteries to enter the base of the tongue deep to the hyoglossus muscle. As it passes between the internal and external carotid arteries, it gives rise to the carotid sinus nerve, which supplies the carotid sinus and carotid body. The carotid body also receives vagal innervation. The superior laryngeal nerve is sensory (through the internal branch) to the laryngopharynx and laryngeal mucosa superior to the vocal cords and is motor (through its external branch) to the cricothyroid muscle, a tensor of the vocal cords. The superior laryngeal is usually medial to the carotid sheath, although the external branch comes in proximity to the superior thyroid artery. Dissection of the external carotid and its branches should stay close to the vessels to avoid injury to the superior laryngeal. Injury to the superior laryngeal may cause voice fatigue.

Endarterectomy (Fig. 9.5)

Technical Points

In most cases, the internal carotid, external carotid, superior thyroid, and common carotid are occluded separately. The internal carotid is clamped before the external or common carotid to minimize the risk for cerebral embolization. It is important to have created adequate exposure of both the internal carotid and common carotid beyond the diseased portions so that the clamps can be safely applied in locations that will not interfere with obtaining adequate end points of the endarterectomy. The arteriotomy can be initiated on either the common carotid or internal carotid in areas away from the most severe disease. The arteriotomy should be performed on the lateral aspect of the internal and common carotid (ie, so that the arteriotomy is directly opposite the orifice of the external carotid) (Fig. 9.5A). Having the incision on this most convex aspect of the vessel reduces the chance of having distortion or kinking after closure. The correct endarterectomy plane is in the outer media, leaving only undiseased circular muscle fibers and the adventitia.

Some surgeons routinely place an indwelling shunt to maintain cerebral perfusion during the endarterectomy (Fig. 9.5B). Only 5% to 10% of patients actually have inadequate collateral flow and experience significant ischemia during the period of clamping. Because placing an indwelling shunt interferes with the endarterectomy and adds a small risk for intimal damage proximal or distal to the endarterectomy site, many surgeons prefer to shunt selectively. Selective shunting requires some form of cerebral perfusion or collateral flow monitoring. The most common forms of monitoring include performing the procedure under regional or local anesthesia so that neurologic testing of the awake patient can be performed, using intraoperative electroencephalogram monitoring, or measuring internal carotid backpressure (with the common and external carotid clamped) as an indicator of adequate collateral flow. I prefer to perform the procedure under a cervical block and insert a shunt only if the patient develops a neurologic deficit with clamping.

Begin the endarterectomy in the proximal internal carotid and completely separate the plaque from the vessel wall proximally before attempting to create the internal carotid end point (Fig. 9.5C). Do not continue in the same plane all the way to the end point because this results in elevation of the more normal intima distally. Usually, the best way to achieve a good end point is to pull the plaque in a proximal direction, allowing the diseased portion to separate (Fig. 9.5D). It may be necessary to remove any residual plaque or intima that is not adherent. Only rarely is it necessary to "tack" the intima distally with sutures.

Create the common carotid end point by elevating the plaque proximally, stopping at a point beyond the most severe disease. The common carotid usually has thickened intima, and the disease does not "feather out" as it does in the internal carotid. Sharply divide the plaque proximally (Fig. 9.5E). Ascertain that the remaining proximal intima is adherent. Although it seems counterintuitive, the proximal end point can elevate despite the apparent direction of blood flow. This lifting of a proximal end-point intimal flap has been observed on ultrasound evaluation and is a potential source of thromboembolism or recurrent stenosis.

External carotid "eversion" endarterectomy is facilitated by having completed the common and internal carotid end points first. Separate the plaque from around the orifice of the external carotid. Then, by simultaneously pulling "out" on the plaque and using the clamp or a forceps to push the distal external carotid "in" toward the orifice, evert the plaque and feather it to a good end point (Fig. 9.5F).

After completing the endarterectomy, remove any loose intimal fronds and check the end points for adherence. There is evidence that patch closure of the endarterectomy site is superior to primary closure with respect to lower postoperative neurologic events and later recurrent stenosis. Patch angioplasty can be performed with either a fabric patch or autologous vein. Begin patch closure distally and complete it with monofilament suture in a continuous fashion (Fig. 9.5G). A single suture can be used or a second suture begun at the proximal end.

Before completing closure, temporarily release each clamp individually to "flush out" any residual debris. Restore flow into the external carotid circulation first (removing the internal carotid clamp last) to minimize the possibility of cerebral embolization of any residual debris or air.

Close the wound in two layers with continuous absorbable suture. The only deep layer that needs to be approximated is the platysmal layer. A continuous subcuticular skin closure with absorbable suture provides an excellent cosmetic result in most patients.

FIGURE 9.5
ENDARTERECTOMY

FIGURE 9.5   **(Continued)**

E

Distal
end point

Proximal
end point

F

G

REFERENCES

1. Abu Rahma AF, Khan JH, Robinson PA, et al. Prospective randomized trial of carotid endarterectomy with primary closure and patch angioplasty with saphenous vein, jugular vein, and polytetrafluoroethylene: perioperative (30 day) results. *J Vasc Surg* 1996;23:998–1006.
2. Barnett HJM, Taylor DW, Eliasziw M, et al. Benefit of carotid endarterectomy in patients with symptomatic moderate or severe stenosis. *N Engl J Med* 1998;339:1415–1425.
3. European Carotid Surgery Trialists' Collaborative Group. Randomised trial of endarterectomy for recently symptomatic carotid stenosis: final results of the MRC European Carotid Surgery Trial (ECST). *Lancet* 1998;351:1379–1387.
4. Executive Committee for the Asymptomatic Carotid Atherosclerosis Study. Endarterectomy for asymptomatic carotid artery stenosis. *JAMA* 995;273:1421–1428.
5. Jackson MR, Clagett GP. Use of vein or synthetic patches in carotid endartectomy. In: Loftus CM, Kresowik TF, eds. *Carotid artery surgery.* 1st ed. New York, Thieme Medical Publishers, 2000:281.
6. Kresowik TF, Bratzler D, Karp HR, et al. Multistate utilization, processes, and outcomes of carotid endarterectomy. *J Vasc Surg* 2001;33:227–235.
7. Kresowik TF, Hoballah JJ, Sharp WJ, et al. Intraoperative B-mode ultrasonography is a useful adjunct to peripheral arterial reconstruction. *Ann Vasc Surg* 1993;7:33–38.
8. Mayberg MR, Wilson SE, Yatsu F, et al. for the Veterans Affairs Cooperative Studies Program 309 Trialist Group. Carotid endarterectomy and prevention of cerebral ischemia in symptomatic carotid stenosis. *JAMA* 1991;273:1421–1428.
9. North American Symptomatic Carotid Endarterectomy Trial Collaborators. Beneficial effect of carotid endarterectomy in symptomatic patients with high-grade carotid stenosis. *N Engl J Med* 1991;325:445–453.

CHAPTER 10

Cervical Lymph Node Biopsy and Scalene Node Biopsy

Lymph node biopsy is performed for diagnostic purposes. Cervical lymph node biopsy should only be performed when a careful examination of the aerodigestive tract has failed to demonstrate a primary carcinoma. Biopsy of a cervical lymph node that is found to contain metastatic carcinoma from a head and neck primary tumor is a grave error because such biopsy contaminates the field should subsequent radical neck dissection be contemplated.

For optimum histologic classification of lymphomas, an entire lymph node with its capsule is needed. Thus, the goal of diagnostic lymph node biopsy is to remove the node intact with minimal trauma.

Scalene node biopsy is performed by removing the fatty node-bearing tissue in the scalene triangle. Formerly performed for diagnosis and staging of lung cancer, it is now occasionally used for other malignancies.

Cervical lymph node biopsy and the closely related scalene node biopsy are discussed in this section, and the major cervical lymph node groups are presented. The anatomy of this region is described in greater detail in Chapter 11.

Major Lymph Node Groups of the Neck (Fig. 10.1)

Technical Points

Lymph nodes are clustered in regions where major vessels converge. In the head and neck, the nodes most commonly selected for biopsy follow the internal jugular vein.

LIST OF STRUCTURES

Platysma muscle
Sternocleidomastoid muscle
Omohyoid muscle
Anterior scalene muscle
Carotid sheath
Thoracic duct
Phrenic nerve
Thyrocervical trunk
Cervical lymph nodes
Scalene lymph nodes

Anatomic Points

Although the position of lymph nodes and the groups of lymph nodes in the neck are relatively constant, the terminology applied to these nodes is not. Here, we follow the terminology of *Nomina Anatomica, 5th edition.*

In general, lymph node groups in the neck can be considered to form a *pericraniocervical ring* (essentially at the head–neck junction), superficial and deep *vertical chains,* and *perivisceral deep nodes.* Lymph node groups in the pericraniocervical ring receive afferent lymph vessels from adjacent head regions or from other groups in the ring. The vertical cervical chains, in addition to receiving afferent lymph vessels from nodes in the pericraniocervical ring, also receive afferents directly from the cranial regions (lymph thus "skips" the immediate regional nodes) and from perivisceral nodes in the neck. The following is a list of most of the regional lymph nodes and what these groups of nodes drain:

Pericraniocervical Node Groups	Afferents From
1. Occipital	Posterior scalp
2. Mastoid (posterior auricular)	Scalp superior to the ear, upper half of the inner aspect of the auricle, posterior wall of the external acoustic meatus
3. Parotid, superficial, and deep	Lateral forehead, temporal region, upper half of the lateral aspect of the auricle, anterior wall of the external acoustic meatus, lateral eyelids, skin over the zygomatic arch, middle ear and mastoid antrum, all the conjunctiva, lateral cheek and skin on the root of the nose, posterior nasal floor, parotid gland, infratemporal region
4. Submental	Central portion of the lower lip, central portion and floor of the mouth, apex of the tongue and frenulum, anterior triangle of the neck superior to the hyoid bone

FIGURE 10.1
MAJOR LYMPH NODE GROUPS OF THE NECK

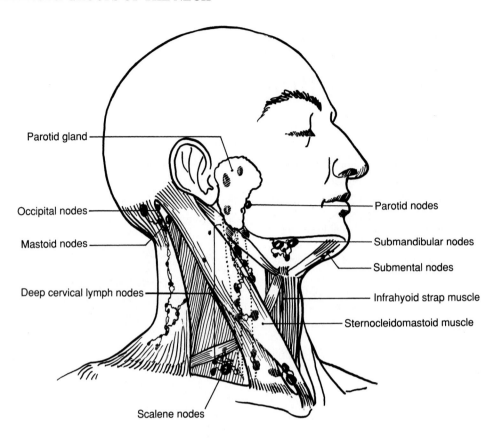

Parotid gland

Occipital nodes

Mastoid nodes

Deep cervical lymph nodes

Scalene nodes

Parotid nodes

Submandibular nodes

Submental nodes

Infrahyoid strap muscle

Sternocleidomastoid muscle

5. Submandibular	Frontal region above the nose, medial eyelids, external nose, cheeks and upper lip, lateral lower lip, oral mucosa, anterior nasal cavity, skin of the root of the nose, gingiva, palate, lateral floor of the mouth, submental nodes
Cervical Node Groups	**Afferents From**
6. Anterior cervical, superficial	Skin of the neck inferior to the hyoid, and deep lower larynx, thyroid gland, cervical trachea
7. Superior deep cervical (including jugulodigastric nodes)	Scalp of the occipital region, auricle, back of the neck, most of the tongue, larynx, thyroid gland, trachea, nasopharynx and nasal cavity, esophagus, and all nodes previously mentioned
8. Inferior deep cervical (including juguloomohyoid nodules)	Scalp of the occipital region, back of the neck, superficial pectoral region, part of the arm, tongue, superior deep cervical nodes, and sometimes, a portion of the superior surface of the liver

Cervical Lymph Node Biopsy (Fig. 10.2)

Technical Points

Position the patient supine with the head turned away from the side on which the biopsy is to be performed. Infiltrate the region of the proposed skin incision with local anesthetic. Make a transverse incision over the palpable node selected for biopsy. Deepen the incision through the platysma, retracting the sternocleidomastoid muscle to expose the node. Place a traction suture of 2-0 silk through the node in a figure-of-eight fashion to facilitate mobilization. This allows the node to be removed intact, with minimal trauma. As dissection progresses, identify the hilum of the lymph node (containing a small artery and vein). Clamp and ligate the hilum.

Sometimes, a matted group of nodes, extending much farther proximally and distally than previously expected, is encountered. If this happens, remove an adequate portion of the accessible surface of the mass rather than attempting complete removal. Attempt to shell out an entire node from the matted, but often still lobulated, mass. Achieve hemostasis in the residual nodal mass by electrocautery or suture ligature.

Close the incision in layers with fine interrupted absorbable sutures. Send the lymph node specimen to the laboratory fresh.

FIGURE 10.2
CERVICAL LYMPH NODE BIOPSY

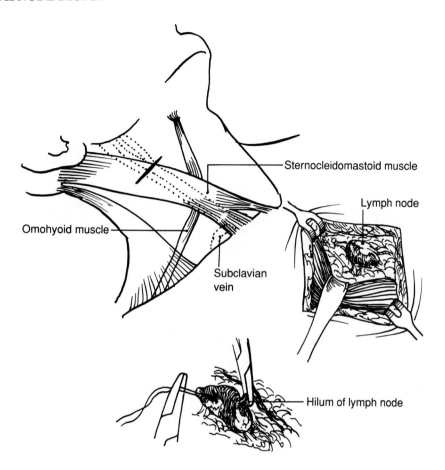

Sternocleidomastoid muscle

Lymph node

Omohyoid muscle

Subclavian vein

Hilum of lymph node

Anatomic Points

Anatomic relationships vary depending on which nodes are to be sampled. Anterior cervical nodes are closely related to terminal filaments of the cervical branch of the facial nerve (VII) and to the anterior jugular vein and its tributaries. The superior deep cervical lymph nodes, including the jugulodigastric node, are closely related to the hypoglossal nerve (XII), accessory nerve (XI), and vagus nerve (X) and its superior laryngeal branch; the cervical, and sometimes marginal mandibular branch of the facial nerve (VII); the superior root of the ansa cervicalis; the external carotid artery and its superior thyroid, occipital, and facial branches; the internal carotid artery; the termination of the common carotid artery; the carotid body and its nerve supply (a branch of the glossopharyngeal nerve); and the internal jugular vein. The inferior deep cervical nodes are most closely related to the internal jugular vein, the common carotid and subclavian arteries, the vagus nerve (X), the thyrocervical trunk and its branches (inferior thyroid, suprascapular, and transverse cervical arteries), the phrenic nerve (C3, C4, and C5), the recurrent laryngeal nerve, the thyroid gland, the inferior root of the ansa cervicalis, parts of the sympathetic trunk, and sometimes, the brachial plexus (C5 to TI).

The occipital nodes are closely related to the occipital artery and to the greater (C2, dorsal ramus) and lesser (C2, ventral ramus) occipital nerves. Mastoid lymph nodes are most closely related to the lesser occipital (C2), posterior auricular (cranial nerve VII), and great auricular (C2 and C3) nerves and to the posterior auricular artery.

Nodes in the posterior triangle lie in relation to the spinal accessory nerve.

Submental nodes are not closely related to neurovascular structures of any consequence. By contrast, submandibular nodes are closely related to the submandibular gland, hypoglossal nerve, marginal mandibular and cervical branches of the facial nerve, and the facial artery and its submental branch.

Scalene Node Biopsy (Fig. 10.3)

Technical Points

In the absence of palpable nodes, do the procedure on the right side to avoid injury to the thoracic duct. Make a transverse incision about one fingerbreadth above the clavicle over the space between the sternal and clavicular heads of the sternocleidomastoid muscle. Place retractors to spread and

FIGURE 10.3
SCALENE NODE BIOPSY

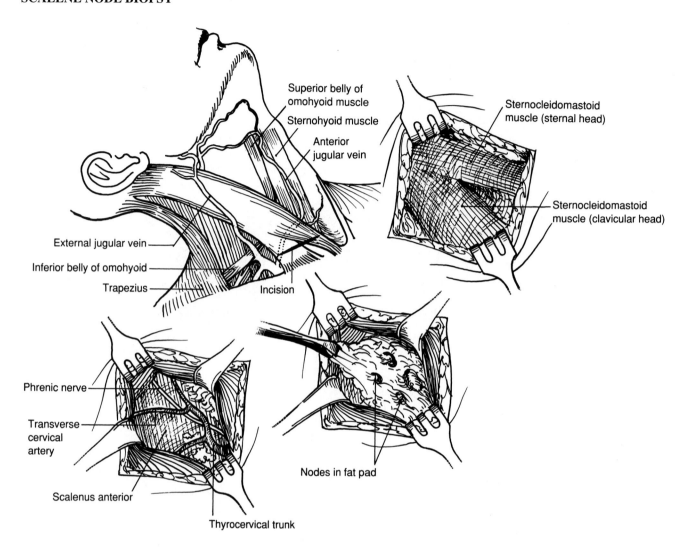

develop the space between the two heads of the sternocleidomastoid, exposing the omohyoid muscle and internal jugular vein. Identify a pad of fatty node-bearing tissue overlying the anterior scalene muscle (which is palpable but not visible), free it up by sharp and blunt dissection, and excise it. Identify and remove any enlarged or palpable nodes. Be careful to avoid the phrenic nerve (running along the anterior scalene muscle deep to the fat pad) and transverse cervical artery.

On the left side, avoid the thoracic duct. If the thoracic duct is injured, milky or opalescent fluid will appear in the operative field. The duct should then be identified and ligated.

Close the incision in layers with interrupted absorbable sutures. Send the fat pad and associated nodes to the laboratory fresh.

Anatomic Points

The scalene triangle, as described, is bounded inferiorly by the clavicle, medially by the sternal head of the sternocleidomastoid muscle, and laterally by the clavicular head of that muscle. Opening this triangle exposes a lymph node–bearing fat pad immediately lateral to the carotid sheath and superficial to the prevertebral fascia, here investing the anterior scalene muscle, phrenic nerve, and lateral branches of the thyrocervical trunk. Gentle retraction of the carotid sheath and its contents medially protects the internal jugular vein, common carotid artery, and vagus nerves. If the dissection is limited posteriorly by the scalene fascia, the phrenic nerve, which closely approximates the direction of the anterior scalene muscle fibers, as well as the lateral branches of the thyrocervical trunk (transverse cervical and suprascapular arteries), should be avoided. On the left side, the thoracic duct enters the neck posteromedial to the common carotid artery. It then arches laterally, passing posterior to the common carotid artery and internal jugular vein, but anterior to the thyrocervical trunk (and its branches) and phrenic nerve to enter the venous system near the junction of the internal jugular and subclavian veins. Again, gentle medial retraction of the carotid sheath and cautious dissection lateral to the sheath should allow this biopsy to be performed with minimal complications.

REFERENCES

1. Hood RM. *Techniques in general thoracic surgery.* Philadelphia: WB Saunders, 1985:145. (Provides an excellent description of scalene node biopsy.)
2. Horowitz NS, Tamimi HK, Goff BA, et al. Pretreatment scalene node biopsy in gynecologic malignancy: prudent or passe? *Gynecol Oncol* 1999;75:238–241. (Reviews current indications and complications in gynecologic practice.)
3. Kierner AC, Zelenka I, Heller S, et al. Surgical anatomy of the spinal accessory nerve and the trapezius branches of the cervical plexus. *Arch Surg* 2000;135:1428–1431.
4. Nason RW, Abdulrauf BM, Stranc MF. The anatomy of the accessory nerve and cervical lymph node biopsy. *Am J Surg* 2000;180:241–243. (Specific tactics for posterior cervical triangle biopsy.)
5. Talmi YP, Hoffman HT, Horowitz Z, et al. Patterns of metastases to the upper jugular lymph nodes (the "submuscular recess"). *Head Neck* 1998;20:682–686.
6. Subcommittees of the International Anatomical Nomenclature Committee. *Nomina Anatomica,* ed 5, Baltimore, Williams and Wilkins Corp, 1983, pp A61.

CHAPTER 11

Radical Neck Dissection

Radical neck dissection is performed to remove lymph nodes in the neck that might harbor metastatic deposits from malignant head and neck tumors. In the classic *radical neck dissection* illustrated here, all soft tissues from the inferior aspect of the mandible to the midline of the neck to the clavicle and posterior to the trapezius muscle are removed *en bloc*. The internal jugular vein, sternocleidomastoid muscle, and portions of the strap muscles are removed with the specimen. The vagus nerve, phrenic nerve, carotid artery, and other important neurovascular structures are protected.

This radical operation has been modified in numerous ways. A standard reporting system divides the cervical lymph node groups into levels (see the Orientation figure). Standard terminology is employed to describe deviations from the extent of dissection performed during standard radical neck dissection. When a nonlymphatic structure such as the internal jugular vein is preserved, the term *modified radical neck dissection* is appropriate. In contrast, a *selective node dissection* means that one or more lymph node groups are preserved, and an *extended radical node dissection* means that additional structures have been resected. References at the end of the chapter detail the standard terminology and some of the variations commonly employed.

Incision and Development of Flaps (Fig. 11.1)

Technical Points

Position the patient supine with the neck in slight extension and the head turned slightly to the contralateral side. Prepare a surgical field that includes the neck, lower face, and upper chest. Elevate the head of the table slightly to reduce venous bleeding.

A variety of incisions have been used for radical neck dissection. All involve elevation of flaps so that the entire area illustrated can be removed *en bloc*. Because many of these patients have received radiation therapy, or may in the future undergo irradiation, viability of skin flaps is especially important. The H-shaped or double-Y–shaped incision shown allows complete lymphadenectomy while preserving good, viable skin flaps. Alternative incisions are also illustrated.

Make an H-shaped incision. Place the vertical arm of the incision so that it does not lie directly over the carotid vessels. Make this limb of the incision vertical, rather than oblique, to place it away from the carotid sheath.

Identify the platysma and include it with the skin flaps. This improves blood supply to the skin flaps and greatly enhances the chances for their survival. Elevate the posterior flaps to the anterior border of the trapezius muscle, the superior flap

LIST OF STRUCTURES

Mandible	Anterior scalene muscle	Cervical branch of facial nerve
Clavicle	Middle scalene muscle	Great auricular nerve
Mastoid process	Internal jugular vein	Transverse cervical nerve
Hyoid bone	Middle thyroid vein	Spinal accessory nerve
Sternocleidomastoid muscle	Facial vein	Brachial plexus
Trapezius muscle	External jugular vein	Phrenic nerve
Platysma muscle	Transverse cervical vein	Hypoglossal nerve
Omohyoid muscle	Carotid sheath	Vagus nerve
Superior belly	Common carotid artery	Ansa cervicalis
Posterior belly	External carotid artery	Descendens cervicalis
Digastric muscle	Internal carotid artery	Descendens hypoglossi
Posterior belly	Thyrocervical trunk	Lingual nerve
Anterior belly	Facial (external maxillary) artery	Submandibular gland
Levator scapulae	Transverse cervical artery	
Mylohyoid muscle	Marginal mandibular nerve	

ORIENTATION

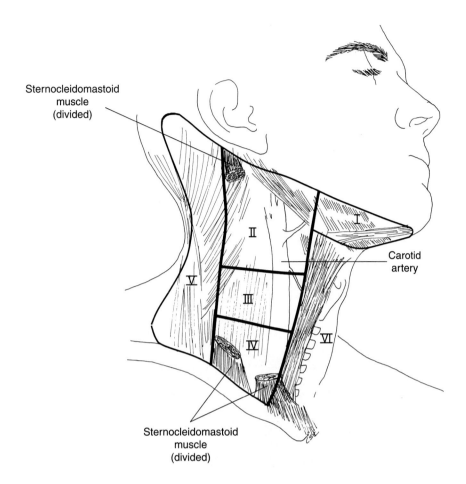

Sternocleidomastoid
muscle
(divided)

Carotid
artery

Sternocleidomastoid
muscle
(divided)

to the mandible, the medial flap to the midline of the neck, and the inferior flap to the clavicle.

The external jugular vein should be visible as it courses obliquely across the midportion of the sternocleidomastoid muscle. As the flaps are raised, be careful to dissect in the adventitial plane of this vein.

At the superior border of the field, divide and ligate the facial (external maxillary) artery and facial vein. Look for and identify the marginal mandibular branch of the facial nerve. Injury to this nerve can occur when flaps are being elevated. It generally is located parallel to and 1 to 2 cm below the lower border of the mandible, crossing superficial to the facial artery and vein. Gentle upward traction on the divided stumps of these vessels will retract the marginal mandibular branch safely up out of the field.

Anatomic Points

The platysma is innervated by the cervical branch of the facial nerve. The nerve courses inferiorly deep to the platysma, with anterior branches supplying the platysma. The skin incision and the subsequent elevation of myocutaneous flaps will, of necessity, denervate all or part of the platysma.

The marginal mandibular branch of the facial nerve is important for cosmetic and functional reasons. This nerve innervates the muscles of the lower lip and chin and can lie as much as 2.5 cm inferior to the ramus of the mandible. It is at risk during development of the upper flap. Begin the incision to raise the superior myocutaneous flap at the mastoid process, then follow a gentle curve inferiorly, about 3 cm inferior to the posterior third of the ramus of the mandible. Then, gently curve the incision superiorly and anteriorly to the mental protuberance of the chin.

Branches of the great auricular nerve, a sensory branch of the cervical plexus bearing fibers from C2 and C3, will be severed during exposure of the upper attachment of the sternocleidomastoid muscle. The vertical limb of the incision almost approximates the course of the external jugular vein, lying immediately deep to the platysma muscle. Be careful to identify this vein and keep the incision superficial to it.

FIGURE 11.1
INCISION AND DEVELOPMENT OF FLAPS

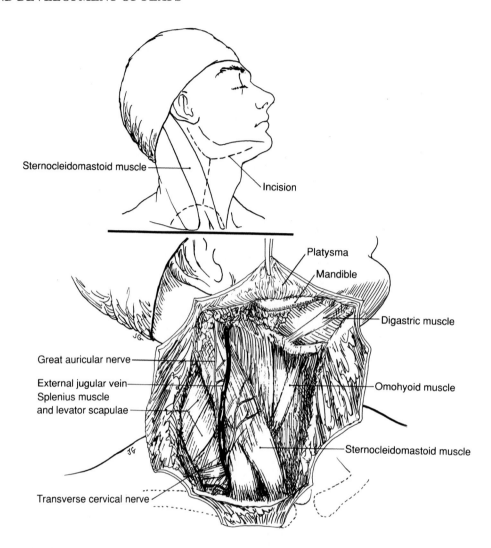

The incision divides branches of the transverse cervical nerve, a sensory branch of the cervical plexus that also carries fibers of C2 and C3.

The inferior limb of the incision is relatively risk free. The supraclavicular nerves (sensory divisions of the cervical plexus carrying fibers of C3 and C4) that supply the skin of the lower neck and extend onto the upper thorax will be encountered and must be cut. The sensory branches of the cervical plexus all emerge from under the middle of the sternocleidomastoid muscle and fan out from this point. Those that supply regions anterior to the sternocleidomastoid muscle cross the superficial surface of that muscle. Several superficial veins will also be encountered deep to the platysma and should be controlled.

Dividing the Sternocleidomastoid Muscle and Beginning the Posterior and Inferior Dissection (Fig. 11.2)

Technical Points

Incise the fascia overlying the anterior border of the trapezius muscle to enter the posterior triangle of the neck. Ligate and divide the transverse cervical artery and vein at the lateral margin of the dissection. Sweep fatty and areolar tissue upward and medially. Identify the spinal accessory nerve, which may be sacrificed or preserved depending on individual preference and the degree of nodal involvement. This nerve is sacrificed in the classic radical neck dissection, but in practice, most surgeons currently preserve it.

Advance the incision medially, just above the clavicle, and by sharp and blunt dissection, expose the external jugular vein. Ligate and divide this vein about 1 cm above the clavicle. Begin to sweep fatty and areolar tissue upward as the dissection progresses medially. Divide the posterior belly of the omohyoid muscle and the medial ends of the transverse cervical artery and vein, which run deep to the omohyoid muscle.

Incise the fascia medial to the sternocleidomastoid muscle and gently elevate it, freeing the muscle from the underlying internal jugular vein. Divide the sternocleidomastoid muscle from its attachments to the clavicle and sternum. Place a Kocher clamp on the divided stump of the sternocleidomastoid muscle and use it to provide upward traction.

FIGURE 11.2
DIVIDING THE STERNOCLEIDOMASTOID MUSCLE AND BEGINNING THE POSTERIOR AND INFERIOR DISSECTION

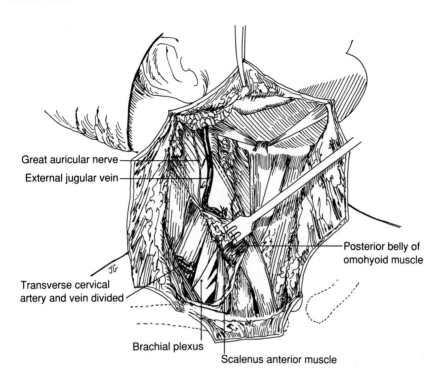

Great auricular nerve

External jugular vein

Transverse cervical artery and vein divided

Brachial plexus

Scalenus anterior muscle

Posterior belly of omohyoid muscle

The brachial plexus, phrenic nerve, anterior scalene muscle, and internal jugular vein should be visible in the floor of the dissection.

Anatomic Points

The fascia investing the sternocleidomastoid muscle, or the investing layer of the deep cervical fascia, also invests the trapezius muscle and that part of the spinal accessory nerve that passes from the sternocleidomastoid muscle to the trapezius muscle. Some surgeons routinely sacrifice this nerve, which crosses the posterior triangle along a line running from slightly superior to the middle of the sternocleidomastoid muscle to the anterior border of the trapezius muscle about 5 cm superior to the clavicle. Others sacrifice it only if a tumor directly invades it. Division of this nerve causes significant disability because elevation, rotation, and retraction of the scapula are all affected, and atrophy of the trapezius muscle presents difficulties when a cervical collar is used.

The external jugular vein crosses the superficial surface of the sternocleidomastoid muscle, passing inferiorly from its beginning in the parotid gland to its junction, just lateral to the clavicular attachment of the sternocleidomastoid muscle, with the subclavian vein. The termination of the subclavian veins and the internal jugular veins is immediately deep to the sternocleidomastoid muscle, as is the end of the thoracic duct on the left and its counterparts—the right lymphatic ducts—on the right.

The omohyoid muscle has two bellies. The inferior belly passes almost horizontally from its origin on the upper border

of the scapula to the intermediate tendon (attached by a fascial sling to the medial ends of the clavicle and first rib), which intervenes between the sternocleidomastoid muscle and the internal jugular vein. The superior belly passes superiorly, and almost vertically, to its attachment on the greater cornu of the hyoid. The inferior belly lies immediately superficial to the supraclavicular part of the brachial plexus, suprascapular and transverse cervical vessels, and phrenic nerve, which lies on the anterior scalene muscle. As the specimen is reflected craniad, the transverse cervical vessels are carefully ligated and divided. The phrenic nerve, crossed superficially by these vessels, must be identified and preserved. It lies deep to the lateral branches of the thyrocervical trunk and superficial to the anterior scalene muscle and is the only longitudinal structure coursing superolaterally to inferomedially in the lower neck.

Dissection in the Carotid Sheath and Ligation of the Internal Jugular Vein (Fig. 11.3)

Technical Points

By sharp and blunt dissection, open the carotid sheath and identify within it the internal jugular vein (Fig. 11.3A). Double-ligate and divide this vein just above the clavicle. Identify the vagus nerve and carotid artery lying posterior to the internal jugular vein. Sweep the internal jugular vein upward with the specimen protecting the vagus nerve and underlying carotid.

Dissection may then proceed relatively rapidly up along the carotid sheath until the carotid bifurcation is reached

FIGURE 11.3
DISSECTION IN THE CAROTID SHEATH AND LIGATION OF THE INTERNAL JUGULAR VEIN

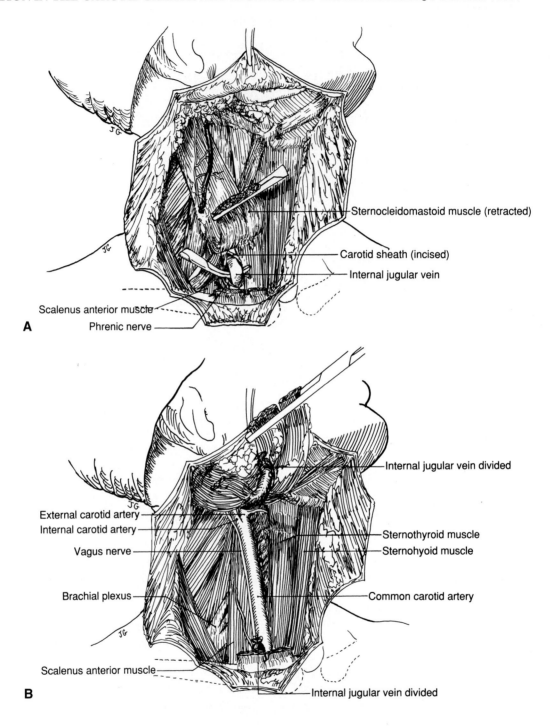

A

Sternocleidomastoid muscle (retracted)

Carotid sheath (incised)

Internal jugular vein

Scalenus anterior muscle

Phrenic nerve

Internal jugular vein divided

External carotid artery

Internal carotid artery

Vagus nerve

Sternothyroid muscle

Sternohyoid muscle

Brachial plexus

Common carotid artery

Scalenus anterior muscle

B

Internal jugular vein divided

(Fig. 11.3B). Proceed slowly past the carotid bifurcation, and identify and protect the hypoglossal nerve. This crosses the internal and external carotid arteries just above their bifurcation and then passes deep to the posterior belly of the digastric muscle.

The bed of the dissection should reveal the medial border of the trapezius muscle, the middle scalene muscle, and the levator scapulae muscle posteriorly (with the spinal accessory nerve, if preserved). The brachial plexus, phrenic nerve, vagus nerve, and common carotid artery should be visible and preserved in the floor of the dissection.

Anatomic Points

Remember the relationships of the structures within the carotid sheath. Just above the medial end of the clavicle, the internal jugular vein is anterolateral, the common carotid artery is anteromedial, and the vagus nerve is posterior, in the groove between these two vessels. As the internal jugular vein is exposed, the middle thyroid vein should be identified, ligated, and divided; this vein, which is present in about half of cases, will be encountered at about the level of the lower and middle third of the thyroid gland. It passes anterior to the common carotid artery.

On the left side, the thoracic duct enters the neck by passing along the left side of the esophagus. It arches (as much as 3 to 4 cm superior to the clavicle) anterior to the thyrocervical trunk, phrenic nerve, and medial border of the anterior scalene muscle and posterior to the left common carotid artery, vagus nerve, and internal jugular vein. From the apex of this arch, the duct descends anterior to the left subclavian artery. It may empty into the junction of the subclavian vein and internal jugular vein or into either of these great veins near their junction, or it may divide into smaller vessels before terminating. On the right, typically, three major lymphatic trunks (right subclavian, right jugular, and right bronchomediastinal trunks) terminate independently on the anterior aspect of the jugulosubclavian junction, the internal jugular vein, the subclavian vein, or any combination of these. If these lymphatic vessels are injured, they should be ligated to prevent development of a chylous fistula.

The sympathetic chain lies immediately posterior to the carotid sheath. Like the phrenic nerve, it lies deep to prevertebral fascia and should be protected. Other than the vagus nerve, which is of substantial size and must be preserved, the only other nerves that should be encountered while dissecting the carotid sheath from its contents are the descendens hypoglossi (typically located on the anterior surface of the carotid sheath) and the descendens cervicalis (generally, lateral or medial to the internal jugular vein, and thus in the lateral wall of the sheath or emerging through the anterior wall). These anastomose to form the ansa cervicalis, which innervates the strap or infrahyoid muscles. These nerves have to be sacrificed, but the descendens hypoglossi should be identified because it leads the surgeon back to the hypoglossal nerve. Other nerves that might be encountered during this dissection include the recurrent laryngeal nerve (the location of which is more variable on the right than on the left) and, much higher, the superior laryngeal nerve with its internal and external branches. Both the superior and the inferior laryngeal nerves lie deep to fascial layers that normally would not be included in the specimen, but their presence is cause for the surgeon to proceed cautiously.

Division of the Sternocleidomastoid Muscle at the Mastoid Process (Fig. 11.4)

Technical Points

Posteriorly, dissect the specimen from the levator scapulae muscle and the splenius capitis muscle. Preserve the spinal accessory nerve. Divide the sternocleidomastoid muscle at its insertion on the mastoid process.

The spinal accessory nerve passes through part of the sternocleidomastoid muscle several centimeters below the

---

FIGURE 11.4
DIVISION OF THE STERNOCLEIDOMASTOID MUSCLE AT THE MASTOID PROCESS

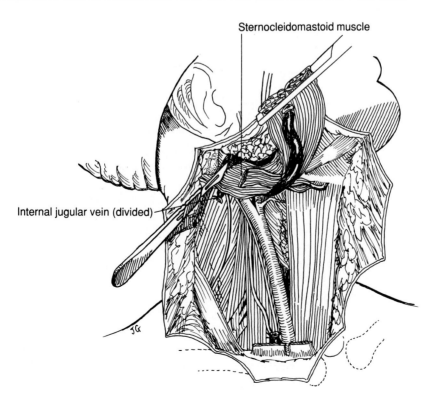

Sternocleidomastoid muscle

Internal jugular vein (divided)

FIGURE 11.5
DIVISION OF THE INTERNAL JUGULAR VEIN

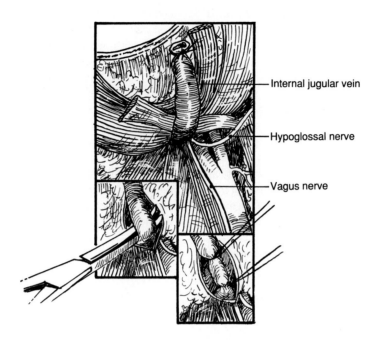

mastoid. Gently tease this nerve out from beneath the cut muscle fibers. Divide the small motor branch to the sternocleidomastoid muscle. Allow the main trunk of the nerve to retract back onto the floor of the dissection. Reflect the specimen medially.

Anatomic Points

As the spinal accessory nerve passes posteriorly, it usually (in 70% of cases) crosses superficial to the internal jugular vein, although in 27% of cases, it passes deep to the jugular vein. It innervates the sternocleidomastoid muscle 4 cm or more inferior to the tip of the mastoid, and then either pierces or passes deep to that muscle to innervate the trapezius muscle. To spare the innervation to the trapezius muscle, carefully detach the sternocleidomastoid from the mastoid process and carefully dissect the nerve free from the deep surface or follow it through the muscle.

Division of the Internal Jugular Vein (Fig. 11.5)

Technical Points

Place a retractor under the posterior belly of the digastric muscle and elevate it to expose the internal jugular vein. Carefully clean the vein to delineate it as separate from the internal carotid artery, hypoglossal nerve, and vagus nerve. Use a high transfixation suture ligature to secure the internal jugular vein. Divide the vein.

Anatomic Points

As the tissue block is reflected superiorly, revealing the superior extent of the internal jugular vein and its tribu-

taries, care must again be taken in ligating and dividing these veins. Branches of the facial nerve, especially the marginal mandibular, should be preserved. In the lateral groove between the internal jugular vein and the internal carotid artery, care should be taken to avoid the descending segment of the hypoglossal nerve, which will curve anteriorly immediately inferior to the occipital artery. In the medial groove between the jugular and carotid, the vagus nerve should be avoided. Again, the key to avoiding these nerves when ligating and dividing is to skeletonize the vein gently, making sure to include only the vein in the clamp or ligature.

Delineation of the Upper Margin of Dissection (Fig. 11.6)

Technical and Anatomic Points

Allow the specimen to fall back down into the bed of the dissection. Identify the marginal mandibular nerve, which was previously located and retracted along with the facial artery and vein. Trace the nerve along the angle of the mandible and preserve it. Divide the soft tissues from the mental process out along the ramus of the mandible.

Superior Aspect of the Dissection and Completion of Procedure (Fig. 11.7)

Technical Points

Reflect the fatty and areolar tissue medially, plainly exposing the anterior belly of the digastric muscle. The submandibular gland is then identified and should be taken with the specimen. Identify and ligate the duct of the submandibular gland,

FIGURE 11.6
DELINEATION OF THE UPPER MARGIN OF DISSECTION

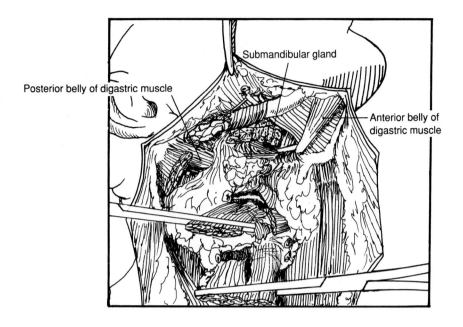

preserving the lingual nerve. Retract the mylohyoid muscle medially to facilitate exposure of the salivary duct. In the depths, identify and preserve the hypoglossal nerve.

Check the field for hemostasis. Place closed-suction drains under both the medial and lateral flaps, and approximate the flaps with care.

Anatomic Points

This part of the dissection is the hardest because many structures are present in a relatively small space. Excision of the submandibular gland necessitates ligation and division of its duct (Wharton's duct). This duct extends anteriorly from the

FIGURE 11.7
SUPERIOR ASPECT OF THE DISSECTION AND COMPLETION OF PROCEDURE

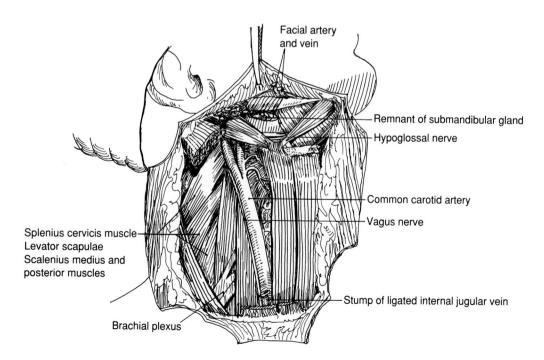

deep surface of the gland, in the interval between the more superficial mylohyoid muscle and the deeper hyoglossal muscle. Here, it lies between the more inferior hypoglossal nerve and the lingual nerve. As the lingual nerve passes forward deep to the mylohyoid muscle, it passes lateral to the duct, gently curves inferiorly, and finally terminates on the medial aspect of the duct by giving off terminal branches. Close to the posterior border of the mylohyoid muscle, pregan-glionic parasympathetic secretomotor fibers diverge from the lingual nerve to synapse with postganglionic fibers in the submandibular ganglion. Postganglionic fibers provide parasympathetic innervation to the submandibular gland; thus, traction on the gland can stretch the lingual nerve. Because of these anatomic relations, it is necessary to skeletonize the submandibular gland gently before ligating and dividing it to ensure that these important nerves are preserved.

SURGICAL REFERENCES

1. Bakamjian VY. Radical neck dissection. In: Malt RA, ed. *Surgical techniques illustrated: a comparative atlas.* Philadelphia: WB Saunders, 1985:848. (Presents a clear description of the use of the McPhee incision.)
2. Beahrs OH. Surgical anatomy and technique of radical neck dissection. *Surg Clin North Am* 1977;57:663. (Offers a detailed description of technique along with an excellent discussion of whether or not to spare the accessory nerve.)
3. Beahrs OH, Kiernan PD, Hubert JP. *An atlas of the surgical techniques of Oliver H. Beahrs.* Philadelphia: WB Saunders, 1985:65. (Provides a summary of this technique as currently practiced.)
4. Clayman GL, Frank DK. Selective neck dissection of anatomically appropriate levels is as efficacious as modified radical neck dissection for elective treatment of the clinically negative neck in patients with squamous cell carcinoma of the upper respiratory and digestive tracts. *Arch Otolaryngol Head Neck Surg* 1998;124:348–352. (Summary of modifications for various head and neck tumors.)
5. Pillsbury HC III, Clark M. A rationale for therapy of the N0 neck. *Laryngoscope* 1997;107:1294–1314. (Extensively referenced; gives both historical context and current philosophy.)
6. Robbins KT, Medina JE, Wolfe GT, et al. Standardizing neck dissection terminology. Official Report of the Academy's Committee for Head and Neck Surgery and Oncology. *Arch Otolaryngol Head Neck Surg* 1991;117:601–605. (Terminology and summary of common variants.)
7. Robbins KT. Classification of neck dissection. Current concepts and future considerations. *Otolaryngol Clin North Am* 1998;31:639–655.
8. Rush BF Jr. Radical neck dissections. In: Nyhus LM, Baker RJ, Fischer JE. *Mastery of surgery.* 3rd ed. Boston: Little, Brown, 1997:373–382.

SPECIAL PROBLEM REFERENCES

1. Bocca E, Pignataro O, Sasaki CT. Functional neck dissection: a description of operative technique. *Arch Otolaryngol* 1980;106:524. (Describes a technique for modified node dissection that spares the spinal accessory nerve, sternocleidomastoid muscle, and internal jugular vein.)
2. Roses DF, Harris MN, Ackerman AB, eds. Diagnosis and management of cutaneous malignant melanoma. Philadelphia: WB Saunders, 1983: 159. (Describes the modification of radical neck dissection for melanomas of the head and neck, including superficial parotidectomy when appropriate.)
3. Rossi RL, Cady B. Surgery of the thyroid gland. In: Cady B, Rossi RL, eds. *Surgery of the thyroid and parathyroid glands.* 3rd ed. Philadelphia: WB Saunders, 1991:187. (Clearly describes the role and extent of radical neck dissection in the treatment of well-differentiated thyroid carcinoma.)

ANATOMIC REFERENCES

1. Beahrs OH, Gossel JD, Hollinshead WH. Techniques and surgical anatomy of radical neck dissection. *Am J Surg* 1955;90:490. (Presents an original detailed description of anatomy.)
2. Branstetter BF 4th, Weissman JL. Normal anatomy of the neck with CT and MR imaging correlation. *Radiol Clin North Am* 2000;38:925–929.
3. Coleman JJ. Complications in head and neck surgery. *Surg Clin North Am* 1986;66:149. (Briefly enumerates the technical complications that can arise, emphasizing anatomy.)
4. Nason RW, Abdulrauf BM, Stranc MF. The anatomy of the spinal accessory nerve and cervical lymph node biopsy. *Am J Surg* 2000;180:241–243.

CHAPTER 12

Operation for Zenker's Diverticulum

Zenker's diverticulum is an outpouching of the cervical esophagus. Mucosa of the esophagus protrudes through an anatomically weak area between the cricopharyngeus inferiorly and the thyropharyngeus, both parts of the inferior pharyngeal constrictor, superiorly. Although this weak spot is posterior, the diverticulum generally is approached through the left neck, where it presents most commonly.

The pathogenesis of Zenker's diverticulum is not fully understood. Spasms of the cricopharyngeus muscle are believed to cause functional obstruction with secondary protrusion of the esophageal mucosa through a weak area. Cricopharyngeal myotomy (division of the muscle) is a critical component of successful repair. When the diverticulum is small, myotomy alone may suffice. However, a large diverticulum generally requires excision of the sac, as well as myotomy. In this chapter, a single-stage diverticulectomy with cricopharyngeal myotomy is discussed.

Position of the Patient and Skin Incision (Fig. 12.1)

Technical Points

Position the patient supine with the head turned slightly to the right. Make an incision along the anterior border of the sternocleidomastoid muscle. An alternative collar-type incision is preferred by some surgeons for an improved cosmetic result. This incision is made at the level of the cricoid cartilage, and skin flaps are elevated to expose the anterior border of the sternocleidomastoid muscle.

Anatomic Points

A pharyngoesophageal (Zenker's) diverticulum is a pulsion diverticulum through the inherently weak area of the hypopharynx and upper esophagus. These diverticula occur most commonly in the region of the cricopharyngeus, a part of the inferior pharyngeal constrictor. A more precise description of the location of such diverticula is impossible owing to the variability in the exact anatomy of the region or to our lack of understanding of the etiology of this disease. Several features of the distal pharynx and proximal esophagus provide an anatomic basis for such pulsion diverticula. Some investigators believe that there is a zone of potential weakness between the cricopharyngeus muscle and the immediately superior thyropharyngeus muscle (again, a part of the inferior constrictor muscle). Other surgeons believe that the zone of weakness is between the superior and inferior parts of the cricopharyngeus itself. (Allegedly, the upper constrictor part is innervated by vagal fibers passing through the pharyngeal plexus, whereas the lower sphincteric part receives its vagal innervation through the recurrent laryngeal nerve.) A third hypothesis is that these diverticula arise in the inverted triangular area bounded laterally by diverging longitudinal esophageal muscle fibers passing to their attachment on the cricoid and superiorly by the inferior border of the cricopharyngeus. In this triangle (the so-called Laimer's area), circular muscle fibers are the sole dynamic covering of the esophagus. Finally, some researchers believe that the diverticulum arises at the point where the pharyngeal branches of the superior or inferior thyroid artery penetrate the pharyngeal wall. Regardless of the exact location of the origin of the diverticulum, most frequently it protrudes toward the left; thus, the initial incision typically is on the left side of the neck.

A skin incision that parallels the anterior border of the sternocleidomastoid muscle will divide twigs of the transverse cervical (anterior cutaneous) nerve, a branch of the cervical plexus containing sensory fibers of C2 and C3. The main trunk of this nerve is located immediately posterior to the middle of the sternocleidomastoid muscle. It bends anteriorly, passing in the plane deep to the platysma and superficial to the sternocleidomastoid muscle, on whose surface it branches to supply most of the skin of the anterior neck. The platysma muscle, innervated by the cervical branch of cranial nerve VII, should be divided in the same direction

LIST OF STRUCTURES

Pharynx	Esophagus	Thyroid gland
Inferior pharyngeal constrictor	Sternocleidomastoid muscle	Thyroid cartilage
Cricopharyngeus	Omohyoid muscle	Middle thyroid vein
Thyropharyngeus	Sternohyoid muscle	Inferior thyroid artery
		Carotid sheath

FIGURE 12.1
POSITION OF THE PATIENT AND SKIN INCISION

A

Sternocleidomastoid muscle

Trapezius muscle

B

Platysma
Thyrohyoid muscle
Omohyoid muscle
Sternohyoid muscle
Sternothyroid muscle
Sternocleidomastoid muscle

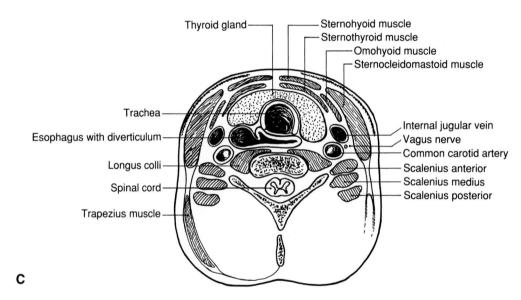

C

Thyroid gland
Sternohyoid muscle
Sternothyroid muscle
Omohyoid muscle
Sternocleidomastoid muscle
Trachea
Esophagus with diverticulum
Internal jugular vein
Vagus nerve
Common carotid artery
Longus colli
Scalenius anterior
Spinal cord
Scalenius medius
Scalenius posterior
Trapezius muscle

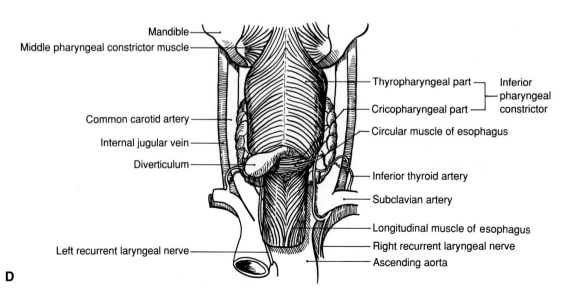

D

Mandible
Middle pharyngeal constrictor muscle
Thyropharyngeal part ⎤ Inferior
Cricopharyngeal part ⎦ pharyngeal constrictor
Circular muscle of esophagus
Common carotid artery
Internal jugular vein
Diverticulum
Inferior thyroid artery
Subclavian artery
Longitudinal muscle of esophagus
Left recurrent laryngeal nerve
Right recurrent laryngeal nerve
Ascending aorta

FIGURE 12.2
EXPOSURE OF THE ESOPHAGUS AND RETROPHARYNGEAL SPACE

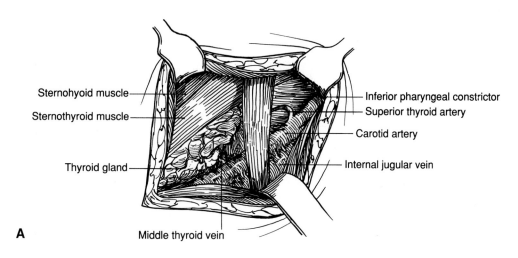

Sternohyoid muscle
Sternothyroid muscle
Thyroid gland
Inferior pharyngeal constrictor
Superior thyroid artery
Carotid artery
Internal jugular vein
Middle thyroid vein

A

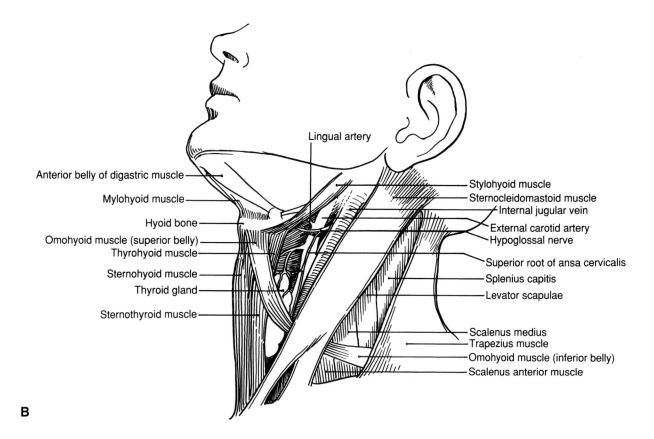

Lingual artery
Anterior belly of digastric muscle
Mylohyoid muscle
Hyoid bone
Omohyoid muscle (superior belly)
Thyrohyoid muscle
Sternohyoid muscle
Thyroid gland
Sternothyroid muscle
Stylohyoid muscle
Sternocleidomastoid muscle
Internal jugular vein
External carotid artery
Hypoglossal nerve
Superior root of ansa cervicalis
Splenius capitis
Levator scapulae
Scalenus medius
Trapezius muscle
Omohyoid muscle (inferior belly)
Scalenus anterior muscle

B

as the skin. An attempt should be made to spare the larger ramifications of the transverse cervical nerve. The alternative, a collar incision, is made through the skin and platysma in a horizontal (transverse) plane. As is the case with any skin incision, those that are parallel to cleavage lines or skin creases tend to produce a more cosmetically acceptable scar. Deep to the platysma, ramifications of the transverse cervical nerve will again be divided, but it should be easy to avoid major divisions of the transverse cervical nerve.

Exposure of the Esophagus and Retropharyngeal Space (Fig. 12.2)

Technical Points

Retract the sternocleidomastoid muscle and the underlying carotid sheath and contents laterally. Divide the omohyoid muscle, if necessary, to improve exposure. Generally, medial retraction of the omohyoid muscle provides sufficient exposure.

Mobilize the thyroid gland by first dividing the middle thyroid vein. Identify the recurrent laryngeal nerve. If necessary, divide the inferior thyroid artery to facilitate retraction of the left lobe of the thyroid medially.

Proceed with blunt dissection in the retropharyngeal space. Palpate the esophagus and place an indwelling esophageal stethoscope and nasogastric tube. The diverticulum is often readily visible in the retropharyngeal space. If it is difficult to locate the sac, ask the anesthesiologist to insufflate air into it through a red rubber catheter, or transilluminate it with a fiberoptic scope. Grasp the sac with an Allis clamp and pull it into the wound, rotating the esophagus to expose its posterior surface. By sharp and blunt dissection, clean the posterior pharyngeal wall to delineate clearly the cricopharyngeus muscle and sac.

Anatomic Points

Retraction of the sternocleidomastoid muscle at its approximate midpoint will expose the midline thyroid and cricoid cartilages, flanked by the sternohyoid and omohyoid muscles. The carotid sheath should be visible in the interval between the retracted sternocleidomastoid muscle and the omohyoid muscle (which crosses superficial to the carotid sheath). If it is necessary to divide the omohyoid muscle to improve exposure, divide this muscle near its insertion on the hyoid bone because this preserves its nerve supply. The carotid sheath and its contents are immediately lateral to the thyroid gland. Before lateral retraction of the carotid sheath, ligate and divide the short and fragile middle thyroid vein, which runs transversely from the thyroid to the internal jugular vein. Further retraction of the carotid sheath and its contents will expose the deeper, transversely oriented, inferior thyroid artery and the longitudinally oriented recurrent laryngeal nerve. Both the middle thyroid vein and inferior thyroid artery tether the thyroid gland to adjacent structures and can be torn if their presence is not anticipated.

The cervical sympathetic chain lies posterior to the carotid sheath. Retraction of the carotid sheath medially would preserve arteries and veins to the thyroid gland but would not provide adequate exposure.

Cricopharyngeal Myotomy (Fig. 12.3)

Technical and Anatomic Points

Retract the diverticulum cephalad. Pass a blunt-tipped, right-angle clamp under the cricopharyngeus muscle and develop the plane between the muscle and the esophageal mucosa. Divide the cricopharyngeus for 3 to 5 cm.

Frequently, after an adequate myotomy, a small, broad-based diverticulum will flatten and become a diffuse bulge. In this case, do not excise the sac. If a large sac remains, diverticulectomy should be performed.

Diverticulectomy (Fig. 12.4)

Technical and Anatomic Points

The diverticulum may be excised and closed by suturing or simply by firing a linear stapler across the base. Here, the suture technique is illustrated.

Pass a number 40 bougie through the mouth into the esophagus and use it as a guide to avoid resecting too much esophagus (optional). Maintain control as you excise the diverticulum by a cut-and-sew technique (Fig. 12.4A). Do not attempt to excise too much tissue; the excess mucosa will flatten when tension is released. Partially transect the neck of the sac. Use the remainder of the neck to maintain exposure as interrupted simple sutures are placed to approximate the esophageal mucosa. Leave the ends of the sutures long and use them for traction sutures. Amputate the sac and complete the closure (Fig. 12.4B).

FIGURE 12.3
CRICOPHARYNGEAL MYOTOMY

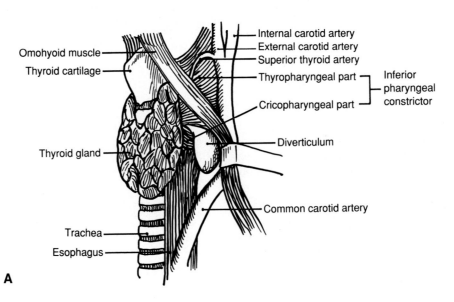

A

Omohyoid muscle
Thyroid cartilage
Internal carotid artery
External carotid artery
Superior thyroid artery
Thyropharyngeal part ⎤ Inferior pharyngeal constrictor
Cricopharyngeal part ⎦
Diverticulum
Thyroid gland
Common carotid artery
Trachea
Esophagus

FIGURE 12.3 (Continued)

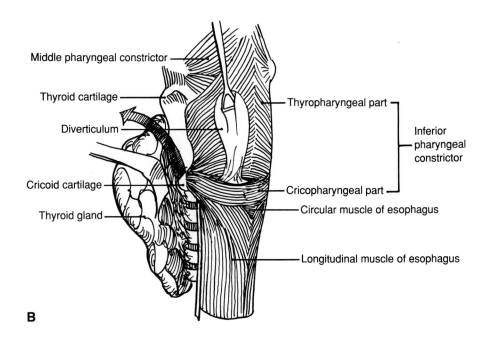

Middle pharyngeal constrictor

Thyroid cartilage

Diverticulum

Cricoid cartilage

Thyroid gland

Thyropharyngeal part

Inferior pharyngeal constrictor

Cricopharyngeal part

Circular muscle of esophagus

Longitudinal muscle of esophagus

B

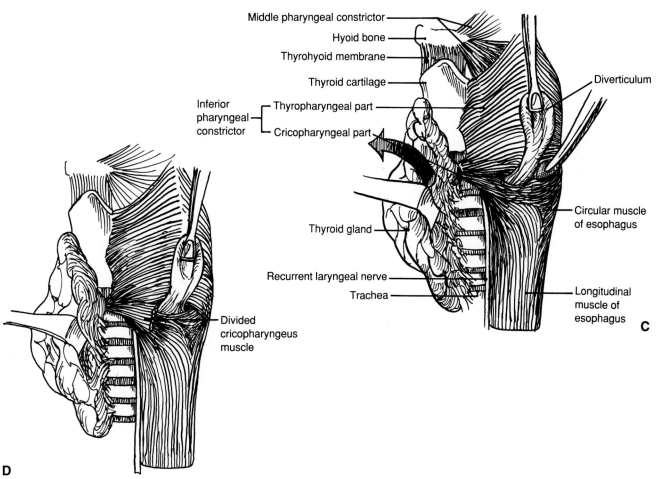

Middle pharyngeal constrictor

Hyoid bone

Thyrohyoid membrane

Thyroid cartilage

Inferior pharyngeal constrictor

Thyropharyngeal part

Cricopharyngeal part

Diverticulum

Thyroid gland

Circular muscle of esophagus

Recurrent laryngeal nerve

Trachea

Longitudinal muscle of esophagus

C

Divided cricopharyngeus muscle

D

FIGURE 12.4
DIVERTICULECTOMY

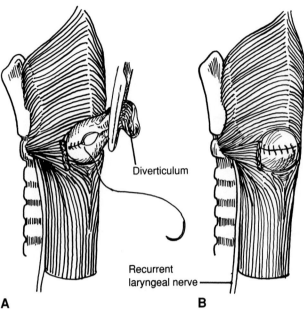

Diverticulum

Recurrent
laryngeal nerve

A　　　　　**B**

FIGURE 12.5
CLOSURE OF ESOPHAGUS

Closure of Esophagus (Fig. 12.5)

Technical and Anatomic Points

Close the muscular layers of the esophagus in a transverse fashion with multiple interrupted sutures. Place a 1/4-inch

Penrose drain (or a soft, closed-suction drain) in the retropharyngeal space.

Close the neck incision by approximating the cervical fascia with interrupted absorbable sutures. Close the skin with a running subcuticular suture.

SURGICAL REFERENCES

1. Crecenzo DG, Trastek VF, Allen MS, et al. Zenker's diverticulum in the elderly: is operation justified? *Ann Thorac Surg* 1998;66:347–350. (Review of complications and outcomes, reaffirms safety and efficacy of procedure.)
2. Payne WS, Clagett OT. Pharyngeal and esophageal diverticula. *Curr Probl Surg* 1965;2:1. (Includes excellent illustrations of diverticula at various levels of the esophagus.)
3. Payne WS, King RM. Pharyngoesophageal (Zenker's) diverticulum. *Surg Clin North Am* 1983;63:815. (Describes myotomy, with and without diverticulectomy.)
4. Rocco G, Deschamps C, Martel E, et al. Results of reoperation on the upper esophageal sphincter. *J Thorac Cardiovasc Surg* 1999;117:28–30.
5. Scott-Conner CEH, ed. *Chassin's operative strategy in general surgery.* 3rd ed. New York: Springer Verlag, in press. (Describes use of linear stapler.)
6. Skinner DB, Belsey RHR. *Management of esophageal disease.* Philadelphia: WB Saunders, 1988:422. (Clearly describes myotomy and diverticulopexy.)
7. Welsh GF, Payne WS. The present status of one-stage pharyngoesophageal diverticulectomy. *Surg Clin North Am* 1973;53:953. (Reviews the procedure in 809 patients.)

ANATOMIC REFERENCES

1. Bonovina L, Khan NA, DeMeester TR. Pharyngoesophageal dysfunctions. *Arch Surg* 1985;120:541. (Includes a discussion of the role of manometry.)
2. Bremner CG. Zenker diverticulum. *Arch Surg* 1998;133:1131–1133. (Reviews anatomy and technique.)
3. Ellis FH. Surgical management of esophageal motility disturbances. *Am J Surg* 1980;139:752. (Describes functional sphincters and esophageal manometry.)
4. Ellis FH, Schlegal JF, Lynch VP, et al. Cricopharyngeal myotomy for pharyngoesophageal diverticulum. *Ann Surg* 1969;170:340.
5. Knuff TE, Benjamin SB, Castell DO. Pharyngoesophageal (Zenker's) diverticulum: a reappraisal. *Gastroenterology* 1982;82:734. (Presents manometric data challenging the concept of dyscoordination of the pharynx and upper esophageal sphincter in patients with Zenker's diverticulum.)

CHAPTER 13

Neck Exploration for Trauma

Timothy Van Natta

Neck exploration is performed in a systematic fashion to evaluate and repair all structures deep to the platysma that have been injured by penetrating trauma. The neck is divided into three zones for the purposes of decision making in trauma surgery.

Zone I lies below the clavicles and comprises the thoracic inlet. Injuries in this region may require sternotomy or thoracotomy (Fig. 13.4) for adequate vascular control. Hemodynamically unstable patients are taken directly to the operating room, whereas stable patients are best evaluated first by arteriography. Chest radiography is done to look for associated hemopneumothorax and injury to the superior aspect of the lung. Significant vascular injury is unlikely, however, if physical examination and chest radiographic findings are negative. Esophageal contrast studies with or without endoscopy, as well as bronchoscopy, are necessary to complete the nonoperative evaluation. Positive findings direct operative repair.

Zone II (between the clavicle and angle of the mandible) includes most of the neck. Injuries to this zone that penetrate the platysma generally warrant exploration, and prompt surgery is required in unstable patients. Massive hemorrhage is likely as a result of an injured common carotid artery or its branches, vertebral artery, jugular vein, or a combination of these. Manual pressure is maintained to control bleeding; blind clamp application for hemorrhage control is to be condemned. Stable patients may be evaluated instead by angiography, followed by radiographic or endoscopic hypopharyngeal and esophageal evaluation. The larynx and trachea must be examined by fiberoptic or rigid endoscopy if appropriate signs or symptoms are present, such as cervical subcutaneous emphysema (by examination or radiography), stridor, respiratory difficulties, hemoptysis, or hoarseness. A selective approach to exploration may be appropriate if diagnostic studies yield negative results.

Zone III extends from the angle of the mandible to the skull base. Patients unstable because of bleeding must be taken expeditiously to the operating room. Meanwhile, manual pressure is applied to the wound to prevent exsanguination. Alternatively, a Foley catheter may be gently inserted into the wound and its balloon inflated to the point of hemorrhage control. If followed by hemodynamic improvement,

preoperative diagnostic and therapeutic arteriography may be possible because attaining distal control near the skull base may be exceedingly difficult if not impossible. When nonoperative evaluation is pursued, fiberoptic endoscopic evaluation of the pharyngeal area should be conducted as well.

Neck exploration can be thought of as a means of systematically inspecting two main compartments in the neck: (a) the vascular compartment, which includes the common carotid, internal carotid, external carotid, and vertebral arteries, as well as the internal jugular vein and its branches; and (b) the visceral tube, which contains the pharynx and esophagus, larynx and trachea, thyroid, parathyroids, and associated structures. Even when preoperative clinical findings or diagnostic studies point to injury of a specific structure, a complete and systematic examination of all structures should be performed.

Positioning of the Patient and Skin Incision (Fig. 13.1)

Technical and Anatomic Points

Position the patient supine with the head turned slightly away from the injury (or kept neutral if cervical spine injury is possible). Prep and drape both sides of the neck and the entire chest. Exploration of the mediastinum through partial or complete median sternotomy or anterolateral thoracotomy may be necessary.

Prepare and drape both groins to allow vascular access and harvest of the saphenous veins in the event they are needed for cervical vessel repair.

Make a long incision along the anterior border of the sternocleidomastoid muscle on the side of injury. Bilateral neck exploration can be accomplished through bilateral incisions. Alternatively, a collar-type incision can be used. However, this incision requires that flaps be raised and thus takes longer than lateral neck incisions. The slightly better cosmetic result achieved with this technique rarely justifies the extra operative time. Control major bleeding by direct digital pressure until proximal and distal control can be achieved. If inadequate, the Foley balloon tamponade technique can be used, which can facilitate skin preparation and draping as well. Always attempt to obtain proximal and distal vascular control before opening any hematoma.

ORIENTATION

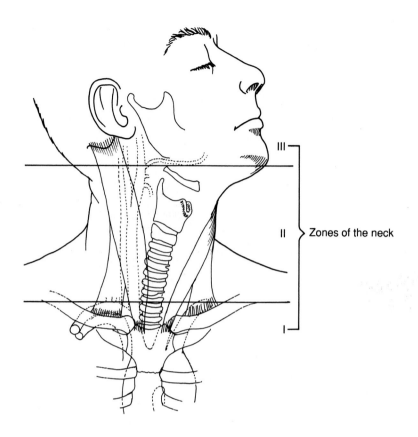

Zones of the neck

III
II
I

FIGURE 13.1
POSITIONING OF THE PATIENT AND SKIN INCISION

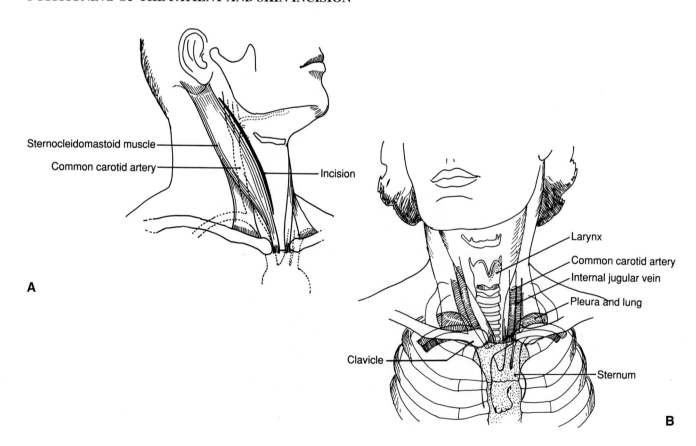

Sternocleidomastoid muscle
Common carotid artery
Incision

Larynx
Common carotid artery
Internal jugular vein
Pleura and lung

Clavicle
Sternum

A

B

FIGURE 13.2
EXPLORATION OF THE VASCULAR STRUCTURES

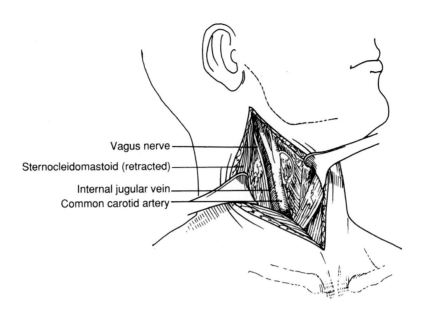

Vagus nerve
Sternocleidomastoid (retracted)
Internal jugular vein
Common carotid artery

Exploration of the Vascular Structures (Fig. 13.2)

Technical and Anatomic Points

Ligate any superficial bleeding vessels. Retract the sternocleidomastoid muscle laterally to expose the carotid sheath. A hematoma involving the carotid sheath requires exploration. Achieve sufficient exposure for proximal and distal control before opening the sheath. Persistent arterial hemorrhage not originating from the common carotid artery or its branches indicates possible injury to the vertebral artery. Such bleeding can be copious. In zone I of the neck, gentle retraction of the carotid sheath contents allows exposure of the more posterior vertebral artery. After proximal and distal control, arterial repair can be effected. If necessary, the vertebral artery can be ligated with a very low risk for stroke. In zones II and III, vertebral artery exposure is much more difficult, generally

FIGURE 13.3
EXPLORATION AND REPAIR OF MIDLINE STRUCTURES

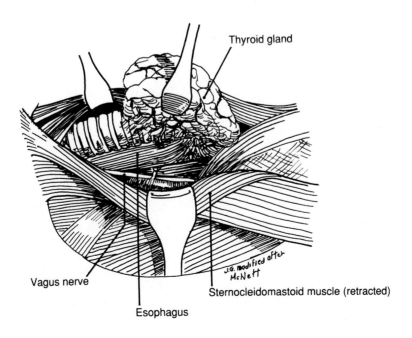

Thyroid gland

Vagus nerve

Esophagus

Sternocleidomastoid muscle (retracted)

J.G. modified after McNett

FIGURE 13.4
ADDITIONAL EXPOSURE FOR INJURIES INVOLVING THE THORACIC INLET

requiring removal of the anterior aspect of the vertebral transverse process, a maneuver that can produce additional hemorrhage. An alternative to direct operative exposure is wound packing followed by therapeutic angiography.

Hemorrhage from within the carotid sheath is often from the internal jugular vein or a large branch thereof. Simple lacerations of the internal jugular vein may be repaired by simple closure with a running monofilament suture (lateral venorrhaphy). For more significant injuries, the vein may be ligated. Avoid bilateral internal jugular vein ligation, if possible, to avoid adverse neurologic complications from venous congestion.

Obtain proximal and distal control before exposing the common, external, and internal carotid arteries. Débride the injury. Repair injuries of the common or internal carotid artery by simple suture (permanent monofilament), vein patch angioplasty, or interposition saphenous vein grafting. Consider using an intraluminal shunt if common or internal carotid artery repair is necessary. As an alternative to interposition vein grafting for proximal internal carotid artery injuries, the uninjured external carotid artery may be transposed, making an anastomosis between it and the distal internal carotid. An injured external carotid artery itself can be ligated with impunity. Inspect the vagus nerve, but handle it minimally to avoid injury to its medially located recurrent laryngeal nerve fibers.

Exploration and Repair of Midline Structures (Fig. 13.3)

Technical and Anatomic Points

Control bleeding from the thyroid gland by direct suture ligature. Such bleeding usually does not respond to cautery. Visualize the recurrent laryngeal nerve if the injury lies close to its position in the tracheoesophageal groove (see Fig. 5.7 in Chapter 5). Expose the trachea from an anterior approach. Close simple tracheal lacerations with interrupted absorbable suture material, tying knots externally to avoid intraluminal granuloma formation. When adjacent injuries to the trachea and esophagus are present, a well-vascularized muscle flap should be interposed between tracheal and esophageal repairs. Laryngeal injuries are similarly repaired but also require endoscopic evaluation of internal laryngeal structures.

The pharynx and esophagus, although in the midline, are approached from the side owing to their posterior location. Full exposure of the cervical esophagus and distal pharynx requires ligation and division of the middle thyroid vein and inferior thyroid artery. The thyroid can then be rotated anteromedially with the trachea as the sternocleidomastoid muscle and carotid sheath are retracted posterolaterally. After appropriate débridement, repair pharyngeal and esophageal injuries using a standard two-layer suture technique. Place a small drain in proximity to the suture line.

Close the wound in layers, approximating the anterior border of the sternocleidomastoid muscle to the divided cervical fascia with absorbable sutures. Bring the drain out through a separate stab wound.

Additional Exposure for Injuries Involving the Thoracic Inlet (Fig. 13.4)

Technical and Anatomic Points

When the exact extent of injury is not known in the unstable patient, median sternotomy provides the best exposure. This incision can be extended superiorly along the anterior border of either sternocleidomastoid muscle as necessary to expose the common carotid artery. Median sternotomy with cervical extension allows excellent exposure and proximal control of the brachiocephalic, proximal right subclavian, and proximal common carotid arteries. A contiguous incision along the right supraclavicular region exposes the more distal right subclavian artery. The very proximal left subclavian artery can be controlled through median sternotomy, but a high left anterolateral thoracotomy (third or fourth interspace) usually provides better proximal exposure. Coupled with a left supraclavicular incision, access to most of the left subclavian artery can be achieved. Rarely, left clavicular division, partial excision, or both may be required. This is justified if vascular control cannot be obtained by other means, but this maneuver is associated with significant morbidity.

REFERENCES

1. Bishara RA, Pasch AR, Douglas DD, et al. The necessity of mandatory exploration of penetrating zone II neck injuries. *Surgery* 1986;100:655.
2. Demetriades D, Chahwan S, Gomez H, et al. Penetrating injuries to the subclavian and axillary vessels. *J Am Coll Surg* 1999;188:290–295. (Contains a wealth of information about dealing with these difficult injuries.)
3. Demetriades D, Asensio JA, Velmahos G, et al. Complex problems in penetrating neck trauma. *Surg Clin North Am* 1996;76:661–683.
4. Dichtel WJ, Miller RH, Woodson GE, et al. Lateral mandibulotomy: a technique of exposure for penetrating injuries of the internal carotid artery at the base of the skull. *Laryngoscope* 1984;94:1140. (Describes division of the mandible to allow significant upward extension of exposure.)
5. Eddy VA, and the Zone I Penetrating Neck Injury Study Group. Is routine arteriography mandatory for penetrating injuries to zone I of the neck? *J Trauma* 2000;48:208–214.
6. Gaspert MG, Lorelli DR, Kralovich KA, et al. Physical examination plus chest radiography in penetrating periclavicular trauma: the appropriate trigger for angiography. *J Trauma* 2000;49:1029–1033.
7. Gilroy D, Lakhoo M, Charalambides D, et al. Control of life-threatening hemorrhage from the neck: a new indication for balloon tamponade. *Injury* 1992;23:557–559.
8. Graham JM, Mattox KL, Feliciano DV, et al. Vascular injuries of the axilla. *Ann Surg* 1982;195:232. (Describes exposure of axillary and subclavian vessels.)
9. Grewal H, Rao PM, Mukerji S, et al. Management of penetrating laryngotracheal injuries. *Head Neck* 1995;17:494–502.
10. Landrenau RJ, Weigelt JA, Megison SM, et al. Combined carotid-vertebral arterial trauma. *Arch Surg* 1992;127:301–304.
11. McIntyre WB, Ballard JL. Cervicothoracic vascular injuries. *Semin Vasc Surg* 1998;11:232–242.
12. Noyes LD, McSwain NE, Markowitz IP. Panendoscopy with arteriography versus mandatory exploration of penetrating wounds of the neck. *Ann Surg* 1986;204:21. (Presents alternative to neck exploration.)
13. Patel AV, Marin ML, Veith FJ, et al. Endovascular graft repair of penetrating subclavian artery injuries. *J Endovasc Surg* 1996;3:382–388. (An alternative to operative management in highly selected cases.)
14. Richardson JD, Martin LF, Borzotta AP, et al. Unifying concepts in treatment of esophageal leaks. *Am J Surg* 1985;149:157.
15. Schenk WG. Neck injuries. In: Moylan JA, ed. *Trauma surgery.* Philadelphia: JB Lippincott, 1988:417. (Describes the management of blunt and penetrating neck injuries.)
16. Shaha A, Phillips T, Scalea T, et al. Exposure of the internal carotid artery near the skull base: The posterolateral anatomic approach. *J Vasc Surg* 1988;8:618. (Provides an excellent description of the exposure obtained through a radical neck–type approach.)
17. Yee LF, Olcott EW, Knudson M, et al. Extraluminal, transluminal, and observational treatment for vertebral artery injuries. *J Trauma* 1995;39:480–486.

SECTION **II**

The Pectoral Region and Chest

The anatomy of the pectoral region and chest will be discussed in three parts: the pectoral region, the mediastinum and midline structures, and the lungs and esophagus.

The basic procedures of subclavian venous catheterization and cutdown on the cephalic vein in the deltopectoral groove will be used to illustrate the anatomy of the subclavian region (Chapter 14). The subclavian vein is the continuation of the axillary vein, and radical mastectomy (and its derivative operation, modified radical mastectomy) has been termed the dissection of the axillary vein. Hence, breast operations are considered next. Both breast biopsy (Chapter 15) and modified radical and classic radical mastectomy (Chapter 16) illustrate the anatomy of the breast, pectoral region, and axilla. For completeness, axillary node biopsy and node dissection (Chapter 17) and sentinel node biopsy for breast cancer (Chapter 18) are included in this section.

The structures of the chest are first discussed by presenting the anatomy of the mediastinum (the "space between"). Mediastinoscopy (Chapter 19) is used to illustrate the topography of the region. A discussion of median sternotomy and thymectomy (Chapter 20) completes the introduction to the anterior mediastinum.

Chapter 21 introduces pulmonary anatomy endobronchially, through fiberoptic and rigid bronchoscopy. Thoracostomy and thoracotomy (Chapter 22) illustrate the anatomy of an intercostal space and the muscles of the chest wall. This is complemented by Chapter 23, which presents the thoracoscopic view. Pulmonary resections—both pneumonectomies (Chapter 24) and lobectomies (Chapters 25 and 26)—complete the discussion of the anatomy of the lungs.

The thoracic outlet is the opening through which major neurovascular structures enter and leave the chest for the neck and upper extremity. The anatomy of this complex space is illustrated in Chapter 27, where surgery for thoracic outlet compression syndromes is considered.

The esophagus, although it is a midline structure, is approached through a thoracotomy incision and hence is discussed with other structures accessed through that approach (Chapter 28 and 29). It provides an introduction to the abdominal region (Section IV).

THE PECTORAL REGION

The pectoral region is described in this section. Structures of importance for venous access include the subclavian and cephalic veins. The approach to the axillary artery is described in Section III (The Upper Extremity), Chapter 30 (Axillobifemoral Bypass). The breast and axilla are included in this section, along with operative descriptions of breast biopsy, mastectomy, and axillary node biopsy, dissection, and sentinel node biopsy for breast cancer.

CHAPTER 14

Venous Access: The Subclavian Vein and the Cephalic Vein in the Deltopectoral Groove

Percutaneous cannulation of the subclavian vein is frequently used for rapid access to the central venous circulation. Because of the relatively constant location of this vein and the bony landmarks that are readily palpable in most individuals, this is a convenient site for cannulation. However, this vein's proximity to other major vascular structures and to the apex of the lung necessitates a thorough understanding of the anatomy so that complications may be avoided when performing this routine procedure.

Performing a cutdown on the cephalic vein in the deltopectoral groove is an alternative means of achieving access to the central circulation. In selected patients, it may be easier or safer than percutaneous methods.

Percutaneous Cannulation of the Subclavian Vein

Positioning the Patient and Identifying Landmarks (Fig. 14.1)

Technical Points

Position the patient supine with arms at the side. Elevate the foot of the bed to a 5- or 10-degree Trendelenburg position. This will increase venous pressure in the central veins,

distending the subclavian vein and rendering the possibility of venous air embolus less likely. Place a vertical roll under the thoracic spine to allow the shoulders to "fall back" slightly, thus opening the angle between the clavicle and the ribs. Inspect both infraclavicular regions for evidence of previous cannulation or local infections. In general, the left subclavian vein is somewhat easier to cannulate and will more reliably provide access to the central circulation than the right subclavian vein. Both, however, are usable.

Identify the constant bony landmarks before cannulation. These include the acromion process, the sternal notch, and the medial third of the clavicle. Prepare and drape a field that includes the medial half of the clavicle. Using your nondominant hand, place the index finger in the sternal notch and the thumb under the clavicle. Identify the place where the curvature of the clavicle begins to change (remember that the clavicle is S-shaped). This should be about one third of the distance from the sternal notch to the acromion and medial to the pulse of the subclavian artery if it is palpable. Use a fine-gauge needle to infiltrate the area with lidocaine without epinephrine. Aspirate as the skin, subcutaneous tissues, and periosteum are infiltrated. "Walk" the needle under the periosteum of the clavicle and aspirate. Free aspiration of venous blood with this fine-gauge needle will help to identify

LIST OF STRUCTURES

Superior vena cava	Aorta	Sternohyoid muscle
Brachiocephalic (innominate) vein	Brachiocephalic artery	Sternothyroid muscle
Internal jugular vein	Subclavian artery	Pectoralis major muscle
Subclavian vein	Thoracic duct	Pectoralis minor muscle
Vertebral vein	Bronchomediastinal lymph trunk	Clavipectoral fascia
Inferior thyroid vein	Subclavian lymph trunk	Prevertebral fascia
Internal thoracic vein	Jugular lymph trunk	Deltopectoral groove
Thymic vein	Acromion process	Deltopectoral triangle
Left superior intercostal vein	Sternal notch	Pleura
Thyroidea ima vein	Clavicle	Thymus
Axillary vein	Sternoclavicular joints	Trachea
Cephalic vein	Anterior scalene muscle	Phrenic nerve
		Vagus nerve

ORIENTATION

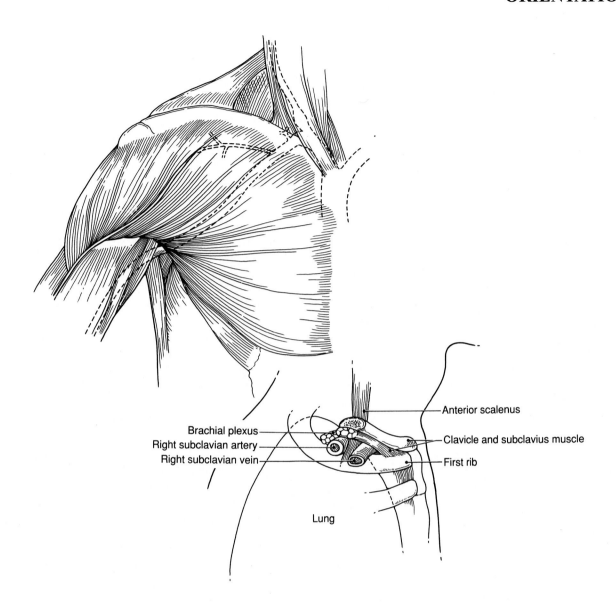

Brachial plexus

Right subclavian artery

Right subclavian vein

Anterior scalenus

Clavicle and subclavius muscle

First rib

Lung

where the subclavian vein lies. Do not inject local anesthesia into the subclavian vein.

After identifying the probable location of the subclavian vein, place an 18-gauge needle on a Luer slip syringe. Maintaining the orientation of the bony landmarks previously described, "walk" the tip of the needle under the clavicle. The point of the needle should be aimed at the sternal notch. The shaft of the needle should remain parallel to the floor at all times. Never point the needle toward the chest wall. You should feel the needle strike the periosteum of the underside of the clavicle and slip under the clavicle; aspirate until free return of venous blood is obtained.

Upon free return of venous blood, use a hemostat to grasp the needle and maintain it in position as the Luer slip syringe is gently removed. Conscious, cooperative patients should

then be asked to perform a Valsalva maneuver before the syringe is disconnected in order to avoid producing a venous air embolus. Immediately place a gloved finger over the hub of the needle so that no air can enter the vein. Introduce the floppy end of the guidewire through the needle. It should pass freely and easily, indicating a central position. Remove the needle, taking care not to lose contact with the guidewire at any time. If resistance is encountered while introducing the wire through the needle, withdraw the needle and guidewire as a unit. Otherwise, withdrawal of the wire through the needle may result in cutting of the wire, which can then embolize to the heart.

If fluoroscopy is available, check the position of the guidewire at this time. Demonstrate by fluoroscopy that the guidewire is centrally located. Use a number 11 blade to

FIGURE 14.1
POSITIONING THE PATIENT AND IDENTIFYING LANDMARKS

Suprasternal notch

enlarge the skin hole around the guidewire and pass a venous dilator and sheath over the guidewire coaxially into the subclavian vein. These should pass easily, although some resistance will be felt as the tissue is dilated. Remove the dilator and wire, leaving the sheath in place. Again, place a gloved finger over the hub of the needle as the wire and dilator are removed to avoid venous air embolus. Introduce the catheter through the sheath; break and peel away the sheath. Confirm the final position of the catheter using fluoroscopy and document, by upright chest radiographic studies, that pneumothorax has not occurred. Secure the catheter in position and place a sterile dressing over the device.

Anatomic Points

The subclavian veins, which represent continuations of the axillary veins, begin at the outer border of the first rib. Posterior to the sternoclavicular joint on each side, the subclavian vein joins the internal jugular vein to form either the right or left brachiocephalic (innominate) vein. The two brachiocephalic veins join posterior to the right side of the sternum, at the level of the first intercostal space, to form the superior vena cava. Both subclavian veins lie more or less posterior to the clavicle and subclavius muscle (although the relationship of the clavicle varies as one progresses from lateral to medial), anterior and slightly inferior to the subclavian artery, and anterior to the anterior scalene muscle. The anterior scalene muscle lies between the subclavian vein (which lies anterior) and the subclavian artery (posterior). Medial to the anterior

scalene muscles, both left and right veins lie on the superior surface of the first rib and then on the dome of the pleura. The fascial relations of the subclavian veins make the threat of an air embolus more than theoretical. Laterally, the vein is firmly attached to the clavipectoral fascia, whereas more medially, it is attached to prevertebral fascia. These attachments prevent collapse of the vein, and during certain movements, such as during inspiration or raising of the arm, they can increase the diameter of the subclavian veins.

The two brachiocephalic veins are quite different in length, orientation, significant tributaries, and relations. Both begin posterior to their respective sternoclavicular joints. The right brachiocephalic vein is usually about 2.5 cm long and is essentially vertical; thus, its axis lies at an angle of almost 90 degrees with respect to the axis of the subclavian vein. As the left brachiocephalic vein joins the right at a point posterior to the right edge of the sternum and superior to the second sternocostal articulation, it is, of necessity, longer (about 6 cm), and its oblique course approaches the horizontal. As a consequence, the axis of the subclavian and brachiocephalic veins is obtuse, approaching 180 degrees. It is the orientation of subclavian and brachiocephalic veins that makes cannulation of the left side easier than cannulation of the right.

In addition to the subclavian and internal jugular veins, tributaries of both brachiocephalic veins typically include vertebral, inferior thyroid, and internal thoracic veins. The left brachiocephalic vein typically also receives the left superior intercostal vein, the thymic veins, and a thyroidea ima vein when the latter is present.

On the right, typically (80% of cases), three lymphatic trunks (right bronchomediastinal, subclavian, and jugular) join the venous system at or near the beginning of the brachiocephalic vein. In about 20% of cases, these trunks join to form a short right lymphatic duct. On the left, these trunks typically join the thoracic duct, which then drains into the venous system as a single vessel at or near the beginning of the brachiocephalic vein.

The anatomic relationships of the brachiocephalic veins are a prime source of morbidity. The right brachiocephalic vein is related anteriorly to the sternohyoid and sternothyroid attachments on the deep aspect of the sternum and, more inferiorly, to the first costal cartilage. Posteriorly, it is related to the pleura and brachiocephalic artery. Medial to it are the brachiocephalic artery and vagus nerve, whereas the pleura and phrenic nerve lie lateral to it. Anterior to the left brachiocephalic vein, the thymus or its remnant separates the vein from the sternum and its related muscles. Posterior to the vein are the arch of the aorta, the roots of all three great arteries, the trachea, the vagus, and the phrenic nerves. Remember that, frequently, a part of the left brachiocephalic vein is superior to the top of the manubrium and, thus can be palpated in the jugular notch.

Cutdown on the Cephalic Vein in the Deltopectoral Groove

Landmarks and Incision (Fig. 14.2)

Technical Points

The cephalic vein runs in a fairly constant position in the deltopectoral groove. Identify the deltopectoral groove

---

**FIGURE 14.2
LANDMARKS AND INCISION**

by palpating the head of the humerus and the muscular heads of the deltoid muscle and the pectoralis major muscle. Prep and drape the field, which includes the lateral half of the pectoralis major muscle, the inferior border of the clavicle, and the medial portion of the head of the humerus. Make a transverse skin incision about two fingerbreadths below the clavicle, just medial to the head of the humerus.

Anatomic Points

The cephalic vein begins on the radial side of the dorsum of the hand and then ascends in the superficial fascia to the deltopectoral triangle, where it pierces the deep fascia, ultimately ending in the axillary vein. In the arm, it is typically located in the groove lateral to the biceps brachii muscle; in the upper arm, this groove and the vein are medial to the anterior edge of the deltoid muscle.

Location of the Vein and Cannulation (Fig. 14.3)

Technical Points

By sharp and blunt dissection, carry the dissection down to the fascia overlying the pectoralis major muscle. Follow this muscle and identify where it lies separate from the adjacent deltoid muscle. This site is identifiable by a slight change in muscle fiber direction. Often, a distinct groove can be found. Spread with a hemostat in the fatty tissue of the groove and identify the cephalic vein. Elevate it into the field and secure it with two loops of 2-0 silk. Make a venotomy on the anterior surface of the vein and introduce the catheter through the venotomy.

The catheter should place easily. Occasionally, the catheter will "hang up" at the angulation between the cephalic vein and the axillary vein. If this happens, move the arm slightly or apply digital pressure in the field to guide the catheter around the bend. Confirm adequate positioning of the catheter by fluoroscopy and tie it in position in the vein. Ligate the distal end of the vein. Close the incision in layers with absorbable suture material.

Anatomic Points

When the cephalic vein reaches the deltopectoral triangle, it pierces the investing fascia covering the pectoralis major and deltoid muscles, continues for a short distance in the plane just deep to that fascia, and then pierces the clavipectoral fascia, just inferior to the clavicle, ending in the axillary vein. Difficulty in locating the vein in the deltopectoral triangle may be attributable to a developmental variation (e.g., absence, hypoplasia) or failure to divide the investing fascia, which will result in looking for the vein in an inappropriate tissue plane. Another variant—a branch that passes anterior to the clavicle and ends in the external jugular vein—could also present problems.

A final point to remember is that, when the cephalic vein ends, its junction with the axillary vein is almost 90 degrees with respect to the latter vein. Further, it tends to terminate

FIGURE 14.3
LOCATION OF THE VEIN AND CANNULATION

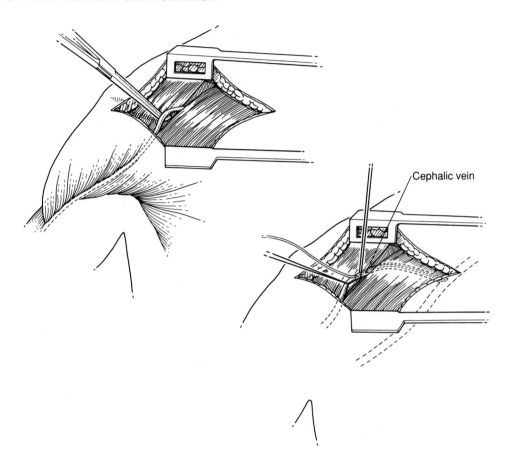

Cephalic vein

on the superior aspect of the axillary vein, so that elevation of the arm may make the angle between the cephalic and axillary veins sharper, thereby making passage of the catheter into the subclavian vein more difficult than need be.

REFERENCES

1. Au FC. The anatomy of the cephalic vein. *Am Surg* 1989;55:638.
2. Hawkins J, Nelson EW. Percutaneous placement of Hickman catheters for prolonged venous access. *Am J Surg* 1982;144:624.
3. Heimbach DM, Ivey TD. Technique for placement of a permanent home hyperalimentation catheter. *Surg Gynecol Obstet* 1976;143:635. (This original technique of placement by cutdown includes a description of catheter placement in the cephalic or internal jugular vein, a procedure that is still applicable when percutaneous subclavian access is contraindicated.)
4. Holland AJA, Ford WDA. Improved percutaneous insertion of long-term central venous catheters in children: the 'shrug' manoeuvre. *Aust N Z J Surg* 1999;69:231–233.
5. Lefrant JY, Cuvillon P, Benezet JF, et al. Pulsed Doppler ultrasonography guidance for catheterization of the subclavian vein. *Anesthesiology* 1998;88:1195–201. (This technique is a useful adjunct in some circumstances.)
6. Muhm M, Sunder-Plassmann G, Apsner R, et al. Supraclavicular approach to the subclavian/innominate vein for large-bore central venous catheters. *Am J Kidney Dis* 1997;30:802–808. (Describes an alternative approach to subclavian.)
7. Sterchi JM, Fulks D, Cruz J, et al. Operative technique for insertion of a totally implantable system for venous access. *Surg Gynecol Obstet* 1986;163:381. (Describes the modification needed for placement of totally implantable devices.)
8. Tan BK, Hong SW, Huang MHS, et al. Anatomic basis of safe percutaneous subclavian venous catheterization. *J Trauma* 2000;48:82–86.
9. Wilson SE, Stabile BE, Williams RA, et al. Current status of vascular access techniques. *Surg Clin North Am* 1982;62:531.

CHAPTER 15

Breast Biopsy and Tylectomy

Small breast masses should be excised in their entirety. Larger masses require incisional biopsy. In cases in which a tumor is suspected on mammographic examination but is not palpable, a biopsy specimen may be obtained after placement of a hook-wire under radiographic or ultrasound guidance (Fig. 15.3).

Choice of Incision (Fig. 15.1)

Technical Points

For most easily palpable lesions that lie within several centimeters of the areola, a circumareolar incision is appropriate for obtaining a biopsy specimen. However, biopsy of ill-defined masses that are not easily reached using this approach should be accomplished through an incision placed directly over the mass. In such cases, the incision should be gently curved in the upper or lower parts of the breast, and should be transverse, or nearly so, in the medial or lateral aspects. This allows the scar to be hidden by clothing or readily incorporated into a mastectomy incision should that procedure be indicated.

Radial incisions, once advocated because they parallel the underlying duct structure of the breast, yield poor cosmetic results and should be used only for very medial or lateral lesions. When planning the incision, remember that the biopsy site will have to be excised with a skin margin should subsequent mastectomy be required. For this reason, inframammary incisions, although cosmetically appealing, should generally be avoided.

Choose a site for incision and infiltrate the area with local anesthetic. If the mass becomes difficult to palpate after the skin preparation has been done, wash the skin of the breast with sterile saline and palpate by sliding gloved fingers over the wet skin.

Anatomic Points

The breast, which is wholly contained within superficial fascia, extends from the second rib superiorly to the sixth rib

LIST OF STRUCTURES

Breast
  Nipple
  Areola
  Axillary tail of Spence

inferiorly, and from the sternum to the midaxillary line. The axillary tail of Spence is an extension of breast tissue into the axilla. The breast is composed of 15 to 20 glandular lobes and adipose tissue arranged radially around the nipple–areolar complex. These are separated by fibrous septa, fibers of which attach to the deep surface of the skin and to the deep layer of the superficial fascia (suspensory ligaments of Spence). The glandular tissue of the lobes, each based on a lactiferous duct that drains at the apex of the nipple, tends to be located more centrally, whereas the adipose tissue tends to be located more peripherally.

A circumareolar incision produces a scar that is almost hidden in the abrupt change in skin pigmentation at the areolar margin. If the location of the lesion makes this impossible, the incision should approximate the direction of the skin cleavage lines. These lines are concentrically arranged around the nipple, although in pendulous breasts, the effects of gravity are superimposed on this pattern. The surgeon should be aware of the underlying radial breast architecture and should restrict the initial incision to the skin.

Biopsy of a Palpable Mass (Fig. 15.2)

Technical Points

Make a circumareolar incision and raise a flap (generally, 0.5 cm in thickness) in the cleavage plane between the subcutaneous tissue and breast. Place retractors to pull the incision closer to the mass. Identify the mass by palpation. If necessary, cut through the overlying breast tissue to expose the mass. Place a traction suture of 2-0 silk in a figure-of-eight fashion through the mass. (Use a curved cutting needle because the tough, fibrous breast tissue will bend a tapered-point needle.) Pull up on the traction suture to elevate the mass into the field. Excise the mass by sharp dissection using a knife or Mayo scissors. Avoid overzealous use of electrocautery on the biopsy specimen because this can invalidate estrogen and progesterone receptor assays. Take care not to violate the pectoral fascia by cutting too deeply because this fascia provides a natural barrier that will help to prevent contamination of the mastectomy field with spilled tumor cells if subsequent mastectomy is performed.

Feel both the excised mass and the residual breast cavity to ascertain that the palpable lesion has been removed. Request that receptor and tumor markers be done if the biopsy is positive for carcinoma. Some laboratories may require that

FIGURE 15.1
CHOICE OF INCISION

FIGURE 15.2
BIOPSY OF A PALPABLE MASS

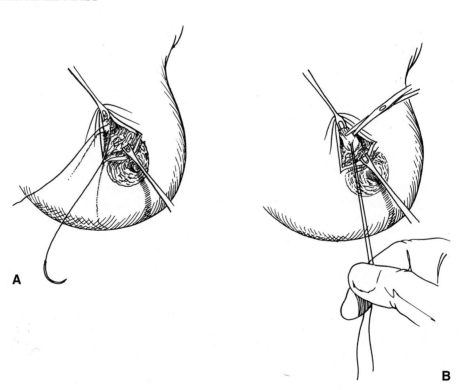

FIGURE 15.3
NEEDLE-LOCALIZED BREAST BIOPSY

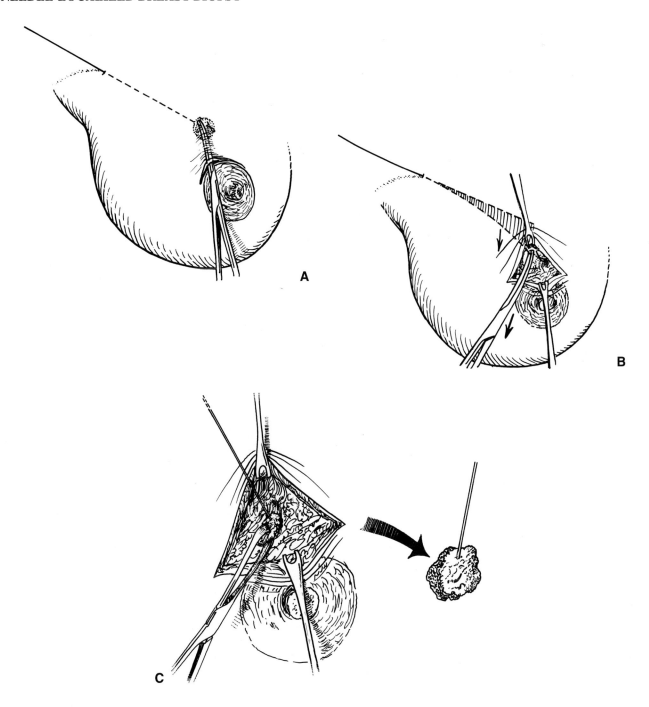

A

B

C

fresh tissue be submitted; know the requirements of your pathologist.

If the mass is ill defined or is located at some distance from the areola, it is safest to make the incision directly over the mass. In such cases, cosmetic considerations should be set aside because the first priority is an accurate diagnosis. Stabilize the mass with the fingers of the nondominant hand and infiltrate the overlying skin with anesthetic. Continue

to hold the mass firmly anchored as you make the skin incision. Place retractors to visualize the underlying breast tissue. Place a traction suture in the mass. The traction suture can then be used to manipulate the mass as it is excised.

Perform local excision (tylectomy) of early breast carcinomas as an excisional biopsy, taking care not to contaminate the biopsy field by cutting into tumor. Remove the lesion along with a generous rim of the surrounding, grossly normal breast tissue, and have the pathologist ink the specimen and check the margins for adequacy of excision. Orient the specimen for the pathologist.

Anatomic Points

In raising a skin flap, one gets the impression that the breast is surrounded by an adipose "capsule" that is prominent everywhere except deep to the nipple and areola. However, throughout this capsule, connective tissue strands connect interlobar and interlobular septa to the deep surface of the dermis. The more prominent connective tissue strands constitute the suspensory ligaments (of Cooper) and tend to be more pronounced on the superior hemisphere than on the inferior hemisphere.

After a skin flap is elevated and the adipose capsule is opened, the breast parenchyma and stroma will be encountered. The glandular parenchyma, organized in pyramidal lobes with their apices toward the nipple, will be recognized by its white color, which contrasts with the yellow-white color of the fat. Although fibrous connective tissue tends to be interlobar and thus radially arranged, the continuity of these septa with interlobular fibers and fibers separating adipose tissue loculi results in an irregular, spongy distribution of this tissue type. Ultimately, the connective tissue septa connect to the fibrous deep layer of superficial fascia. Deep to this fascial layer, a thin layer of loose connective tissue with a small amount of retromammary fat separates the breast from the pectoral fascia, the deep or investing fascia of the muscles of the pectoral region. This loose areolar tissue should warn you of impending exposure of pectoral fascia.

Needle-Localized Breast Biopsy (Fig. 15.3)

Technical and Anatomic Points

Close communication between the mammographer or ultrasonographer and surgeon is essential. Review the prelocalization and postlocalization radiographic films with the radiologist and be certain that you understand the three-dimensional relationship between the skin entry site, the shaft of the wire, the thickened portion of the shaft, the hooked tip of the wire, and the target lesion.

Remove the dressing from the breast with care because the wire can become dislodged if pulled too hard. Prepare the entire breast and the wire. Gently tug on the exposed wire while feeling the underlying breast along the projected course of the needle. Often, the site of the target lesion can be identified by noting the region of the breast that moves slightly as the wire is tugged. Plan an incision that is cosmetically acceptable yet close to the tip of the wire. It may be possible to use a circumareolar incision; however, most of the time, it is preferable to make the incision as close as possible to the terminal 2 to 3 cm of wire. Generally, the incision should not be made over the skin entry site of the wire, which is commonly at some distance from the areola and also far from the target lesion.

FIGURE 15.4
CLOSURE OF THE INCISION

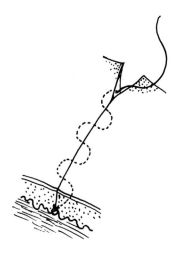

Elevate a flap toward the wire and expose it. If dissection becomes difficult, use a knife because scissors can cut the wire. Identify the wire by the tactile sensation of the steel on steel and by noting motion of the exposed wire as you probe. Anchor the distal wire with a hemostat so that it is not inadvertently pulled out, and then deliver the proximal end of the wire into the wound by pulling it back through the skin. Periodically verify, by gentle traction on the wire, the probable location of the tip. Dissect down parallel to, but 1 to 2 cm distant from, the wire. Start the dissection behind the wire and work toward the tip. Often, a previously nonpalpable target lesion becomes palpable as dissection progresses.

Terminate the dissection by cutting well past the tip of the wire. Remember that the best chance to excise the target lesion is at the first pass. Once the wire has been removed, orientation is lost. Submit the wire and specimen for radiographic study, returning the mammograms with the specimen for comparison. Feel the cavity for any residual abnormal tissue. Excise and submit for specimen radiography any palpably abnormal residual tissue in the biopsy cavity.

Close the incision after receiving confirmation that the target area was included in the specimen. If the lesion was missed, a review of localization films and specimen radiographs will frequently provide a clue as to which portion of the cavity wall undergoing biopsy is likely to contain the area of interest.

Closure of the Incision (Fig. 15.4)

Technical and Anatomic Points

Achieve complete hemostasis in the biopsy incision by irrigating it to remove blood clots and then sequentially grasping portions of the cavity wall with an Allis clamp and pulling them up for inspection.

Do not place sutures deep in the breast to close the cavity or to attempt to "reconstruct" the breast. Such sutures create a deformity by tethering the normally mobile, fluid breast tissue. Place several interrupted fine absorbable sutures to approximate the subcutaneous fat just under the skin and close the skin incision with a subcuticular suture. Drains are rarely used. Either a pressure dressing or, preferably, a light dressing held by a snugly fitting brassiere will help to prevent hematoma formation.

REFERENCES

1. Bloomston M, D'Angelo P, Galliano D, et al. One hundred consecutive advanced breast biopsy instrumentation procedures: complications, costs and outcome. *Ann Surg Oncol* 1999;6:195–199. (Describes alternative method of securing large biopsy of nonpalpable lesion.)
2. Hughes LE, Webster DJT, Mansel RE. Operations. In: Hughes LE, Mansel RE, Webster DJT, eds. *Benign disorders and diseases of the breast: concepts and clinical management.* 2nd ed. London: WB Saunders, 2000:265–289. (Presents clear description of techniques for excision of various benign breast lesions, including ductal excision.)
3. Kwasnik EM, Sadowsky NL, Vollman RW. An improved system for surgical excision of needle-localized nonpalpable breast lesions. *Am J Surg* 1987;154:476. (Description of technique of needle localization.)
4. Margolese R, Poisson R, Shibata H, et al. The technique of segmental mastectomy (lumpectomy) and axillary dissection: a syllabus from the National Surgical Adjuvant Breast Project workshops. *Surgery* 1987;102:828. (Provides an excellent description of adequate excision of breast cancer by lumpectomy.)
5. Velanovich V, Lewis FR Jr, Nathanson SD, et al. Comparison of mammographically guided breast biopsy techniques. *Ann Surg* 1999;229:625–633.

CHAPTER 16

Mastectomy: Total (Simple), Modified, and Classic Radical

Total (sometimes called *simple*) mastectomy removes all the glandular tissue of the breast. It is sometimes required for treatment of extensive ductal carcinoma *in situ*. In combination with reconstructive surgery, bilateral total mastectomy is sometimes used for breast cancer prophylaxis in carefully selected patients.

Modified radical mastectomy adds the removal of the node-bearing tissue of the axilla while preserving the muscular contours of the upper chest wall. The operation was modified from the original or classic radical mastectomy to enhance the cosmetic result without compromising control of disease. Many modifications of the original classic radical mastectomy have been described. They differ in the extent of tissue removed and the completeness of axillary dissection. The modification described here combines a thorough axillary dissection with preservation of muscle contour. Other modified radical mastectomy techniques are detailed in the references.

Classic radical mastectomy is still used in those rare circumstances in which wider excision of the pectoral muscles might enhance local control.

Total and Modified Radical Mastectomy

Position of the Patient and Skin Incision (Fig. 16.1)

Technical and Anatomic Points

The operation is performed under general anesthesia. After the initial intubation, muscle relaxants are avoided so that nerve function can be assessed. Position the patient supine, with the ipsilateral arm extended on an armboard. If necessary, place a small, folded sheet under the shoulder, to improve exposure. Avoid hyperextending the shoulder because this can cause neuropraxia. Drape the arm free so that it can be moved during the course of the dissection.

Plan a generally transverse incision, defining an ellipse of skin that includes both the nipple–areolar complex and the biopsy scar. Allow 5 cm on each side of the biopsy incision. Very high medial or lateral biopsy sites may require oblique incisions. The biopsy cavity is considered to be contaminated by tumor cells and frequently contains gross residual disease. It must be excised in its entirety as dissection progresses. Therefore, if the biopsy is performed through an incision located at some distance from the mass, a correspondingly larger amount of skin should be sacrificed. Do not compromise the skin incision because of fear of difficulty in closure. A skin graft will heal well over the underlying muscle and may be used if necessary.

Development of Flaps (Fig. 16.2)

Technical Points

Incise the skin and subcutaneous tissue. Visualize the breast as lying encapsulated in a separate layer of subcutaneous fat that lies 0.5 to 1.0 cm below the skin. Often, this layer can be defined as the skin incision is made. Place Lahey clamps on the dermal side of the upper flap and have an assistant place these under strong upward traction. Apply countertraction by downward traction on the breast with a lap sponge. Avoid manipulating the breast overlying the biopsy site. Develop flaps by sharp dissection using a shaving motion with a sharp knife. Change blades frequently. Dissection in the proper plane is surprisingly bloodless. A network of large

LIST OF STRUCTURES

Pectoralis major muscle	Thoracodorsal nerve	Internal thoracic (mammary) vein
Pectoralis minor muscle	Long thoracic nerve	Axillary lymph nodes
Subclavius muscle	Axillary artery	**Landmarks**
Clavipectoral fascia	Axillary vein	Clavicle
Coracoid process	Thoracoacromial artery	Anterior rectus sheath
Lateral pectoral nerve	Thoracodorsal vein	Latissimus dorsi muscle
Medial pectoral nerve	Internal thoracic (mammary) artery	Sternum

FIGURE 16.1
POSITION OF THE PATIENT AND SKIN INCISION

A

B

subcutaneous veins is often visible on the underside of the flap. Ligate occasional bleeders on the underside of the flap. (Use electrocautery with caution on the flap because it can burn through the thin flap to damage the overlying skin surface.) Confirm the thickness of the flap by palpation as the dissection progresses.

In the axilla, the skin flap will be crossed by hair follicles and apocrine glands. Divide these sharply. Raise flaps to the level of the clavicle superiorly, the midline medially, the anterior rectus sheath inferiorly, and the anterior border of the latissimus dorsi muscle laterally. Of these, the lateral border of the latissimus dorsi is generally the most difficult to find. Identify this muscle by palpation of a longitudinal ridge of muscle tissue. Dissect sharply down to confirm its identity by visualizing longitudinal muscle fibers. Trace the muscle up toward the axilla. Check the upper flap for hemostasis and place a moist laparotomy pad under the flap.

Place Lahey clamps on the inferior skin incision and develop the inferior flap by the same technique. The plane between breast and subcutaneous tissue is frequently less well defined inferiorly, and unless care is taken, the inferior flap may be cut too thick. Guard against this by constant palpation

of the thickness of the flap. If white fibrous tissue (breast or Cooper's ligaments) is seen, the flap is too thick and must be cut thinner.

Draw a line around the margins of the dissection by incising the fascia at the perimeter of the field with electrocautery. This will prevent your dissecting too far in any direction. Recheck both flaps for hemostasis and place warm moist lap pads under them. Take care throughout the operation not to allow the subcutaneous fat of the underside of the flaps to become exposed and desiccated.

Anatomic Points

The breast is a conical ectodermal derivative limited to superficial fascia. The base of the breast overlies the chest wall from the second rib to the sixth, and from the edge of the sternum to the midaxillary line. A lateral tongue of breast tissue—the axillary tail of Spence—extends into each axilla from the otherwise conical breast. This tail sometimes passes through the deep fascia of the axilla and approaches the pectoral group of axillary lymph nodes. Superficial to the breast is the superficial layer of the superficial fascia, whereas deep to the breast is the deep layer of superficial fascia. The

FIGURE 16.2
DEVELOPMENT OF FLAPS

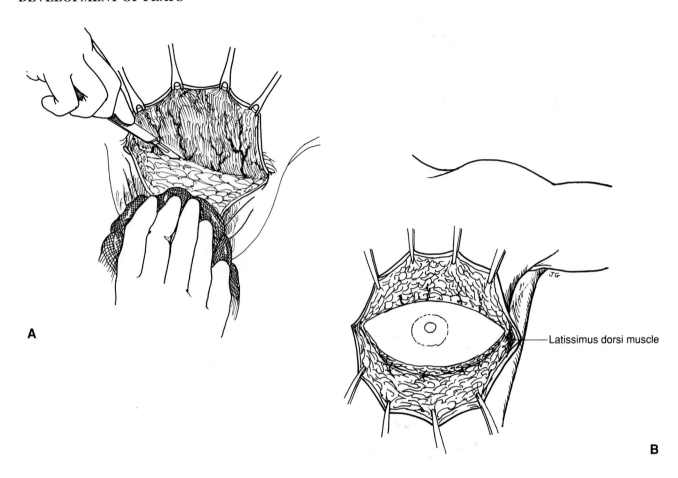

A

B

Latissimus dorsi muscle

subcutaneous fat lobules are small and easy to differentiate from the larger fat lobules of the breast itself.

As the skin flaps are developed, the suspensory ligaments (of Cooper) must be severed. These ligamentous bands traverse the fat of the gland and attach to the deep layer of superficial fascia and dermis. They are especially well developed in the upper portion of the breast.

Because the extent of the skin flaps can be related to musculoskeletal structures, the anatomy of these structures should be reviewed. The clavicle extends laterally from the superolateral corner of the manubrium to the acromion process of the scapula. Those muscles that attach to the clavicle and are palpable include a part of the pectoralis major muscle (medial half), the deltoid muscle (lateral third), and the sternocleidomastoid muscle (medial third). Most of the breast lies on the pectoralis major muscle. This muscle forms the anterior wall of the axilla. Its free lower edge is the muscular framework for the anterior axillary fold. In addition to its clavicular part, it also has a sternocostal part and an abdominal part. The sternocostal part originates from the anterior surface (essentially to the midline) of the sternum (manubrium and body), and from the cartilage of all true ribs. The abdominal part arises from the aponeurosis of the external abdominal oblique mus-

cle. From this wide origin, the fibers converge on a flat tendon inserted into the lateral lip of the intertubercular sulcus of the humerus. Thus, fibers of the clavicular part pass obliquely inferiorly and laterally, those of the sternocostal part pass horizontally or superolaterally, and those of the abdominal part ascend almost vertically.

The rectus abdominis attaches to the costal cartilage of ribs five through seven. It is covered superficially by the anterior rectus sheath, here composed only of external oblique aponeurosis. The lateral edge of the upper rectus (and hence, the rectus sheath) lies at the midclavicular line.

The latissimus dorsi forms the muscular basis for the posterior axillary fold. It originates either directly or through an aponeurosis from all vertebrae between T5 and the coccyx, the lower three to four ribs, the inferior angle of the scapula, and the iliac crest. From this origin, fibers pass laterally to converge on a tendon that inserts on the medial wall and floor of the intertubercular groove of the humerus. The most superior fibers pass almost horizontally, and the lower fibers ascend at an increasingly oblique angle toward the humerus. Thus, fibers originating from the iliac crest, especially the more anterior ones, have an almost vertical course. The latter fibers contribute to the posterior axillary fold. The

FIGURE 16.3
REMOVAL OF BREAST FROM THE PECTORALIS MAJOR MUSCLE

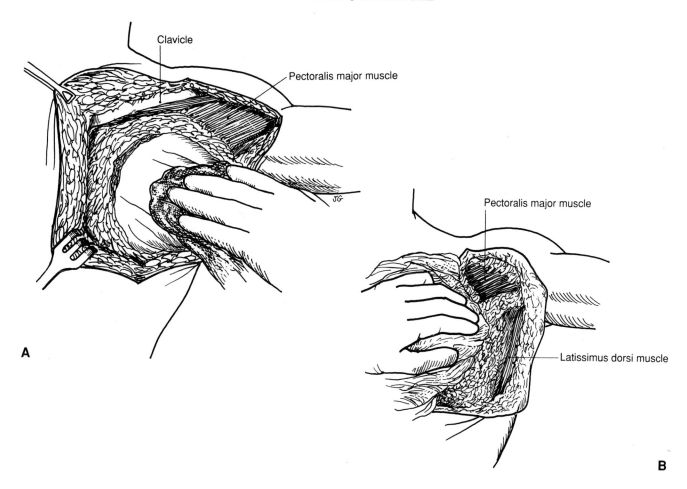

direction of muscle fibers is the key to their identification during surgery.

Removal of Breast from the Pectoralis Major Muscle (Fig. 16.3)

Technical Points

Place retractors in the medial aspect of the upper and lower flaps to expose the midline. Place Allis clamps on the pectoral fascia as breast and pectoral fascia are removed medially to laterally. Look for, and carefully ligate and divide, a series of perforating branches of the internal thoracic (mammary) artery and vein; these will be encountered as dissection progresses past the sternum. Generally, these are located within 1 to 2 cm of the edge of the sternum, one at each interspace. Use a knife to remove pectoral fascia cleanly with the breast. Only the exposed fibers of the pectoralis major muscle should remain. If tumor is locally fixed to the pectoralis major muscle, excise a portion of the muscle with the specimen. Progress from medial to lateral until the lateral border of the pectoralis major muscle is seen. Clean this lateral border, allowing the attached breast to fall laterally.

If the operation is planned as a total mastectomy, the breast is then excised from the underlying axillary tissues with electrocautery. Axillary node dissection is not performed.

Anatomic Points

The blood supply of the breast is derived from axillary, internal thoracic (mammary), and intercostal arteries. The branches of the axillary artery that supply the breast include the thoracoacromial, lateral thoracic, and subscapular branches. The internal thoracic (mammary) artery, a branch of the subclavian, usually supplies the breast through comparatively large perforating arteries in the second, third, and fourth intercostal spaces; of these, the one in the second space is typically the largest. Finally, the anterior intercostal arteries provide small perforators that are distributed to the deep aspect of the breast. Thus, the principal blood supply of the breast enters the gland superolaterally (axillary branches) and superomedially (internal thoracic branches).

Pectoral fascia is the deep fascia associated with the pectoralis major muscle. Although it is typically quite thin, it increases in thickness laterally, where it forms the floor of the axilla; it then becomes continuous with the latissimus

FIGURE 16.4
DISSECTION UNDER THE PECTORALIS MAJOR MUSCLE AND REMOVAL OF THE PECTORALIS MINOR MUSCLE

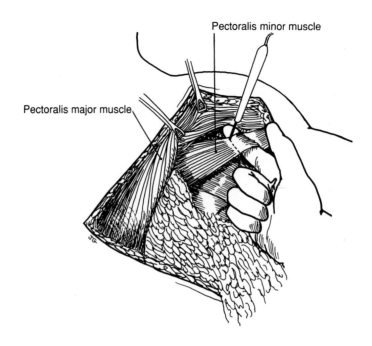

dorsi fascia and fascia of the arm. The fascial layer, of which the pectoral fascia is one regional expression, is distinct and superficial to the clavipectoral fascia. The latter fascial layer is associated with the pectoralis minor muscle.

Dissection Under the Pectoralis Major Muscle and Removal of the Pectoralis Minor Muscle (Fig. 16.4)

Technical Points

Subsequent complete axillary dissection is greatly facilitated by relaxing the pectoral muscles by elevating the arm. Have an assistant lift the arm and hold it up and over the chest wall. Place Allis clamps on the lateral edge of the pectoralis major muscle and have the assistant elevate it. Clean the underside of the pectoralis major muscle by removing fatty, areolar, node-bearing tissue and exposing the underlying pectoralis minor muscle.

Identify and preserve the medial and lateral pectoral nerves that innervate the pectoralis major and minor muscles. The lateral pectoral nerve pierces the clavipectoral fascia, whereas the medial pectoral nerve pierces the pectoralis minor muscle to enter the pectoralis major muscle relatively medially. Sacrifice of these nerves causes atrophy of the pectoralis major muscle. The muscle then becomes a fibrous cord, at which point it is both a cosmetic and a functional liability.

Incise the clavipectoral fascia on both sides of the pectoralis minor muscle in the superior portion of the field. Pass a finger behind this muscle. Look underneath to confirm that the underlying fascia is intact and that no major structures

were inadvertently raised with the muscle. If visualization under the muscle is difficult, divide the muscle using electrocautery, thus detaching it from the coracoid process.

Anatomic Points

Innervation of the pectoralis major muscle is provided by the lateral and medial pectoral nerves. These nerves are named according to their respective origins from the lateral and medial cords of the brachial plexus, not on the basis of their relative location on the anterior thoracic wall. They carry fibers of spinal cord levels C5 to C7 and C5 to T1, respectively. The lateral pectoral nerve crosses anterior to the first part of the axillary artery and vein (that segment which is proximal to the pectoralis minor muscle), and there sends an anastomotic branch to join the medial pectoral nerve. The main ramus pierces the clavipectoral fascia with the thoracoacromial artery and is distributed to the pectoralis major and minor muscles along with the pectoral branches of this artery. The medial pectoral nerve arises from the medial cord somewhat more distally than the lateral pectoral nerve—that is, at the level of the second part of the axillary artery (that segment which is posterior to the pectoralis minor muscle). Typically, this nerve pierces the pectoralis minor muscle (providing innervation to the muscle), and then ramifies on the deep surface of the pectoralis major muscle. In addition, it usually gives off two or three branches that accompany the lateral pectoral artery along the inferior border of the pectoralis minor muscle and that ultimately are distributed to the pectoralis major muscle.

Pectoralis minor muscle

Pectoralis major muscle

FIGURE 16.5
IDENTIFICATION OF THE AXILLARY VEIN AND INITIAL AXILLARY DISSECTION

Highest point of
axillary dissection

Pectoralis minor muscle

In addition to the variably developed natural separation between the clavicular and sternocostal parts of the pectoralis major muscle, there is a difference in innervation of the two parts. The lateral pectoral nerve innervates the clavicular part of the pectoralis major muscle and frequently also innervates the superior part of the sternocostal portion. The medial pectoral nerve has several branches, some of which enter the pectoralis minor muscle and innervate it. Some of these branches continue through the pectoralis minor muscle and, in addition to branches passing around the inferior border of this muscle, supply most of the sternocostal and all of the abdominal parts of the pectoralis major muscle.

Reflection or retraction of the pectoralis major muscle is done to allow access to lymph nodes that lie posterior to this muscle, ultimately including all axillary nodes.

Identification of the Axillary Vein and Initial Axillary Dissection (Fig. 16.5)

Technical Points

Incise the fascia under the pectoralis minor muscle and look carefully for the underlying axillary vein. It is often lower than expected, particularly if the pectoralis major muscle has been divided. Dissect medially in the anterior adventitial plane of the vein to the surgical apex of the axilla. Divide the few small vessels that cross over the vein.

The highest axillary nodes are the subclavian nodes, which lie in the medial apex of the field. Remove them by sharp and blunt dissection and sweep all fatty node-bearing tissue down as the chest wall is exposed. Remove the pectoralis minor

muscle with the specimen by dividing its attachments to the chest wall using electrocautery.

Cleanly dissect the chest wall, progressing from medial to lateral. Ribs and intercostal muscles should be well exposed. Sweep fatty tissue and the pectoralis minor muscle laterally, with the breast.

Anatomic Points

Clavipectoral fascia is that fascia which invests the pectoralis minor muscle. Inferior to the muscle, it is continuous with serratus anterior fascia and with the so-called axillary fascia (primarily derived from pectoralis major muscle fascia). Superomedially, it blends with intercostal fascia, whereas superolaterally, it continues as a dense sheet, splitting to invest the subclavius muscle. When splitting this fascia, care should be taken not to damage either the thoracoacromial artery or the lateral pectoral nerve, both of which pierce the fascia superior to the pectoralis minor muscle.

Division of the pectoralis minor muscle allows exposure of all three parts of the axillary artery and vein. The axillary vein is the most inferior (or medial) of the major neurovascular structures in the axilla. Components of the brachial plexus are closely associated with the axillary artery; thus, nerves will lie in the interval between vein and artery, where appropriate. The axillary sheath, in continuity with scalene fascia, surrounds the artery and nerves but not the vein.

Exposure of the axillary vessels provides complete access to axillary lymph nodes (chiefly those of the central and apical group), which are located adjacent to the second and first part of these vessels, respectively.

On average, there are 35 axillary lymph nodes, which are loosely arranged in groups associated with the major arteries and veins. Although major anatomy texts frequently list five groups, perhaps the best classification system is that of Haagensen, who maintains that there are six groups, as follow:

1. *External mammary nodes:* an average of 1.7 nodes lying deep to the lateral edge of the pectoralis major muscle and being associated with the lateral thoracic artery. Lymphatic drainage from these nodes passes to the central or subclavicular nodes.

2. *Interpectoral (Rotter's) nodes:* an average of 1.4 nodes that are associated with the pectoral branches of the thoracoacromial artery. These nodes are located in the areolar tissue between the pectoralis major muscle and the clavipectoral fascia that envelops the pectoralis minor muscle. Lymphatic drainage from these nodes passes to the central or subclavicular nodes.

FIGURE 16.6
DISSECTION OF THE AXILLARY VEIN AND IDENTIFICATION OF NERVES

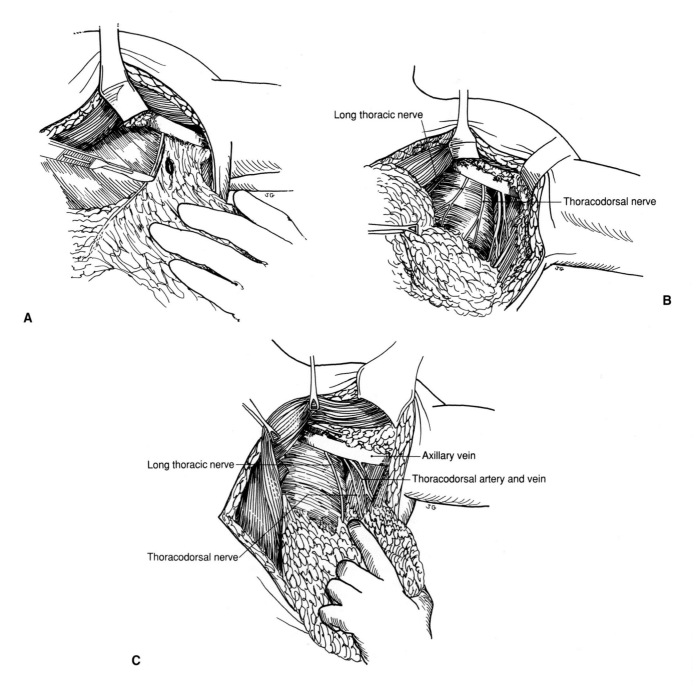

3. *Scapular nodes:* an average of 5.8 nodes that are associated with the subscapular vessels and their thoracodorsal branches. Because the intercostobrachial and thoracodorsal nerves pass through this group of nodes, these nerves may have to be sacrificed to allow removal of the nodes. Lymphatic drainage from these nodes passes to the central nodes.

4. *Central nodes:* an average of 12.1 nodes lying in fat in the central axilla, about halfway between the anterior and posterior axillary folds. Frequently, one or more of these nodes is located between the skin and superficial fascia. Lymphatic drainage from these nodes passes to the axillary nodes.

5. *Axillary nodes:* an average of 10.7 nodes that are closely associated with the axillary vein from the tendon of the latissimus dorsi muscle to the termination of the thoracoacromial vein. Lymphatic drainage from these nodes passes to the subclavicular nodes.

6. *Subclavicular nodes:* an average of 3.5 nodes that are associated with the axillary vein proximal to the termination of the thoracoacromial vein. These nodes, then, are located in the apex of the axilla, and are primarily posterior to the subclavius muscle, which is enveloped by the clavipectoral fascia. Access to the nodes is facilitated by division of the pectoralis minor muscle and its enveloping clavipectoral fascia. This group of nodes receives lymphatics from all other axillary nodes. Lymphatic drainage from these nodes passes into the inferior deep cervical nodes or directly into the venous system in the vicinity of the jugulosubclavian junction. These nodes are considered to be the highest, or apical, lymph nodes, at least from the standpoint of the breast surgeon.

Dissection of the Axillary Vein and Identification of Nerves (Fig. 16.6)

Technical Points

Follow the axillary vein laterally, dividing any small vessels that cross over it and any venous tributaries that pass inferiorly. As the chest wall starts to curve down away from you, look for the long thoracic nerve just under the fascia. Identify it as a long straight nerve. Incise the fascia and confirm the identity of the nerve by gentle mechanical stimulation with a forceps or with an electrical nerve stimulator. Extend the incision of the overlying fascia inferiorly and gently push the nerve down against the chest wall and posterior axilla.

Continue dissecting laterally in the anterior adventitial plane of the axillary vein. Look for a large venous tributary, the thoracodorsal vein. Ligate and divide this vein. It is a landmark for the second important nerve in the region, the thoracodorsal nerve. The thoracodorsal artery and nerve pass about 1 cm deep to the plane of the axillary vein. The thoracodorsal nerve lies in close proximity to, and generally just deep to, the thoracodorsal artery. Confirm the identity of this nerve by gentle stimulation.

Sweep the axillary contents downward, keeping both nerves in view and preserving them. The thoracodorsal artery can be ligated, and the thoracodorsal nerve can be sacrificed, if necessary, if it is involved by tumor. The long thoracic nerve should be preserved, however, because significant functional and cosmetic liabilities accompany its sacrifice.

Remove the specimen by rapidly dividing the remaining attachments inferiorly.

Anatomic Points

A triangular surgical field, which almost corresponds to the anatomic axilla, is accessible when the pectoral muscles are retracted or divided. This surgical field is limited superolaterally by the axillary vein, inferolaterally by the latissimus dorsi muscle, medially by the serratus anterior muscle, and posteriorly by the subscapular, teres major, and latissimus dorsi muscles. The apex of this triangle is superomedial, deep to the clavicle. Here, the dominant feature of immediate concern is the axillary vein.

The long thoracic nerve is formed in the posterior triangle of the neck by anastomosis of the branches of brachial plexus roots C5 to C7. It enters the field deep to the vein and parallels the curvature of the thoracic wall, being on the axillary surface of the serratus anterior muscle. It descends into the axilla posterior to the brachial plexus, the first part of the axillary vessels, and all other neurovascular structures. It then continues its descent along the superficial (axillary) surface of the serratus anterior muscle, supplying each digitation of this muscle in its course. The long thoracic nerve can be

FIGURE 16.7
CLOSURE OF THE WOUND

located at the point where the axillary vein passes over the second rib. Injury of the nerve impairs the serratus anterior muscle, whose prime function is to protract the scapula, especially its inferior angle. Without rotation of the scapula, it is impossible to raise the arm above the level of the shoulder. In addition, the serratus muscle holds the vertebral border of the scapula to the trunk; therefore, loss of function of the serratus muscle results in "winging" of the scapula. Thus, injury to this nerve can be both disabling and disfiguring.

The thoracodorsal or middle subscapular nerve carries fibers from C6 to C8. It originates from the posterior cord of the brachial plexus posterior to the second part of the axillary vessels and accompanies the thoracodorsal branch of the subscapular artery along the posterior axillary wall to supply the latissimus dorsi muscle. The nerve lies on the subscapular and teres major muscles. Damage to this nerve that is sufficient to paralyze the latissimus dorsi muscle weakens adduction, inward rotation, and extension of the arm (as in a swimming stroke). It also hinders the ability to depress the scapula, a function that is important when using crutches to support the weight of the body.

Closure of the Wound (Fig. 16.7)

Technical and Anatomic Points

Achieve careful hemostasis and irrigate the field to remove debris and loose bits of fat. Use sterile water as the final irrigating solution to lyse any stray tumor cells.

Place closed-suction drains under upper and lower flaps. Excise redundant skin and "dog ears," but remember that extra skin may be an asset to the plastic surgeon if postmastectomy reconstruction is planned. Close the skin with multiple fine interrupted sutures, skin clips, or a subcuticular suture.

Classic Radical Mastectomy

Surgical Technique (Fig. 16.8)

Technical and Anatomic Points

Make the incision and raise flaps exactly as described previously. Because classic radical mastectomy is generally used for more advanced lesions, a larger amount of breast skin may need to be sacrificed. Prepare and drape a thigh in case a skin graft is needed.

Place retractors in the medial aspect of both flaps and shave the pectoralis major muscle off the chest wall from medial to lateral. Take care to identify and ligate the perforating branches of the internal thoracic (mammary) artery and vein, which at this point will be seen to emerge directly from the interspaces. Secure any vessels that "retract" into an interspace by suture-ligature. Take care not to poke the tips of a hemostat into the interspace because it is extremely easy to enter the chest inadvertently.

As the pectoralis major muscle is elevated from the chest wall, the pectoralis minor muscle will be encountered. It should likewise be shaved off. Divide the attachments of the

FIGURE 16.8
SURGICAL TECHNIQUE

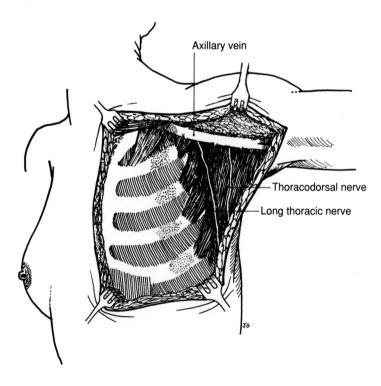

Axillary vein

Thoracodorsal nerve

Long thoracic nerve

pectoralis major muscle to the clavicle and the humerus superiorly and laterally. Divide the pectoralis minor muscle at its attachment to the coracoid process, as previously described. Allow the breast and the muscles to fall laterally.

Dissect the axillary vein, identifying nerves as previously described (Figs. 16.5 and 16.6). Closure of the wound at the conclusion of the operation is similar to that for modified mastectomy. If a large amount of skin has been removed and the flaps will not come together without excessive tension, close the medial and lateral portions of the incision partially, leaving an elliptical defect centrally. Change gown and gloves and use new instruments to harvest a split-thickness skin graft. Place the graft over the elliptical defect, suturing the graft to the flaps and anchoring both to the underlying chest wall. A tie-over stent is often useful. Generally, the graft will take well to the muscle of the chest wall. Certainly, a well-placed graft is preferable to closure of flaps under tension, with the attendant risk for subsequent flap necrosis.

REFERENCES

1. Bland KI, O'Neal B, Weiner LJ, et al. One-stage simple mastectomy with immediate reconstruction for high-risk patients. An improved technique: the biologic basis for ductal glandular mastectomy. *Arch Surg* 1986;121:221. (Provides a clear and concise description of a cosmetic yet biologically sound prophylactic mastectomy.)
2. Carlson GW, Bostwick J III, Styblo TM, et al. Skin-sparing mastectomy: oncologic and reconstructive considerations. *Ann Surg* 1997;225:570. (Provides an excellent description of an increasingly popular alternative, particularly for early lesions.)
3. Haagenson CD. *Diseases of the breast.* Philadelphia: WB Saunders, 1986. (Presents a clear description of classic radical mastectomy.)
4. Hidalgo DA. Aesthetic refinement in breast reconstruction: complete skin-sparing mastectomy with autogenous tissue transfer. *Plast Reconstr Surg* 1998;102:63.
5. Hoffman GW, Elliott LF. The anatomy of the pectoral nerves and its significance to the general and plastic surgeon. *Ann Surg* 1987;205:504. (Presents a brief review of relevant anatomy.)
6. Moosman DA. Anatomy of the pectoral nerves and their preservation in modified mastectomy. *Am J Surg* 1980;139:883. (Reviews the variant anatomy of pectoral nerves.)
7. Patey DH. A review of 146 cases of carcinoma of the breast operated on between 1930 and 1943. *Br J Cancer* 1967;21:260. (This is the original description of the Patey technique, with resection of the pectoralis minor muscle.)
8. Roses DF, Harris MN, Gumport SL. Total mastectomy with axillary dissection: a modified radical mastectomy. *Am J Surg* 1977;134:674. (Describes a modified technique involving division of the sternal head of the pectoralis major muscle for wide exposure of the apex of the axilla.)
9. Slavin AS, Schnitt SJ, Duda RB, et al. Skin-sparing mastectomy and immediate reconstruction: oncologic risks and aesthetic results in patients with early-stage breast cancer. *Plast Reconstr Surg* 1998;102:49.

CHAPTER 17

Axillary Node Biopsy and Axillary Node Dissection

Biopsy of a palpable enlarged axillary node is performed when other means, such as fine-needle aspiration cytology, have failed to yield a diagnosis. As in the neck and groin, axillary node biopsy contaminates the field and may make subsequent radical lymphadenectomy more difficult. It should, therefore, be performed only when necessary.

Axillary lymphadenectomy is most commonly performed in conjunction with mastectomy. Sentinel node biopsy (Chapter 18) may have preceded the procedure. Occasionally, however, the procedure is done alone, for example, for malignant melanoma. The surgical anatomy of the axilla is detailed in Figs. 16.4 to 16.6 in Chapter 16. This chapter discusses the technical modifications required when axillary node dissection is done alone.

The final section of this chapter describes a more limited axillary node sampling procedure that is performed for staging of breast carcinomas. The aim of this more limited procedure is to remove a sampling of group I and group II axillary nodes.

Axillary Node Biopsy (Fig. 17.1)

Technical Points

Position the patient supine with the ipsilateral arm extended out on an armboard. If necessary, place a small folded sheet under the shoulder to improve exposure.

LIST OF STRUCTURES

Lymph node groups
Anatomic
  Pectoral
    External mammary
    Interpectoral
  Scapular
  Central
  Axillary
  Subclavicular (apical)
Topographic
  Group I
  Group II
  Group III

Palpate the node and plan a transverse incision below the hair-bearing region of the axilla. Make the incision a bit low and raise a flap, if necessary, to avoid this area.

Infiltrate the area with local anesthetic and incise the skin. Raise flaps as necessary to expose the node. Place a traction suture through the node and excise it as described for cervical node biopsy.

Anatomic Points

The incision should be made as close as possible to the palpable node. For cosmetic reasons, here as elsewhere, Langer's lines should be followed. In the region of the axilla, these lines are approximately transverse. Corresponding to the relaxed skin tension lines of Kreissl, they are perpendicular to the line of action of underlying muscle fibers. Avoid the hair-bearing area of the axilla—not for cosmetic reasons, but rather to avoid the morbidity associated with its moist and bacteria-laden environment.

Discrete superficial and deep fascia is not encountered in the axilla. Instead, the axillary fascia (derived from the fascia of the pectoralis major, latissimus dorsi, and serratus anterior muscles as well as the fascia investing the muscles of the arm) is adherent to the superficial fascia and is, in the hollow of the armpit, along with the suspensory ligament of the axilla, a continuation of the clavipectoral fascia.

The axillary lymph nodes are predominantly located on the medial side of the axillary neurovascular bundle, although some lie on the medial axillary wall. For convenience, these are described by anatomists in five groups. Terms in parentheses indicate the approximate equivalent in Haagensen's system. The *lateral group* (axillary), on the third part of the axillary neurovascular bundle, drains the upper limb. The *subscapular* (scapular) or posterior group, located around the subscapular artery and vein, drains the shoulder and posterior thorax. The *pectoral* (external mammary) group, which is associated with the lateral thoracic vessels along the inferolateral border of the pectoralis major muscle, drains and receives lymph from the anterior thoracic wall, including the lateral breast. These three groups drain into the *central group* of (central) lymph nodes, which is located approximately on the second part of the axillary neurovascular bundle. The *apical group* (subclavian), associated with the first part of the axillary neurovascular bundle, receives lymphatics from the

FIGURE 17.1
AXILLARY NODE BIOPSY

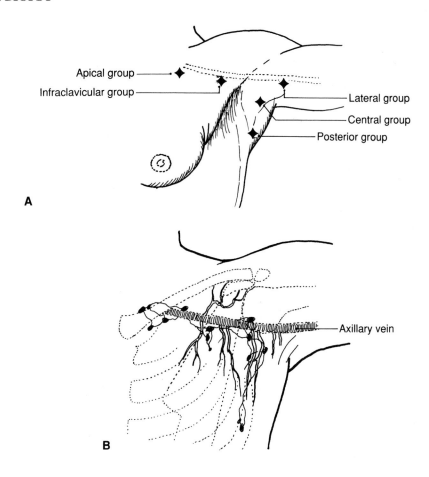

central group as well as from the upper outer quadrant of the mammary gland.

Surgeons commonly use a different terminology (topographic) for axillary lymph nodes. Topographic group I nodes include the pectoral, subscapular, and lateral nodes. Topographic group II nodes are central nodes, whereas topographic group III nodes are apical nodes.

Axillary Node Dissection

Choice of Incision and Elevation of Flaps (Fig. 17.2)

Technical Points

Position the patient as for modified radical mastectomy (see Fig. 16.1 in Chapter 16). An incision along the lateral border of the pectoralis major muscle provides excellent access to the axilla. Alternatively, a more cosmetically appealing transverse incision may be used. This transverse incision should be planned to lie below the hair-bearing portion of the axilla. Raise flaps to expose the subcutaneous tissues shown.

FIGURE 17.2
CHOICE OF INCISION AND ELEVATION OF FLAPS

FIGURE 17.3
EXPOSURE OF THE AXILLARY VEIN

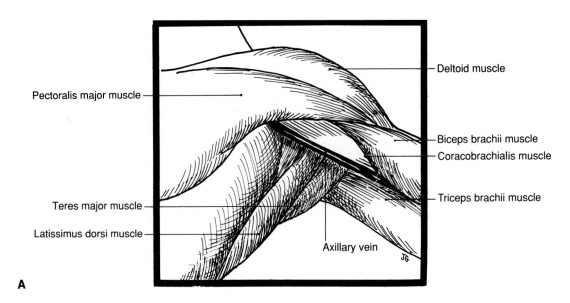

Pectoralis major muscle

Teres major muscle

Latissimus dorsi muscle

Deltoid muscle

Biceps brachii muscle

Coracobrachialis muscle

Triceps brachii muscle

Axillary vein

A

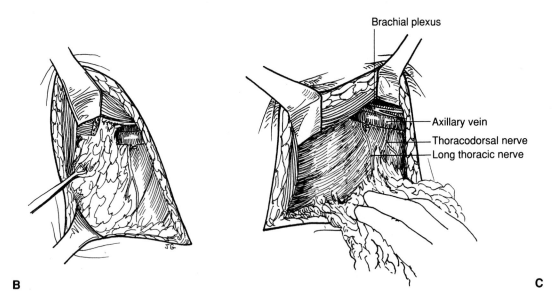

Brachial plexus

Axillary vein

Thoracodorsal nerve

Long thoracic nerve

B

C

Exposure of the Axillary Vein (Fig. 17.3)

Technical Points

Identify the lateral border of the pectoralis major muscle and clean the fatty tissue from the underside of the muscle. Take care to preserve the nerve to the pectoralis major muscle. Place a retractor under this muscle. Identify the pectoralis minor muscle and incise the clavipectoral fascia on each side of this muscle. Divide the pectoralis minor muscle to gain access to the axillary vein. If necessary, sacrifice the pectoralis minor muscle to improve access to the subclavian nodes, as described for modified radical mastectomy (see Fig. 16.4 in Chapter 16). Then remove the fatty node-bearing tissue of the axilla medially to laterally, cleaning the axillary vein and identifying the long thoracic and thoracodorsal nerves exactly as previously described.

The specimen consists of axillary contents and should be marked to assist the pathologist in orientation of node groups. By convention, group I nodes lie below the pectoralis minor muscle. Group II nodes lie deep to the pectoralis minor muscle, whereas group III nodes (the highest axillary nodes) lie medial to this muscle. Each node group may be tagged for identification. Alternatively, the corners of the usually triangular specimen may be marked medial, lateral, and inferior. Close communication with the pathologist will help to ensure the most accurate reporting of nodal involvement.

FIGURE 17.4
INCISION AND EXTENT OF DISSECTION

A

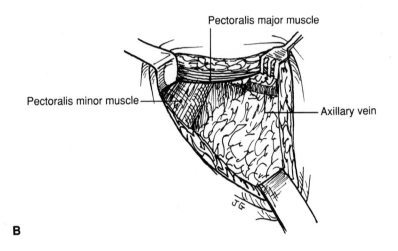

Pectoralis major muscle

Pectoralis minor muscle

Axillary vein

B

Recheck hemostasis and place two closed-suction drains under the flaps. Close the incision with fine interrupted skin sutures, with skin staples, or with a subcuticular suture.

Anatomic Points

Be aware that the innervation of the pectoralis major muscle is provided by the lateral and medial pectoral nerves. These nerves, named according to their origin on the lateral and medial cords of the brachial plexus (not on the basis of their relative location on the anterior thoracic wall), carry fibers of spinal cord levels C5 to C7 and C8 to T1, respectively. The lateral pectoral nerve crosses anterior to the first part of the axillary artery and vein (that segment which is proximal to the pectoralis minor muscle), there sending an anastomotic branch to join the medial pectoral nerve. The main ramus pierces the clavipectoral fascia with the thoracoacro-mial artery and is distributed to the pectoralis major and minor muscles along with the pectoral branches of this artery. The medial pectoral nerve arises from the medial cord somewhat more distally than the lateral pectoral nerve, that is, at the level of the second part of the axillary artery (that segment which is posterior to the pectoralis minor muscle). Typically, this nerve pierces the pectoralis minor muscle (providing innervation to the muscle); it then ramifies on the deep surface of the pectoralis major muscle. In addition, it usually gives off two or three branches that accompany the lateral pectoral artery along the inferior border of the pectoralis minor muscle and that ultimately are distributed to the pectoralis major muscle.

Clavipectoral fascia is that fascia which invests the pectoralis minor muscle. Inferior to the muscle, it is continuous with the serratus anterior fascia and with the so-called axillary fascia (primarily derived from the pectoralis major fascia), whereas superomedially, it blends with intercostal fascia, and superolaterally, it continues as a dense sheet, splitting to invest the subclavius muscle. When splitting this fascia, care should be taken not to damage either the thoracoacromial artery or the lateral pectoral nerve, both of which pierce the fascia superior to the pectoralis minor muscle.

Division of the pectoralis minor muscle allows exposure of all three parts of the axillary artery and vein. This improves access to the axillary lymph nodes (chiefly those of the central and apical group) located adjacent to the second and first part of these vessels, respectively. When removing the node-bearing axillary tissue, one should remember that the long thoracic nerve, formed in the posterior triangle of the neck by anastomosis of branches of brachial plexus roots C5 to C7, descends into the axilla posterior to the brachial plexus and the first part of the axillary vessels. It continues its descent along the superficial (axillary) surface of the serratus anterior muscle, supplying each digitation of this muscle in its course. Damage to this nerve that is sufficient to cause paralysis of the serratus anterior muscle is manifested by "winging" of the scapula and an inability to elevate the arm above the horizontal. Thus, care should be taken to avoid this nerve when removing lymph nodes or fascia from the serratus anterior muscle.

Likewise, surgeons should identify the thoracodorsal (middle subscapular) nerve, which carries fibers from C6 to C8. This nerve originates from the posterior cord of the brachial plexus posterior to the second part of the axillary vessels, accompanying the thoracodorsal branch of the subscapular artery along the posterior axillary wall to supply the latis-simus dorsi muscle. Damage to this nerve that is sufficient to result in paralysis of the latissimus dorsi muscle weakens adduction, inward rotation, and extension of the arm (as in a swimming stroke), and aids in depression of the scapula. The latter function is important in enabling one to support the weight of the body on crutches placed in the armpit. For this reason, the nerve should be saved if at all possible.

Axillary Node Sampling

Incision and Extent of Dissection (Fig. 17.4)

Technical and Anatomic Points

Make an incision similar to that shown in Fig. 17.2, but make it shorter. Raise flaps to expose the area indicated. Begin at the lateral border of the pectoralis major muscle to sweep fatty tissue laterally and out of the axilla. Place a retractor under the pectoralis major muscle to aid in exposure of the pectoralis minor muscle. The aim of the dissection is to remove a representative sampling of group I and group II axillary nodes. These nodes lie lateral to the breast up to, but not beyond, the medial border of the pectoralis minor muscle. Remove fatty tissue down to the level of the pectoralis minor muscle, but do not dissect under this muscle. Sweep the fatty node-bearing tissue laterally out of the axilla. Do not carry the dissection as far posteriorly as would be appropriate for a formal node dissection. Nerves are generally not formally identified; hence, the dissection must remain relatively superficial.

Check hemostasis and place a small closed-suction drain under the flaps. Close the incision with a subcuticular suture.

REFERENCES

1. Cox CE, Bass SS, Ku NN, et al. Sentinel lymphadenectomy: a safe answer to less axillary surgery? *Recent Results Cancer Res* 1998;152: 170.
2. Gumport SL, Lyall D, Zimany A. A radical axillary lymph node dissection for malignancy. *Arch Surg* 1961;83:227.
3. Harris MN, Gumport SL, Maiwandi H. Axillary lymph node dissection for melanoma. *Surg Gynecol Obstet* 1972;135:936. (Describes division of the sternal head of the greater pectoral muscle for wide exposure of the apex of the axilla; also discusses incontinuity wide excision of melanoma.)
4. Luini A, Zurrida G, Galimberti V, et al. Axillary dissection in breast cancer. *Crit Rev Oncol Hematol* 1999;30:63.
5. Margolese R, Poisson R, Shibata H, et al. The technique of seg-mental mastectomy (lumpectomy) and axillary dissection: a syllabus from the National Surgical Adjuvant Breast Project workshops. *Surgery* 1987;102:828. (Describes axillary dissection through a small, separate incision when done as part of breast conservation surgery.)
6. McNeil C. Endoscopy removal of axillary nodes gains ground abroad, toehold in US. *J Natl Cancer Inst* 1999;91:582. (Presents an alternative technique that is under development.)
7. Morrow M. Lumpectomy and axillary dissection. *Surg Rounds* 1991;753. (Describes axillary dissection for carcinoma of the breast.)
8. Roses DF, Harris MN, Ackerman AB. *Diagnosis and management of cutaneous malignant melanoma*. Philadelphia: WB Saunders, 1983:169. (Describes wide and deep excision with incontinuity axillary node dissection.)

CHAPTER 18

Sentinel Node Biopsy for Breast Cancer

Peter R. Jochimsen

Identification of involved lymph nodes in patients with breast cancer has several purposes. Lymph node involvement is the most important predictor of patient prognosis and may also be the most critical factor in deciding the need to treat with adjuvant chemotherapy or hormonal therapy. Removing involved lymph nodes may significantly reduce the subsequent development of axillary disease that is difficult to control even by surgical means. Finally, removal of the involved lymph nodes has the potential, in some finite percentage of patients, to remove the last vestige of disease.

Unfortunately, axillary lymphadenectomy also has detrimental consequences, which vary greatly in degree. Some patients will experience little or no morbidity, whereas others will be frustrated by persistent numbness of the axillary skin due to division of the intercostobrachial nerves. Other patients may suffer from swelling (edema) of the extremity, thought to be related to division of the lymphatic channels. The degree of edema may be minimal to massive. Persistence of this edema can lead to repeated and frequent bouts of cellulitis or other forms of infection. Eventually, especially in association with radiation to breast and axilla, secondary lymphangiosarcoma may appear.

Accurate staging of the axilla in a manner that avoids unnecessary surgery in those patients whose lymph nodes do not harbor tumor but that provides the needed surgery for those whose lymph nodes do have metastases has been long sought. Sentinel node biopsy attempts to provide this staging by identifying the node to which tumor will have spread first, the so-called sentinel node. If this node is negative, the remainder of the lymph nodes are presumed to be negative, and axillary dissection is omitted. If the sentinel node is positive, axillary lymphadenectomy is performed.

Several national and international trials are underway to prove unequivocally that sentinel node biopsy is without serious tradeoffs in terms of morbidity and mortality in the breast cancer population. In advance of these definitive proofs, the technique has been widely adopted by the surgical community.

Historically, this technique evolved after demonstration of its utility in cutaneous melanoma (Chapter 88). Initially, a dye, isosulfan blue (Lymphazurin Blue) was injected around the tumor, as used in melanoma patients. Subsequently, it was demonstrated that one could better identify the sentinel node using both dye and technetium-labeled sulfur colloid, and this has become the technique most commonly employed.

Some have recommended that the isotope be administered the day before surgery, others 2 to 4 hours before surgery. The number of nodes is time dependent, and some point out not only that lengthy delay increases the number of nodes identified but also that those nodes are not true sentinel nodes. The absolute answer to this question of timing has yet to be determined. Some controversy exists as to whether the colloid should be filtered or unfiltered; ideally, such patients should be entered into a trial and the detailed protocol of that trial followed. Whether the surgeon or nuclear medicine physician performs the injection is subject to local variation and must be similarly worked out. A uniformly acceptable protocol needs to be agreed on and followed.

The radioisotope injection is performed at least 3 to 4 hours before the surgical procedure, and a lymphoscintogram is obtained. Generally, 0.5 to 1.0 mCi of a technetium-labeled radiopharmaceutical is injected into the tissue surrounding the breast cancer mass or the biopsy cavity in a volume of 10 mL. To put this dose of radiation into perspective, this amounts to between $1/20$ and $1/40$ of the amount used in a standard bone scan.

Injection of Tracer and Dye (Fig. 18.1)

Technical Points

Sentinel node biopsy is done only in those patients in whom a breast carcinoma has been identified. If diagnosed by fine-needle aspiration cytology, the mass will still be present. If a previous open biopsy has been performed, a palpable mass will usually remain at the biopsy site.

Preoperative injection of isotope: Anesthetize the skin of the proposed injection sites. Inject 10 mL of diluted isotope (0.5 to 1.0 mCi) at four or five locations around the palpable

LIST OF STRUCTURES

Axillary lymph nodes
Axillary fascia
Breast

FIGURE 18.1
INJECTION OF TRACER AND DYE

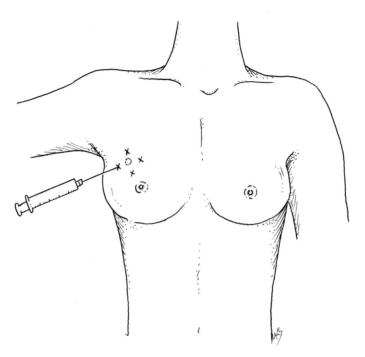

mass (tumor or biopsy cavity), in equal aliquots. Some suggest that a very small amount of this isotope can and should be injected subdermally directly over the lesion. If the lesion is nonpalpable, radiographic needle localization is used to guide injection in four quadrants around the identified mass. Take care to avoid getting isotope on the skin of the breast or anywhere else but in the peritumoral tissue. Obtain a lymphoscintogram $1^1/_2$ to 2 hours later.

Injection of blue dye: In the operating room, the patient is prepared for surgery and anesthetized. Inject isosulfan blue, 5 mL, in the four quadrants around the tumor and make an additional small (0.5 mL) subdermal injection over the tumor. A very small percentage of patients will have an adverse reaction to the dye, and it is imperative that the anesthesiologist be aware of that possibility. Gently massage the breast for 5 minutes, and prepare the skin of the breast and axilla in the usual way.

Use of the Gamma Probe (Fig. 18.2)

Technical and Anatomic Points

It is imperative that the surgeon be familiar with the use of the handheld gamma probe. Various devices are on the market. These differ somewhat in instrumentation and in the directionality of the probe itself. A unit that is very directional is best because it allows for precise localization.

Pass the probe gently over the skin of the axilla and identify the hottest area. A useful way to do this is with the detector on both the audio mode and the 1-second count mode. This allows both qualitative and quantitative evaluation. Once a "hot" area is discovered, advancing the detector into the soft

tissue should lead to an increased rate of emissions as the node comes closer to the detector head.

The very hot spot in the breast created by injection of the isotope may overshadow the node by its close proximity. Several maneuvers can be employed to separate the two foci. First, the lymphoscintogram may demonstrate the number and location of the nodes in relation to the point of injection. Retracting the breast away from the axilla by pulling it down and medially may facilitate identification of the node using the detector. Finally, varying the angle at which the probe approaches the axilla and using a highly directional probe may assist in identifying the node.

Identification and Removal of the Sentinel Node (Fig. 18.3)

Technical and Anatomic Points

Mark the skin over the hot spot and make an incision in a natural skin line over the node. Obtain careful hemostasis in this incision.

Divide the axillary fascia with cutting cautery and dissect with the palpating finger in the loose areolar tissue. Place retractors and seek a blue lymphatic channel or lymph node. If none is seen, use the detector to localize the most active area. Visualize the node and transfix it with a suture or hold it with a clamp. Excise it using cautery or ligating clips. After removing the hottest area, seek other areas with the gamma probe. Remove these additional areas if the count is at least 10% of the count of the hottest node.

After removal, the detector in the axilla should generally be quiet, with few emissions identified. If enlarged nodes are encountered, remove these even if not hot or "blue."

FIGURE 18.2
USE OF THE GAMMA PROBE

FIGURE 18.3
**IDENTIFICATION AND REMOVAL OF THE
SENTINEL NODE**

Send the tissue to pathology for touch-prep analysis. In about 20% of patients with truly positive nodes, the touch-prep will be negative, and completion axillary dissection will need to be performed in a second procedure. Frozen-section evaluation of the lymph nodes is not done unless the pathologist believes it to be appropriate.

Close the wound in layers with subcutaneous absorbable sutures and the skin with either a subcuticular absorbable suture or a running nylon stitch. No drain is required.

Attention is then turned to the breast; the tumor is removed by mastectomy or wide local excision, if not previously performed at the time of excisional biopsy.

If the sentinel node is found to harbor metastatic disease, completion axillary dissection (Chapter 17) is always recommended.

Technique using blue dye alone: If sentinel node biopsy is done with dye alone, it is recommended that injection be performed as described previously. This may be done within minutes of the search for the node. Be aware that it will take longer for the dye to reach the axilla if the tumor is in a more distant location (e.g., the lower inner quadrant).

Make a transverse incision just below the hair-bearing axillary skin. Perform blunt dissection until the blue stain is identified either in a node or a lymphatic channel. Follow the channel toward the point of injection to be certain that no more proximal node is identified, and then away from the breast until a blue node is identified.

The remainder of the operation proceeds as noted previously.

REFERENCES

1. Borgstein PJ, Pijpers R, Comans EF, et al. Sentinel lymph node biopsy in breast cancer: guidelines and pitfalls of lymphoscintigraphy and gamma probe detection. *J Am Coll Surg* 1998;186:275–283.
2. Guiliano AE, Kirgan DM, Guenther JM, et al. Lymphatic mapping and sentinel lymphadenectomy for breast cancer. *Ann Surg* 1994;220:391–401.
3. Veronesi U, Paganelli G, Galimberti V, et al. Sentinel node biopsy to avoid axillary dissection in breast cancer with clinically negative lymph nodes. *Lancet* 1997;349:1864–1867.

MEDIASTINAL STRUCTURES AND THE MEDIAN STERNOTOMY APPROACH

The mediastinum is the "thoracic space" between the two pleural sacs, the root word originally meaning septum. The mediastinum extends from the thoracic inlet cephalad to the superior surface of the diaphragm. The undersurface of the mediastinum is bounded posteriorly by the anterior longitudinal spinal ligament (dorsal) and the posterior mantel of the sternum anteriorly (ventral). Although lesions of the paravertebral region (costovertebral sulci) are traditionally classified as mediastinal in nature, this area is not formally within the mediastinum.

Multiple surgical and radiologic subdivisions within the mediastinum have been described in the literature. Most commonly, the mediastinum has been divided either into four compartments (superior, anterior, middle, and posterior) or three compartments (anterosuperior, middle or visceral, and posterior).

For the purpose of the following chapters, we have chosen a commonly used classification as laid out by Hardy in 1983. His three-compartment model, defined previously, is the one most commonly used among thoracic surgeons.

The anterior mediastinum can be defined as the area bounded by the thoracic inlet superiorly, the sternum anteriorly, and the pericardium and vertebral column inferiorly (see Orientation figure). Each compartment extends to the diaphragm inferiorly and is bounded laterally by the mediastinal surface of the respective parietal pleura.

Within the subdivisions of the mediastinum are numerous structures that are of frequent surgical interest. The anterosuperior compartment contains multiple lymph node stations and the thymus. Additionally, it can be the site of displaced parathyroid tissue, ectopic thyroid tissue, and other benign and malignant tumors.

The regional lymph nodes can give rise to primary tumors or pathologic processes or, more commonly, can be regionally (or systemically) involved with malignant lesions. Additional structures within this compartment include the trachea, great vessels, and their proximal tributaries. The middle, or visceral, compartment contains the heart, proximal great vessels, proximal pulmonary arteries and veins, lymph nodes, and the pericardium. The posterior mediastinum contains the azygos and hemiazygos veins, sympathetic trunks, esophagus, thoracic duct, lymph nodes, and the descending aorta.

In this chapter, the anatomy of the mediastinum is explored through a series of operative procedures. Cervical mediastinoscopy, anterior mediastinoscopy, and mediastinotomy (Chamberlain's procedure) (Chapter 19) are diagnostic maneuvers used to gain access to mediastinal lymph nodes.

Median sternotomy (Chapter 20) provides wide access to the anterior mediastinum and heart. It is used for major cardiac surgery, some pulmonary surgery, exposure of the thymus gland, great vessel and proximal upper vascular exposure, and occasionally, improved hepatic exposure. The posterior mediastinum is most easily approached laterally, through

ORIENTATION

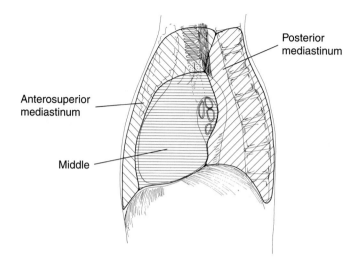

a thoracotomy incision, because the heart, lungs, and great vessels form a barrier limiting adequate access from the front.

The esophagus is a mediastinal structure. However, because of its posterior location, it is approached either through a thoracotomy incision or through combined cervical and abdominal approaches. Hence, the thoracic esophagus can be included in the next part (The Lungs and Structures Approached Through a Thoracotomy Incision).

CHAPTER 19

Mediastinoscopy and Mediastinotomy

Phillip C. Camp and M. Victoria Gerken

The surgeon is frequently called on to evaluate mediastinal lymph nodes. This may be done for diagnosis of an isolated mediastinal mass or significant mediastinal adenopathy. Examples include cases of sarcoidosis (more than 90% of which will show noncaseating granulomas within the hilar or scalene lymph nodes) or with lymphoma (isolated mediastinal disease is more commonly Hodgkin's). With helical scanning and robust increases in computing power, computed tomography (CT) of the chest permits good visualization of these nodes and related thoracic structures. However, the precision of CT with lesions and nodes smaller than 1 cm drops off. Multiple modalities are being investigated to interrogate the mediastinum and thorax noninvasively. These include positron-emission tomography (PET) scanning, magnetic resonance imaging (MRI), octreatide-based imaging, and antibody-based imaging. Individually and in combination, these scans have increased the ability to screen the mediastinum, but no noninvasive test has matched the sensitivity and specificity of lymph node sampling. Many thoracic surgeons routinely use cervical (and anterior where indicated) mediastinoscopy as an initial invasive diagnostic procedure. It is our practice to use mediastinoscopy routinely as a staging intervention in the workup of thoracic malignancies. Lymph nodes from zones II, IV, and VII, as well as from zone V, can be safely sampled using mediastinoscopy.

Mediastinoscopy

Mediastinoscopy is performed to evaluate pretracheal and paratracheal lymphadenopathy. It involves the creation of a tunnel or a space just anterior to the trachea and posterior to the aortic arch. As such, it does not provide access to the retrosternal space, the subcarinal space, or the left hilum.

The procedure is performed under general anesthesia. In special circumstances, local anesthesia may be used; however, this will significantly increase the difficulty and risk of the operation.

Skin Incision and Exposure of the Pretracheal Fascia (Fig. 19.1)

Technical Points

Good head position allows adequate exposure. The neck should be in full extension with the shoulders elevated. The entire neck and chest should be prepared into the surgical field should a more extensive exposure be quickly required. As with any neck scar, asymmetry leads to an unaesthetic result, and marking the intended site often results in a more pleasing closure. Make the skin incision about two finger-breadths cephalad to the suprasternal notch. The incision need only be 2 to 3 cm long, enough to accommodate the mediastinoscope, extending only to the anterior borders of

LIST OF STRUCTURES

Trachea	Aorta	Pleura
Pretracheal fascia	Brachiocephalic (innominate) artery	Left recurrent laryngeal nerve
Carina	Left common carotid artery	Right recurrent laryngeal nerve
Thyroid	Left subclavian artery	Esophagus
Sternum	Superior vena cava	Paratracheal lymph nodes
Manubrium	Azygos vein	Tracheobronchial lymph nodes
Clavicle	Anterior jugular vein	Scalene nodes
Sternoclavicular joint	Inferior thyroid vein	Perichondrium
Sternocleidomastoid muscle	Thymus	Periosteum
Right pulmonary artery	Brachiocephalic (innominate) vein	Internal thoracic (mammary) artery

FIGURE 19.1
SKIN INCISION AND EXPOSURE OF THE PRETRACHEAL FASCIA

the sternocleidomastoid muscle. Carry the incision down by electrocautery through the subcutaneous tissue to the level of the strap muscles. Sizable veins (anterior jugular veins) can run in this tissue and may require formal ligation with silk ties. Identify the midline as a fine, pale-yellow line. Incise this connective tissue with electrocautery or Metzenbaum scissors superiorly and inferiorly, and retract the strap muscles vertically. Divide the connective tissue of the midline by sharp dissection or electrocautery until the trachea is encountered. Incise the pretracheal fascia to allow access to the correct tissue plane, just anterior to the trachea itself.

Anatomic Points

When making the incision, the trachea will be exposed at about the same location as in tracheostomy, caudal to the thyroid. The inferior thyroid vein can often pass cephalad in the midline and requires careful mobilization and lateral retraction.

As the surgeon's finger passes under the manubrium, the back of the aortic arch is palpated just as it gives off the brachiocephalic (innominate) artery. Place a pulse oximeter on a finger of the patient's right hand to monitor compression of this artery during the procedure.

Development of the Mediastinal Tunnel and Passage of the Mediastinoscope (Fig. 19.2)

Technical Points

Moisten your index finger with saline and carefully introduce it into the superior mediastinum, staying directly on the cartilage rings of the anterior trachea. Take care to keep the dorsal aspect of the finger (fingernail) against the trachea as a guide against dissection into the wrong plane. As the tip of your finger passes under the manubrium, palpate laterally. Enlarged deep scalene nodes will be palpable in this region, even if they were not appreciated on physical examination. Continue blunt dissection downward very gently, staying on the *anterior* aspect of the trachea and introducing your finger as far as it will reach. When the finger is fully introduced, the pulsations of the aortic arch (anterior to the left main bronchus) and brachiocephalic (innominate) artery takeoff (anterior and to the right of the midtrachea) are easily appreciated on the volar aspect of the finger. Careful palpation may identify lesions but is *rarely* very accurate in predicting the yield with the mediastinoscope. Occasionally, an enlarged node will adhere to the dorsum of the aortic arch; careful palpation can help to determine whether biopsy of the node can be accomplished safely. Continued gentle blunt dissection with the finger should be undertaken to widen the channel to either side of the trachea. Never force areas of dense adhesion or induration because this can result in significant vascular injury and major bleeding.

Withdraw your finger and introduce the saline-moistened mediastinoscope with the light source connected. Dim the overhead lights in the operating room because the glare may hamper visualization through the scope. Pass the scope only through that tunnel which has already been created by your digit. It should pass easily. Allow the tip of your scope to glide along the surface of the trachea. Difficulty passing the scope should lead to scope removal and additional blunt digital dissection.

FIGURE 19.2
DEVELOPMENT OF THE MEDIASTINAL TUNNEL AND PASSAGE OF THE MEDIASTINOSCOPE

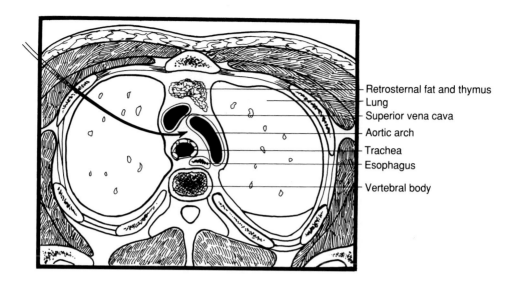

- Retrosternal fat and thymus
- Lung
- Superior vena cava
- Aortic arch
- Trachea
- Esophagus
- Vertebral body

Anatomic Points

It is of paramount importance to remember the anatomic relationships of the trachea. Anteriorly, between the trachea and manubrium, are thymic remnants, the left brachiocephalic (innominate) vein, the aorta with two of its branches (brachiocephalic or innominate artery and left common carotid artery), and the deep cardiac plexus. Posteriorly and somewhat to the left is the esophagus. To the right are the mediastinal pleura, right vagus nerve, brachiocephalic (innominate) artery, right brachiocephalic vein, arch of the azygos vein, and the superior vena cava. To the left are the mediastinal pleura, the left recurrent laryngeal nerve, the arch of the aorta, and the left common carotid and subclavian arteries. Paratracheal lymph nodes are found on either side of the trachea, and tracheobronchial lymph nodes are located caudal to the bifurcation of the trachea. A good three-dimensional awareness of the anatomy will avoid injury and improve lymph node recovery.

Identification of Structures and Biopsy of Nodes (Fig. 19.3)

Technical Points

Keep the field dry with the long blunt metal (Jackson) suction tip and use it for minor blunt dissection around the lymph nodes. It is imperative to clean the lymph node adequately with the suction tip and then to identify the anatomic structures. This is critical because the dark-blue color of veins can mimic the anthracotic color of lymph nodes under the light limitations of the mediastinoscope. A combination of digital "palpation," gentle blunt dissection with the suction tip, and careful anatomic identification will help to determine which structures lend themselves to safe biopsy. Several authors suggest routine aspiration of structures before biopsy. We do not use aspiration unless the anatomy is unclear and

the patient has had no resultant bleeding complications. The biopsy forceps used should be fairly sharp so that they easily bite into the node. The lymph node should be dissected well enough that the jaw of the biopsy forceps easily engages the tissue. Blind biopsies are fraught with peril and should not be attempted. Tugging with dull forceps in an attempt to tear off part of the nodes can be disastrous because an inflammatory process may have resulted in dense adhesions of the node to major vessels deep in the mediastinum. Usually, the first one or two bites of the forceps simply clear away the node capsule. Patiently continue with safe, small bites of clearly identified nodal tissue, and you will eventually accomplish your goal.

The superior tracheobronchial (level IV), paratracheal (level II), and the inferior tracheobronchial (subcarinal, level VII) lymph nodes are accessible by this technique. The right paratracheal lymph nodes are proximal to the azygos vein and are located outside the investing paratracheal fascia. The mediastinal pleura lies just lateral to this lymph node station and should be preserved to avoid pneumothorax. Superior tracheobronchial nodes are at and along the tracheobronchial angle and are slightly distal to the azygos vein. Careful dissection with the sucker tip to protect the azygos vein (right) and recurrent laryngeal nerve (left) is indicated.

The inferior tracheobronchial (subcarinal) nodes require passing between the trachea (inferior) and the right main pulmonary artery (superior). This dissection requires patience and careful tissue manipulation to avoid bleeding.

Hemostatic packing material (such as Gelfoam or Surgicel) should be available during these procedures for local, persistent hemorrhage.

In this procedure, especially, better is the enemy of good. Your aim is merely to perform a biopsy, not to resect the nodes. Once adequate biopsy specimens have been obtained,

FIGURE 19.3
IDENTIFICATION OF STRUCTURES AND BIOPSY OF NODES

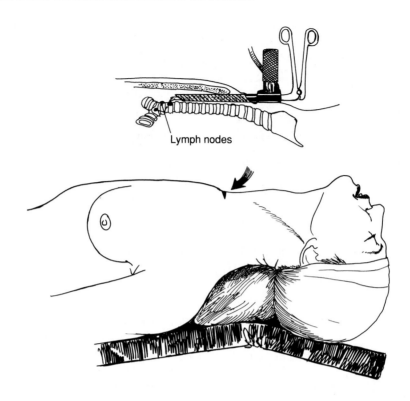

Lymph nodes

the temptation to keep "nibbling away" on the node should be resisted because no further information will be obtained, and the risk of the procedure will be substantially increased. Likewise, if a node cannot be exposed satisfactorily to allow safe biopsy, it is better not to obtain a biopsy specimen than to proceed with an unanticipated emergent median sternotomy.

At the completion of this procedure, gently irrigate the biopsy site with saline. Unexpected air bubbles in the saline or disappearance of the irrigant into the wound is predictive of an unrecognized pleural injury. Hemostasis can be achieved with electrocautery if the suction device is so equipped; alternatively, it can be accomplished by packing the area as noted previously.

Close the cervical incision in layers, approximating the strap muscles in the midline. Reapproximate the platysma or subcutaneous tissue with interrupted stitches. A running subcuticular closure with an absorbable stitch yields a cosmetically acceptable scar. Obtain a postoperative chest radiograph to exclude the rare complication of pneumothorax.

Anatomic Points

There are several blood vessels within the reach of the biopsy forceps. As a result, the brachiocephalic (innominate) artery, pulmonary artery, azygos vein, and aortic arch have all yielded biopsy specimens in the past, with inevitably disastrous results. However, if the surgeon carefully dissects and identifies the target node before reaching for the biopsy forceps, lymph node biopsy in this area can be both rewarding and safe.

The pleura lies lateral to the operative field, and anthracotic lung behind the pleura can look like a lymph node. Again, cleaning the supposed node off with the suction tip will reveal its true identity.

Anterior Mediastinoscopy and Mediastinotomy (Chamberlain's Procedure)

There are several clinical situations that cannot be answered by a cervical mediastinoscopic approach. Suspicious nodes or lesions of lymph node stations V and VI and staging of lymph nodes for left upper lobe lesions require an anterior approach to the mediastinum from the left side. We presently use this approach routinely for staging purposes.

Although the traditional anterior approach is through a mediastinotomy, requiring a large incision and resection of costal cartilage, adequate lymph node sampling can generally be obtained by inserting a mediastinoscope into the second intercostal space after blunt digital dissection. This less invasive approach can be extended to a formal mediastinotomy (Chamberlain's procedure) if additional exposure is required.

Mediastinotomy (Chamberlain's Procedure) (Fig. 19.4)

Technical Points

The incision should provide adequate exposure to the second intercostal space and the third rib. The angle of Louis is a good

FIGURE 19.4
MEDIASTINOTOMY (CHAMBERLAIN'S PROCEDURE)

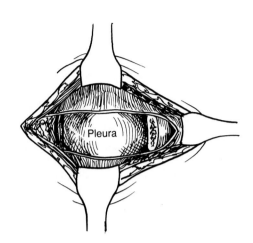

landmark. The placement of a scope requires a very small incision, enough to accommodate a mediastinoscope, your finger, or both. A mediastinotomy, essentially a mini anterior thoracotomy, consists of an extension of the scope site for access to structures inaccessible to the mediastinoscope.

Examine the chest films carefully to determine which costal cartilage should be resected to yield the most information. The second, third, and fourth costal cartilages on the right and the second and third on the left are all amenable to Chamberlain's procedure.

The patient is first anesthetized and intubated. The anterior chest is then prepared widely enough to permit chest tube insertion, if indicated. (This procedure often follows a cervical mediastinoscopy.) Incise the skin over the third costal cartilage, extending the incision from the edge of the sternum for a distance of 3 to 4 cm. Carry the incision down by means of electrocautery through the subcutaneous tissue and through the pectoralis major muscle to expose the superior aspect of the costal cartilage. Score the fascia and divide the intercostal muscles along the superior surface of the cartilage with cautery, taking care to stay medial to the internal mammary artery (IMA). The IMA is generally preserved with a scope approach. Digital blunt dissection allows lateral mobilization of the mediastinal pleura. The finger then sweeps along the inferior aspect of the arch, ultimately dissecting between the ascending aorta and arch and the pulmonary artery. Often, the nodes can be palpated if firm or enlarged. The mediastinoscope is gently inserted in a 10- to 11-o'clock position. Gentle dissection using a long blunt metal (Jackson) suction tip along the aorta and pulmonary artery allows identification of lymph nodes. As with cervical mediastinoscopy, careful dissection and identification of lymph nodes allows for safe biopsy.

Our experience has demonstrated high success with this approach, with no recent need to convert to a formal Chamberlain's procedure. If needed, score the perichondrium along the anterior surface of the cartilage with cautery, carrying it back onto the bony rib. Elevate the perichondrium and periosteum off the cartilaginous and bony rib with a periosteal elevator. Then transect it laterally at an appropriate site and disarticulate it medially. Open the posterior perichondrium with a scalpel to reveal the pleura. Identify and divide the internal thoracic (mammary) vessels between silk ligatures. Gently tease the pleura off the mediastinum with a "peanut" dissector.

Place a Tuffier retractor ("pediatric rib spreader") into the opening and widen it to its limits. Place a narrow Deaver retractor laterally to hold the pleural contents out of harm's way. Explore the anterior mediastinum and hilum by gentle blunt dissection. Biopsy or resection of the nodes in this area can be accomplished at this time. Occasionally, it may be necessary to enter the pleural space to allow further access to the hilum. Generally, exposure is quite good, but occasionally, a tumor may encase the hilum, preventing safe biopsy as a result of the limited exposure. An experienced surgeon may not need to obtain tissue to confirm a clinical impression of unresectability, but tissue for diagnosis and staging and for the oncologist is generally advantageous.

At the completion of the procedure, withdraw the retractors. If the pleura was opened, place a medium-sized, red rubber catheter (about 16 French) into the pleural space. Close the perichondrium with a running absorbable stitch, bringing the red rubber catheter out at one end. Close the pectoral fascia in similar fashion. Place a stitch around the site where the red rubber tube exits, but do not tie it down yet. Connect the tube to wall suction. While the anesthesiologist slightly hyperinflates the lung, quickly withdraw the tube and tie the last suture securely down. In this way, any pneumothorax that may be present is evacuated without the morbidity of an indwelling chest tube. Obtain a chest radiograph in the recovery room to confirm the absence of pneumothorax. If purulent material is encountered during the biopsy, or if a pleural effusion was already present, an indwelling chest tube can easily be placed at the time of the biopsy.

The mediastinoscopy approach does not require any deep tissue approximation.

The subcutaneous tissue and the skin are reapproximated according to the preference of the surgeon.

Anatomic Points

A posteroanterior chest film is helpful in planning the operative site. Tracing the ribs anteriorly will allow you to predict fairly accurately the exposure gained by resection of that cartilage. Resection of the second costal cartilage will expose the superior hilar structures, whereas resection of the third costal cartilage will expose the middle to lower hilum. Resection of the fourth cartilage on the left generally places you directly over the ventricular surface of the heart, with poor exposure to the hilum.

On the right, the inferior vena cava can be easily identified medial to the wound. The pulmonary artery can likewise be identified at the depths of the operative field. The mediastinum is entered by removing a segment of rib and costal cartilage. By going through the bed of the rib (within the superior and inferior boundaries of the perichondrium and periosteum), the intercostal neurovascular bundles, which are present both above and below a rib (the inferior bundles are the larger), are avoided. However, it is important to remember that the internal thoracic (mammary) artery, from which the anterior intercostal arteries of the upper spaces arise, lies approximately 1 to 1.5 cm lateral to the sternum, and is just deep to the perichondrium.

REFERENCES

1. Carlens E. Mediastinoscopy: a method for inspection and tissue biopsy in the superior mediastinum. *Dis Chest* 1959;36:343. (This is the original description of mediastinoscopy.)
2. Foster ED, Munro DD, Dobell ARC. Mediastinoscopy: a review of anatomical relationships and complications. *Ann Thorac Surg* 1972;13:273. (Presents good discussion of potential pitfalls.)
3. Hardy JD, Ewing HP. The mediastinum. In Glenn WWL, ed. *Thoracic and cardiovascular surgery.* 4th ed. Norwalk, CT: Appleton-Century-Crofts, 1983.
4. Lewis RJ, Sisler GE, Mackenzie JW. Repeat mediastinoscopy. *Ann Thorac Surg* 1984;37:147. (Describes technique of reoperation.)
5. McNeill TM, Chamberlain JM. Diagnostic anterior mediastinotomy. *Ann Thorac Surg* 1966;2:532. (This is the original description of the technique that now bears Chamberlain's name.)
6. Paneth M, Goldstraw P, Hyams B. Mediastinoscopy. In: *Fundamental techniques in pulmonary and oesophageal surgery.* New York: Springer-Verlag, 1987:2.
7. Shields TW. Primary tumors and cysts of the mediastinum. In Sheild TW, ed. *General thoracic surgery.* Philadelphia: Lea & Febiger, 1972.

CHAPTER 20

Median Sternotomy and Thymectomy

M. Victoria Gerken and Phillip C. Camp

Median Sternotomy

The median sternotomy allows rapid, excellent exposure to the anterior or middle mediastinum and is ideal for cardiac, thymic, and bilateral pleural procedures. Bilateral pulmonary resections, such as bullae or metastases, can be performed; however, it can be difficult to perform a formal lobectomy through this incision. Sternotomy, including partial or upper sternotomy, can allow for thymectomy and provides access to the trachea to the level of the carina. As an extension of a cervical incision, a partial or complete sternotomy can provide adequate exposure for resection of an enlarged substernal goiter. Only limited exposure of the posterior mediastinum (esophagus and descending aorta) is obtained. The sternum is generally stable on closure, and dehiscence of this incision occurs only rarely. It also offers the distinct advantage of being less painful than the standard posterolateral thoracotomy and is very well tolerated in all age groups. Respiratory status is only minimally impaired after this approach.

Incision (Fig. 20.1)

Technical Points

Mark the midline of the skin before incising, ensuring that the skin incision is in the midline. Extend it from the sternal notch to a point roughly 1 to 2 cm below the tip of the xiphoid. Using electrocautery, divide the connective tissue until the sternum is reached. Occasionally, there is a thin layer of decussating pectoral muscle in the midline over the sternum. Divide this and score the external periosteum of the sternum with electrocautery. Carefully palpate the lateral edges of the sternum with the thumb and index finger of your nondominant hand so that the incision can be kept directly in the midline. At the angle of Louis (sternomanubrial junction), use a snap or forceps to identify the lateral margins of the sternum. This is advised because the pectoralis muscles do not universally delineate the center of the sternum. Straying off the midline will later cause the sternal retractor to "kick up" on the thinner side and can adversely affect healing of the sternal bone.

Score the periosteum caudally to the tip of the xiphoid. Divide the abdominal fascia in the midline for a short distance, taking care not to enter the peritoneum. Superiorly, score the periosteum to the sternal notch and carefully feel for a tough ligamentous structure on the posterior aspect of the notch. Divide this ligament with great care using cautery. (The electric sternal saw frequently will jam or bog down on tissue of this type.) Introduce your index fingers under the sternum from both the sternal notch and the xiphoid. Gentle dissection here will facilitate detachment of the underlying structures from the back of the sternum before the sternum is divided. Ask the anesthesiologist to deflate the lungs fully to allow the pleura to fall posteriorly as much as possible. Bisect the sternum with the sternal saw starting from either end. Pull gently up and forward with the saw during this maneuver, again to reduce the risk for injury to underlying structures. Obtain hemostasis by cauterizing the periosteum along the lower edge of the sternum. Because the soft tissue will slightly retract after sternal division, be sure to cauterize several millimeters back along the undersurface of the cut sternum. The divided edge of the sternum often oozes from the marrow. Application of a paste containing thrombin, Gelfoam, or a similar material will promote hemostasis and keep your field clean.

Place folded green towels along the divided edges of the sternum and insert the sternal retractor. When you place the sternal spreader, remember that the more cephalad the

LIST OF STRUCTURES

Sternum	Interclavicular ligament	Left and right brachiocephalic
Gladiolus (body)	Sternocleidomastoid muscle	(innominate) veins
Manubrium	Pectoralis major muscle	Internal thoracic (mammary) arteries
Xiphoid process	Aponeuroses of internal and external	Pericardium
Angle of Louis	oblique muscles	Pleura
	Brachiocephalic (innominate) artery	Thymus

FIGURE 20.1
INCISION

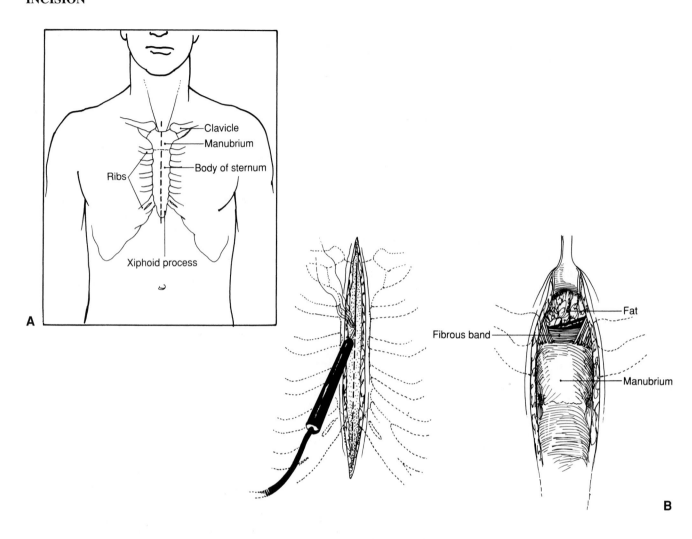

A

B

Clavicle
Manubrium
Body of sternum
Ribs
Xiphoid process

Fibrous band
Fat
Manubrium

retractor is placed, the greater the risk for injury to the bra-chial plexus. In the situation of a tight or limited exposure, modest additional division of the midline abdominal fascia (extraperitoneal) may be beneficial.

Anatomic Points

A median sternotomy incision exactly in the midline should not sever any muscle fibers anterior to the sternum. Should the incision stray from the midline, however, it is possible to divide some fibers of the sternocleidomastoid muscle (orig-inating from the manubrium), the pectoralis major muscle (originating from the manubrium and body), and the aponeu-roses (linea alba) of the internal and external oblique mus-cles (attached to the xiphoid process). A true midline divi-sion of the sternum likewise should not involve any muscle fibers attached to the deep surface of the sternum. However, slightly lateral to the midline, the sternohyoid and sternothy-roid muscles originate from the manubrium, and the slips of the transversus thoracis originate from the body. Frequently,

slips of the diaphragm originate from the sides of the xiphoid process.

More significant than the muscles attached to the sternum is the relationship of the sternum to mediastinal structures. From cranial to caudal, the following structures could be encountered in the midline: (a) interclavicular ligament; (b) brachiocephalic (innominate) artery, sometimes just deep to the inferior thyroid vein (and thyroidea ima artery, if present); (c) left brachiocephalic (innominate) vein; (d) thy-mus; (e) right pleural sac and lung; (f) pericardial sac and as-cending aorta; (g) right atrium and ventricle; (h) diaphragm; and (i) peritoneal cavity and left lobe of the liver. The left margin of the sternum is related, cranial to caudal, to (a) the left lobe of the thyroid gland, (b) the left brachiocephalic vein overlying the left common carotid artery, (c) the thymus overlying the pericardium and ascending aorta, (d) the left pleural sac and lung, (e) the pericardial sac overlying the left and right ventricles, (f) the diaphragm, and (g) the peritoneal cavity and left lobe of the liver. From cranial to caudal, the right sternal margin is related to (a) the right lobe of the

FIGURE 20.2
STERNOTOMY CLOSURE

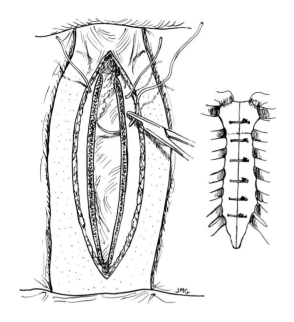

thyroid, (b) the thymus, (c) the right brachiocephalic (innominate) vein, (d) the right pleural sac and lung overlying the superior vena cava, (e) the right pleural sac and lung overlying the pericardial sac and right atrium, (f) the diaphragm, and (g) the falciform ligament, peritoneal cavity, and left lobe of the liver.

Sternotomy Closure (Fig. 20.2)

Technical Points

At the completion of the procedure, place one or two chest tubes into the anterior mediastinum. Chest tubes should leave the mediastinum deep to the midline fascia, then tunnel through the fascia, bringing them out slightly lateral to the midline. Place the tip of each tube low enough so that it will not press on the brachiocephalic (innominate) vein when the sternum is reapproximated.

Close the sternotomy with number 5 stainless steel wire. Although wires must pierce through manubrial bone, for best results, place the wires around the sternum, rather than through it, because the latter would reduce the stability of the closure. The advantage of this is the strength of the cortical bone, promoting better stability and lower risk for sternal dehiscence. Care, however, should be taken to hug the sternal bone so as not to endanger the internal thoracic (mammary) vessels. Place two wires through the manubrium and five figure-of-eight wires around the body of the sternum. The uppermost figure-of-eight should cross over the sternomanubrial junction or joint. Tighten the wires and trim them to an appropriate length. Bury the tips in the soft tissue. Many surgeons choose to use only simple sternal wires (three manubrial, five sternal). However, we believe that the figure-

of-eight technique substantially reduces the risk for sternal dehiscence.

Abdominal fascia should be reapproximated with figure-of-eight heavy absorbable suture up through the level of the xiphoid. Approximate the edges of the pectoral fascia over the turned-in wires using a heavy absorbable suture. Carry this stitch down to reapproximate the linea alba in the midline. Reapproximate the subcutaneous tissue and skin edges.

Anatomic Points

The brachiocephalic (innominate) vein lies deep to the strap muscles directly underlying the manubrium. The pericardium lies behind the gladiolus, or body of the sternum. It is uncommon to injure either one of these structures unless the median sternotomy is a reoperation, in which case injury to either is quite possible. This approach should never be used for a redo sternal incision.

The pleura can be injured upon either opening or closing, but such injuries seldom cause much of a problem. If a small hole is made in either pleural sac, it is advantageous to open it widely so that any air can be evacuated through the anterior mediastinal chest tubes. The tip of the mediastinal tubes can be deviated into the open pleural space to prevent pneumothorax.

The brachiocephalic (innominate) and left common carotid arteries run just lateral to the manubrium and can be injured during closing if the surgeon chooses to place the wires around the manubrium, rather than through it.

The relationship of the sternum to mediastinal structures has already been discussed in Fig. 20.1. At this point, it is necessary to mention that the internal thoracic (mammary) arteries—branches of the subclavian arteries—descend deep to the costal cartilages about 1 cm lateral to the sternal margin. This distance is variable, however.

Thymectomy

Thymic resection is usually performed for either myasthenia gravis or thymic neoplasms. In treating myasthenia, some surgeons resect the thymus gland through a cervical incision to avoid entering the chest of an already weakened patient. However, recent discussions of surgical failures with thymectomy in the treatment of myasthenia gravis have focused more and more on possibly inadequate resections. For this reason, transsternal resection is once again considered to be the procedure of choice.

Thymic Resection (Fig. 20.3)

Technical Points

Open the chest through a median sternotomy incision. After placement of the sternal spreader, the thymus gland is usually readily identifiable. In the older patient, the thymus is frequently largely replaced with fat. Adequate resection of what may grossly appear to be nothing more than fat is essential.

FIGURE 20.3
THYMIC RESECTION

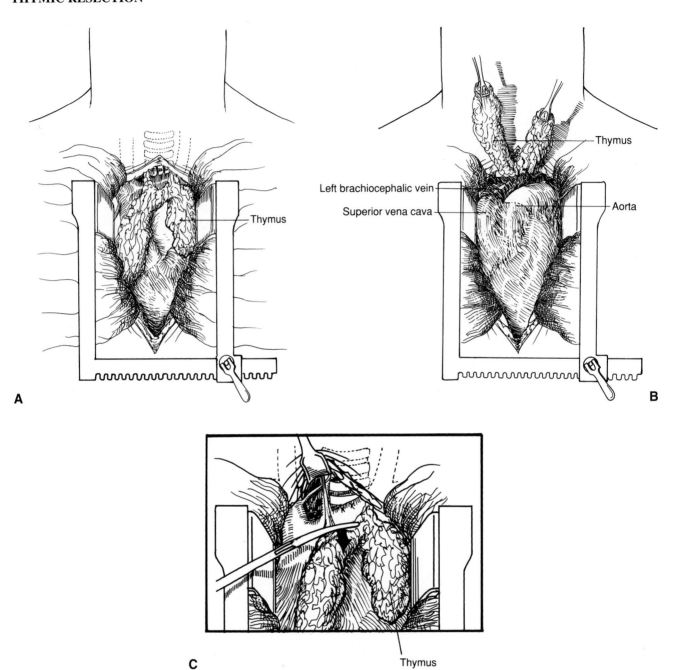

Identify the caudal tips of the lower lobes of the thymus and dissect each off the pericardium by either sharp dissection or electrocautery. This often will track down to the level of the diaphragm. One cannot help but notice an unusual but characteristic odor to the thymus ("salmon fishcakes") if it is transected with electrocautery. When the lateral margin is not well defined, resect all soft tissue, including the pleura, over to the phrenic nerve on each side. Great care should be taken to identify the phrenic nerve repeatedly and to avoid use of

electrocautery with 2 cm. Sharp and gentle blunt dissection will suffice. Phrenic injury and paralysis of the diaphragm can be catastrophic in a patient with myasthenia gravis. After both lower lobes are freed up inferiorly, elevate the gland superiorly and dissect the back of the thymus free from the pericardium. As the dissection is carried carefully cephalad, identify the posterior venous attachments from the gland to the brachiocephalic (innominate) vein. Control these short delicate veins with either silk ligature or clips. Avulsion of one of these branches off the brachiocephalic (innominate) vein can cause significant hemorrhage. Trace the lobes superiorly well up into the neck where they eventually change into attenuated fibrotic cords. At this point, they should be divided and ligated.

Many surgeons recommend that the anterior surface of the pericardium should be cleaned from phrenic nerve to phrenic nerve in order to resect all thymic tissue. In doing so, the pleura is commonly inadvertently opened on either or both sides. This is not serious if you recognize that it has happened and if you are careful to suction all irrigation fluid from the pleural cavity. If the pleural opening is small, open it more widely so that any air that is present can be evacuated by the mediastinal chest tubes. In younger patients with no pleural breach, or no evidence of air leak, we have used flexible drains (Blake, Jackson-Pratt) as an alternative method of drainage.

Anatomic Points

The thymus lies over the anterior surface of the pericardium and extends over the anterior surface of the left brachiocephalic (innominate) vein, to which it is connected posteriorly by one to four small veins. The arterial supply of the thymus is partially derived from very tiny branches from the internal thoracic (mammary) arteries. These vessels are so small that they require no attention during the dissection. Additional branches are derived from the inferior thyroid arteries.

The thymus, an immune and endocrine organ, develops from endodermal tissues primarily of the third pharyngeal pouch, which gives rise to the inferior parathyroids. Sometimes, the fourth pouch, which gives rise to the superior parathyroids, also gives rise to some thymic tissue. From this bilateral cervical origin, the thymus descends into the mediastinum, "dragging" the inferior parathyroid glands with it.

The size of the thymus in relation to body weight is greatest in the first 2 years of life, when the gland weighs 10 to 15 g. However, it reaches its maximal size during puberty, when it weighs about 30 to 40 g. After this, the gland is infiltrated and gradually replaced by adipose tissue, although functional thymic tissue is always present.

In the adult, the thymus gland, which usually has a distinct capsule, lies in the anterior mediastinum, extending from the root of the neck to the level of the fourth costal cartilage. Typically, a thyrothymic ligament attaches the thymus and thyroid glands.

The thymus is related anteriorly to the sternothyroid and sternohyoid muscles, the sternum, and usually the parietal pleura forming the costomediastinal recesses. Posteriorly, it is related to the trachea, left brachiocephalic vein, arch of the aorta and its branches, and pericardium. Its blood supply is principally derived from branches of the internal thoracic (mammary) artery, with additional branches from the inferior thyroid arteries. The venous drainage is primarily through one or two comparatively large veins emptying into the anterior surface of the left brachiocephalic (innominate) vein, with additional tributaries to the internal thoracic and inferior thyroid veins.

The surgeon should be aware of other normal or variant locations of thymic tissue. In about 75% of patients, thymic tissues are located in the mediastinal connective tissue outside of the capsule. In addition, one or both lobes of the gland may (about 6% of cases) lie posterior to the left brachiocephalic vein. Ectopic thymic tissue has been reported superior to or in association with the thyroid gland (thymic tissue possibly derived from the fourth pharyngeal pouch), in the left main-stem bronchus, in the lung parenchyma, in the posterior mediastinum, and in the lung hilum. Because of the normal location of the gland, and given the potential sites for ectopic tissue, a median sternotomy has become the approach of choice for complete removal of the thymus.

REFERENCES

1. Austin EH, Olanow CW, Wechsler AS. Thymoma following transcervical thymectomy for myasthenia gravis. *Ann Thorac Surg* 1983;35:548. (Discusses inadequate excision through the transcervical route.)
2. Hankins JR, Mayer RF, Satterfield JR, et al. Thymectomy for myasthenia gravis: 14 year experience. *Ann Surg* 1985;201:618. (The discussion following this article provides a good description of a cosmetic inframammary incision for median sternotomy in young women.)
3. Johnston MR. Median sternotomy for resection of pulmonary metastases. *J Thorac Cardiovasc Surg* 1983;85:516. (Includes a discussion of mobilization of the lungs when this approach is used.)
4. Masaoka A, Nagoaka Y, Kotake Y. Distribution of thymic tissue in the anterior mediastinum. *J Thorac Cardiovasc Surg* 1975;70:747. (Presents the anatomic rationale for performing median sternotomy rather than using the transcervical approach.)
5. Urschel HC, Razzuk MA. Median sternotomy as a standard approach for pulmonary resection. *Ann Thorac Surg* 1986;41: 130.
6. Yasuura K, Okamoto H, Morita S, et al. Results of omental flap transposition for deep sternal wound infection after cardiovascular surgery. *Ann Surg* 1998;227:455–459.

THE LUNGS AND STRUCTURES APPROACHED THROUGH A THORACOTOMY INCISION

Bronchoscopy (Chapter 21) continues the discussion of the anatomy of the tracheobronchial tree begun in Chapters 2 and 3 and introduces the segmental anatomy of the lungs. Following this, the lateral chest wall, associated muscles, and the anatomy of an intercostal space are described as the procedures of tube thoracostomy and thoracotomy (Chapter 22) are detailed. The anatomy of the lungs is discussed further in chapters that follow, where pulmonary resections are illustrated. A discussion of one common operative approach to the thoracic outlet syndrome presents additional anatomy relevant to both the chest and neck (Chapter 27). Finally, the thoracic esophagus, a mediastinal structure approached from the side, is included in this section (Chapters 28 and 29).

Major thoracic vascular operations, thoracoscopy, resection of posterior mediastinal tumors, and less common esophageal procedures are described in the references listed at the end of this section.

CHAPTER 21

Bronchoscopy

M. Victoria Gerken and Phillip C. Camp

Fiberoptic Bronchoscopy

Introduction of the Bronchoscope (Fig. 21.1)

Technical Points

Anesthesia is crucial for successful fiberoptic bronchoscopy. There are certain situations in which it is expedient to perform this procedure under general anesthesia (ie, when the patient cannot tolerate topical anesthesia, when the patient is anesthetized for another reason, or before a thoracotomy that is being performed to resect a small, peripheral nodule). Although general anesthesia does allow the endoscopist to examine the periphery closely without having to deal with coughing, the proximal trachea and the cords cannot be examined in an intubated patient. This is especially pertinent when one is evaluating central lung lesions and when there is a possibility of involvement of the recurrent laryngeal nerve. However, more than half of the life-threatening complications stemming from bronchoscopy are related to hypoxemia, hypercapnia, respiratory depression (oversedation), and medication side effects. Each clinical scenario should be carefully considered.

Most diagnostic bronchoscopy procedures are performed using topical anesthesia. However, all too often, the inexperienced endoscopist fails to achieve adequate anesthesia and ends up with an incomplete bronchoscopy because the patient is coughing and is clearly dyspneic. With an adequate balance of sedation (ie, with diazepam or midazolam hydrochloride), adequate analgesia and antitussive management (meperidine, morphine), and adequate topical anesthesia of the naris, the posterior pharynx, the aryepiglottic folds, and the cords, the average patient will be able to tolerate the procedure with little or no coughing, dyspnea, or agitation.

Place viscous lidocaine jelly on a series of cotton-tipped applicators and use these to anesthetize the naris, progressing slowly to the back of the nasopharynx as an anesthetic effect is achieved. Anesthetize the rest of the airway by connecting an atomizer filled with 4% lidocaine to a high-flow oxygen system with a Y connector. The anesthetic can then be sprayed gently over the mucous membranes with good control.

The use of intravenous sedation, careful monitoring of pulse oximetry, adequate topical anesthesia, and antisialagogues (atropine, glycopyrrolate) when indicated will allow careful and systematic examination of the proximal tracheobronchial tree. With the fiberoptic bronchoscope, you should be able to reach, without difficulty, the orifices of the third order of bronchi in all lobes.

Introduce the fiberoptic bronchoscope through the anesthetized naris. Pass the instrument into the back of the oropharynx and identify the larynx and vocal cords. Ask the awake patient to speak in order to confirm equal and full movement of the true cords. You may wish to inject additional topical anesthetic at this point to ensure its direct application to the cords. Under direct visualization, pass the fiberoptic bronchoscope through the cords into the proximal trachea. Inspect the area for neoplasms (both tumors and granulomas), excessive collapse of the trachea (tracheomalacia), points of external compression, and injuries

LIST OF STRUCTURES

Inferior nasal meatus
Nasopharynx
Oropharynx
Pharynx
Laryngeal aditus
Larynx
Vocal cords
Cricoid cartilage
Aryepiglottic folds
Trachea

Carina
Right main-stem bronchus
    Bronchus intermedius (intermediate
      bronchus)
Left main-stem bronchus
Right lung
    Right upper lobe
    Right middle lobe
    Right lower lobe

Left lung
    Left upper lobe
      Lingula
    Left lower lobe
Bronchopulmonary segments
Left and right vagus nerves
Stomach
Cardioesophageal junction
Spleen
Gastrosplenic (lienogastric) ligament

FIGURE 21.1
INTRODUCTION OF THE BRONCHOSCOPE

airway is about 11 cm long and 2 to 2.5 cm wide. It is narrowest at its beginning, where the only complete cartilaginous ring, the cricoid cartilage, is located. From there on, it assumes an inverted U shape owing to the signet-ring–shaped cartilages. The mucosa of the posterior wall, which widens as the carina is approached, has distinct longitudinal corrugations. The endoscopist should note that, during inspiration, the posterior membrane in the thorax moves posteriorly, whereas during expiration, it moves anteriorly in response to interairway pressure changes.

The carina, located at the end of the trachea and between the left and right main bronchi, is normally vertical, sharp, and narrow at its center, widening as its anterior and posterior limits are approached (normally, it is widest anteriorly). Although the normal orientation of the carina is vertical, it can vary from the perpendicular by as much as 45 degrees.

Examination of the Bronchial Tree (Fig. 21.2)

Technical Points

It is always advisable to "go where the money is" first. If chest radiographic studies show a mass on the left, examine that side first in case the patient develops dyspnea and the procedure needs to be terminated before a complete examination can be performed.

If the patient's condition allows, proceed to examine the entire tracheobronchial tree systematically. Develop a routine so that, in the excitement of identifying pathologic changes, you do not forget to examine the entire tree. The routine described here examines the right side first, then the left.

When looking down the right main-stem bronchus, the orifice to the upper lobe usually will be seen to be in a very lateral location. However, there is some variability to this finding (in contrast to the anatomy of the rest of the right lung). Occasionally, the orifice will lie directly opposite the carina, but usually it lies 2 to 3 cm distally. Herein lies one of the strong advantages of fiberoptic bronchoscopy over rigid bronchoscopy: the tip of the scope must be flexed fairly sharply to be able to look into the right upper lobe bronchus (clearly not possible with a rigid instrument). When looking up the right upper lobe bronchus, the three segmental bronchial orifices can easily be identified.

Just past the takeoff of the right upper lobe, you enter the bronchus intermedius. The anatomy here rarely varies. Anteriorly, a bronchial orifice will be seen that leads to the middle lobe. Down this orifice, the two segmental orifices that quickly branch further can usually be identified without difficulty. Directly posterior (and typically directly opposite the middle lobe orifice) is the orifice of the superior segment of the lower lobe. Between these two orifices is the bronchus leading to the four basilar segments of the right lower lobe.

The left main-stem bronchus branches much less acutely, with division into the upper and lower lobes. The upper lobe orifice lies superior to and slightly lateral to the lower lobe orifice. The upper lobe bronchus quickly bifurcates to go to the upper lobe and the lingula. The superior segment bronchial

(erosions, trauma, hematoma, disruption). The U shape of the tracheal cartilages and the comparatively flat, softer, membranous posterior wall make easy landmarks for maintaining proper orientation. The carina should appear to have a very acute angle with a sharp edge. Blunting of this angle can be seen with disease involving the subcarinal lymph nodes.

Anatomic Points

The fiberoptic bronchoscope should be advanced through the nose by way of the inferior nasal meatus (below the inferior nasal concha) because this is the widest passageway. As the bronchoscope is advanced into the nasopharynx, the tip should be directed 60 to 90 degrees caudally because this is the angle of the pharyngeal cavity with respect to the nasal cavity.

An alternative approach is to pass the flexible bronchoscope orally through an oral (bite block) specifically designed to allow passage of a scope. The advantage of this approach allows easier removal and reinsertion than when cleaning or unplugging of the scope's channels is required.

After the bronchoscope is advanced through the laryngeal aditus, the trachea should be clearly visible. This part of the

FIGURE 21.2
EXAMINATION OF THE BRONCHIAL TREE

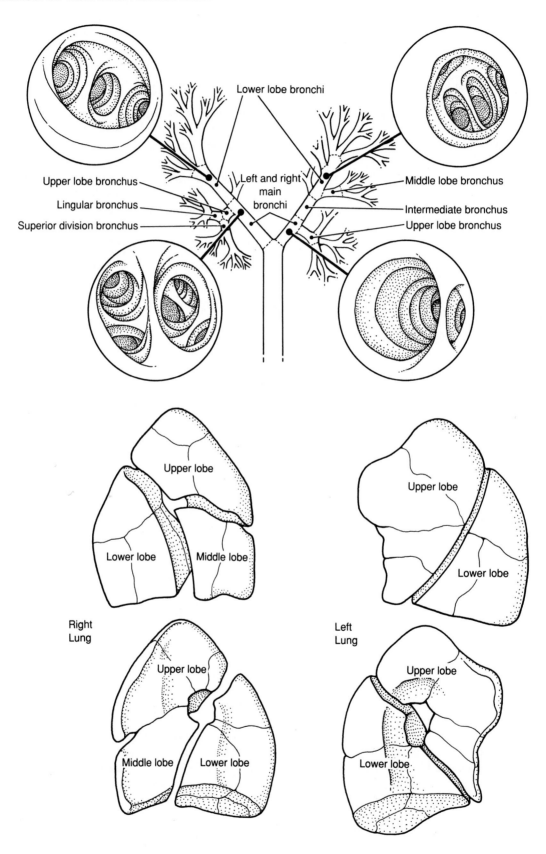

orifice is clearly seen posterior to the bronchus to the basal segments of the lower lobe.

One caveat pertains to the excessive use of suction. The ability to suction blood or mucus is critical to adequate visualization. However, the inexperienced endoscopist can unwittingly leave a finger on the suction port throughout the entire procedure. This virtually guarantees hypoxia and should be avoided.

Anatomic Points

Successful fiberoptic bronchoscopy demands knowledge of the bronchopulmonary segments. These segments, supported by third-order (segmental) bronchi, are the surgical units of the lung because there is little or no communication between segments. Each segment is based on the ramifications of a segmental bronchus and the accompanying ramifications of the pulmonary and bronchial arteries. Tributaries of the pulmonary vein, on the other hand, are intersegmental.

The right lung has 10 segments, whereas the left lung has 8 segments (although in the British literature, 10 segments are recognized on the left). As seen endoscopically, the 10 segments of the right lung and the relative positions (related to a clock face) of the orifices of their bronchi are as follows:

Upper lobe
    Apical segment (B I)—orifice at 4 o'clock
    Anterior segment (B II)—orifice at 12 o'clock
    Posterior segment (B III)—orifice at 8 o'clock
Middle lobe
    Lateral segment (B IV)—orifice at 3 o'clock to 6 o'clock
    Medial segment (B V)—orifice at 9 o'clock to 12 o'clock
Lower lobe
    Superior segment (B VI)—orifice at 5 o'clock, immediately past the middle lobe bronchus
    Medial basal segment (B VII)—orifice at 9 o'clock, usually more proximal than other basal segments
    Anterior basal segment (B VIII)—orifice at 1 o'clock
    Lateral basal segment (B IX)—orifice at 3 o'clock
    Posterior basal segment (B X)—orifice at 6 o'clock

It should be noted that, in more than half of patients, there is a subapical segment in the lower lobe, the bronchus of which is posterior. This tertiary bronchus can arise anywhere along the lower lobe bronchus from the opening of the superior segment to the final division of the lobar bronchus.

In a similar fashion, the bronchopulmonary segments of the left lung, and the relative location of the openings of their bronchi, are as follows:

Upper lobe
    Upper division—orifice at 8 o'clock
        Apicoposterior segment (B I + III)
        Anterior segment (B II)
    Lingular division—orifice at 2 o'clock
        Superior segment (B IV)—orifice at 10 o'clock
        Inferior segment (B V)—orifice at 2 o'clock
Lower lobe
    Superior segment (B VI)—orifice at 6 o'clock, shortly past the origin of the lower lobe

    Anteromedial basal segment (B VIII + VII)—orifice at 12 o'clock
    Lateral basal segment (B IX)—orifice at 9 o'clock
    Posterior basal segment (B X)—orifice at 5 o'clock

Rigid Bronchoscopy

Rigid bronchoscopy, the only technique available before the development of the fiberoptics that have revolutionized endoscopy, still has much to offer. True, fiberoptic bronchoscopy does allow manipulation within the bronchial tree, permitting much improved visualization of the distal tree (especially the right upper lobe), and it is well tolerated by the awake patient. However, rigid bronchoscopy is preferable for retrieval of foreign bodies, for severe hemoptysis, and for suctioning and hyperexpansion of an atelectatic lung. Additionally, rigid bronchoscopes are designed to allow concurrent ventilation, accept Hopkins telescopes, accommodate large biopsy forceps without obstructing the view, and allow passage of flexible bronchoscope.

Positioning the Patient and Manipulating the Scope (Fig. 21.3)

Technical and Anatomic Points

This procedure is usually done using general anesthesia, providing concurrent ventilation through the scope's side port. Much of the technique is a matter of personal preference. Just as there are anesthesiologists with varying ideas as to how the head of a patient should be positioned for intubation, so, too, do thoracic surgeons vary in their bronchoscopic techniques. A single, rolled towel under the patient's shoulders creates a very slight hyperextension of the neck and chin extension, facilitating exposure. Marked hyperextension will make exposure much more difficult.

Introduce the scope through the mouth, elevating the epiglottis with the tip of the lubricated scope and passing the instrument through the glottis and the cords and into the upper trachea. Alternatively, a laryngoscope can be used to expose the posterior oropharynx and vocal cords. Always place the scope through the cords under direct visualization. Care must be taken to continuously support the rigid bronchoscope and to prevent sudden or jarring motions. The rigid scope can cause significant trauma when not manipulated in a coordinated fashion.

Give the ventilation port to the anesthesiologist for continued ventilation of the patient during the procedure. While viewing through the glass-covered eyepiece, advance the scope along the tracheobronchial tree until the desired area is reached.

It is extremely important to communicate and work well with the anesthesiologist. Wedging the scope into a lobar bronchus (especially if it is obstructed by a foreign body) may not allow adequate ventilation. Having an experienced anesthesiologist monitoring the ventilator bag, the pulse oximeter, and the CO_2 monitor will ensure early detection of potential problems.

FIGURE 21.3
POSITIONING THE PATIENT AND MANIPULATING THE SCOPE

A

Carina

B

C

Extraction of foreign bodies, although challenging, is often an interesting endeavor. A variety of grasping forceps are made for this purpose. Occasionally, one will find it useful to pass a Fogarty catheter past the offending object and then, with the Fogarty balloon inflated, to draw back on it until it is impacted in the end of the bronchoscope. At this time, the bronchoscope, with the entrapped foreign body, is removed to allow for adequate ventilation through the anesthesia mask. It is advisable in this circumstance to then reintroduce the cleaned bronchoscope to check for any remaining remnants of the foreign body. (Peanuts are notorious for fracturing during removal.)

When performing this procedure on children, many endoscopists administer racemic epinephrine (by nebulizer), dexamethasone (Decadron), or both, in an attempt to reduce further swelling of the small airway.

In cases of severe hemoptysis, examination of the tracheobronchial tree can be performed better with the rigid scope because it permits much better suctioning through larger suction catheters. In the setting of airway hemorrhage, an obstructing balloon catheter can be purposefully directed and inflated quickly, protecting the remainder of the airway. If the hemorrhage is massive, the rigid bronchoscope can then be introduced into the main-stem bronchus of the unaffected side to allow ventilation through it during a subsequent thoracotomy. However, this is rarely done any more because the fit is seldom tight enough to rule out spillage of blood into the "good" side around the bronchoscope. Use of a Robert-Shaw or Carlens tube tends to be much more satisfactory.

REFERENCES

1. Oho K, Amemiya R. *Practical fiberoptic bronchoscopy.* Tokyo: Igaku-Shoin, 1980.

CHAPTER 22

Tube Thoracostomy, Thoracotomy, Wedge Resection, and Pleural Abrasion

M. Victoria Gerken and Phillip C. Camp

In this chapter, the basic procedure of tube thoracostomy is used to introduce chest wall anatomy. The basic thoracic surgery incision—posterolateral thoracotomy—is described in detail. Two common, simple, thoracic surgery procedures—wedge resection and pleural abrasion—are then described.

Tube Thoracostomy

Placement of a Tube Thoracostomy (Fig. 22.1)

Technical Points

The relatively simple procedure of tube thoracostomy demands careful attention to detail. Poor performance will cause patient discomfort and underlying lung injury, and may even necessitate open thoracotomy or laparotomy for correction.

In the past, chest tubes placed for pneumothoraces were inserted in the anterior chest, causing much unnecessary discomfort for the patient and substantially increasing the risk for hemorrhage from the anterior chest wall. Current practice dictates that chest tubes for uncomplicated pleural effusions, hemothoraces, or pneumothoraces be placed between the anterior axillary line and the midaxillary line, resulting in best results and minimum pain to the patient. Loculated collections of fluid or air may often require variations in technique that will not be discussed in this chapter.

Adequate analgesia is key to successful, uncomplicated tube thoracostomy. Create a 2- to 3-cm skin wheal with 0.5% to 1.0% lidocaine about one interspace width below the planned thoracic entrance site. Subsequent or serial injections of lidocaine (5 mg/kg maximum dose), including the rib periosteum, intercostal muscles, and chest wall pleura, will greatly improve the ease of the procedure and patient comfort.

Prepare the skin widely and drape the area. For most purposes, chest tube insertion at the sixth interspace is adequate and safe. To prevent pneumothorax at the time of tube removal, plan to make the skin incision a full interspace lower than where you intend to enter the chest. In this way, the tube will pass through a subcutaneous tunnel measuring 2 to 3 cm in length between the skin and the entry site between the ribs. Thus, the skin incision should be made at the seventh interspace.

Incise the skin with the scalpel and then create the subcutaneous tunnel with a long curved clamp. Repetitive gentle spreading to a width equal to your finger and the chest tube will allow adequate access. Identify the top of the rib with the clamp and spread the intercostal muscle just over it, carefully hugging the superior surface. Control the clamp carefully so that when you "pop" through the pleura, the tip of the clamp does not injure underlying tissue. While the clamp is still in, spread the tips to widen the intercostal defect. Place your index finger through this incision into the chest and "sweep" down any adhesions, feeling for rind on the lung, pleural

LIST OF STRUCTURES

Pleura
Pleural space
Intercostal space
External intercostal muscles
Internal intercostal muscles
Innermost intercostal muscles
Intercostal neurovascular bundle
    Intercostal vein
    Intercostal artery
    Intercostal nerve

Diaphragm
Costal margin
Xiphoid process
Serratus anterior muscle
Endothoracic fascia
Latissimus dorsi muscle
Scapula
Trapezius muscle

Triangle of auscultation
Rhomboideus major muscle
Erector spinae muscles (paraspinous
    muscles)
Long thoracic nerve

ORIENTATION

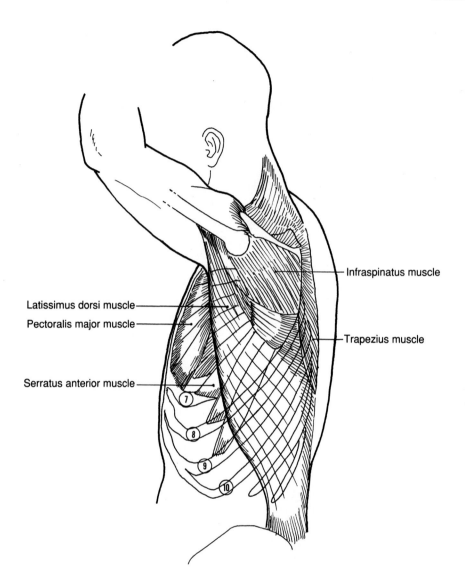

Infraspinatus muscle

Latissimus dorsi muscle

Pectoralis major muscle

Trapezius muscle

Serratus anterior muscle

7

8

9

10

implants, and blood clots. Confirm the intrathoracic placement of a low chest tube by palpating the superior surface of the diaphragm.

Grasp the tip of the chest tube with the tip of a curved clamp and introduce it into the chest as shown (Fig. 22.1A). Inset the tube just far enough so that the last drainage hole is well within the chest cavity. An alternative method is to leave your finger in the tunnel and feed the tube next to it. The fingertip is blunt and allows the tube to be directed in a more specific direction. Either way, spinning the tube in a counterclockwise direction while advancing will help keep the tube from kinking and being misplaced into a fissure.

Secure the tube at the skin level with a heavy silk suture. The suture should be a U stitch or a single horizontal mattress stitch, which will allow skin approximation at the time of

closure (Fig. 22.1B). Connect it to a chest drainage and suction device, such as a Pleurovac. Dress the site appropriately.

Removal of the tube is best accomplished by two people. Prepare an occlusive dressing by placing a petroleum jelly gauze on 4 × 4s. Expose the chest tube site and mobilize the stitch. Ask the patient to hold his or her breath in full inspiration. Place the dressing over the site with petroleum jelly apposing the incision. Quickly withdraw the tube, secure the suture, and tape the dressing tightly down while holding it firmly to the chest wall.

Anatomic Points

One of the potential hazards of tube thoracostomy—inadvertent placement of the tube below the diaphragm—

FIGURE 22.1
PLACEMENT OF A TUBE THORACOSTOMY

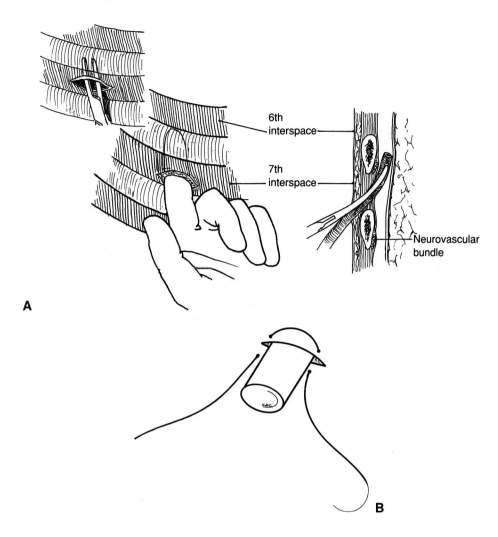

can be avoided by analyzing the structure and morphology of the diaphragm. This muscle has a circumferential origin and divides the thoracic cavity from the abdominal cavity. Posteriorly, the diaphragm takes its origin from the anterolateral surfaces of the upper two or three lumbar vertebrae. It has a costal origin from the internal surfaces of the lower six ribs and costal cartilages at the costal margin; hence, as one progresses anteriorly, the origin of the diaphragm becomes progressively more cranial. Anteriorly, it has two small slips of origin from the deep surface of the xiphoid process. From this origin, the muscular fibers insert on the expansive, aponeurotic central tendon.

The upper limits of the diaphragm are at the level of the nipple, or fourth intercostal space, so that it is dome shaped. As a consequence, the peripheral part of the thoracic cavity becomes progressively attenuated inferiorly, resulting in a sharp, narrow costophrenic recess. In the midclavicular line, the reflection of parietal pleura from body wall to diaphragm is at the level of the eighth rib, whereas in the midaxillary line,

this reflection is at the level of the tenth rib. Because of this reflection and the dome shape of the diaphragm, incisions below the level of the eighth rib may not enter the pleural cavity and can easily pass through the diaphragm into the abdominal cavity. The sharp costophrenic recess is precisely why excellent clamp control when popping into the chest is mandatory. Overly aggressive entry can easily continue on through the adjacent diaphragm and into the abdomen. The slippery dome has been known to be confused with the diaphragm. Digitally palpating the diaphragm and lung wall helps confirm accurate location.

The other main hazard is injury to the intercostal neurovascular bundle. Each major intercostal neurovascular bundle is located in the costal groove (on the inferior surface of the rib), which helps to protect it. From superior to inferior, the arrangement of neurovascular structures is *vein— artery—nerve*. The nerve, lying lowest, is most susceptible to iatrogenic injury. To avoid this neurovascular bundle, make the intercostal incision close to the superior margin of the lower rib, rather than along the inferior margin of the upper rib.

In the midaxillary line, muscle fibers that must be divided before entering the intercostal neurovascular plane include those of the serratus anterior, external intercostal, and internal intercostal muscles. The neurovascular bundle lies in the plane between the deep innermost intercostal muscle layer and the more superficial internal intercostal layer. Deep to the innermost intercostal layer is the endothoracic fascia, a thin layer to which the costal pleura is adherent.

Standard Posterolateral Thoracotomy

Position of Patient and Incision (Fig. 22.2)

Technical Points

Correct patient positioning is mandatory for the safe performance of this procedure. To have the patient roll slightly forward or backward during the procedure is, at best, extremely frustrating, and, at worst, dangerous.

Place the patient in the lateral decubitus position with a roll under the dependent axilla to protect the shoulder and the axillary contents. In general, the diameter of the roll should approximate the diameter of the upper arm. The roll remains parallel to and just caudal to the dependent arm, which is flexed 90 degrees at the shoulder. The roll should prop up the chest wall, allowing the shoulder to drop down, thus relieving pressure on the brachial plexus. A common misperception is that the roll is tucked into the axilla, which is incorrect. Fold a soft pillow double and place it over this arm. Drape the superior arm over the pillow or onto a sling cephalad to the dependent arm.

A vacuum-activated "beanbag," previously placed under the patient, should be molded to the patient's dependent half of the torso and hips and aspirated until rigid. Alternatively, place a 10-lb sandbag just anterior to the patient's abdomen, supporting any panniculus. Leave the lower, dependent leg straight. Flex the upper leg 90 degrees at both the hip and the knee. Support the calf with two pillows. A strip of wide tape will help stabilize the patient in this position. The tape should extend from the table edge over the buttocks and hip and down the length of the flexed thigh to the table edge on the opposite side. Take care not to place the tape over the fibular head on the upper leg where it may press on the common peroneal nerve. In addition, avoid undue force in applying the tape because this may cause a counter–pressure point.

Once the patient has been securely positioned, prepare the hemithorax extending across the midline both anteriorly and posteriorly. The prep should extend up to the prominent spine of the seventh cervical vertebra and over the exposed shoulder and should include the nipple on the operative side. Extend the prep down to the iliac crest inferiorly.

FIGURE 22.2
POSITION OF PATIENT AND INCISION

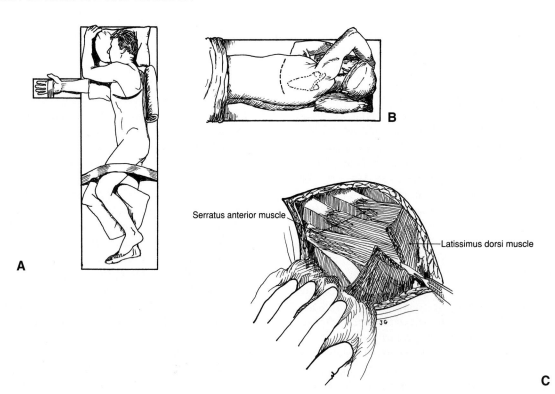

Stand at the patient's back. Draw an incision beginning at the anterior axillary line at the level of the inframammary fold in a woman, or at a point about 6 cm inferior to the nipple in a man. Extend the incision laterally so that it passes 2 to 3 cm inferior to the inferior angle of the scapula and then curves gently cephalad, ending midway between the spine of the scapula and the thoracic vertebral column. Incise the skin.

Use electrocautery to divide the subcutaneous tissue down to the level of the muscles. Expose and divide the latissimus dorsi muscle with electrocautery. Posteriorly, expose the lateral edge of the trapezius muscle and divide it in the same way. Identify the auscultatory triangle, which is just inferior and posterior to the inferior angle of the scapula, and divide its thin connective tissue. Slip your hand under the posterior edge of the serratus anterior muscle.

Divide the serratus anterior muscle with electrocautery or identify and divide its attachments to the chest wall, exposing these attachments by retracting the inferior edge of the divided latissimus dorsi muscle with a sharp-pronged rake retractor.

Posteriorly, divide the lateral edge of the rhomboideus major muscle with cautery. Slide your hand up under the scapula to identify the ribs. The first rib can seldom be felt; hence, the identification process usually begins with the second rib, the outer aspect of which has a characteristic, flattened surface. A helpful marker of the second rib is the insertion of the subclavius and anterior scalene muscles.

In general, enter the chest in the third, fourth, or fifth interspace depending on the operation being performed. Very seldom is it necessary to resect a rib; this is done almost exclusively when there is dense pleural disease or when the rib is needed for a bone graft.

Divide the external and internal intercostal muscle, staying just superior to the lower rib in order to avoid the neurovascular bundle. As you approach the parietal pleura, ask the anesthesiologist to "drop the lung," or to deflate the lung to reduce the risk for injury to the underlying pulmonary parenchyma. Using the tip of a hemostat or careful, delicate strokes with a scalpel, pop into the pleura. Place an index finger or a plastic Yankauer suction catheter into the pleural cavity and advance the intercostal incision anteriorly, keeping the cautery on your finger (or suction catheter) in order to protect the underlying lung. Stay directly on the superior edge of the lower rib. If the intercostal space is so narrow as to be uncomfortable on your finger, place the blade of the smallest available Richardson retractor in the intercostal space and use it to widen the space. Posteriorly, extend the intercostal incision, using cautery, to the anterior border of the paraspinous muscles. *Do not divide the paraspinous muscles;* these define the posterior extent of your soft tissue dissection. Identify and score the anterior margin of these muscles with electrocautery. Using a large periosteal elevator, elevate the muscle off the outer surface of the ribs and slide a small Army-Navy elevator in to keep this outer surface exposed.

Place the rib spreader in such a way as to "catch" or trap the tip of the scapula to prevent its protruding into your line of vision. Open the intercostal space along its length, taking care not to divide the internal mammary artery about 1 to 2 cm from the most anteromedial aspect of the rib. Dividing the intercostal muscles under direct vision (through the spreader) without dividing the overlying muscles of the thoracic cage allows excellent exposure, typically avoids deliberate division of the rib for exposure, and minimizes unplanned rib fractures.

Anatomic Points

Here, as elsewhere, knowledge of surface anatomy is important in planning the incision. The anterior axillary fold is formed by the inferolateral border of the pectoralis major muscle, whereas the posterior axillary fold is formed by the lateral margin of the latissimus dorsi muscle. Between these two muscles, the thoracic wall is covered by the interdigitating costal attachments of the serratus anterior and external oblique muscles. In men and in women with small breasts, the nipple typically overlies the fourth intercostal space. The inferior angle of the scapula usually overlies the eighth rib, whereas the root of the spine of the scapula is located at about the third intercostal space.

After skin incisions have been made, the muscles related to the posterior thoracic wall and scapula are identified next. Adjacent to the posterior midline and for a variable distance laterally, the most superficial muscle fibers, directed superolaterally, are those of the inferior border of the trapezius, a muscle that originates from the superior nuchal line of the occipital bone and the spinous processes of all cervical and thoracic vertebrae and that inserts on the spine of the scapula and lateral clavicle. The lower trapezius fibers overlie the essentially horizontal upper fibers of the latissimus dorsi, a muscle whose broad origin includes the lower six thoracic vertebral spines, all lumbar and sacral spines, and the posterior iliac crest by way of its attachment to the thoracolumbar fascia, and the iliac crest lateral to the erector spinae muscles. The latissimus dorsi fibers converge to form a flat tendon of insertion onto the lateral floor of the humeral intertubercular sulcus.

Division of the lower trapezius fibers and upper latissimus dorsi fibers effectively increases the size of the triangle of auscultation, a triangle bounded by the upper border of the latissimus dorsi muscle, the lower lateral border of the trapezius muscle, and the vertebral border of the scapula. Division of the trapezius and latissimus dorsi fibers allows increased mobility of the lower part of the scapula. A margin of 2 to 3 cm inferior to the inferior angle of the scapula should be maintained to allow adequate closure and to not disrupt the local capsule.

The anatomic relationships of the serratus anterior muscle are potentially confusing. This muscle arises from muscular digitations of the anterolateral aspect of the upper 8 to 10 ribs, and then passes posteriorly between the thoracic wall and scapula to insert along the entire length of the vertebral border of the scapula. It is innervated by the long thoracic nerve, which originates from roots (C5 to C7) of the brachial plexus and descends on the external surface of the serratus muscle deep to the fascia covering this muscle, approximately in the posterior axillary line. The long thoracic nerve is accompanied, especially low in its course, by branches from the subscapular artery. Higher up in the axilla, behind the pectoralis minor muscle, the nerve passes posterior to the origin of the lateral thoracic artery, an anatomic relation that can be used to identify this nerve.

Some difficulty may be encountered in counting ribs deep to the scapula. Here, as anteriorly, it is easiest to start counting with the second rib. This rib can be identified by palpating the insertion of the serratus posterior superior muscle because this is the highest rib to which this muscle is attached.

The term *paraspinous muscles,* as used here, refers to the erector muscles of the spine. These muscles are divisible into a medial spinalis muscle column adjacent to spinous processes, an intermediate longisimus column occupying the interval between the spinalis muscle column and the angles of the lower ribs, and a lateral iliocostalis column, attached to the angles of ribs. Division of iliocostal or longissimus fibers should not affect the function of these muscular columns because their innervation, through branches from the posterior primary divisions of spinal nerves, is segmental. However, division of these muscle groups is rarely required and should be avoided if possible.

Closure of Thoracotomy (Fig. 22.3)

Technical Points

At the completion of the procedure, ask the anesthesiologist to inflate the lung fully. This is the best time to expand any lung that may have become atelectatic intraoperatively; atelectasis is difficult enough to treat postoperatively without starting the problem in the operating room.

At this time, instill bupivacaine hydrochloride into the posterior intercostal spaces for two or three spaces above and below the incision. This strategy helps to control postoperative pain if regional anesthesia or analgesia is not being used.

At the completion of the case, place one or two chest tubes into the hemithorax; these should exit caudal on the chest wall, anterior to the midaxillary line, for greatest patient comfort. If two tubes are used, place a right-angled tube in the posterior position to promote batter basilar fluid drainage. Place the anterior chest tube with the tip in the apex of the pleural space. Secure the tubes to the skin with heavy silk.

Use six to eight figure-of-eight "pericostal" stitches of heavy absorbable suture material to approximate the ribs. A nice method to minimize accidental punctures is to use a large "liver" needle (blunted tip, large 180-degree curve) to place the intercostal sutures. We have found this to be quick and rather safe. After placing the sutures, fully inflate the lung and approximate the ribs. Again, take care to avoid the

FIGURE 22.3
CLOSURE OF THORACOTOMY

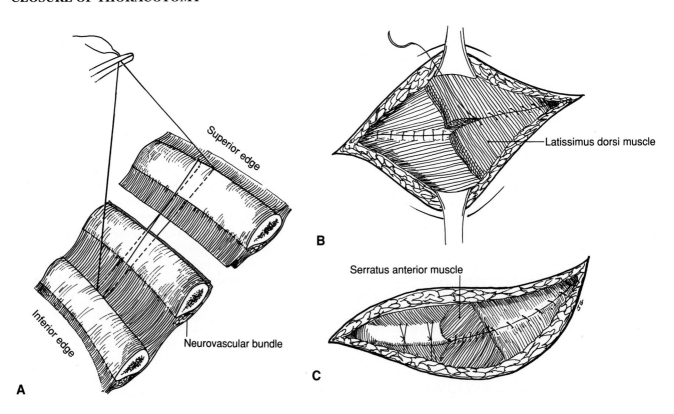

intercostal neurovascular bundles. Although some surgeons prefer to use the Bailey rib approximator to appose the ribs while tying these sutures, a slipknot permits snug approximation of the ribs without endangering the intercostal vessels. Individually reapproximate the serratus anterior, rhomboideus, latissimus dorsi, and trapezius muscles anatomically with heavy absorbable suture material.

Approximate the subcutaneous tissue with absorbable suture, after which the skin edges should be approximated, either with skin staples or a subcuticular running monofilament suture.

Anatomic Points

The use of a local analgesic injected two to three spaces above and below the incision is partially based on the anatomic principles of segmental innervation. Seemingly, only the interspace of the incision should require analgesia because it should be wholly within a dermatome. However, there is overlap of dermatomes, which means that about half of a segment is at least partially innervated by the nerve preceding that for the given segment and about half is at least partially innervated by the nerve succeeding the segment.

When the anterior chest tube is placed, the tube should be in the apex, about 2.5 cm cephalad to the medial third of the clavicle. The lower chest tube is placed just anterior to the posterior axillary line. If this is placed as low as possible, it

will be in the eighth or ninth intercostal space. Again, caution should be exercised to prevent trauma to the diaphragm or the abdominal contents.

Muscle-Sparing Thoracotomy (Fig. 22.4)

Technical Points

The division of the latissimus dorsi muscle causes severe postoperative pain, which often leads to splinting of the chest wall and a long recovery period and which can hinder good pulmonary function and toilet in the postoperative period. For intrathoracic operations not requiring maximal exposure (pleural abrasions, wedge resections, biopsies), a procedure associated with less morbidity—a muscle-sparing thoracotomy—can be performed in many cases.

Use the same skin incision as for the standard thoracotomy, but do not make it as long posteriorly. Divide the subcutaneous tissue and free it up from the fascia of the latissimus dorsi muscle superiorly to the scapula and inferiorly to the iliac crest. Mobilize the anterior edge of the latissimus dorsi muscle and free the undersurface. Free the serratus muscle in a similar fashion so that the latissimus dorsi can be freely retracted posteriorly and the serratus anteriorly to expose the ribs.

Enter the chest in the intercostal space as described previously. Use two smaller rib-spreader retractors: the first for separating the free edges of the latissimus dorsi and serratus

---

FIGURE 22.4
MUSCLE-SPARING THORACOTOMY

FIGURE 22.5
WEDGE RESECTION

A   B

muscles, and the second for placement in the usual intercostal space. This creates a window through which the procedure can be performed.

At the completion of the procedure, place the chest tubes and the pericostal stitches as described previously. Place a flat suction drain under the muscle flaps, bringing it out through a separate stab wound. Approximate the subcutaneous tissue and close the skin.

Anatomic Points

Again, be aware that the intercostal bundle, containing the intercostal vein, artery, and nerve, runs medial and inferior to the lower edge of the corresponding rib. This unfortunately makes it a structure that is easy to injure during chest closure.

Wedge Resection (Fig. 22.5)

Technical Points

Many procedures are easily approached by thoracoscopy, but often the nature of the lesion, the stability of the patient, or the tolerance of single-lung ventilation will favor open approaches. Pulmonary procedures generally begin with exploration of the hemithorax. Just as the peritoneal cavity should be explored before proceeding with a formal hemicolectomy, so, too, should an examination of the hilum of the lung, the entire lung, the pleural surfaces, and the anterior and posterior mediastinum be performed before proceeding with lobectomy, segmentectomy, or wedge resection. Wedge resections of lung tissue for diagnostic purposes (e.g., diffuse infiltrative disease, acute respiratory distress syndrome) allow for a minimal incision but will, by their size, limit complete thoracic exploration. This approach will help to determine the appropriateness of curative versus palliative resection, compared with a simple biopsy.

For small subpleural (peripheral) masses, grasp the lung on either side with lung clamps. Elevate these regions to "tent up" the lesion. Use a stapling device to divide under the lesion. Bolstering stapled margins with bovine pericardium can be advantageous and minimize postoperative.

Air leak: This approach also can be somewhat stronger when wedging out thicker portions of tissue. For lesions that are large or that lie deep within the parenchyma, it may be necessary to fire the stapler twice to "wedge out" the lesion. In such cases, it is extremely important to remember the segmental anatomy of the lung. It is possible, and quite disastrous, to resect a wedge in such a fashion that the bronchial or vascular communication of the remaining lung is compromised. This leaves nonaerated, nonperfused lung behind to serve as a septic source. After performing a wedge resection, deflate the remaining lung and then have the anesthesiologist reinflate it to confirm the adequate function of all remaining lung.

Anatomic Points

The segmental anatomy of the lung is of crucial importance. It is discussed in detail in the chapters devoted to bronchoscopy (Chapter 19) and lobectomy (Chapter 22). Because a nonanatomic wedge resection crosses subsegmental boundaries, aeration of the adjacent pulmonary parenchyma must be confirmed at operation.

Pleural Abrasion (Fig. 22.6)

Technical and Anatomic Points

Recurring spontaneous pneumothoraces usually occur in otherwise healthy young people. After the second occurrence, most surgeons recommend thoracostomy or thoracotomy. This chapter discusses the open approach.

FIGURE 22.6
PLEURAL ABRASION

This is an ideal situation for muscle-sparing thoracotomy. Open the chest in the fifth or sixth intercostal space and examine the lung parenchyma carefully for subpleural blebs. These occur at the apex of the upper lobe, along the apical edge of the superior segment of the lower lobe, and rarely, along the fissures. If any are visualized, exclude them with the stapling device. It is not necessary to resect much tissue if a minimal amount of parenchyma is involved. Fill the hemithorax with sterile saline and inflate the lung to a pressure of 30 to 40 cm H_2O. Anything more than minimal air leaks should be addressed by oversewing the staple line or restapling.

Suction all saline from the chest. Abrade the parietal pleura by rubbing briskly with a dry laparotomy sponge. As the sponge becomes moistened with serous fluid, replace it with a dry one. An alternative approach is to use an abrasive pad (we use the disposable pad designed for electrocautery cleaning) to cause numerous microlacerations in the pleural surface. The key to successful pleural abrasion is causing significant inflammation between the two pleural surfaces, thus obliterating the potential space.

In the setting of apical blebs causing the recurrent pneumothorax, we will physically excise the apical pleural cap from within the thorax. This is a more aggressive maneuver but will definitely scar in the problematic portion of the lung. It is important that all pleura be abraded to the point of mild hemorrhage to ensure success. Include the diaphragm and the apex of the chest. Just before closing, 5 g of talc poudrage should be evenly applied to the inner thoracic surface.

Place two chest tubes in the usual positions and close the chest. It is imperative that the chest tubes be kept patent and suctioned; the visceral and parietal pleural surfaces must be kept in direct apposition if adhesions are to form as desired.

TUBE THORACOSTOMY REFERENCES

1. Daly RC, Mucha P, Pairolero PC, et al. The risk of percutaneous chest tube thoracostomy for blunt thoracic trauma. *Ann Emerg Med* 1985;14:865.
2. Millikan JS, Moore EE, Steiner E, et al. Complications of tube thoracostomy for acute trauma. *Am J Surg* 1980;140:738.
3. Peters J, Kubitschek KR. Clinical evaluation of a percutaneous pneumothorax catheter. *Chest* 1984;86:714. (Describes the "dart" percutaneous technique for simple pneumothoraces.)
4. Silver M, Bone RC. The technique of chest tube insertion. *J Crit Illness* 1986;1:45.

THORACOTOMY REFERENCES

1. Moore FA, Moore EE. Care of the surgical patient. In: Wilmore DW, Brennan MF, Harken AH, et al, eds. *Part I. Emergency care; Part II. Trauma resuscitation.* New York: Scientific American, 1991:7. (Describes tube thoracostomy for trauma, as well as emergency "slash" thoracotomy for thoracic trauma.)
2. Paneth M, Goldstraw P, Hyams B. Left thoracotomy. In: *Fundamental techniques in pulmonary and oesophageal surgery.* New York: Springer-Verlag, 1987:8.

CHAPTER 23

Thoracoscopy, Thoracoscopic Wedge Resection

Kemp Kernstine

A thoracotomy incision is traumatic and painful and frequently leaves the patient with a cosmetically unappealing scar. Two percent of thoracotomy patients have incapacitating pain that lasts for more than a year, 4% have upper extremity disability, and 40% have persistent mild-to-moderate discomfort. Reducing the incision size appears to reduce the trauma, pain, and disability. Endoscopic thoracic surgery appears to accomplish these goals.

Three types of thoracic endoscopic procedures can be performed:

Pleuroscopy usually involves a single puncture wound and portal for visualization, biopsy, and dissection. Visualization is either directly through an open scope, such as a Pilling or Storz mediastinoscope, or indirectly with a digital scope. The direct scope gives a limited view but is very efficient in that it allows visualization and manipulation through the same port. Pleuroscopy is ideally suited to evaluate and treat pleural effusions or pleural masses. It may also assist in placement of pleural drains. Although this pleuroscopy is done most frequently under general anesthesia, it may also be performed using fairly mild sedation with local anesthesia, if the planned procedure is brief with minimal manipulation or biopsy.

Thoracoscopy involves two or more portals through which the visualization, dissection, and resection are performed.

Video-assisted thoracoscopic surgery (VATS) employs multiple ports. All the dissection that would be performed through an open thoracotomy is performed by endoscopic visualization. A non–rib-spreading incision may be necessary to dissect and extract the surgical specimen. To minimize, pain retractors are not used. Thoracoscopy and VATS are used for a wider variety of procedures: lung biopsies; wedge resections; resections of thoracic masses; intrapleural, extrapleural, hilar, and mediastinal masses; and resection of lesions within the esophagus, portions of the esophagus, and myotomies.

It is essential to obtain a chest computed tomography (CT) scan before performing any form of endoscopic thoracic surgery. This allows three-dimensional operative planning and appropriate positioning of the surgical ports. The most appropriate patients for the thoracoscopic or video-assisted procedure are those whom have had no prior thoracotomy, have a large thoracic cavity, are not ventilator dependent, and are not obese. Lesions most suitable for access through this approach are smaller than 3 cm and are peripherally located. Preoperative pulmonary function testing is very helpful in assisting intraoperative and postoperative management.

Anesthetic intubation management is dependent on the procedure planned. All three procedures may be performed using (a) single-lumen intubation with apnea or CO_2 insufflation, (b) double-lumen intubation, or (c) bronchial blocker. For brief, pleurally-based procedures, apnea may be appropriate. Ventilator-dependent patients may require CO_2 insufflation. Single-lung ventilation by either double-lumen tube technique or bronchial blocker is desirable because it improves intrathoracic visibility, minimizes respiratory motion, reduces pulmonary parenchymal bleeding, and decreases the damage to the lung and the pulmonary vasculature. The greater the complexity of the intended endoscopic procedure, the greater these factors must be realized.

Patient Position and Port Placement (Fig. 23.1)

Technical Points

Patients are typically placed in the lateral decubitus position, although the supine or prone position may be necessary. Always have radiologic studies available for intraoperative review, and ensure that view boxes are available in the operating room.

Incisions of 5 mm to 1 cm are then placed. In the case of pleuroscopy, especially in those situations where malignant mesothelioma or other locally recurrent tumors are likely, a single port should be placed in the fifth to seventh intercostal space at the anterior axillary line. The port site must be planned in anticipation of an extrapleural pneumectomy resection, which would include the chest wall area in which this port site is placed. Use the chest wall topical anatomy, such as the tip of the scapula, the manubriosternal junction, and the xiphoid process and the landmarks on the chest computed tomography (CT) scan as they relate to the intended surgical target. For particularly small masses, those smaller

FIGURE 23.1
PATIENT POSITION AND PORT PLACEMENT

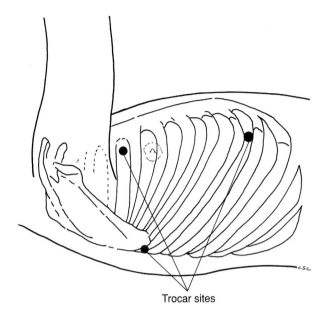

Trocar sites

than 5 mm and deeper than 1 to 2 cm from the pleural surface, preoperative, CT-guided wire localization may prove useful.

When more than one port is used, we usually place the first port in the low anterior chest wall in the anterior axillary line and pass a straight or 30-degree angled thoracoscope. For single ports, an open direct visualization scope, such as is used for mediastinoscopy, may be used when there is a limited view, as described earlier. Further ports may be placed as necessary, especially when performing complex procedures. For thoracoscopy, portal arrangement is placed as a baseball diamond, with the video port placed at home plate, grasping and biopsy portals at first and third bases, and the region of interest at second base.

The instrumentation is dependent on the planned procedure. Plastic and rubber portals can be used when instrumentation must be repeatedly changed to prevent injury to the chest wall and intercostal nerves. Grasping, retracting, dissecting, suturing, and clip-applying equipment are all available. We prefer to grasp the lung with ring clamps. Endoscopic stapling equipment is very beneficial to seal the lung after resection.

Lung Biopsy (Fig. 23.2)

Technical Points

The chest CT scan is used to identify the most diseased portion of the lung. Ports are placed to reach the diseased lung. It is essential that the lesion be either palpable or easily visualized. If this is not likely, perform preoperative CT-guided wire localization and resection with fluoroscopic assistance (Fig. 23.2A).

Enlarge the axillary port and insert a finger to palpate the lung, using an opposing operative grasping clamp to bring the lung into range (Fig. 23.2B). Take all adhesions down bluntly, or use electrocautery if the adhesions are dense. Biopsy may be performed with a forceps or by performing a wedge resection using a standard stapling device. If possible, biopsy the most cephalad portion of the lung or a portion adjacent to an edge in order to obtain an adequate sample and reduce the

FIGURE 23.2
LUNG BIOPSY

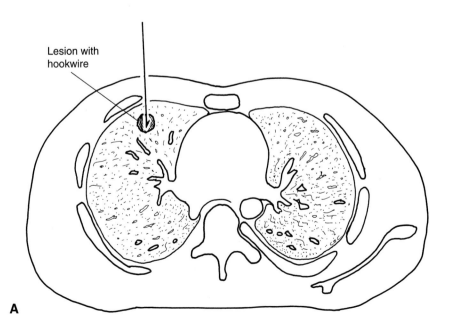

Lesion with hookwire

A

FIGURE 23.2 (Continued)

Nodule

B

likelihood for postoperative air leak. Typically, there is no need to cauterize any bleeding sites along the staple line. For particularly friable lung, we use a reinforced stapler (staplers may be reinforced with pericardium or synthetic material). Staple lines that appear weak or that are bleeding may be reinforced with a knife-lacking stapler.

Chest tube drainage is optional and depends on the health of the lung and the patient. We tend to be very conservative and leave a chest tube in place when there is any question rather than place a chest tube postoperatively.

Spontaneous Pneumothorax (Fig. 23.3)

Technical Points

Three ports are placed in the following locations: low anterior axillary line for the video port, third to fourth intercostal space in the midaxillary line, and high middle back between the scapula and the posterior spinous process. Thoroughly inspect the pulmonary space for bullous disease because missed bullae represent one of the most common causes of recurrence. Bullous disease is most common at the apex of the upper lobe, followed by the superior segment of the lower lobe, the tail of the right middle lobe, and the base of the lower lobe adjacent to the inferior pulmonary ligament. The diseased lung must be treated as well as the pleural space to achieve optimal results.

After all bullous disease has been identified, judicious resection (using the stapling device) is performed. In most young patients, the apex of the lung is all that is necessary to be resected, although we have been referred recurrent

FIGURE 23.3
SPONTANEOUS PNEUMOTHORAX

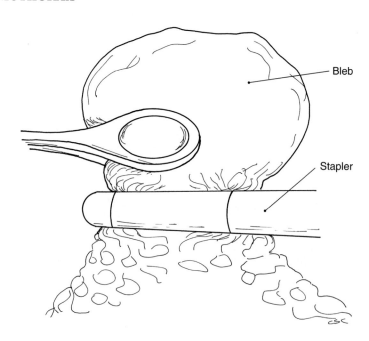

Bleb

Stapler

pneumothorax patients with disease in the other locations who were successfully treated with repeat thoracoscopy.

After resecting all bullous disease, remove or abrade the apical parietal pleural. We prefer to remove the parietal pleura from the fourth rib level to the apex.

Place a chest tube to the apex. Leave this tube on suction for 48 hours for maximal adherence of the lung to the exposed intrapleural chest wall. Patients rarely require chest tube suctioning for more than 3 days. The recurrence rate should be less than 2% to 3%.

REFERENCES

1. Deshmukh SP, Krasna MJ, McLauglin JS. Video assisted thoracoscopic biopsy for interstitial lung disease. *Int Surg* 1996;81:330–332.
2. Kakuda J, Omari B, Renslo R, et al. CT guided needle localization for video thoracoscopic resection of pulmonary nodules. *Eur J Med Res* 1997;2:340–342.
3. Loddenkemper R. Thoracoscopy: state of the art. *Eur Respir J* 1998; 11:213–221.
4. Yim AP, Liu HP. Video assisted thoracoscopic management of primary spontaneous pneumothorax. *Surg Laparosc Endosc* 1997;7:236–240.

CHAPTER 24

Right and Left Pneumonectomy

M. Victoria Gerken and Phillip C. Camp

Pneumonectomy is most commonly performed for carcinoma of the lung or for removal of trapped and necrotic lung following cavitary diseases. In this chapter, the operations of right and left pneumonectomy are described, and the hilar anatomy of the right and left lung is illustrated.

Right Pneumonectomy

Exposure of the Hilum and Division of the Pulmonary Artery (Fig. 24.1)

Technical Points

Enter the chest in the fourth or fifth intercostal space, using a standard posterolateral thoracotomy incision. Examine the mediastinum and hilum to confirm that the diseased area does not extend into the mediastinum, chest wall, or apex and is thus resectable. Retract the lung inferiorly to reveal the superior hilum. Inferior to the azygos vein, dissect the pleura carefully at the apex with Metzenbaum scissors or electrocautery.

Identify and mobilize the main pulmonary artery by careful blunt dissection with a "peanut" dissector. Pass a large right-angled clamp carefully around the artery in preparation for double ligation. For security, first tie the proximal pulmonary artery with heavy silk (usually number 1). Place a transfixion suture ligature (usually one size smaller than the freehand tie) just distal to the freehand tie. Control the distal end of

the artery (specimen side) with a freehand tie and divide the pulmonary artery. Alternatively, a linear stapler with vascular staples is an expedient way to secure the proximal side of this large, fragile vessel.

Anatomic Points

Review the location of mediastinal structures and the relationships of major structures in the root of the lung before surgery. Mediastinal structures of concern include the azygos vein, superior vena cava, phrenic and vagus nerves, and esophagus. The unpaired azygos vein provides a reliable landmark, for the superior aspect of the right hilum. This vein, lying on the side of the thoracic vertebral bodies, drains the right intercostal spaces and receives the termination of the hemiazygos vein on the left, then arches anteriorly to enter the superior vena cava immediately superior to the hilum of the lung. The right bronchial vein, which drains the lung parenchyma, also empties into the azygos vein. Division of the azygos vein, if necessary, is permissible owing to the abundant collateral venous return of the chest wall.

The right pulmonary artery lies immediately anterior to the right main-stem bronchus and is the first hilar structure to be encountered as dissection proceeds from above downward. The superior vena cava, just inferior to the termination of the azygos vein, is still extrapericardial. It is immediately anterior to the right pulmonary artery.

LIST OF STRUCTURES

Mediastinum	Right lung	Left lung
Azygos vein	Right pulmonary artery	Inferior pulmonary ligament
Hemiazygos vein	Right main-stem bronchus	Left pulmonary artery
Accessory hemiazygos vein	Right superior pulmonary vein	Left superior pulmonary vein
Superior vena cava	Right inferior pulmonary vein	Left inferior pulmonary vein
Phrenic nerve	Bronchial arteries	Left main-stem bronchus
Pericardiophrenic artery	Right bronchial vein	
Vagus nerve		
Recurrent laryngeal nerve		
Esophagus		
Aorta		
Pericardium		

ORIENTATION

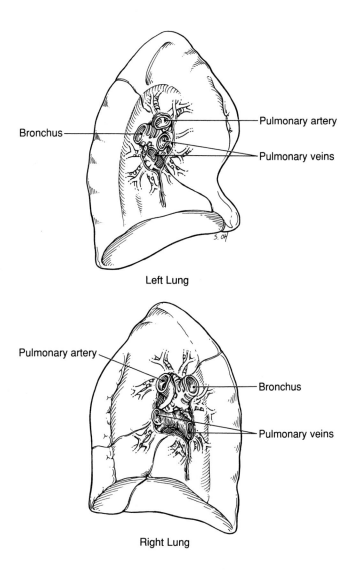

Bronchus — — Pulmonary artery

— Pulmonary veins

Left Lung

Pulmonary artery —

— Bronchus

— Pulmonary veins

Right Lung

Division of the Superior and Inferior Pulmonary Veins (Fig. 24.2)

Technical Points

Attention is now directed to the anterior mediastinum. Divide the pleura sharply as it reflects on the lung. This line of dissection should be well posterior to the phrenic nerve. With careful blunt dissection, clean off the superior pulmonary vein. Place a large clamp around the vein close to the pericardium. Again, use either staples or suture to ligate the vein securely. The vascular stapler allows the advantage of making a single pass around the vessel to create a division. Distal control must frequently be obtained at the level of the branches in order to leave enough space for division of the vessel (Fig. 24.2C).

Retract the lung anteriorly and superiorly to identify the inferior pulmonary ligament. Incise this carefully up to the level of the inferior pulmonary vein; secure and divide this vein in a manner similar to that used for the superior vein. Division of this ligament with retraction of the lung superiorly will yield exposure of the distal esophagus. Obtain hemostasis by means of electrocautery.

Anatomic Points

The right phrenic nerve and accompanying pericardiophrenic artery lie in the mediastinal adventitia adherent to the superior vena cava and pericardial sac. They are the only longitudinal structures passing anterior to the root of the lung. Careful retraction of the lung and its associated tissues should

FIGURE 24.1
EXPOSURE OF THE HILUM AND DIVISION OF THE PULMONARY ARTERY

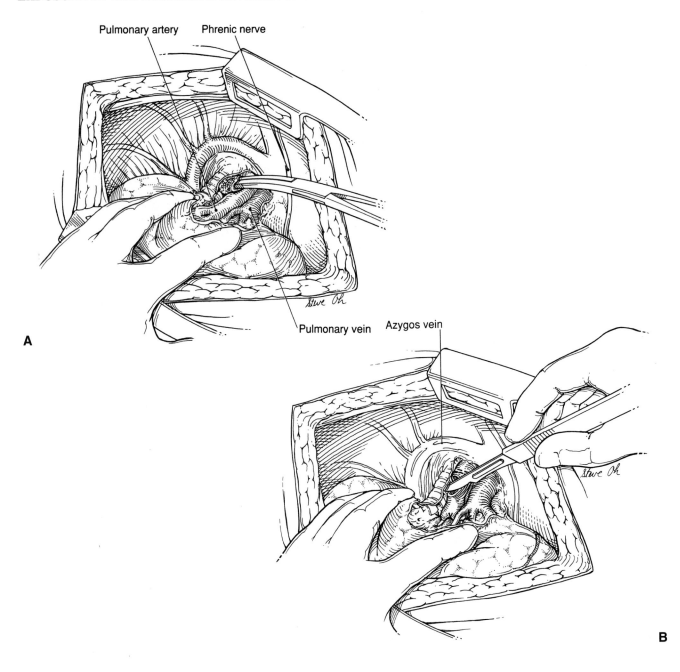

A

B

not include the phrenic nerve because it is in a different tissue plane.

The vagus nerve in the superior mediastinum is closely associated with the trachea. In the vicinity of the tracheal bifurcation, the main part of this nerve passes posteriorly to continue through the mediastinum in association with the esophagus. It could conceivably be damaged if the azygos vein is divided because it lies between the azygos vein and trachea/left bronchus. In addition, the initial retraction of the lung, which is necessary to gain adequate access to the hilum

of the lung, can cause "tenting" of the vagus secondary to vagal contributions to the pulmonary plexuses.

The esophagus and the accompanying right vagus nerve are posterior to the hilum. Inferior to the hilum, the mediastinal side of the pulmonary ligament is immediately anterior to the esophagus.

The pulmonary vessels—both arteries and veins—are comparatively fragile. Abundant lymph nodes, loose connective tissue, and autonomic nerve fibers surround the major tubular structures in the hilum. The bronchial arteries,

FIGURE 24.2
DIVISION OF THE SUPERIOR AND INFERIOR PULMONARY VEINS

A

Inferior pulmonary vein

B

C

which supply the lung parenchyma and bronchi, will probably not be identified, but the fact that they and their ramifications are closely associated with the bronchial tree should be remembered.

Within the hilum of the right lung, pulmonary veins are most anterior, and their identification is facilitated by the fact that their course is predominately inferomedial. The course of the intermediately disposed pulmonary artery is predomi-

nately transverse, and the course of the bronchus, most posterior in the hilum, is superolateral.

Division of the Bronchus (Fig. 24.3)

Technical Points

Incise the rest of the pleural reflection inferiorly and posteriorly. This will reveal the bronchus as the only remaining

FIGURE 24.3
DIVISION OF THE BRONCHUS

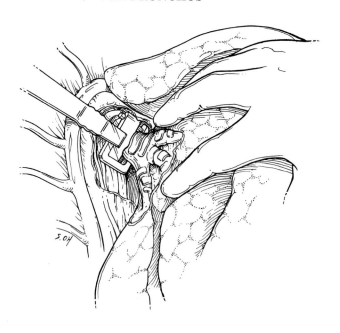

connection. To seal the bronchus securely, clean most adhering connective tissue off by means of blunt sweeping and modest electrocautery. Avoid excessive cleaning of the bronchus because this may cause devascularization of the stump. Moreover, the complications of dehiscence and bronchopleural fistula may result. Silk suture closure of the bronchus has been used successfully for years; however, the marked reduction in the incidence of bronchopleural fistulas that has accompanied the introduction of the stapling device makes the latter the technique of choice. The apposition of the curved bronchial cartilage squarely against the membranous bronchus is key to a successful bronchial closure. Test the stapled bronchial closure for adequacy by filling the hemithorax with sterile saline and inflating the other lung to a pressure of 30 to 40 cm H_2O. Any air leak from the bronchial stump must be addressed by reclosure and patching with a muscle flap.

If possible, stitch a small flap of pleura over the bronchial closure. After irrigation and hemostasis, close the chest without chest tubes. Place a small catheter into the chest, and remove air that is extubated. This allows equalization of pressures. Obtain a "stat" chest film to ensure that the mediastinal structures are indeed in the midline. If much purulence is encountered within the chest, or if hemostasis is difficult owing to coagulopathy (e.g., from trauma), it may be necessary to drain the hemithorax. In these cases, connect the chest tubes to a "balanced suction" system (usually a three-bottle setup) to control carefully the amount of negative suction exerted on the hemithorax throughout the respiratory cycle in order to keep the mediastinal contents in the midline.

Occasionally, the proximity of tumor or the presence of an inflammatory disease may dictate exposure of the pulmonary vessels within the pericardium before they can be safely ligated. To do this, open the pericardium just anterior to the hilum and posterior to the phrenic nerve. This will provide excellent exposure of the vessels, which can then be ligated individually.

Anatomic Points

The azygos vein is very constant in position as it crosses from the posterior mediastinum to the superior vena cava just cephalad to the hilum. This vessel was used as a landmark by the thoracic surgeons in the days of tuberculosis surgery; they relied on it to "predict" the pulmonary artery as they dissected the dense adhesions in the apex.

The phrenic nerve runs on the surface of the pericardium anterior to the hilar structures of the lung. The vagus runs in the posterior mediastinum, usually lying directly on the esophagus.

Left Pneumonectomy

Anatomy of the Left Lung and Left Pneumonectomy (Fig. 24.4)

Technical Points

Enter the left chest in the fourth or fifth intercostal space and place retractors. Examine the diseased area for resectability, and then retract the lung inferiorly to reveal the superior hilum. Divide the pleura and clean the pulmonary artery by means of blunt dissection. Divide the artery with a stapler, or suture as described previously. Retract the lung posteriorly and divide the anterior pleura, staying posterior to the phrenic nerve. Clean the superior vein, ligate it, and divide it.

With retraction of the lung superiorly, place tension on the inferior pulmonary ligament and divide it to the level of the inferior pulmonary vein. Next, divide the inferior pulmonary vein. The bronchus is then well exposed. Clean it to a satisfactory (but not excessive) degree, and divide it with a stapler. Check the stapled closure for adequacy by filling the hemithorax with sterile saline and inflating the remaining lung with air to a pressure of 30 to 40 cm H_2O. Address any air leak from the bronchial closure. The pleura can frequently be closed over the hilar structures after hemostasis has been obtained.

As described earlier, after closure of the chest, aspirate air from the hemithorax to preclude a shift of the mediastinum away from midline.

Anatomic Points

Mediastinal structures of note on the left include the accessory hemiazygos and hemiazygos veins and their connections, the vagus nerve and its recurrent laryngeal branch, the phrenic nerve, the aorta, and the esophagus. Note, on the left, there is no azygos vein crossing superior to the hilum. Upon examination, the hemiazygos vein can be identified, although its course differs from that of the azygos vein. Remember that, in the left chest, the longitudinal veins that drain the intercostal spaces and receive the bronchial veins are part of the hemiazygos and accessory hemiazygos system. In addition to communicating with the azygos vein on the right, there usually is a large communication with the left superior intercostal vein at a level approximating the roots of the left common carotid and subclavian arteries. This venous system provides no landmark for the surgeon. The left vagus nerve, lying in the interval between the left common carotid artery and subclavian artery, should be identified and followed inferiorly to cross the left side of the arch of the aorta. On the underside of the arch, its recurrent laryngeal branch, which is closely associated with the ligamentum arteriosum, should also be noted. In this location, it can be injured during left pneumonectomy, especially if care is not taken in cleaning the pulmonary artery before placement of the vascular stapler. The left vagus then runs inferiorly between the left pulmonary artery and the aorta, ultimately passing out of the operative field by associating with the esophagus, which here is posterior to the pericardium and to the right of the aorta. It can be avoided with a minimum of difficulty. The descending aorta is readily apparent and easily avoided during pneumonectomy.

FIGURE 24.4
ANATOMY OF THE LEFT LUNG AND LEFT PNEUMONECTOMY

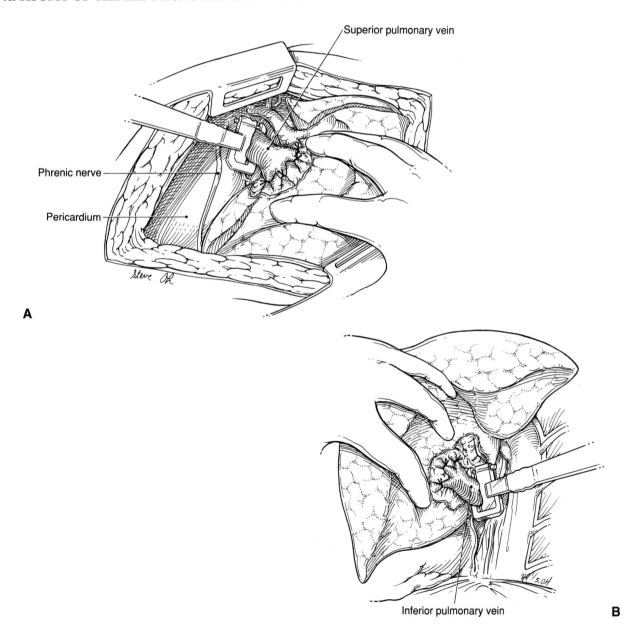

A

B

FIGURE 24.4 (Continued)

C

Recurrent laryngeal nerve

Vagus nerve

D

The esophagus can frequently be identified after division of the inferior pulmonary ligament.

The phrenic nerve, which is anterior to the common carotid artery and thus anterior to the vagus nerve, is closely associated with perivascular tissue and adventitia of the pericardium, not with adventitia of the lung. It is well anterior to the necessary dissection. Like its counterpart on the right, it is the only longitudinal structure that is anterior to the root of the lung.

A review of structures in the hilum of the lung again should be prefaced by noting the abundance of hilar lymph nodes,

autonomic nerve fibers, and adventitia. The small bronchial arteries, associated with the peribronchial adventitia, should also be noted.

In the hilum of the lung, the main pulmonary artery is superior to the bronchus and pulmonary vein. On this side, it is quite evident that the pulmonary artery is initially anterior and then curves over the bronchus before it divides. The pulmonary veins, like those on the right, are anterior and inferior in the hilum, whereas the bronchus is posterior. As on the right side, it should again be noted that pulmonary arteries and veins are comparatively fragile.

REFERENCES

1. Hood RM. *Techniques in general thoracic surgery.* Philadelphia: WB Saunders, 1985.
2. Ravitch MM, Steichen FM. *Atlas of general thoracic surgery.* Philadelphia: WB Saunders, 1988.
3. Sabiston DC, Spencer FC, eds. *Gibbon's surgery of the chest.* 4th ed. Philadelphia: WB Saunders, 1983.

CHAPTER 25

Lobectomy

Phillip C. Camp and M. Victoria Gerken

Pulmonary lobectomies are most commonly performed for carcinoma. Resection of a more limited amount of pulmonary tissue allows preservation of the maximum amount of lung function. Even more limited segmental and subsegmental resections are possible and are described in the references at the end.

Right Upper Lobectomy

Ligation of the Pulmonary Arteries (Fig. 25.1)

Technical Points

Secure the left endobronchial double-lumen tube, allowing single-lung ventilation for the duration of the resection. Place the patient in the left lateral decubitus position and make a right posterolateral thoracotomy. A muscle-sparing thoracotomy is a feasible alternative but should never be allowed to hinder the resection.

Retract the lung inferiorly and posteriorly and divide the pleura around the hilum.

Identify the superior pulmonary vein and dissect along it distally up to the lung parenchyma. Mobilize around the vessel in the appropriate plane. Identify and preserve the middle lobe vein, which typically enters the superior pulmonary vein. Be alert to aberrant venous drainage, including occasional direct connections to the vena cava.

The pulmonary artery lies just posterior and superior to the vein (Fig. 25.1A). Gently develop the appropriate plane, and dissect proximally and distally. The pulmonary artery is an extremely delicate and unforgiving vessel. Great care and attention to detail will aid in successful mobilization. Mobilize circumferentially and place an umbilical tape loosely around it to provide proximal control should bleeding occur.

Distal dissection will identify the truncus anterior (apicoanterior) branch. Dissection should be circumferential and should avoid spreading of surrounding tissue. Gently passing a blunt curved clamp can help define planes. *Never* pass the clamp against resistance. "Peanut" dissection is often useful for better defining the anatomy once you are in the correct plane. Free the pulmonary artery from the upper lobe branches and any attachments to the azygos vein.

Retract the lung anteriorly and incise the pleura overlying the bifurcation of the upper lobe bronchus and bronchus intermedius. Careful use of electrocautery will control small bronchial vessels in this area. Reliably, a lymph node is located at this point and is swept anteriorly. Anterior to the lymph node is the superior segment branch of the pulmonary artery to the lower lobe, which is much better seen from this aspect than by the anterior approach. Once you have identified this branch, any intact portion of the posterior aspect of the major fissure can be completed (divided) with staplers.

LIST OF STRUCTURES

Right main pulmonary artery
  Superior branch
  Posterior segmental artery
Right superior pulmonary vein
  Branches to anterior and apical
    segments
  Posterior segmental vein
Right inferior pulmonary vein
Right upper lobe bronchus
Intermediate bronchus
  Middle lobe bronchus
  Right lower lobe bronchus

Major fissure
Minor fissure
Middle lobe
Inferior pulmonary ligament
Left pulmonary artery
  Arteries to the apicoposterior
    segment
  Anterior segmental artery
  Lingular artery
  Branch to the superior segment of
    the lower lobe
  Basilar segmental artery

Left inferior pulmonary vein
Left superior pulmonary vein
  Apicoposterior segmental vein
  Lingular segmental veins
  Anterior basal segmental vein
Left lower lobe bronchus
Left upper lobe bronchus

ORIENTATION

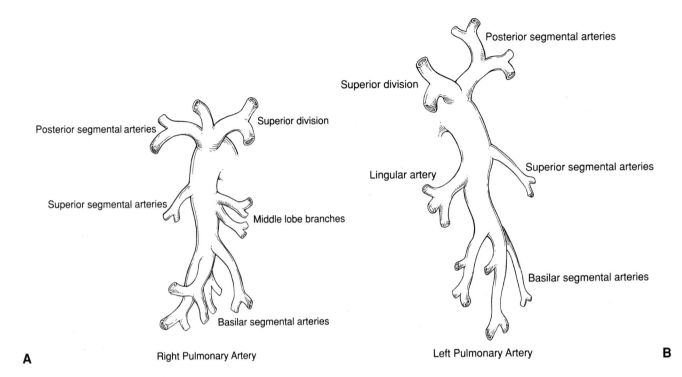

Posterior segmental arteries

Superior division

Posterior segmental arteries

Superior division

Superior segmental arteries

Lingular artery

Middle lobe branches

Superior segmental arteries

Basilar segmental arteries

Basilar segmental arteries

A   Right Pulmonary Artery

Left Pulmonary Artery   **B**

This posterior approach to the superior segment branch greatly improves the anatomic division and is rather efficient (Fig. 25.1B).

Divide the apical segmental vein, crossing the anterior segmental artery, either with vascular staples or with suture ligatures.

Mobilize and divide the superior arterial trunk with a vascular stapler or suture ligature. Ligate apical and segmental branches.

Anatomic Points

Remember that the azygos vein arches from posterior to anterior immediately superior to the root of the right lung, and that, at least conceptually, the plane of the major pulmonary veins is anterior to that of the arteries. The right pulmonary artery, at the point where it leaves the pericardial sac, is anterior and somewhat inferior to the right main-stem bronchus. It enters the minor fissure and passes inferolaterally anterior to the upper lobe bronchus. Slightly before it enters the minor fissure, it gives off a superior branch from its superior aspect, which can supply all three segments of the upper lobe. Frequently, however, the superior trunk supplies only the apical and anterior segments, whereas the posterior segment is supplied by an ascending artery that branches off the superior aspect of the main pulmonary artery, somewhat distal to the superior branch.

Division of Remaining Vascular Attachments (Fig. 25.2)

Technical Points

Next, divide the superior pulmonary vein with a vascular stapler or suture ligatures. With the vein divided, the distal pulmonary artery is readily visualized posteriorly. Identify the middle lobe branch and posterior segment branches of the pulmonary artery. Using these as landmarks, identify the (usually poorly defined) minor fissure and divide it with a linear stapler.

The remaining pulmonary artery branch, the posterior ascending branch (present in 90% of cases), can be approached from multiple directions but most easily in a retrograde fashion.

Anatomic Points

Remember that there is a superior and inferior pulmonary vein draining the right lung and emptying independently into the left atrium. Sometimes, the middle lobe vein can open independently into the left atrium, although it usually empties into the inferior aspect of the superior pulmonary vein.

As the superior pulmonary vein lies anterior to the pulmonary artery, it is most easily visualized anteriorly. It always drains the apical and posterior segments of the upper lobe, and usually drains the anterior segment. However, the anterior segmental vein can drain into the middle lobe vein.

FIGURE 25.1
LIGATION OF THE PULMONARY ARTERIES

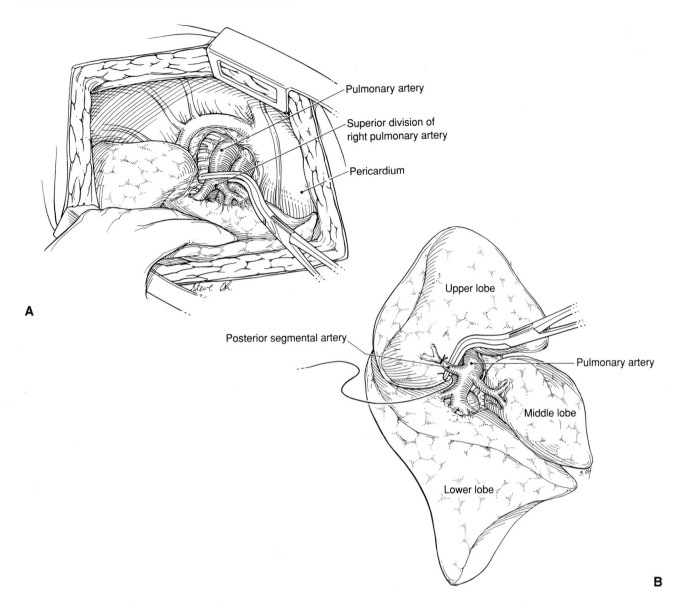

The superior division is the first branch of the pulmonary artery; it divides to form the branches to the apical and anterior segments. The posterior is the next branch and is usually about 1 to 2 cm above the branches to the middle lobe and the superior segment of the lower lobe.

The superior pulmonary vein drains both the upper and the middle lobes. Its branching is not always constant, but the variations are easily seen and handled.

Division of Bronchus and Remaining Vascular
Pedicle (Fig. 25.3)

Technical Points

Retract the lung anteriorly. Divide branches of the vagus nerve to the upper lobe. Dissect the upper lobe bronchus free from surrounding tissue, recalling that the remaining arterial

branch is just deep to the bronchus. The bronchus can then be divided with a linear stapler loaded with a 4.8-mm cartridge. With the divided upper lobe bronchus gently retracted upward, the posterior ascending artery is gently dissected free of areolar tissue and divided. The remaining intact fissures are then divided between linear staplers. Anchor the middle lobe to the lower lobe to avoid torsion, a potentially disastrous complication. Divide the inferior pulmonary ligament to allow the remaining lobes to fill the thoracic cavity.

After hemostasis has been achieved, examine the stapled bronchial closure for adequacy by filling the hemithorax with sterile saline and inflating the lungs to a sustained pressure of about 30 to 40 cm H_2O. Small air bubbles arising from the parenchyma along the fissure are acceptable, but a major air loss from the bronchus, although rare, must be addressed by reclosure of the bronchial stump or use of a muscle flap. Place

FIGURE 25.2
DIVISION OF REMAINING VASCULAR ATTACHMENTS

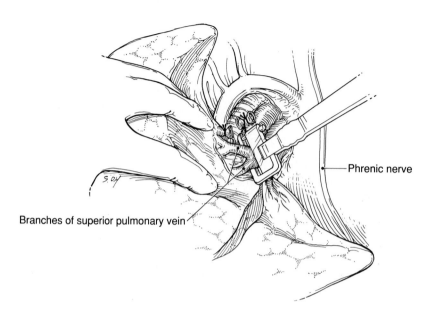

Phrenic nerve

Branches of superior pulmonary vein

two chest tubes. Place the anterior tube with the tip almost in the apex of the chest. Place the posterior tube (usually a right-angled tube) in such a way as to drain the posterior sulcus. Close the chest in standard fashion.

Anatomic Points

The bronchus to the upper lobe is at almost a 90-degree angle to the main stem. This makes appropriate placement of the linear stapler easy.

The major fissure is usually complete, but occasionally, there will be adhesion of the superior segment of the lower lobe to the upper lobe. The minor fissure is more variable, with incomplete development being relatively common.

In the mediastinum and hilum of the lung, the bronchi are the most posterior major structures; the small bronchial arteries and veins are intimately related to the posterior surface of the bronchial apparatus. Care must be taken when dividing the pleural reflection to expose the bronchial tree because the right vagus nerve, associated with the esophagus, is just

FIGURE 25.3
DIVISION OF BRONCHUS AND REMAINING VASCULAR PEDICLE

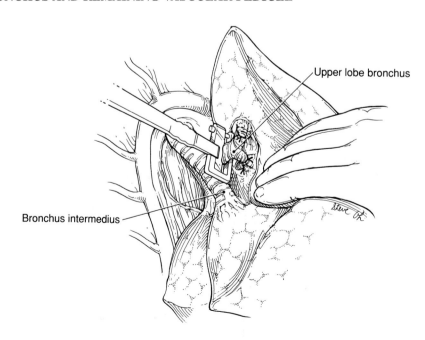

Upper lobe bronchus

Bronchus intermedius

posterior to the line of pleural division. The upper lobe bronchus arises laterally, at about a 90-degree angle, from the main bronchus. The main bronchus, past this point, is referred to as the *bronchus intermedius* and gives rise to the middle and lower lobe bronchi.

Right Middle Lobectomy

Right Middle Lobectomy (Fig. 25.4)

Technical Points

It is rarely necessary to perform a middle lobectomy as a sole procedure. In the preantibiotic era, middle lobectomy was often performed for bronchiectasis. Middle lobectomy is now most often performed in conjunction with resection of the right upper or lower lobe as a bilobectomy for malignant disease.

Enter the right chest in the fifth intercostal space. Begin dissection at the confluence of the major and the minor fissures. Here, the pulmonary artery is readily identified, and the middle lobe branch directly opposes the branch to the superior segment of the lower lobe. Occasionally, there will be two branches to the middle lobe coming directly off the pulmonary artery. However, more commonly, there is only one, which quickly bifurcates. Divide and ligate this. Retract the lung posteriorly and divide the anterior mediastinal pleura posterior to the phrenic nerve. Visualize the superior pulmonary vein. Identify, ligate, and divide the branches draining the middle lobe.

Examine both fissures. Usually, the major fissure is quite well developed and needs only minimal dissection to separate the middle from the lower lobe. The minor fissure is frequently incomplete, however, and must be developed with the TA-60 or the TA-90 linear stapler. With a finger, create a hole for passage of the stapler from the area of arterial dissection through to the anterior mediastinum. Take great care to avoid the upper lobe branches of the superior pulmonary vein, which are in close proximity.

Clean the bronchus, and then place the stapler and close it. Before firing the stapler, fully inflate the lung to ensure that the position of the stapler will not interfere with aeration of the basal segments. Secure the upper and lower lobes with one or two silk ties.

FIGURE 25.4
RIGHT MIDDLE LOBECTOMY

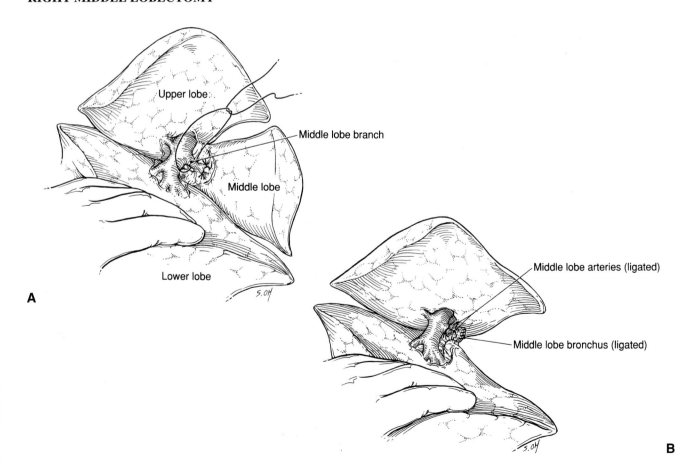

A

B

Obtain hemostasis and check the bronchial closure for adequacy, as described earlier. Place chest tubes and close the chest.

Anatomic Points

The arterial supply is easily identified rising anteriorly off the pulmonary trunk. Although it is usually a single vessel, it may occasionally arise directly off the pulmonary artery as two or three branches. Gentle distal dissection will readily provide adequate exposure.

The pulmonary venous branches draining the middle lobe flow into the superior pulmonary vein. This vein is at greatest risk for injury not during ligation of the appropriate branches, but rather during development of an incomplete minor fissure with the stapler.

Right Lower Lobectomy

Right Lower Lobectomy (Fig. 25.5)

Technical and Anatomic Points

Right lower lobectomy is probably the easiest type of lobectomy to perform. Enter the right chest in the fifth or sixth intercostal space. Begin the dissection at the confluence of the fissures, and identify the pulmonary artery. The interlobular artery lies deep in the region of the confluence of the oblique and horizontal fissures. Exposure is augmented by superior retraction of the upper lobe and inferior retraction of the lower lobe. Stapled completion of the fissures is to be avoided before identifying the artery. The visceral pleura is opened over the interlobular artery, and the pulmonary artery is mobilized. The superior segmental branch lies directly across from the

FIGURE 25.5
RIGHT LOWER LOBECTOMY

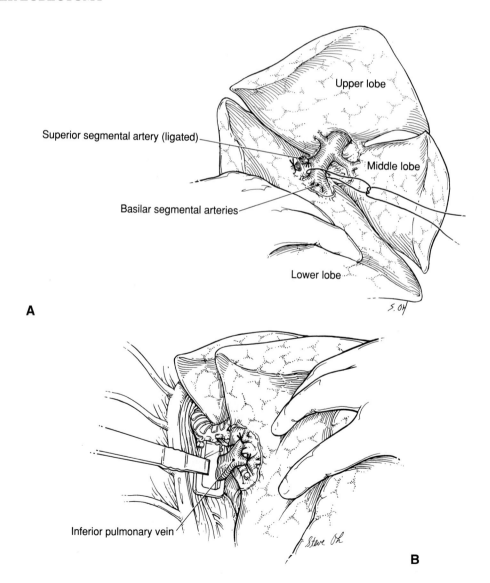

middle lobe branch and, hence, must be separately ligated and divided. After this, the basilar segmental artery can usually be ligated and divided as a unit. Perform ligation with a freehand silk tie and transfixion stitch or with the TA-30 vascular stapler.

Next, retract the lung anteriorly and superiorly. Mobilize and divide the inferior pulmonary ligament. Divide the pleural reflection along the inferior half of the hilum to expose the inferior pulmonary vein and bronchus intermedius. Mobilize and divide the inferior pulmonary vein at the pericardial reflection. Take care not to leave a stump of vein because this may promote left atrial clot formation.

Open the posterior mediastinal pleura and identify the bronchus. Clean it and divide it with the stapler, checking before firing to ascertain that the position of the stapler does not interfere with aeration of the middle lobe. Rarely, it may be necessary to protect the middle lobe by stapling the bronchus to the superior segment of the lower lobe separately.

Occasionally, it may be necessary to complete the major fissure with the stapler. As with the upper lobectomy, the minor fissure must then be checked to rule out potential torsion of the middle lobe. Silk stitches can be placed to anchor the two lobes; however, this is seldom necessary.

After adequate hemostasis has been obtained and bronchial closure is found to be airtight, place chest tubes, and close the chest.

Left Upper Lobectomy

Left Upper Lobectomy (Fig. 25.6)

Technical Points

Left lobectomies are performed under left single-lung ventilation. Place the patient in a right lateral decubitus position and approach the lung through a left posterolateral

FIGURE 25.6
LEFT UPPER LOBECTOMY

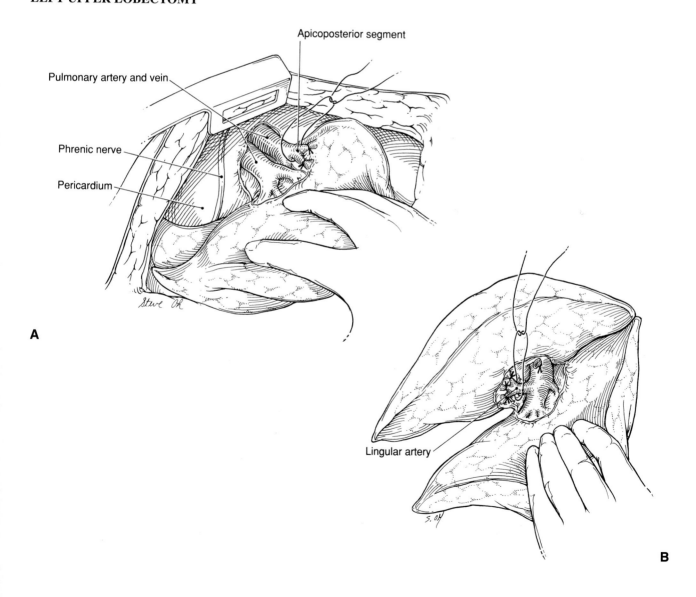

Apicoposterior segment

Pulmonary artery and vein

Phrenic nerve

Pericardium

A

Lingular artery

B

thoracotomy. As with the right-sided approach, a muscle-sparing technique can frequently be used for left pulmonary resections but should never be allowed to hamper the safety of the surgical resection.

Retract the lung inferiorly and open the pleura over the superior hilum to expose the left main pulmonary artery. Proximal control of the pulmonary artery is recommended. Incise the pleura over the medial aspect of the superior pulmonary vein lateral to the pericardium. Posteriorly, the vagus nerve will indicate the posterior-most aspect of the pleural incision.

Gently mobilize the main pulmonary artery from surrounding areolar tissue and define the plane between the artery and the superior pulmonary vein. Following gentle digital dissection, pass a blunt curved clamp around the pulmonary artery and secure an umbilical tape.

Retract the upper lobe anteriorly. Mobilize and divide the pleural reflection along the oblique fissure to expose the pulmonary artery. If the posterior aspect of the oblique fissure is incomplete, use a linear stapler to divide the remaining intact parenchyma. With this done, the pulmonary artery and its branches are exposed.

As the midportion of the exposed artery is gently dissected, the posterior segmental arteries are noted opposite the superior segmental artery. Furthermore, more distal dissection along the pulmonary artery exposes the lingular artery (which may be multiple). Dissection along the artery is adequate once the basilar segmental branches to the lower lobe are clearly identified.

Continued upper lobe superior retraction allows adequate exposure. The lingular branches are then mobilized, double-ligated, and divided. Gentle clockwise rotation of the upper lobe then leads to mobilization, ligation, and division of the posterior segmental arteries in a similar fashion. Occasionally, the row of vessels can be group-ligated with an endoscopic vascular stapler.

Attention is finally drawn to the apicoposterior segmental branches arising from the convex surface of the proximal pulmonary artery. The branches are often quite short but can often be successfully divided with a vascular stapler. If not, then careful double ligation and sharp division will suffice. Roll the pulmonary artery away from the bronchus to rule out any aberrant vascular branches.

Retract the lung posteriorly. Identify the superior pulmonary vein and clean it for an appropriate length. The proximal end can be ligated safely with a vascular stapler, but the distal branches should be ligated with silk before division of the vessel.

Retract the upper lobe anteriorly to expose the bronchus, which should be in clear view. Apply the stapler, inflating the lung after closure of the stapler jaws. Delay its firing until the left lower lobe bronchus is checked by adequate inflation of the lung.

Divide the inferior pulmonary ligament with electrocautery, allowing free expansion of the lower lobe to fill the hemithorax.

Test the bronchial closure by filling the hemithorax with sterile saline and inflating the lungs to a pressure of 30 cm H_2O. Significant air leaks must be repaired. After adequate hemostasis is attained, place chest tubes and close the chest.

Anatomic Points

Unlike on the right side, the most superior major structure in the root of the lung is the pulmonary artery. Visualization of this artery requires division of the superior aspect of the pleural reflection; care must be taken to avoid the phrenic nerve, which runs anterior to the root of the lung, and the left vagus and its recurrent branch, which lies very close to the pulmonary artery. The main-stem bronchus is posteroinferior to the artery, whereas the superior pulmonary vein is anteroinferior to the artery, and just anterior to the bronchus. However, as on the right side, the inferior pulmonary vein is the most inferior major structure in the root of the lung.

The number of arteries supplying the upper lobe varies between three and seven. The most common pattern is three branches arising from the left pulmonary artery. The branch to the anterior segment arises near the anterior surface of the mediastinum, whereas the branch to the apicoposterior segment and the branch to the two lingular lobes lie near the interlobar pleura and are best visualized posteriorly. Because the anatomy is so variable, it is important to examine the length of the pulmonary artery carefully before stapling the bronchus in order to identify any aberrant arteries that may remain unligated.

Because the veins are anteriorly located, the best approach for visualization is anterior. The veins tend to parallel the arteries and are dispersed on a vertical line near the surface of the anterior root of the lung. Typically, the apicoposterior segmental vein is single and drains independently into the superior pulmonary vein, as does the anterior segmental vein. By contrast, the lingular segmental veins usually unite before emptying into the superior pulmonary vein. The surgeon should be aware that a vein draining the anterior basal segment might drain into a lingular vein rather than into the inferior pulmonary vein. The superior pulmonary vein on the left is a mixed blessing. Because the lingula is not a separate lobe, the vessel may be ligated close to the heart without the necessity of dissecting individual branches, as must be done on the right. However, the superior pulmonary vein lies directly on the bronchus and in close proximity to the origin of the left pulmonary artery. In the presence of a dense inflammatory process, great care must be taken in cleaning off this vessel if disaster is to be avoided.

The upper lobe bronchus, like its corresponding lobar bronchus on the right, arises from the main bronchus at approximately right angles. Anterior retraction of the upper lobe facilitates visualization of this bronchus because the bronchial tree is the most posterior major structure in the hilum. It should be remembered that the small bronchial arteries and veins are intimately associated with the posterior surfaces of the major bronchi.

As on the right, the phrenic and vagus nerves can usually be easily identified well away from the dissection site. The recurrent laryngeal nerve is at risk for injury (as discussed in the section on left pneumonectomy in Chapter 24).

Left Lower Lobectomy

Left Lower Lobectomy (Fig. 25.7)

Technical Points

In the setting of a complete oblique fissure, the left lower lobectomy is likely the simplest of all the pleural resections. Retract the lung anteriorly, allowing incision of the pleura from the bronchus to the level of the inferior pulmonary ligament. Divide the inferior pulmonary ligament with electrocautery superiorly to the level of the inferior pulmonary vein.

Retract the lower lobe posteriorly and inferiorly while the upper lobe is retracted anteriorly and superiorly. As described in the previous section (left upper lobe resection), divide any remaining fused lung parenchyma along the oblique fissure with a linear stapler.

Carefully open the sheath of the pulmonary artery, and gently mobilize the vessels to the lower lobe. The superior segmental artery arises from posterolateral aspect of the interlobular pulmonary artery, roughly adjacent to the posterior segmental artery of the upper lobe. Dissection is carried down to the level of the basilar arteries.

Doubly tie and divide the superior segmental and basilar arteries, or use a vascular stapler. Take care not to impinge on the vessels to the upper lobe.

Next, mobilize the inferior pulmonary vein, dividing the pleura along the pericardial reflection. Divide the vein with a vascular stapler along its most medial aspect to decreases potential dead space for left atrial clot formation.

After the stapler is applied but not yet fired, check for compromise of the rest of the bronchial tree by inflating the remaining lung. Rarely, it may be necessary to staple

FIGURE 25.7
LEFT LOWER LOBECTOMY

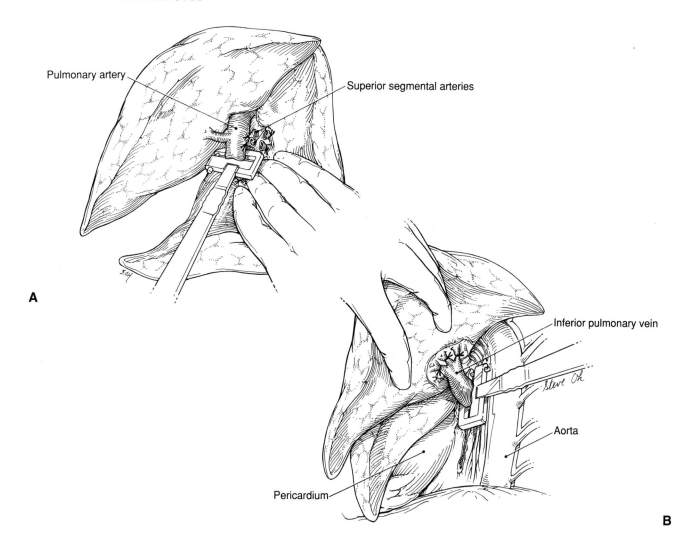

Pulmonary artery

Superior segmental arteries

A

Inferior pulmonary vein

Aorta

Pericardium

B

the bronchus to the superior segment separately and then to staple the bronchus to the basilar segments, in order not to compromise the airway to the lingula.

Examine the hilum and chest for hemostasis, test for bronchial closure as described earlier, and place chest tubes. Then proceed with chest closure.

Anatomic Points

The pulmonary artery is best visualized in the major fissure. Here, the arteries to the upper lobe arise from the superior aspect of the pulmonary artery, whereas those to the lower lobe branch from the inferior and distal aspect of the artery. The branch to the superior segment is almost always separate from the branches to the basal segment and is significantly more proximal than the latter. It usually lies opposite the apicoposterior segmental branch. Either the basal segmental arteries branch from a common trunk or the main artery divides into two trunks, one to the anterior basal segment and the other to the lateral and posterior basal segments. Other arrangements are possible, but these two are the most frequent patterns.

Division of the pulmonary ligament to visualize the inferior pulmonary vein is safer on the left than on the right because the phrenic nerve is at a safe distance anteriorly and the esophagus and aorta are relatively distant posteriorly. Because the inferior pulmonary vein is completely separate from the superior vein, it can be divided rapidly and safely.

The bronchus, as before, is best visualized posteriorly. However, it is immediately posterior to the superior pulmonary vein, which crosses at about a right angle.

REFERENCES

1. Ravitch MM, Steichen FM. *Atlas of general thoracic surgery.* Philadelphia: WB Saunders, 1988.

2. Sabiston DC, Spencer FC, eds. *Gibbon's surgery of the chest.* 4th ed. Philadelphia: WB Saunders, 1983.

CHAPTER 26

Thoracoscopic Lobectomy, Segmentectomy, or Pneumonectomy

Kemp Kernstine

Thoracoscopic lobectomy or other anatomic thoracoscopic lung resections are performed as described for the other thoracoscopic procedures (see Chapter 23). Allow an extra 30 to 60 minutes for a thoracoscopic approach. The learning curve is significant, and these procedures should only be attempted with a surgeon experienced in this approach. Ideal patients are those with tumor diameters less than 3 cm, tumor not involving the hilar vessels, and minimal hilar scarring and nodal disease. In patients with significant adhesions, poor visibility, and chest wall or hilar-invading tumors, the open technique should be used for resection.

Port Placement (Fig. 26.1)

Technical and Anatomic Points

Typically, five ports are required. The resected specimen is removed through the axillary port, which is usually extended to 4 to 5 cm once the decision to perform a thoracoscopic procedure has been made. We place two posterior ports that are used for retraction and three anterior ports for dissection and visualization, although any of the ports can be used for dissection, retraction, or visualization. The lower three anterior ports are placed along the anterior axillary line; the first is a video port placed at the sixth to seventh intercostal space and the second in the midchest level. The third and most superior port is placed in the midaxillary line at the axillary hair line, typically at the second to third intercostal space. It is through this port that the specimen will be delivered, and it may need to be enlarged to perform this function. The two posterior ports are placed 10 to 15 cm apart and are in the line of the middle distance between the posterior portion of the scapula and the posterior spinous processes. For upper lobes, these posterior ports are somewhat higher than for inferior lobes. After the ports are placed, any of them can be used for video examination or dissection.

Dissection of Hilar Structures (Fig. 26.2)

Technical Points

The venous drainage is identified first, regardless of which portion of the lung is to be removed. It is essential to ascertain that venous drainage to the rest of the lung is normal and adequate. Although it is rare, some patients may have venous anatomy that is insufficient for the remaining lung. Once this has been determined, dissect the vein free, close to the pericardium. Pass a Semb dissector around the vein, taking great care to avoid injury to the pulmonary artery beneath it for upper and middle lobes, and cephalad to it for lower lobes. Next pass a silk tie around the vein to hold the dissected area open for the later passage of a vascular endoscopic stapling device.

Divide the vein with an endoscopic linear stapler loaded with 2.5-mm staples.

We use a plastic Yankauer suction device and an endoscopic "peanut" to dissect the adjacent pulmonary artery. Through the posterior ports, place ring forceps or endoscopic retracting instruments to retract the lung parenchyma and place the pulmonary artery on stretch. Exercise great care because too much retraction may avulse the pulmonary artery. After identifying the branches of the pulmonary artery, encircle it with Semb clamp, and then silk tie as previously noted. Use an endoscopic vascular stapler to divide the pulmonary artery. Clips are not recommended because they can get caught in the stapling devices, resulting in staple misfiring. Once the vessels have been resected, resect the associated lymph nodes with an endoscopic peanut dissector and shears.

Anatomic Points

Variations in the arterial anatomy must be considered when performing the arterial resections. For the right upper lobe, the bifurcation of the upper lobe artery and the intermedius artery can occur well within the hilum in about 5% to 10% of patients. Thus, the main pulmonary artery may be accidentally resected when attempting to resect the right upper lobe artery. Avoid this problem by resecting the vein first, as described. It is mandatory that the intermedius artery be identified. Identify and divide the recurrent branch separately lest it be avulsed during the division of the fissure or cause significant bleeding at the parenchymal staple line.

For the left upper lobe, identify the lingular vessels anteriorly along the course of the main, intrahilar pulmonary artery, distal to the superior segment artery.

177

FIGURE 26.1
PORT PLACEMENT

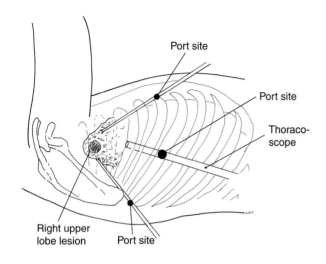

Port site

Port site

Thoraco-
scope

Right upper
lobe lesion

Port site

Completion of Resection (Fig. 26.3)

Technical and Anatomic Points

If the fissure is incomplete, dissect adjacent parenchyma from the vasculature to the remaining lung using the Yankauer suction tip and endoscopic peanut dissector. Then divide the fissure with an endoscopic linear stapler.

It is very easy to lose the three-dimensional perspective at this point. Take extreme care to ensure that the appropriate lung is being resected. In the case of segmentectomy, we pass a TA-60 stapler with a 4.8-mm load to resect the segment. Finally, approach the bronchus. It is easy to divide the wrong bronchus during thorascopic surgery; therefore, it is essential to avoid misidentification by performing both of the following two maneuvers. First, visualize the appropriate bronchus through the endotracheal tube (Fig. 26.3A). The transilluminated segment should be visible through the thoracoscope.

Second, position and close the endoscopic stapler at the proposed point of bronchial transection, but do not fire it.

FIGURE 26.2
DISSECTION OF HILAR STRUCTURES

Right upper
lobe (RUL)

RUL pulmonary
vein

A

B

FIGURE 26.3
COMPLETION OF RESECTION

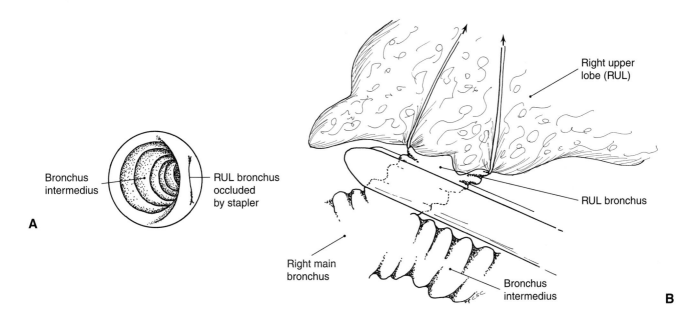

Have the anesthesiologist inflate the lung on the side to be resected. The segment to be resected should not inflate, but the remaining lung should both inflate and deflate without difficulty. It is surprising how easy it is to confuse a main bronchus with a lobar bronchus when performing the final resection. Divide the bronchus using a 3.5-mm stapler for a lobe or 4.1-mm stapler for a main bronchus or thickened airway (Fig. 26.3B).

Carefully dissect all the nodal tissue adjacent to the bronchus away from vital structures and remove it. When dissecting around the bronchial stump, take care to avoid and protect the posterior blood supply to the airway. Do not disturb the integrity of the staple line.

We usually place a single 28- to 32-French chest tube to the apex after lobectomies and segmentectomies. For lower lobectomies and segmentectomies, we also place a right-angled chest tube of the same diameter. Minimal to no suction is placed on these tubes. We do not routinely place chest tubes after pneumonectomies. In cases in which there is a significant amount of mediastinal dissection or there is concern that the chest cavity may fill too rapidly, we place a chest tube overnight—rarely longer.

REFERENCES

1. McKenna R Jr. VATS lobectomy with mediastinal lymph node sampling or dissection. *Chest Surg Clin North Am* 1995;5(2):223–232.

2. Lewis JR, Caccavale RJ. Video-assisted thoracic surgical non-rib spreading simultaneously stapled lobectomy (VATS(n)SSL). *Semin Thorac Cardiovasc Surg* 1998;10(4):332–339.

CHAPTER 27

First Rib Resection for Thoracic Outlet Syndrome

M. Victoria Gerken and Phillip C. Camp

First rib resection is a controversial solution to a complex problem. The term *thoracic outlet syndrome* refers to a variety of symptoms that are usually neurologic but are on occasion vascular and that result from any of a number of anatomic situations. Most patients with thoracic outlet syndrome improve significantly with physical therapy and repetitive behavior avoidance. Only a small number of patients require surgical intervention. When such intervention is indicated, resection of the first rib is the most common approach but is not the only possible procedure. Some authors recommend subperiosteal resection of the first rib in order to reduce the risk for injury to the neurovascular contents; however, leaving the periosteum intact can lead to reformation of a rudimentary rib, which can cause recurrence of the symptoms. In this chapter, complete resection of the first rib and its periosteum is described. For further discussion of the etiology and treatment of this complex condition, the reader is referred to the references. This uncommon procedure is included because it illustrates regional anatomy well.

Position of the Patient and Skin Incision (Fig. 27.1)

Technical Points

Place the patient in the lateral decubitus position, as for standard thoracotomy. Your assistant should support the superior arm at a 90-degree angle from the torso. Flex the patient's arm at the elbow to make it easier for the assistant to support it comfortably. Allow the assistant to relax the position of the arm periodically during the case to prevent undue stress to its neurovascular supply (and to the assistant).

Make a skin incision just under the axillary hairline (usually over the third rib), extending it from the pectoral to the latissimus dorsi muscles. Carry the dissection down to the chest wall. Identify and protect the intercostobrachial nerve.

Anatomic Points

The skin incision described runs from the anterior axillary fold, which is formed by the lower edge of the pectoralis major muscle, to the posterior axillary fold, which is formed by the lateral edge of the latissimus dorsi muscle. The intercostobrachial nerve—the lateral branch of the second intercostal nerve (T2)—pierces the serratus anterior muscle about midway between the anterior and posterior walls of the axilla. It runs laterally across the axilla to join the medial brachial cutaneous nerve and is distributed to the upper part of the medial and posterior arm. Frequently, there are two or three intercostobrachial nerves. When present, these originate from the third and fourth intercostal nerves (T3, T4) and have a similar distribution to the branch arising from T2.

The medial wall of the axilla is formed by the serratus anterior muscle, fascicles of which arise from the first eight or nine ribs. The muscle inserts along essentially the entire

LIST OF STRUCTURES

Anterior axillary fold	Intercostal muscles	Sibson's fascia
Posterior axillary fold	Intercostobrachial nerve	Carotid sheath
Pectoralis major muscle	Medial brachial cutaneous nerve	Sympathetic trunk
Latissimus dorsi muscle	Long thoracic nerve	Axillary artery
Serratus anterior muscle	Phrenic nerve	Thyrocervical trunk
Anterior scalene muscle	Brachial plexus	Suprascapular artery
Middle scalene muscle	Axillary vein	Transverse cervical artery
Posterior scalene muscle	Subclavian vein	Thoracic duct
Smallest scalene muscle	Internal jugular vein	
Subclavius muscle	Cervical fascia	

ORIENTATION

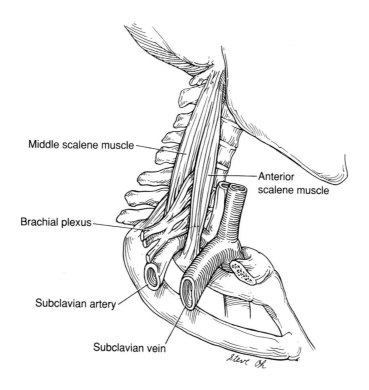

Middle scalene muscle

Anterior
scalene muscle

Brachial plexus

Subclavian artery

Subclavian vein

vertebral border of the scapula. It receives its innervation by the long thoracic nerve, which arises in the neck from roots C5 to C7 of the brachial plexus. From this origin, the nerve passes through or posterior to the middle scalene muscle to pass along the outer surface of the serratus anterior muscle, about midway between the origin and insertion of the individual fascicles, giving branches to the individual fascicles as it crosses them. Denervation of the serratus anterior muscle is debilitating to the patient because it results in "winging" of the scapula and an inability to abduct or flex the arm beyond the horizontal.

Division of Muscles and the First Rib (Fig. 27.2)

Technical Points

Bluntly dissect the fascia to separate carefully the axillary contents from the thoracic outlet. Identify the anterior scalene muscle between the axillary vein and artery. Place a right-angled clamp around this tendon with great care, and sharply divide the tendon. The phrenic nerve travels on the anterior surface of the anterior scalene muscle in the neck. At this level, it is usually medial to the muscle. Be careful to avoid injuring this nerve during division of the anterior scalene tendon.

Identify the subclavius tendon anterior to the axillary vein and sharply divide it. The middle scalene muscle lies posterior

to the brachial plexus. Bluntly detach it from the first rib extraperiosteally. Division of this muscle endangers the long thoracic nerve, which runs on the anterolateral aspect of the middle scalene muscle.

Separate the intercostal muscle (which runs between the first and second ribs) extraperiosteally from the first rib. Carefully resect the first rib anteriorly across the costal cartilage and posteriorly close to the transverse process using right-angled rib shears. Smooth the cut surfaces to prevent injury to the neurovascular structures or to the apex of the parietal pleura. To perform this rib resection safely, it may be necessary to cut the rib midlength and then divide it anteriorly and posteriorly, removing it in two pieces. This usually allows increased maneuverability of the rib segments, thereby maximizing exposure. Resect all sharp bony shards.

After resection of the first rib, the anterior scalene muscle is retracted back into the field. Occasionally, there will be a fibrous connection or band between this muscle and the middle scalene muscle. It is imperative to check for this and to resect it if it exists. Irrigate the wound and check for hemostasis. Ease tension on the arm and approximate the subcutaneous tissue. Close the skin with an absorbable running subcuticular stitch.

If the parietal pleura was violated during the operation, place a small red rubber catheter into the hole. After placing the subcuticular running stitch, but before tying it, connect the

FIGURE 27.1
POSITION OF THE PATIENT AND SKIN INCISION

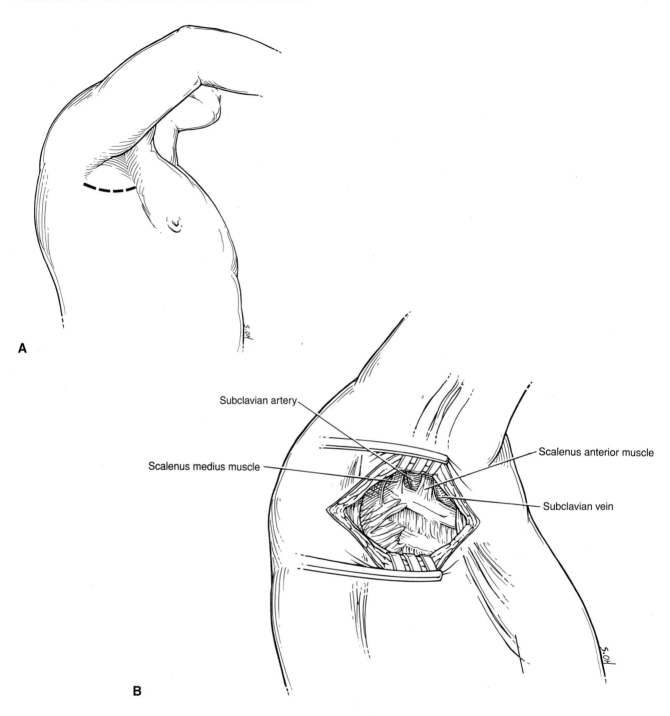

A

B

Subclavian artery

Scalenus medius muscle

Scalenus anterior muscle

Subclavian vein

red rubber catheter to suction and have the anesthesiologist fully inflate the lung. Tie the subcuticular stitch while the first assistant quickly withdraws the catheter from the chest.

Anatomic Points

The scalene muscles (anterior, middle, and posterior) are landmarks for this procedure. All three muscles arise from transverse processes of several cervical vertebrae. From this origin, the muscles diverge to attach to the upper one or two ribs, thus forming a muscular dome surrounding the apex of the lung. The anterior scalene fibers form a tendon inserted on the scalene tubercle of the first rib, posterior to the groove of the subclavian vein and anterior to the groove of the subclavian artery. The middle scalene muscle inserts onto the first rib posterior to the groove of the subclavian artery.

FIGURE 27.2
DIVISION OF MUSCLES AND THE FIRST RIB

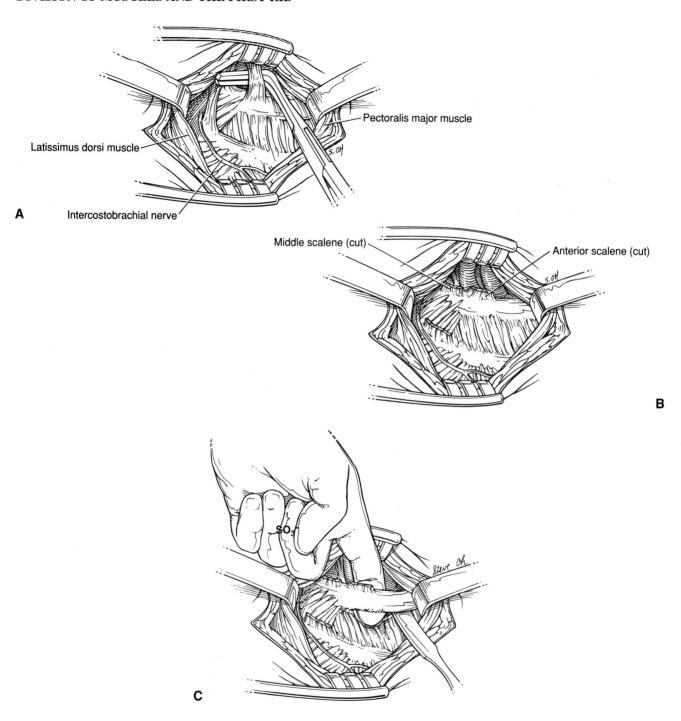

The posterior scalene muscle, which frequently is inseparable from the middle scalene muscle, inserts on the outer surface of the second rib, posterior to the origin of the upper part of the serratus anterior muscle. These three muscles, as well as some neurovascular structures, are invested with scalene fascia, a continuation of the prevertebral fascia of the neck. The fascia covering the inner surface of the scalenes (i.e., that which is in contact with the cervical pleura) is somewhat thicker than that found elsewhere and has been referred to as *Sibson's fascia.*

The subclavian vein crosses the first rib, making a shallow groove in this rib just anterior to the insertion of the anterior scalene muscle. Lying on the muscle fibers of the anterior scalene, and thus deep to the scalene fascia, is the phrenic nerve. This nerve passes from superolateral to inferomedial so that, at the insertion of the anterior scalene muscle, the nerve is just medial to its insertion. The sympathetic trunk lies more medially and posterior to the carotid sheath. It has been confused with the phrenic nerve because it parallels the latter. Crossing the anterior scalene muscle and phrenic nerve transversely, but above the level of the subclavian vein, are the suprascapular and transverse cervical arteries, both of which are branches of the thyrocervical trunk. The thyrocervical trunk itself ascends close to the medial edge of this muscle. Finally, on the left side only, the thoracic duct arches forward medial to the anterior scalene muscle and lateral to the carotid sheath. At about the level of the suprascapular artery, it passes across the anterior scalene muscle, superficial to the muscle, phrenic nerve, and suprascapular artery, and drains into the venous system about at the junction of the internal jugular and subclavian veins.

Posterior to the anterior scalene muscle, in the interval between it and the middle scalene muscle, are the roots of the brachial plexus and the subclavian artery. Of these, the subclavian artery is lowest, causing a groove to be formed posterior to the insertion of the anterior scalene muscle. Lateral to the insertion of the middle scalene muscle, and posterior to the brachial plexus is the long thoracic nerve, which supplies the serratus anterior muscle.

Frequently (about two thirds of the time), the smallest scalene muscle is present. This muscle, apparently a detached portion of the anterior scalene muscle, inserts independently into the first rib. This insertion is always posterior to the subclavian artery and anterior to at least part of the brachial plexus.

Important relationships of the posterior scalene muscle include the long thoracic nerve as it descends on its anterior surface to innervate the serratus anterior muscle. Remember that this nerve is posterior to the brachial plexus.

Finally, mention must be made of the subclavius muscle. This muscle arises from the first rib near its costochondral junction. Fibers fan out laterally to insert along most of the lower border of the clavicle. This muscle can be hard to visualize, both because it is concealed by the more anterior pectoralis major muscle and the clavicle and because it is invested by the clavipectoral fascia. The subclavian vessels and the brachial plexus lie immediately posterior to this small muscle.

REFERENCES

1. Jochimsen PR, Hartfall WG. Per axillary upper extremity sympathectomy: technique reviewed and clinical experience. *Surgery* 1972;71:686. (Describes technique of transaxillary sympathectomy.)
2. Leffert R. Discussion. In: Grillo HC, Eschappase H, eds. *International trends in general thoracic surgery. Vol. 2: Major challenges.* Philadelphia: WB Saunders, 1987:356. (Presents general review of issues involved.)
3. Mercier C. Thoracic outlet syndrome: anatomy, clinical syndrome, diagnosis, and conservative treatment. In: Grillo HC, Eschappase H, eds. *International trends in general thoracic surgery. Vol. 2: Major challenges.* Philadelphia: WB Saunders, 1987:343. (Provides good general review.)
4. Pollak EW. Surgical anatomy of the thoracic outlet syndrome. *Surg Gynecol Obstet* 1980;150:97. (Discusses relevant anatomy.)
5. Roos DB. The place for scalenectomy and first-rib resection in thoracic outlet syndrome. *Surgery* 1982;92:1977.
6. Roos DB. Thoracic outlet syndrome: surgical management. In: Grillo HC, Eschappase H, eds. *International trends in general thoracic surgery. Vol. 2: Major challenges.* Philadelphia: WB Saunders, 1987:359.
7. Roos DB. Transaxillary first rib resection for thoracic outlet syndrome: indications and techniques. *Contemp Surg* 1985;26:55.
8. Sanders RJ, Raymer S. The supraclavicular approach to scalenectomy and first rib resection: description of technique. *J Vasc Surg* 1985;2:751. (Describes alternative approach.)
9. Scher LA, Veith RJ, Samson RH, et al. Vascular complications of thoracic outlet syndrome. *J Vasc Surg* 1986;3:565.
10. Thevenet A. Discussion. In: Grillo HC, Eschappase H, eds. *International trends in general thoracic surgery. Vol. 2: Major challenges.* Philadelphia: WB Saunders, 1987:370.

CHAPTER 28

Esophageal Resection: Esophagogastrectomy and the Ivor Lewis Approach

Lesions of the lower to middle third of the esophagus are approached through a thoracotomy in conjunction with laparotomy. The lower esophagus is easily reached through the left chest, but the middle esophagus is inaccessible through this approach. Esophagogastrectomy (resection of the lower esophagus and upper stomach) is employed for carcinoma of the cardioesophageal junction. Lesions that extend above this level are better managed by an Ivor Lewis (laparotomy and right thoracotomy) type of resection, which provides access to the entire thoracic esophagus. Alternative surgical approaches, such as esophagectomy without thoracotomy and minimally invasive esophagectomy, are described in the references.

Esophagogastrectomy

Incision and Initial Exploration (Fig. 28.1)

Technical Points

Position the patient in a modified left thoracotomy position. Place the hips of the patient flat on the operating table. Raise the left shoulder and support the left arm. Ideally, the shoulders should be in an almost full thoracotomy position, while the pelvis is flat. Patients with less flexible spines may not

be able to tolerate this position. In such cases, the patient's pelvis should be allowed to rotate with the upper trunk.

Plan a thoracoabdominal incision that extends in a straight line from the eighth intercostal space to a point just above and slightly beyond the umbilicus. Mark the line of the proposed skin incision. Make your initial incision through just the abdominal portion of this incision and assess resectability of the tumor before proceeding into the chest.

Incise the fascial and muscular layers of the abdominal wall in a direct line with the incision. Use electrocautery to control bleeding as you pass through the muscular layers of the abdominal wall. Continue the skin incision up several centimeters over the costal margin, but do not yet divide the costal margin.

Assess resectability by palpating the tumor at the cardioesophageal junction and assessing its mobility. Check the liver and other intraabdominal viscera for metastatic deposits. Palpable nodes along the celiac axis do not necessarily preclude resection, which will provide the best palliation for a lesion in this area. If the lesion is believed to be resectable, extend the incision up into the chest. Divide the costal cartilage and excise a 1-cm piece of it. After opening the left chest in the eighth intercostal space and attaining hemostasis in the intercostal muscles, place a self-retaining or Finochietto-type retractor and spread the ribs.

LIST OF STRUCTURES

Esophagus	Short gastric vessels	Aorta
Diaphragm	Spleen	Azygos vein
Phrenic nerve	Left gastroepiploic vessels	Thoracic duct
Internal thoracic (mammary) artery	Right gastroepiploic vessels	Internal jugular vein
Musculophrenic artery	Gastroduodenal artery	Sternocleidomastoid muscle
Superior epigastric artery	Gastrocolic ligament	Omohyoid muscle
Rectus abdominis muscle	Greater omentum	Middle thyroid veins
Inferior pulmonary ligament	Lesser omentum	Recurrent laryngeal nerve
Inferior pulmonary vein	Right gastric artery	
Stomach	Left gastric artery	
Pylorus	Coronary vein	
Cardia	Inferior phrenic artery	

ORIENTATION

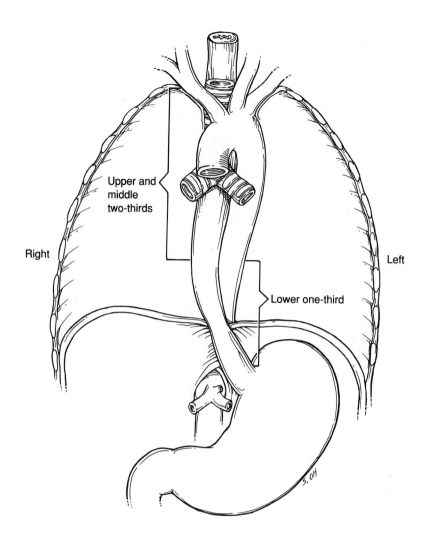

Divide the diaphragm with a curvilinear lateral incision that is planned to avoid the phrenic nerve. Sharply divide the inferior pulmonary attachments and reflect the left lung upward. An indwelling nasogastric tube or esophageal stethoscope should be palpable in the esophagus.

Anatomic Points

When planning a thoracoabdominal incision, make sure that the thoracic part of the incision is through the appropriate intercostal space. The first rib cannot be palpated because of the clavicle; hence, one must start counting with the second rib, which articulates with the sternum at the sternal angle of Lewis. The incision should be inferior to the pectoralis major and minor muscles. As in any thoracic incision, divide the intercostal muscles along the superior margin of the lower rib to avoid the intercostal neurovascular bundle. Remember that the anterior portion of the costal margin is formed by the union of costal cartilages of the eighth through tenth ribs articulating with the cartilage of the rib above, and that the

lowest costal cartilage articulating with the sternum is that of the seventh rib.

The combined thoracoabdominal incision divides the terminal branches of the internal thoracic (mammary) artery. One of these branches—the musculophrenic artery—passes inferolaterally behind the seventh to ninth costal cartilages. The other—the superior epigastric artery—is divided when the rectus abdominis muscle is divided. Both arteries have free anastomoses with other arteries.

Division of the diaphragm must take into account the location of the phrenic nerve and its three major branches. The left phrenic nerve enters the muscular part of the right hemidiaphragm just lateral to the left cardiac surface. As it traverses the diaphragm, it divides into (a) a sternal branch that runs anteromedially toward the sternum, (b) an anterolateral branch that passes laterally anterior to the central tendon, and (c) a posterior branch that runs posterior to the central tendon and that supplies crural fibers to the left of the esophageal hiatus, regardless of whether the esophageal hiatus is entirely surrounded by right crus or by both left and right crura.

FIGURE 28.1
INCISION AND INITIAL EXPLORATION

A

B

The mediastinal root of the pulmonary ligament is anterior to the esophagus. Division of this ligament allows the lung to be retracted superiorly, exposing the distal esophagus in the left chest. Caution must be exercised, however, because the fragile inferior pulmonary vein lies at the top of the pulmonary ligament.

Mobilization of the Stomach and Pyloromyotomy (Fig. 28.2)

Technical Points

Mobilize the stomach by creating a window along the greater curvature. The spleen may be taken with the specimen. The mobilization is essentially the same as that described for total gastrectomy (see Chapter 48). Preservation of the omentum will allow some omentum to be wrapped around the anastomosis at the conclusion of the surgery, thus ensuring a good blood supply for the stomach. Fully mobilize the stomach from the pylorus to the cardioesophageal junction.

Perform a Kocher maneuver to mobilize the duodenum. Do this by incising the peritoneum lateral to the duodenum and elevating the duodenum off the retroperitoneum by sharp and blunt dissection. This should be an avascular plane that allows the duodenum to rotate toward the midline. The head of the pancreas will come up with the duodenum.

Perform a pyloromyotomy. Place two stay sutures of 2-0 silk about 1 cm apart on the pylorus. Lift up on these and incise the muscular ring of the pylorus for a distance of about

2 cm. Completely divide the muscle of the pylorus, taking care to leave the mucosa intact. At the conclusion of the pyloromyotomy, the ring of the pylorus should be palpable as a broken (no longer intact) ring. If the mucosa is inadvertently entered during this dissection, convert the pyloromyotomy to a pyloroplasty. To do this, completely incise all layers of the pylorus as well as a section a short distance proximal along the stomach and distal along the duodenum. Achieve hemostasis in the edges of this incision. Close this longitudinal incision in a transverse fashion with multiple interrupted sutures of 2-0 silk. Place sutures to invert the edges slightly, ensuring accurate approximation of the edges and a watertight seal.

Anatomic Points

Mobilization of the stomach along the greater curvature will require division, between ligatures, of the short gastric and left gastroepiploic vessels (from the splenic vessels). The right gastroepiploic vessels, arising from the gastroduodenal vessels, must be preserved. Division of the gastrocolic ligament will require division, again between ligatures, of the omental branches; care should be taken, however, to *preserve the ligament's blood supply* so that it can be used to wrap the anastomosis. In addition, care should be taken to avoid injury to the middle colic artery, which is in close proximity to the right gastroepiploic artery.

Mobilization along the lesser curve requires division of the lesser omentum. When this is done, the right gastric artery,

FIGURE 28.2
MOBILIZATION OF THE STOMACH AND PYLOROMYOTOMY

arising from the hepatic artery or one of its derivatives, should be preserved. Variant hepatic branches from the left gastric artery should also be divided. Division of the left gastric artery should be done, between ligatures, as close to its origin as possible to ensure preservation of a collateral blood supply.

Esophageal vessels at the hiatus must also be divided.

These include the coronary vein, esophageal branches from the left gastric artery, and frequently (in as many as 56% of cases), a sizeable branch of the inferior phrenic artery.

The Kocher maneuver provides adequate mobilization of the duodenum, allowing the pylorus and distal stomach to rotate up, thereby increasing the length of stomach that can be pulled into the chest. The anatomic rationale for this

FIGURE 28.3
MOBILIZATION OF THE ESOPHAGUS

A

B

procedure is to develop the avascular plane posterior to the duodenum and pancreas that resulted from fusion and degeneration of the mesoduodenum and serosa with parietal peritoneum. A pyloromyotomy or pyloroplasty is performed because resection of the esophagus, of necessity, also results in a bilateral truncal vagotomy.

Mobilization of the Esophagus (Fig. 28.3)

Technical Points

Reflect the left lung upward until the left inferior pulmonary vein is visible. This forms the superior boundary of the exposure attained by this approach. This limited exposure explains why only lesions of the cardioesophageal junction can be treated by esophagogastrectomy. Palpate the esophagus above the tumor in the mediastinum. Incise the pleural

covering overlying the esophagus and develop flaps of pleura. By sharp and blunt dissection, mobilize the esophagus above the tumor and surround it with a Penrose drain. Then, with full mobilization of the stomach and with the esophagus surrounded above the tumor, resect the tumor from the mediastinum by sharp and blunt dissection. Remove any lymph nodes in the mediastinum that are in proximity to the tumor along with the specimen. When the tumor is fully mobilized, you are ready for resection.

Anatomic Points

The esophagus can be exposed by reflection of the pleura posterior to the mediastinal root of the pulmonary ligament. Because the pulmonary ligament does not extend to the diaphragm, the pleura will have to be reflected inferiorly, past the termination of the ligament.

FIGURE 28.4
RESECTION

A

B

Mobilization of the esophagus may disrupt some esophageal vasculature. Although the distal esophagus receives most of its blood supply from esophageal branches of the left gastric artery, it also has branches arising directly from the aorta.

Resection (Fig. 28.4)

Technical and Anatomic Points

Have the anesthesiologist pull back the nasogastric tube into the proximal esophagus, well above the operative field. Place a TA-90 linear stapling device across the upper third of the stomach to divide it. Use Kocher clamps on the portion of the stomach that is to be removed with the specimen. Select the region on the proximal esophagus that is to be used for anastomosis. Place stay sutures of 2-0 silk on each side of the esophagus. Sharply divide the esophagus. Remove the specimen.

Check the mediastinum and the bed of the stomach carefully for hemostasis before proceeding with the anastomosis.

Anastomosis (Fig. 28.5)

Technical and Anatomic Points

The use of the EEA stapling device, as described later, has greatly facilitated esophageal anastomosis. Alternatively, a standard hand-sewn, two-layered anastomotic technique may be used.

Check to make sure that the stomach will reach comfortably up to the stump of the esophagus without tension. Place a pursestring suture of 2-0 Prolene in a whipstitch fashion on the proximal esophageal stump. The epithelium of the esophagus will tend to retract; hence, one must be careful to include the epithelium with each bite. Handle the epithelium as little as possible to avoid shredding it.

Calibrate the esophagus with EEA sizers to determine the size of stapling device that it will accommodate. Make a stab wound in the fundus of the stomach and introduce the EEA stapler without the anvil. Poke the spike of the device up through the proximal stomach and place the anvil back on the device. Gently place the anvil of the stapler within

FIGURE 28.5
ANASTOMOSIS

A

Esophagus

B

the esophageal stump and snugly tie the pursestring suture. Close the EEA stapler, taking care to make sure that the esophagus and stomach are well inverted within the stapling device. Fire the EEA stapler and then open it. Place two stay sutures of 2-0 silk in a Lembert fashion across the anastomosis and tie these. Leave them long and use them for traction. Pull on these sutures to elevate the anterior wall of the anastomosis away from the stapling device as the stapler is retracted. This will help to avoid trauma to the anastomosis as the EEA stapler is withdrawn.

Gently remove the EEA stapler using a twisting and pulling motion. Check to make sure that there are two intact donuts of tissue. Reinforce the staple line by rolling stomach up around it with multiple interrupted 3-0 silk Lembert sutures. Close the gastrotomy with a single application of a linear stapling device.

An alternative stapling technique, using the GIA stapler, provides a wider esophagogastric anastomosis. This technique is especially useful when the esophagus is small and will not accommodate a large EEA stapler. A more detailed description of this technique may be found in the articles by Chassin.

Closure of the Incision (Fig. 28.6)

Technical Points

Recheck hemostasis. Place omentum around the anastomosis. Place two large chest tubes in a dependent portion of the left chest. Bring these out through separate stab wounds below the main incision. Place two closed-suction drains in the vicinity of the hiatus through the abdominal incision. Bring these out through separate stab wounds. Close the abdominal portion of the incision in the usual fashion.

Reapproximate the diaphragm with multiple figure-of-eight sutures of number 1 Mersilene. Close the hiatus comfortably around the stomach but do not constrict the stomach. Tack the stomach to the hiatus with multiple interrupted 3-0 silk sutures. Pass the nasogastric tube through the anastomosis and down to the region of the pylorus. Control its passage through the anastomosis by palpating it within the chest. Confirm that it is in a good position and have the anesthesiologist secure it in place.

Have the anesthesiologist reinflate the left lung. Place warm saline in the left chest and check for air leaks. Close the thoracotomy incision with multiple figure-of-eight pericostal sutures of number 1 Vicryl. Close the muscular layers of the chest wall with running number 1 and 0 Vicryl. Secure drains and chest tubes in place and close the skin.

Anatomic Points

Again, remember that intercostal neurovascular bundles lie inferior to a rib, not superior to it. Hence, division of intercostal muscles is best accomplished along the top of a rib.

FIGURE 28.6
CLOSURE OF THE INCISION

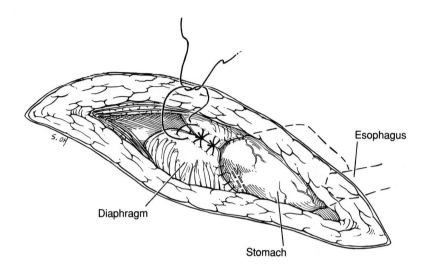

Esophagus

Diaphragm

Stomach

Ivor Lewis Type of Resection

Position of the Patient (Fig. 28.7)

Technical Points

Position the patient with the hips supine and the right chest slightly elevated in a modified thoracotomy position. The Ivor Lewis resection is performed through an upper midline incision and a right thoracotomy. The upper abdomen should be angled about 30 degrees from supine, and the chest should be angled at as close to 90 degrees as is possible. Positioning

FIGURE 28.7
POSITION OF THE PATIENT

is limited by the mobility and flexibility of the patient's spine; be especially careful when positioning elderly patients.

Prepare and drape the right neck for possible cervical esophagogastric anastomosis.

Make an upper midline abdominal incision and assess the abdomen for the presence of metastatic disease. Extensive metastatic disease within the abdomen precludes resection. Mobilize the stomach as described in Fig. 28.2, and perform a pyloromyotomy.

Anatomic Points

The upper midline incision, as opposed to the thoracoabdominal incision described previously, does not involve division of any major branches of the superior epigastric artery.

Thoracotomy and Esophageal Mobilization (Fig. 28.8)

Technical Points

Make a right thoracotomy in the fifth intercostal space. Achieve hemostasis in the muscular layers of the chest wall and place a self-retaining rib spreader in the incision. Assess the lesion for mobility. Incise the pleura over the esophagus. Palpate the indwelling nasogastric tube or esophageal stethoscope and the tumor.

Identify the azygos vein in the upper mediastinum. Incise the pleura overlying the azygos vein and mobilize the right lung upward and medially. Double-ligate and divide the azygos vein.

Surround the esophagus above the tumor with a Penrose drain. With mobilization of the proximal esophagus, carefully dissect the tumor from the mediastinum, taking all visible tumor and palpable nodes with the specimen. Once full mobilization of the tumor is achieved, a decision can be made as to whether the anastomosis should be done in the chest or in the neck. Performance of the anastomosis in the neck

FIGURE 28.8
THORACOTOMY AND ESOPHAGEAL MOBILIZATION

allows a higher resection to be done and is safer for the patient because leakage from the anastomosis will occur in the neck rather than entering the chest. Presently, this approach is preferred by most surgeons.

Divide the stomach with a TA-90 stapling device. If the anastomosis is to be done in the chest, place two stay sutures of 2-0 silk on the proximal esophagus and divide it. After removing the specimen, check the mediastinum for hemostasis. Pull the stomach up into the chest. It should easily reach to the upper chest, or even the neck, without tension. If there is tension on the stomach, recheck to see that the duodenum is adequately kocherized. Perform the anastomosis in a similar fashion to that described for esophagogastrectomy.

If anastomosis in the neck is selected, make a separate incision in the right neck and expose the esophagus. The approach to the cervical esophagus was previously described in Chapter 11.

Follow the esophagus down into the chest, establishing a communication between the chest wound and the neck incision. Divide the esophagus. Pull the stomach up into the neck wound and perform an anastomosis. Generally, a hand-sewn, two-layer anastomosis is performed. Place a small Penrose drain in the vicinity of the anastomosis and bring it out through the inferior pole of the cervical incision. Close the abdominal incision and the thoracotomy incision in the usual fashion.

Anatomic Points

As usual, make the thoracotomy incision along the top, rather than the bottom, of a rib. This prevents injury to the intercostal neurovascular bundle, which lies in the costal groove on the lower side of each rib.

As the right mediastinum is approached, recall that major longitudinal vascular structures on this side, as opposed to the left thorax, are all venous. Posteriorly, along the bodies of the vertebrae, lies the azygos vein, which drains the intercostal spaces of the right side. Immediately superior to the root of the lung, the azygos vein curves anteriorly to enter the superior vena cava. At the beginning of this terminal part of the azygos, tributaries draining the superior two or three intercostal spaces can be observed.

Incision of the pleura and mobilization of the lung to expose the esophagus and azygos vein will necessitate division of the pulmonary ligament inferiorly because this pleural fold is immediately anterior to the esophagus. Care must be taken at the superior aspect of the pulmonary ligament because the

inferior pulmonary vein lies at the upper limits of the ligament. Division of the pleura is best accomplished posterior to the root of the lung, which necessitates reflection of the lung anteriorly and medially.

Division of the azygos vein must be done between secure ligatures and in the terminal segment that arches over the root of the lung. This maneuver, along with incision of mediastinal pleura along the right mediastinum, will expose the esophagus from the thoracic inlet almost to the diaphragm. Extensive venous collaterals in this area ensure that there are no ill effects from azygos vein division.

Mobilization of the intrathoracic esophagus obviously necessitates division of most of the blood supply of the esophagus. Inferiorly, the esophagus is supplied by esophageal branches of the left gastric artery, one or more branches from the aorta, and frequently, a branch from the left inferior phrenic artery. In its midportion, the blood supply to the esophagus is derived from one or more additional branches from the aorta and esophageal branches of the bronchial arteries.

A potential complication of esophageal mobilization is disruption of the thoracic duct, which lies posterior to the esophagus through most of its mediastinal course. However, this delicate duct is most closely associated with the aorta and lies in the tissue between the aorta and the azygos vein; at the level of the arch of the aorta, it ascends into the neck along the medial side of the left subclavian artery. In the neck, it turns laterally, posterior to the common carotid artery and internal jugular vein, then arches inferiorly, in front of the subclavian artery, to open into the venous system in the region where the left subclavian and internal jugular vein join. Hence, if mobilization of the esophagus is done carefully, staying as close as possible to the esophagus, the thoracic duct should not be endangered. However, if it is injured, it can be ligated because extensive collateral lymphatic pathways exist.

Exposure of the cervical esophagus involves an incision along the anterior border of the right sternocleidomastoid muscle, followed by division of the omohyoid muscle and middle thyroid veins. Care must be taken to avoid both the right and left recurrent laryngeal nerves, which lie in the vicinity of the tracheoesophageal groove. The right recurrent nerve is quite variable in its location, having been reported to be as much as 1 cm lateral to the tracheoesophageal groove. The left recurrent laryngeal nerve is more often located in the groove, but its location, too, may vary. In the cervical region, the blood supply of the esophagus is derived from both left and right inferior thyroid arteries.

REFERENCES

1. Akiyama H, Miyazono H, Tsurumaru M, et al. Use of the stomach as an esophageal substitute. *Ann Surg* 1978;188:606. (Includes photographs of injected specimens showing blood supply.)
2. Belsey R, Hiebert CA. An exclusive right thoracic approach for cancer of the middle third of the esophagus. *Ann Thorac Surg* 1974;18:1. (Describes elegant technique of mobilization through the chest.)
3. Bolton JS, Fuhrman GM, Richardson WS. Esophageal resection for cancer. *Surg Clin North Am* 1998;78:773–794.
4. Chassin JL. Esophagogastrectomy: data favoring end-to-side anastomosis. *Ann Surg* 1978;188:22. (Describes technique using GIA stapler to create wide lumen.)
5. Chassin JL. Stapling technic for esophagogastrostomy after esophagogastric resection. *Am J Surg* 1978;136:399.

6. Donahue PE, Nyhus LM. Exposure of the periesophageal space. *Surg Gynecol Obstet* 1981;152:218.

7. Ellis FH. Esophagogastrectomy for carcinoma: technical considerations based on anatomic location of lesion. *Surg Clin North Am* 1980;60:265.

8. Fiocco M, Krasna MJ. Thoracoscopic lymph node dissection in the staging of esophageal carcinoma. *J Laparoendosc Surg* 1992;2:111. (Discusses thoracoscopy used to stage extent of tumor involvement before resection.)

9. Fisher RD, Brawley RK, Kieffer RF. Esophagogastrostomy in the treatment of carcinoma of the distal two-thirds of the esophagus: clinical experience and operative methods. *Ann Thorac Surg* 1972;14:658.

10. Furst H, Hartl WH, Lohe F, et al. Colon interposition for esophageal replacement: an alternative technique based on the use of the right colon. *Ann Surg* 2000;231:173–178.

11. Gavriliu D. Aspects of esophageal surgery. *Curr Probl Surg* 1975;12:1. (Advocates reversed gastric tube for reconstruction.)

12. Gray SW, Rowe JS, Skandalakis JE. Surgical anatomy of the gastroesophageal junction. *Am Surg* 1979;45:575.

13. Loinaz C, Altorki NK. Pitfalls and complications of colon interposition. *Chest Surg Clin North Am* 1997;7:533–549.

14. May IA, Samson PC. Esophageal reconstruction and replacements. *Ann Thorac Surg* 1969;7:249.

15. Merendino KA, Johnson RJ, Skinner JJ, et al. The intradiaphragmatic distribution of the phrenic nerve with particular reference to the placement of diaphragmatic incisions and controlled segmental paralysis. *Surgery* 1956;39:189. (Provides excellent review of pertinent anatomic considerations.)

16. Nguyen NT, Schauer P, Luketich JD. Minimally invasive esophagectomy for Barrett's esophagus with high-grade dysplasia. *Surgery* 2000;127:284–290.

17. Orringer MB, Marshall B, Iannettoni MD. Transhiatal esophagectomy: clinical experience and refinements. *Ann Surg* 1999;230:392–400.

18. Ratzer ER, Morfit HM. Cervical esophagostomy. *Surg Clin North Am* 1969;49:1413.

19. Robinson JC, Isa SS, Spees EK, et al. Substernal gastric bypass for palliation of esophageal carcinoma: rationale and technique. *Surgery* 1982;91:305.

20. Sicular A. Direct septum transversum incision to replace circumferential diaphragmatic incision in operations on the cardia. *Am J Surg* 1992;164:167. (Describes alternative diaphragmatic incision.)

21. Skinner DB. Esophageal reconstruction. *Am J Surg* 1980;139:810.

22. Swanstrom LL, Hansen P. Laparoscopic total esophagectomy. *Arch Surg* 1997;132:943–947.

23. Williams DB, Payne WS. Observations on esophageal blood supply. *Mayo Clin Proc* 1982;57:448.

CHAPTER 29

Thoracoscopic Surgery of the Esophagus

This chapter describes two procedures: thoracoscopic esophagomyotomy and esophageal mobilization for resection. These are used to illustrate the thoracoscopic appearance of the mediastinum. As with open esophageal surgery (see Chapter 28), only the distal one third of the esophagus is accessible through the left chest. Access to the proximal two thirds requires a right thoracoscopic approach and is preferred for resection. Both are described here, and references at the end give information about other procedures.

A thoracoscopic schematic view of the left posterior mediastinum is shown in part A of the orientation figure. Generally, only the lower part is accessed for esophageal surgery. Part B of the orientation figure shows the corresponding view of the right posterior mediastinum.

Thoracoscopic Esophagomyotomy: Initial Exposure and Mobilization of Esophagus (Fig. 29.1)

Technical Points

After adequate single-lung ventilation has been achieved, place the patient in the thoracotomy position with the left side up. Place thoracoports as shown (Fig. 29.1A).

Divide the inferior pulmonary ligament with ultrasonic shears and retract the collapsed lung cephalad with a lung retractor. Take care not to extend this incision up into the lower lobe pulmonary vein.

Incise the mediastinal pleura between pericardium and aorta to expose the esophagus (Fig. 29.1B). Have an assistant pass an esophagogastroscope into the esophagus. Gentle deflection of the tip will elevate the esophagus from the groove behind the pericardium and facilitate dissection (Fig. 29.1C).

Completely encircle the esophagus and place a short segment of Penrose drain around it to facilitate subsequent retraction. Apply cephalad traction to the Penrose drain to elevate the gastroesophageal junction above the esophageal hiatus.

Anatomic Points

The inferior pulmonary ligament is simply the reflected pleura and helps tether the lung. As it ascends, the inferior pulmonary ligament divides to encircle the hilum of the left lung. Therefore, the lower lobe pulmonary vein is encountered at the cephalad border of this ligament. Mediastinal pleura invests the pericardium, aorta, and esophagus.

The esophagus is accessible not only at the inferior aspect of the mediastinum, where it is approached for esophagomyotomy, but also in the extreme upper aspect of the mediastinum. Two esophageal triangles define the space within which the esophagus is encountered from the left chest. At the inferior aspect, Truesdale's triangle is bounded inferiorly by the diaphragm, superiorly by the pericardium, and inferiorly by the descending aorta. In the superior mediastinum, the second esophageal triangle has its base on the vertebral bodies, and its two approximately equal sides are formed by the arch of the aorta inferiorly and the left subclavian artery.

The blood supply of the distal esophagus in the left chest comes from descending branches of the esophageal arteries, which arise directly from the aorta. Additional vessels ascend from branches of the inferior phrenic, left gastric, and splenic arteries. Generally, the distal esophagus can be encircled near the diaphragmatic hiatus without encountering any vessels.

LIST OF STRUCTURES

Esophagus
Vagus nerves
Inferior pulmonary ligament
Mediastinal pleura
Lower lobe pulmonary vein
Diaphragm
  Muscular portion
  Central tendinous portion

Hiatus
Pericardium
Aorta
  Arch of aorta
  Left subclavian artery
  Bronchial arteries
  Inferior phrenic nerve

Phrenoesophageal membrane
  Endothoracic fascia
  Phrenoesophageal fascia
  Transversalis fascia
  Peritoneum
Azygos vein
Hemiazygos vein
Thoracic duct

ORIENTATION

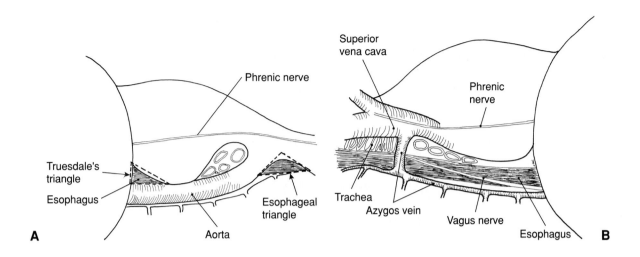

A
- Phrenic nerve
- Truesdale's triangle
- Esophagus
- Esophageal triangle
- Aorta

B
- Superior vena cava
- Phrenic nerve
- Trachea
- Azygos vein
- Vagus nerve
- Esophagus

FIGURE 29.1
THORACOSCOPIC ESOPHAGOMYOTOMY: INITIAL EXPOSURE AND MOBILIZATION OF ESOPHAGUS

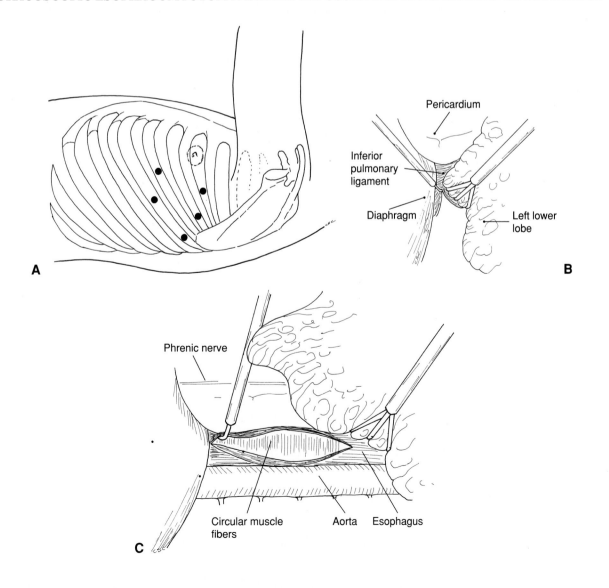

A

B
- Pericardium
- Inferior pulmonary ligament
- Diaphragm
- Left lower lobe

C
- Phrenic nerve
- Circular muscle fibers
- Aorta
- Esophagus

From above, the diaphragm is seen to comprise a central tendinous region and more lateral muscular portion. The inferior phrenic nerve crosses near the hiatus on the abdominal surface of the diaphragm and is not visible from above. The phrenoesophageal membrane forms a tight seal between pleural and peritoneal spaces. It comprises pleura, endothoracic fascia, phrenoesophageal fascia, transversalis fascia, and peritoneum. It provides a rough guide to the location of the esophagogastric junction but is often attenuated or distorted in patients with hiatal hernias.

Thoracoscopic Esophagomyotomy: Performance of Myotomy (Fig. 29.2)

Technical Points

Begin the myotomy on a convenient location in the midportion of the thickened segment of esophagus. Take care to avoid the left vagus nerve, visible as a thick white cord on the anterior surface of the esophagus. Spread the outer longitudinal fibers to expose the thickened circular muscle. Elevate and divide this with hook cautery (Fig. 29.2A). Observe the

---

FIGURE 29.2
THORACOSCOPIC ESOPHAGOMYOTOMY: PERFORMANCE OF MYOTOMY

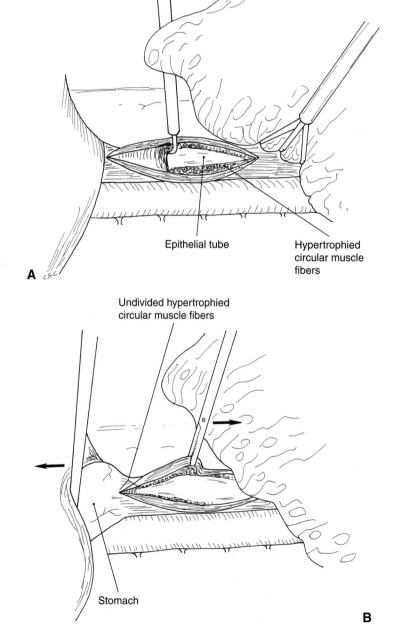

Epithelial tube

Hypertrophied circular muscle fibers

A

Undivided hypertrophied circular muscle fibers

Stomach

B

epithelial tube, which will protrude into the lumen. Ensure that this myotomy extends down onto the proximal stomach 1 to 1.5 cm. Continue cephalad until the hilum of the left lung is reached (Fig. 29.2B).

Fill the chest with warm saline and use the esophagogastroscope to insufflate the lumen of the esophagus. Confirm, by absence of bubbles, that no perforation has occurred.

Anatomic Points

In the distal esophagus, the esophageal vagal plexus coalesces into the anterior and posterior vagal trunks. Although only one trunk may be visible, numerous small twigs still exist at this level and may generally be disregarded.

Esophageal Resection: Exposure of Esophagus (Fig. 29.3)

Technical Points

After adequate single-lung ventilation has been achieved, place the patient in the thoracotomy position with the right side up. Insert thoracoports as shown (Fig. 29.3A). Incise the inferior pulmonary ligament with ultrasonic shears and retract the right lung cephalad and medial to expose the entire posterior mediastinum.

Divide the mediastinal pleura overlying the azygos vein (Fig. 29.3B). Gently mobilize the vein and divide it with an endoscopic linear stapler loaded with a vascular cartridge (Fig. 29.3C).

Continue the pleural incision proximal and distal to expose the esophagus.

Anatomic Points

Mediastinal pleura covers the azygos vein and esophagus and divides to cover the pulmonary hilum, extending inferiorly as the less prominent inferior pulmonary ligament. In the hilum of the right lung, the lower pulmonary vein is again the first structure encountered from below.

The azygos vein arches over the esophagus to drain into the posterior aspect of the superior vena cava. Abundant collaterals ensure that no ill effect comes from this ligation.

FIGURE 29.3
ESOPHAGEAL RESECTION: EXPOSURE OF ESOPHAGUS

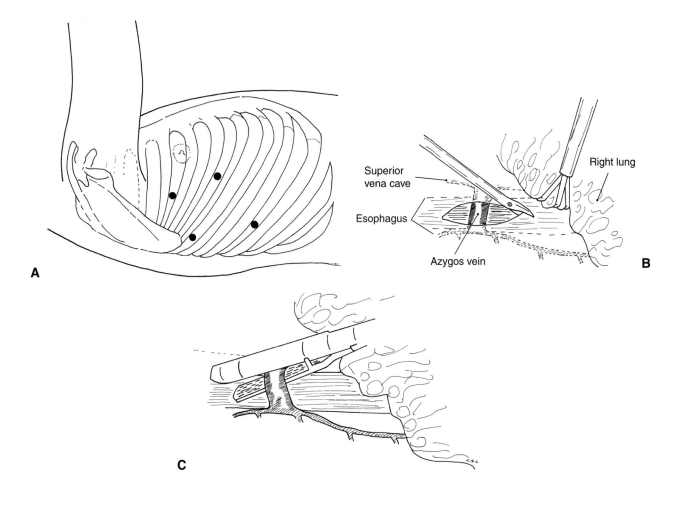

FIGURE 29.4
MOBILIZATION OF ESOPHAGUS IN RIGHT CHEST

Mobilization of Esophagus in Right Chest (Fig. 29.4)

Technical Points

Encircle the esophagus with a Penrose drain, and use this to elevate it, facilitating subsequent dissection. Work gently in the groove between esophagus and mediastinum using ultrasonic shears until the entire length of thoracic esophagus is mobilized. Numerous lymph nodes are found in the region of the esophagus and tracheobronchial tree. These should be excised with the specimen.

Anatomic Points

The blood supply of the upper thoracic esophagus comes primarily from branches that arise from the subclavian artery or a lower branch of the inferior thyroid artery. Less commonly, an anterior esophagotracheal artery arises from the aortic arch. The midthoracic esophagus derives its blood supply from ascending or descending branches of bronchial arteries. These vessels may arise directly from the aortic arch. Less common sources include the right internal thoracic artery, the right costocervical trunk, or the right subclavian artery. Although many vessels are listed as potential sources for esophageal arteries, the blood supply to the esophagus is generally fairly sparse and typically consists of only one or two major vessels.

Venous drainage of the upper two thirds of the esophagus goes to the systemic circulation, through small vessels that may drain into the azygos or hemiazygos vein. The lower one third drains into the portal circulation through the left gastric vein, splenic vein, or left inferior phrenic vein.

Lymphatic drainage of the upper two thirds goes to peritracheal, hilar, subcarinal, paraesophageal, periaortic, and pericardial lymph nodes. The distal one third drains to nodes along the lesser curvature of the stomach, the left gastric artery, and the celiac axis. Drainage patterns are extremely unreliable.

At the level of T6 to T7, the thoracic duct, which has been ascending on the right side of the esophagus and initially at some distance from it, crosses behind the esophagus to continue its ascent on the left side of the esophagus. It is rarely actually seen, but may be injured during esophageal mobilization. Leakage of clear or milky fluid into the operative field should prompt a search for an injured thoracic duct, which can cause chylothorax if not identified and ligated.

Below the azygos vein, the esophagus lies posterior to the carina and right main-stem bronchus. Above that level, the esophagus and posterior wall of the trachea are in close apposition, and care must be taken not to injure the trachea.

REFERENCES

1. Chevallier JM, Vitte E, Derosier C, et al. The thoracic esophagus: sectional anatomy and radiosurgical applications. *Surg Radiol Anat* 1991;13:313–319.
2. Gossot D, Fourquier P, Celerier M. Thoracoscopic esophagectomy: technique and initial results. *Ann Thorac Surg* 1993;56:675–670.
3. McAnena OJ. Oesophagectomy. In: Walker WS, ed. *Video-assisted thoracic surgery.* Oxford, UK: Isis Medical Media, 1999:189–199.
4. McAnena OJ, Rogers J, Williams NS. Right thoracoscopically assisted oesophagectomy for cancer. *Br J Surg* 1994;81:236–238.
5. Skandalakis JE, Ellis H. Embryologic and anatomic basis of esophageal surgery. *Surg Clin North Am* 2000;80:85–155. (Provides exhaustive review of anatomy.)
6. Zucker KA. Minimally invasive surgery for achalasia. In: Zucker KA, ed. *Surgical laparoscopy.* 2nd ed. Philadelphia: Lippincott Williams & Wilkins, 2001:467–491.

SECTION III

The Upper Extremity

This section continues the anatomy of some structures that were first introduced in Section II. The extraanatomic vascular bypass procedure—axillobifemoral bypass (Chapter 30)—describes the axillary artery and completes the discussion of the major neurovascular structures of the region.

The remaining sections describe those areas of upper extremity anatomy that are likely to be encountered in the operating room by the general surgeon or surgery resident. References at the end include texts of hand and orthopedic surgery that give greater detail on these procedures as well as information about other operations.

Vascular anatomy of the arm and hand is explored further in Chapters 31 and 32, in which the radial artery, ulnar artery, brachial artery, and associated veins are described. Two specialized procedures–tendon repair (Chapter 33) and carpal tunnel release (Chapter 34)—are included because they are commonly performed or observed and because they illustrate well the regional anatomy of the tendons and nerves of the hand.

CHAPTER 30

Axillobifemoral Bypass

Kenneth B. Simon

Axillobifemoral bypass is one of the most commonly performed extraanatomic bypasses in vascular surgery today. This procedure is generally performed in the following types of patients:

1. Patients who have undergone previous multiple intraabdominal procedures
2. Poor-risk patients with impending limb loss who are not candidates for aortic reconstruction by the transabdominal or retroperitoneal approach
3. Patients with intraabdominal sepsis
4. Patients with infected aortic grafts that must be removed

The vascular conduit created by this procedure provides adequate inflow to the lower extremities.

In this chapter, the procedures of axillofemoral and axillobifemoral bypass (the more common of the two) are illustrated and used to introduce the anatomy of the axillary artery. By necessity, some anatomy of the femoral region is included as well; this topic is presented in greater detail in Chapters 86 and 100.

Position of the Patient and Exposure of the Axillary Artery (Fig. 30.1)

Technical Points

Evaluate each upper extremity to assess the quality of pulses and blood pressure. Generally, the right axillary artery is used for the bypass; however, if there is a discrepancy in either the pulse or blood pressure in the upper extremities, use the extremity with the strongest pulse or greatest blood pressure. Place the patient in a supine position with the donor arm abducted to no greater than 90 degrees. Place a small roll under the flank on the side of the bypass to ensure that the graft tunnel will cross the costal margin in the midaxillary line.

Make a 10-cm transverse incision along the inferior margin of the clavicle, extending it from the proximal one third of the clavicle medially to the deltopectoral groove laterally (Fig. 30.1A). Expose the fascia of the pectoralis major muscle by dissection through the subcutaneous fat. Incise the fascia and muscle fibers of the pectoralis major muscle and divide these along the direction of their fibers. Continue

LIST OF STRUCTURES

Axillary region
Thyrocervical trunk
  Suprascapular artery
  Transverse cervical artery
Axillary artery
  Highest (superior) thoracic artery
  Thoracoacromial artery
    Pectoral branch
    Acromial branch
    Clavicular branch
    Deltoid branch
  Lateral thoracic artery
  Subscapular artery
First anterior intercostal artery
Clavicle
Scapula
  Coracoid process

Deltopectoral groove
Pectoralis major
Pectoralis minor
Pectoral fascia
Deltoid muscle
Subclavius muscle
Clavipectoral fascia
Sternoclavicular joint
Axillary vein
  Cephalic vein
Brachial plexus
Supraclavicular nerves (medial, intermediate, and lateral)
Sternocleidomastoid muscle
Platysma muscle

Femoral region
Anterosuperior iliac spine
Inguinal ligament
Fossa ovalis (saphenous hiatus)
Femoral vein
  Superficial circumflex iliac vein
  Superficial epigastric vein
  Greater saphenous vein
Inguinal lymph nodes (superficial and deep)
Femoral artery
  Superficial femoral artery
  Profunda femoris artery
Pectineus muscle
Adductor longus muscle

ORIENTATION

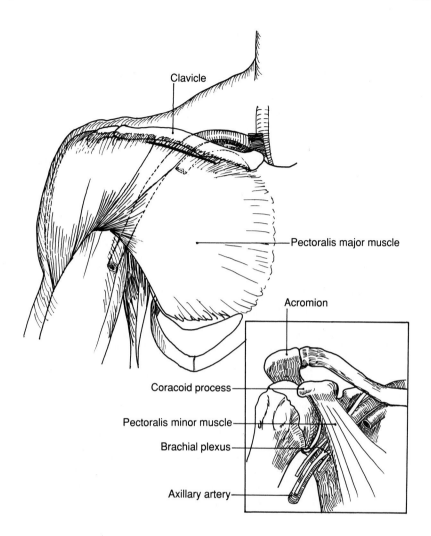

the dissection laterally to the medial border of the pectoralis minor muscle.

The subpectoral space contains the axillary artery and vein and the brachial plexus. The axillary artery is bounded by the axillary vein anteriorly and the brachial plexus posteriorly. Carefully expose the axillary artery from the highest thoracic artery medially to the medial border of the pectoralis minor muscle laterally. If necessary, ligate and divide the highest thoracic artery to facilitate exposure of the axillary artery. Encircle the artery with Silastic vessel loops to facilitate exposure of its inferior surface (Fig. 30.1B).

Anatomic Points

The skin overlying the clavicle is innervated by the medial, intermediate, and lateral supraclavicular nerves. These nerves, which arise as a common trunk from the cervical plexus,

contain fibers from C3 and C4. They emerge from the posterior border of the middle of the sternocleidomastoid muscle and descend under cover of the platysma muscle. They supply the skin over the clavicle and anterior thoracic wall to the level of the second rib. These nerves are accompanied by small branches of suprascapular or transverse cervical arteries, branches of the thyrocervical trunk.

The subclavian artery crosses over the first rib to become the axillary artery. Like the subclavian, the axillary artery is divided into three parts by an overlying muscle, in this case the pectoralis minor muscle. The first part of the axillary artery runs from the inferior border of the first rib to the medial margin of the pectoralis minor muscle. Its only branch is the highest (superior) thoracic artery (Fig. 30.1C). The second portion of the axillary artery lies deep to the pectoralis minor muscle. Its branches are the thoracoacromial artery and the lateral thoracic artery. The third part of the axillary artery

FIGURE 30.1
POSITION OF THE PATIENT AND EXPOSURE OF THE AXILLARY ARTERY

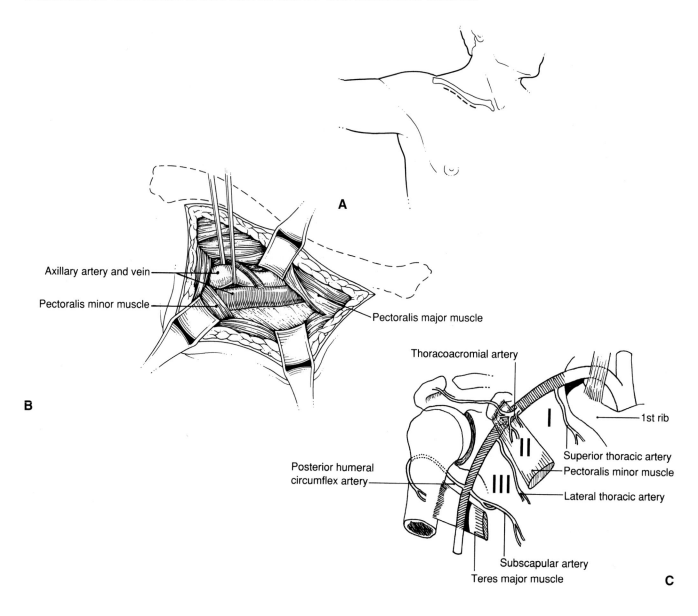

extends from the lateral border of the pectoralis minor muscle to the inferior margin of the teres minor muscle (where the axillary artery exits the axilla to become the brachial artery).

In addition to the arteries accompanying the supraclavicular nerves, other arteries present in the area include the perforating branches of the first anterior intercostal artery and branches of the thoracoacromial artery. The thoracoacromial artery, a branch of the second part of the axillary artery, pierces the clavipectoral fascia and divides into four branches (pectoral, acromial, clavicular, and deltoid). The pectoral branch runs between the two pectoral muscles and supplies them and the breast; the acromial branch crosses the coracoid process deep to the deltoid and supplies this muscle; the clavicular branch ascends medially between the clavicular part of the pectoralis major muscle and the clavipectoral fascia, supplying the subclavius muscle and sternoclavicular joint; and the deltoid branch accompanies the cephalic vein in the del-

topectoral triangle, supplying the deltoid and pectoralis major muscles. Carefully split the clavicular fibers of the pectoralis major muscle to expose the medial border of the pectoralis minor muscle to identify and control these branches.

Exposure of the medial border of the pectoralis minor muscle will allow visualization of the first part of the axillary artery, the axillary vein, and part of the brachial plexus. At this level, the axillary artery has only one branch, the highest (superior) thoracic artery. This small artery arises from the axillary artery near the inferior border of the subclavius muscle and then runs anteromedially above the medial border of the pectoralis minor muscle. It supplies the two pectoral muscles and the upper thoracic wall, anastomosing with branches of the intercostal arteries and the internal thoracic artery. The next branch of the axillary artery is the thoracoacromial artery (whose branches have already been described), which arises posterior to the insertion of the pectoralis minor muscle.

The axillary artery itself, at this level, is posterior to the axillary vein. In addition, it is surrounded by cords of the brachial plexus. The lateral cord lies lateral to the axillary artery, the medial cord lies medial to the artery, and the posterior cord is posterior to the artery. Slightly more proximal (retroclavicular), the axillary artery is related to the inferior divisions (i.e., the anterior and posterior divisions of the inferior trunk) of the brachial plexus. Here, the artery lies anterior to these divisions. Remember that all posterior divisions contribute to the posterior cord (primarily, the radial and axillary nerves), whereas the most inferior anterior divi-

sion contributes to the medial cord (primarily, the ulnar and medial head of the median nerve).

Exposure of Femoral Vessels (Fig. 30.2)

Technical Points

The groin dissection is often performed concurrently by a second surgeon as the axillary dissection progresses. Make a longitudinal skin incision overlying the femoral vessels (Fig. 30.2A). The incision should extend from 2 to 3 inches above the inguinal ligament to about 3 inches below the

FIGURE 30.2
EXPOSURE OF FEMORAL VESSELS

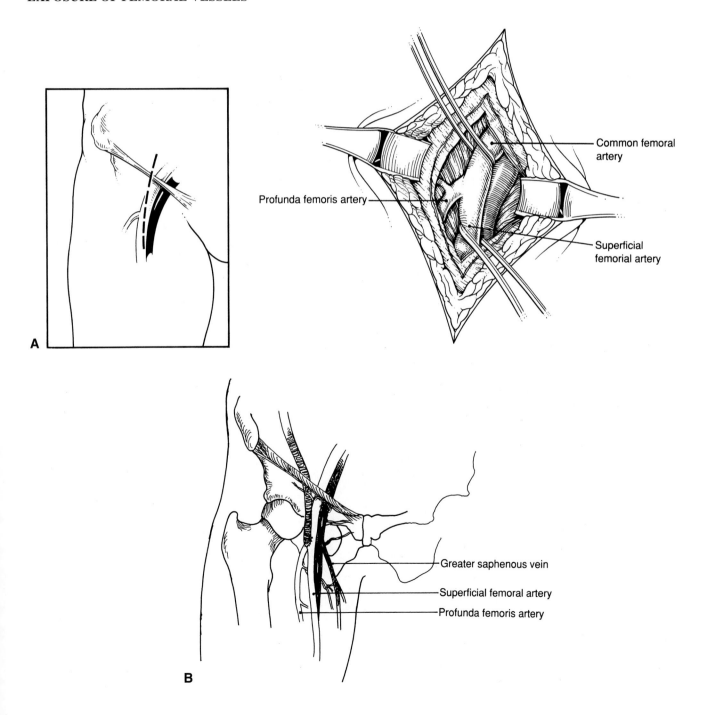

inguinal ligament. Be careful to avoid injury to the lymphatic channels and lymph nodes in the area. Carefully dissect the common femoral, profunda femoris, and superficial femoral artery using meticulous technique. Obtain proximal and distal control of each vessel using Silastic loops.

Prepare a tunnel along the midaxillary line extending from the subpectoral space to the groin incision for placement of the graft (Fig. 30.2B). Pass a Rob DeWeese tunneler or a long blunt-ended straight clamp through the subpectoral space laterally down to the groin incision. Make a counterincision midway between the axillary and groin incision to facilitate completion of this tunnel. The tunnel created will be medial to the anterosuperior iliac spine. Tie an umbilical tape to the tunneler and leave this in the tract as a guide for placement of the graft.

Anatomic Points

The longitudinal groin skin incision, with subsequent dissection through the superficial and deep fascia of the subinguinal region, should be made directly over the femoral artery. An incision in this location will necessitate division of the superficial circumflex iliac vein and, possibly, the superficial epigastric artery and vein. These vessels, located in the superficial fascia, can be ligated with impunity. The surgeon should be aware that the superficial (horizontal) group of inguinal lymph nodes lies in the superficial fascia, paralleling the inguinal ligament. The efferent lymph vessels from these nodes pass through the saphenous hiatus (fossa ovalis of the thigh), along with the greater saphenous vein, to drain into the deep inguinal lymph nodes lying medial to the femoral vein.

Divide the fascia lata and femoral sheath to expose the so-called common femoral artery and its two major branches, the superficial femoral artery and the profunda femoris artery. The profunda femoris artery arises from the posterolateral aspect of the femoral artery, about 3.5 cm distal to the inguinal ligament. Initially, it lies lateral to the superficial femoral artery; then, it passes posterior to the artery and femoral vein to pass distally posterior to the long adductor muscles.

Proximal Anastomosis (Fig. 30.3)

Technical and Anatomic Points

Ask the anesthesiologist to heparinize the patient fully (100 units/kg intravenously). Place an 8- or 10-mm graft into the tunnel tract. Achieve proximal and distal control of the exposed axillary artery using Silastic loops. Make a longitudinal arteriotomy about 2 cm long along the inferior surface of the artery. Sew an 8-mm woven Dacron graft with a beveled end to the axillary artery using a 5-0 polypropylene running stitch. Loosen the Silastic loop controlling the distal portion of the axillary artery to allow retrograde flow into the graft; then, release the proximal vessel loop. Clamp the graft below the anastomosis to reestablish flow to the upper extremity. Milk the graft free of blood. Tie the end of the graft to the umbilical tape and pass it through the tunnel. Mark the anterior aspect of the graft to ensure proper alignment of the graft when passed through the tunnel. Pull the end of the graft gently to avoid laxity and redundancy. Do not allow the axillary artery to kink or buckle as a result of straightening of the graft because this may lead to early thrombosis at the anastomotic site.

FIGURE 30.3
PROXIMAL ANASTOMOSIS

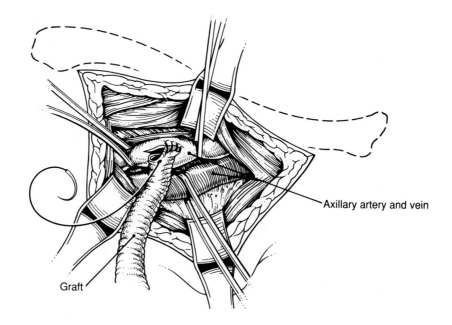

Axillary artery and vein

Graft

FIGURE 30.4
DISTAL ANASTOMOSIS AND AXILLOBIFEMORAL BYPASS

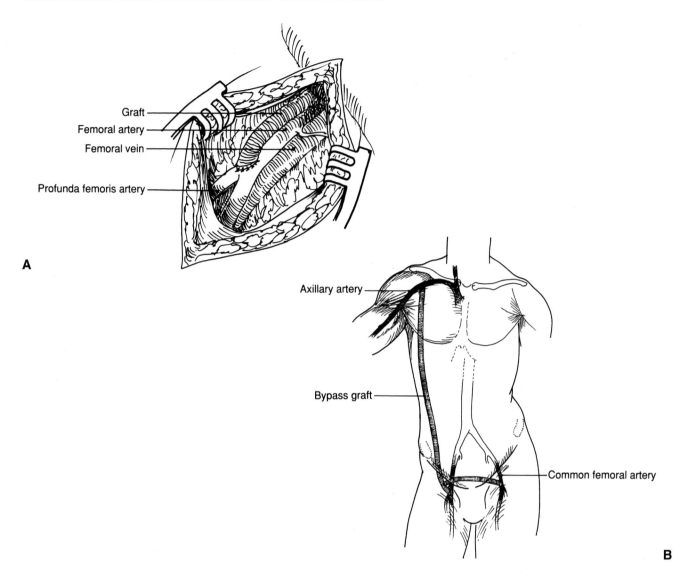

A

B

Distal Anastomosis and Axillobifemoral Bypass (Fig. 30.4)

Technical and Anatomic Points

Control the femoral vessels with vessel loops. Make an arteriotomy measuring 2 cm in the common femoral artery, extending it onto the deep femoral artery (Fig. 30.4A). Tailor the end of the graft and sew it to the femoral artery in an end-to-side fashion using 5-0 polypropylene. Release the axillary vascular clamp just before completion of the anastomosis to flush the graft of air and clot. Place a vascular clamp proximal to the femoral anastomosis. Release the vessel loops on the deep femoral and superficial femoral arteries to assess the anastomosis. Once hemostatic control is achieved at the anastomotic site, release all remaining vascular control. Assess the graft for proper alignment. Irrigate all wounds with antibiotic

solution. Close the subcutaneous tissue of each wound in two layers using absorbable suture. Close the skin with either staples or nylon suture.

Axillobifemoral Bypass

Perform the axillary dissection as previously described for axillofemoral bypass and perform bilateral groin dissections. After completing the axillofemoral anastomosis, use a Satinsky clamp to occlude partially the distal portion of the femoral limb of the graft.

Make an arteriotomy 1.5 to 2 cm long on the anteromedial surface of the distal portion of the graft. Tailor an 8-mm Dacron graft and anastomose it to the graft in an end-to-side fashion using a running 5-0 polypropylene suture. Tunnel this graft through the suprapubic subcutaneous tissue to the opposite groin. Sew the graft to the common femoral artery in an end-to-side fashion using 5-0 polypropylene (Fig. 30.4B).

Irrigate all wounds with antibiotic-containing irrigant. Close the subcutaneous tissue in two layers using absorbable suture. Close the skin using staples or nylon suture.

REFERENCES

1. Calligaro KD, Ascer E, Veith FJ, et al. Unsuspected inflow disease in candidates for axillofemoral bypass operations: a prospective study. *J Vasc Surg* 1990;11:832.
2. Ascer E, Veith FJ, Gupta SK, et al. Comparison of axillounifemoral and axillobifemoral bypass operations. *Surgery* 1985;97:169.
3. Cina C, Ameli FM, Kalman P, et al. Indications and role of axillofemoral bypass in high risk patients. *Ann Vasc Surg* 1988;2:237–241.
4. Rashleigh-Belcher HJ, Newcombe JF. Axillary artery thrombosis: a complication of axillo-femoral bypass grafts. *Surgery* 1987;101:373–375.

CHAPTER 31

Radial Artery Cannulation

The radial artery is cannulated for monitoring purposes. A catheter in the radial artery can be used for direct measurement of arterial pressure and for sampling arterial blood for blood gas determinations. It is almost always possible to cannulate the radial artery percutaneously, particularly if Doppler ultrasound guidance is used in difficult cases. Under rare circumstances, a patient with significant vascular disease or shock may require direct cutdown on the artery, with subsequent introduction of the catheter under direct vision. Both procedures are described in this chapter.

Position of the Extremity and Identification of Landmarks (Fig. 31.1)

Technical Points

Before inserting an indwelling radial artery catheter, perform an Allen test to assess the adequacy of collateral circulation of the ulnar artery across the palmar arch. Because the arch is variable, the adequacy of circulation must be checked in each individual and in each extremity. Instruct the patient to clench the fist tightly. Use both of your hands to occlude both the radial and ulnar arteries. Then have the patient open the fist, which should be blanched. Release pressure on the ulnar artery and note the time required for the hand to become pink. The hand should become pink within 3 seconds after release of occlusion. Alternatively, a Doppler ultrasound stethoscope may be used as a more objective means of determining the adequacy of circulation. Place the Doppler stethoscope over the palmar arch and do the test as previously described. In this case, use the appearance of Doppler flow in the palmar arch as evidence of collateral flow by the ulnar artery.

Place the patient's hand on an armboard with a roll under the wrist and secure the hand in a slightly wrist-cocked position. Palpate the radial pulse. Prepare the area over the radial pulse with povidone-iodine (Betadine) about 1 to 2 cm proximal to the crease in the wrist. Infiltrate the area with 1% lidocaine (Xylocaine). Palpate the patient's pulse with the fingers of your nondominant hand while gently introducing an over-the-needle catheter at an angle of about 45 degrees. As soon as pulsating arterial blood is obtained from the needle, slide the catheter over the needle into the artery. Pulsating blood should exit the catheter freely after the needle is removed. To stop the flow, simply occlude the radial artery proximal to the catheter entry site. Secure the catheter in place and secure the extremity.

Anatomic Points

To perform radial artery cannulation and cutdown successfully and safely, it is necessary to understand the relationships of skin creases, bony landmarks, and neurovascular structures at the wrist and to ascertain the blood supply and collateral circulation in the hand.

Typically, the flexor surface of the wrist has a proximal, middle, and distal skin crease. The proximal wrist crease does not correspond to any palpable landmarks. The middle wrist crease corresponds approximately to the styloid processes of both the radius and ulna as well as to the proximal extent of the common flexor synovial sheath. The consistent distal wrist crease is the most important of the three. From the radial to ulnar sides of the wrist, it overlies the tip of the styloid process, is just proximal to the tuberosity of the scaphoid, crosses the distal part of the lunate, and terminates just proximal to the pisiform. Furthermore, it marks the proximal border of the flexor retinaculum. The palmaris longus tendon bisects the distal skin crease and overlies the median nerve.

LIST OF STRUCTURES

Radial artery	Ulnar artery	Brachioradialis tendon
Superficial palmar radial artery	Deep palmar artery	Tendon of the flexor carpi radialis
Principal artery of the thumb	Superficial palmar arch	Tendons of the flexor digitorum
Radial artery of the index finger	Common palmar digital arteries	superficialis
Deep palmar arch	Radius	Tendon of the flexor carpi ulnaris
Palmar metacarpal arteries	Styloid process	Median nerve
	Ulna	Ulnar nerve
	Palmaris longus tendon	

FIGURE 31.1
POSITION OF THE EXTREMITY AND IDENTIFICATION OF LANDMARKS

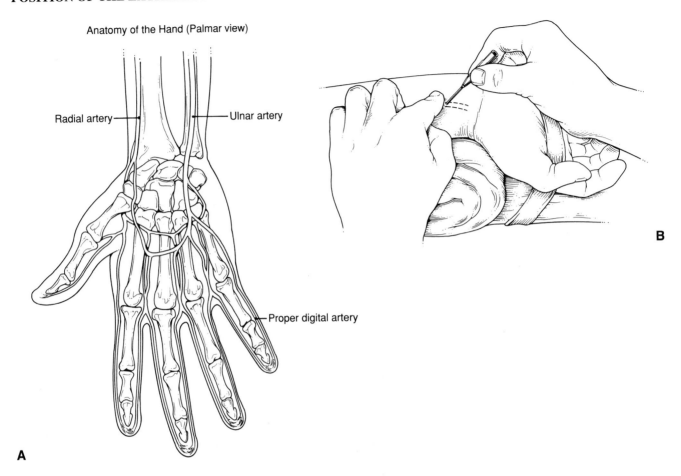

Anatomy of the Hand (Palmar view)

Radial artery

Ulnar artery

Proper digital artery

A

B

Identification of palpable structures at the wrist enables identification of the radial artery. The most lateral tendon is the brachioradialis tendon. The radial artery, identified by its pulsations, lies between this tendon and the tendon of the flexor carpi radialis muscle. Medial to this muscle is the palmaris longus tendon overlying the median nerve. The palmaris longus tendon is absent in about 10% of cases. Medial to this tendon (or centrally, if it is absent), tendons of the flexor digitorum superficialis can be palpated. Medial to this is the ulnar artery, accompanied (on its medial aspect) by the ulnar nerve. The most medial palpable structure is the tendon of the flexor carpi ulnaris.

The Allen test is used to determine whether the superficial palmar arterial arch, principally derived from the ulnar artery, is complete. The ulnar artery, always located superficial to the flexor retinaculum, gives off a small deep palmar artery, which passes deeply between the hypothenar muscles to contribute to the deep palmar arterial arch. The continuation of the ulnar artery past this point is the superficial palmar arterial arch, lying just deep to the palmar aponeurosis and curving laterally. The apex of this arch is located approximately at the level of the distal base of the extended thumb, or close to the proximal palmar skin crease. In about 88% of

hands examined, it anastomoses with an artery derived from the radial artery, such as the small superficial radial artery (35%), the principal artery of the thumb, or the radial artery of the index finger. In its course through the hand, the superficial arch gives off four common digital arteries; typically, these digital arteries are joined by a palmar metacarpal artery derived from the deep palmar arterial arch.

The deep palmar arterial arch is the major continuation of the radial artery. After the radial artery gives off its small superficial palmar branch, it wraps around the lateral aspect of the wrist, passing through the anatomic snuffbox, to lie on the dorsum of the hand. At the base of the first intermetacarpal space, this artery dives between the muscles of this space to enter the hand and becomes known as the *deep palmar arterial arch.* This arch runs medially across the palm of the hand in the interval between the long flexor tendons and the metacarpal bones with their attached interosseous muscles and usually is completed by anastomosing with a small derivative of the ulnar artery. Branches of the distal radial artery/deep palmar arterial arch include the principal artery of the thumb, the radial artery of the index finger (in 13%, this was found to arise solely from the superficial arch), the carpal arteries, and the metacarpal arteries.

FIGURE 31.2
RADIAL ARTERY CUTDOWN

Radial Artery Cutdown (Fig. 31.2)

Technical Points

Perform the Allen test, as previously described, to confirm adequacy of the ulnar collateral circulation. A transverse incision that is parallel to the wrist crease and 1 to 2 cm proximal to it may be used. Infiltrate the area with lidocaine and make an incision through the skin only. Use a hemostat to spread gently in a longitudinal direction as you look for the radial artery, which will lie just medial to the radius. Generally, it is identifiable by pulsations that, although they may not have been palpable before the wrist was open, will be palpable once the artery is exposed. The artery is exposed and then cannulated by direct puncture, as previously described. Close the incision loosely around the cannula.

Anatomic Points

Remember that the radial artery lies between the brachioradialis tendon laterally and the tendon of the flexor carpi radialis medially. It is worthwhile to note that the superficial radial nerve, which accompanies the radial artery proximally, is lateral (dorsal) to the brachioradialis tendon at the wrist. Likewise, the median nerve is medial to the tendon of the flexor carpi radialis muscle. Consequently, there is no nerve accompanying the radial artery at the wrist, although branches of the lateral antebrachial cutaneous nerve (a continuation of the musculocutaneous nerve) are located in the superficial fascia over the radial artery. Because no nerves actually accompany the radial artery at this level, iatrogenic nerve injuries are virtually nonexistent.

REFERENCES

1. Allen EV. Thromboangiitis obliterans: methods of diagnosis of chronic occlusive arterial lesions distal to the wrist with illustrative cases. *Am J Med Sci* 1929;178:237. (This is the original description of the test that bears the author's name.)
2. Brodsky JB. A simple method to determine patency of the ulnar artery intraoperatively prior to radial artery cannulation. *Anesthesiology* 1975;42:626.
3. Clakr VL, Kruse JA. Arterial catheterization. *Crit Care Clin* 1992;8: 687–698. (Excellent review includes alternative sites.)
4. Cronin KD. Radial artery cannulation: the influence of method on blood flow after decannulation. *Anaesth Intens Care* 1986;14:400.
5. Diz JC, Ares X, Tarrazo AM, et al. Bilateral superficial radial artery at the wrist. *Acta Anaesthesiol Scand* 1998;42:1020.
6. Durbin CG Jr. Radial arterial lines and sticks: what are the risks? *Respir Care* 2001;46:229–231. (Presents review of complications.)
7. Ejrup B, Fischer B, Wright IS. Clinical evaluation of blood flow to the hand: the false positive Allen test. *Circulation* 1966;33: 778.
8. Gellman H, Botte MJ, Shankwiler J, et al. Arterial patterns of the deep and superficial palmar arches. *Clin Orthop Relat Res* 2001;383:41–46. (Provides thorough review of anatomy and anomalies.)
9. Goldenheim PD, Kazemi H. Cardiopulmonary monitoring of critically ill patients. Part II. *N Engl J Med* 1984;311:776.
10. Jones RM. The effect of method of radial artery cannulation on postcannulation blood flow and thrombus formation. *Anesthesiology* 1981;55:76.

11. Kamienski RW, Barnes RW. Critique of the Allen test for continuity of the palmar arch assessed by Doppler ultrasound. *Surg Gynecol Obstet* 1976;142:861.

12. Mandel MA, Dauchot PJ. Radial artery cannulation in 1,000 patients: precautions and complications. *J Hand Surg* 1977;2:482.

13. Mozersky DJ. Ultrasonic evaluation of the palmar circulation. *Am J Surg* 1973;126:810.

14. Pyles ST. Cannulation of the dorsal radial artery: a new technique. *Anesth Analg* 1982;61:876. (Describes cannulation of the radial artery in the anatomic snuffbox.)

15. Slogoff S, Keats AS, Arlund C. On the safety of radial artery cannulation. *Anesthesiology* 1983;59:42.

16. Venus B, Mallory DL. Vascular cannulation. In: Civetta JM, Taylor RW, Kirby RR, eds. *Critical care.* Philadelphia: JB Lippincott, 1992:149.

CHAPTER 32

Vascular Access for Hemodialysis

Beth A. Ballinger

The creation of an arteriovenous fistula is a common procedure for surgeons involved in dialysis programs. The goal of this procedure is to create an accessible, high-flow (300 mL/min) conduit that can withstand repeated puncture by large-bore (16-gauge) needles and yet remain patent and uninfected. The most common access procedures are performed in the forearm. The Brescia-Cimino arteriovenous fistula is the preferred form of access because it is constructed from the patient's own tissue, making it durable and resistant to infection. When a fistula cannot be constructed, an arteriovenous hemodialysis graft using polytetrafluoroethylene (PTFE) is then created.

Incision and Identification of a Suitable Vein (Fig. 32.1)

Technical Points

The radial artery and the cephalic vein may be exposed through a single incision placed 1 cm lateral to the longitudinal axis of the radial artery. The nondominant upper extremity is preferred for dialysis access, presuming the vessels are of good quality because this allows freedom of movement for the dominant hand during the considerable hours spent undergoing hemodialysis.

Establish the position of the wrist joint crease by inspecting the skin folds of the flexed wrist. Place a tourniquet above the elbow to facilitate inspection of the distended veins of the forearm. When available, preoperative duplex Doppler ultrasound provides useful information regarding quality and patency of venous conduits. Phlebitic, occluded, or stenotic veins, whether at the forearm, brachial, or axillosubclavian level, will mandate selection of an alternate site. Large

side-branch tributaries of the cephalic vein may be identified on ultrasound; these should be ligated to promote fistula maturation. A straight vein that is confined to the anterior surface of the arm and has few tributaries is ideal for the creation of a fistula.

Place the incision proximal to the mobile areas of the wrist to prevent normal joint motion from affecting the anastomosis. A longitudinal incision, placed parallel to the vessels, allows the vein to be dissected far enough distally to reach the artery easily. Sharp dissection will minimize adventitial loss and destruction of the vasa vasorum when dissecting the vein. Bathing the vein in a dilute papaverine solution minimizes vasospasm and allows more accurate assessment of conduit quality and size.

Anatomic Points

The goal of this procedure is to anastomose the cephalic vein, located in the superficial fascia lateral (or dorsal) to the brachioradialis tendon, to the radial artery, located deep to the deep fascia and medial to the brachioradialis tendon. An incision 1 cm lateral to the axis of the radial artery, or directly over the brachioradialis tendon, will provide access to both of these vessels. A longitudinal incision carries less risk of dividing the sensory nerves in this area, which are branches of the superficial branch of the radial nerve. These branches frequently communicate with branches of the lateral antebrachial cutaneous nerve, a sensory branch of the musculocutaneous nerve. This incision can also easily be extended. The cephalic vein begins on the dorsum of the hand over the anatomic snuffbox, draining the lateral aspect of the dorsal venous arch. At approximately the junction of the distal and

LIST OF STRUCTURES

Radial artery	Brachial artery	Superficial radial nerve
Cephalic vein	Median nerve	Lateral antebrachial cutaneous nerve
Basilic vein	Biceps brachii tendon	Medial antebrachial cutaneous nerve
Superficial fascia	Bicipital aponeurosis	Musculocutaneous nerve
Median basilic vein	Brachioradialis tendon	Anatomic snuffbox
Median cephalic vein	Supinator muscle	
Median antebrachial vein	Radial nerve	

FIGURE 32.1
INCISION AND IDENTIFICATION OF A SUITABLE VEIN

FIGURE 32.2
EXPOSURE OF THE RADIAL ARTERY AND ITS VENAE COMITANTES

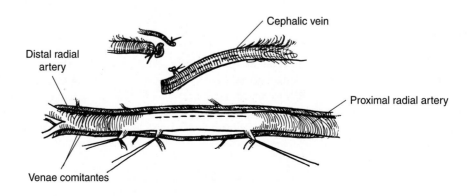

medial thirds of the forearm, it courses from the lateral aspect of the forearm to lie on its anterolateral surface. Distal to the cubital fossa, it has a wide communication with the median cubital vein, which is an oblique communication with the basilic vein. In the cubital region, there is typically a large communication between the superficial cephalic or median cubital vein and the deep venous drainage in the cubital fossa. The cephalic vein usually is accompanied by branches of the superficial radial nerve.

Exposure of the Radial Artery and its Venae Comitantes (Fig. 32.2)

Technical Points

Expose the radial artery by division of the forearm fascia. Mobilize a sufficient length of artery to allow proximal and distal control as well as construction of an anastomosis that is 6 to 10 mm long. Sharply dissect the venae comitantes from the artery in order to maintain a bloodless field for anastomotic control. Avoid ligating branches of the radial artery. Place a Silastic tourniquet or small atraumatic vascular clamp around these vessels, removing them at the end of the procedure.

Anatomic Points

The deep fascia of the forearm is continuous with the deep fascia of the arm and cubital fossa proximally, and also with the subcutaneous fascia of the hand. It is thicker proximally, where muscle fibers are seen to originate from it, and is attached to the epicondyles of the humerus and the olecranon process. Distally, it is thin except where it thickens to form the superficial and deep divisions of the flexor retinaculum; here, it is attached to the distal portions of the radius and ulna. Division of this fascia over the brachioradialis tendon, with reflection anteromedially, will expose the radial artery, which at this location emerges from under cover of the belly of the brachioradialis muscle and lies immediately deep to the deep fascia. Several branches of the radial artery may be seen near the wrist. Because most of these communicate with branches derived directly or indirectly from the ulnar artery, these branches should be controlled for hemostasis.

Again, remember that this artery, which in the proximal forearm was accompanied by the radial nerve, in the distal forearm at the wrist has no nerve accompanying it. Lateral to the cubital fossa, the radial nerve divides into deep and superficial branches. The deep branch pierces fibers of the supinator muscle to gain access to the posterior forearm, where it continues distally in the plane between superficial and deep extensors. The superficial branch, which is all sensory, leaves the company of the radial artery in the distal third of the forearm, passing dorsally deep to the tendon of the brachioradialis muscle and becoming superficial (i.e., piercing the deep fascia) near the dorsum of this wrist. This course places the main trunk of the superficial radial nerve out of the dissection field.

FIGURE 32.3
BRESCIA-CIMINO FISTULA (SIDE-TO-END ANASTOMOSIS)

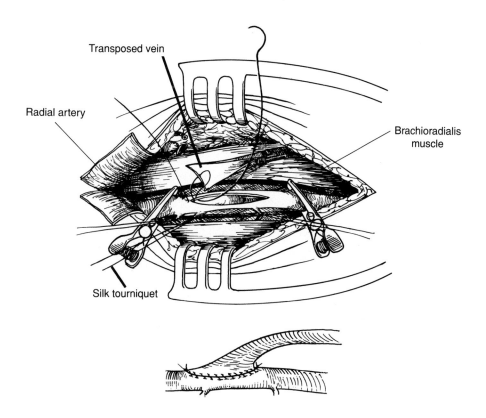

Transposed vein

Radial artery

Brachioradialis muscle

Silk tourniquet

FIGURE 32.4
ARTERIOVENOUS HEMODIALYSIS ACCESS WITH PROSTHETIC GRAFT

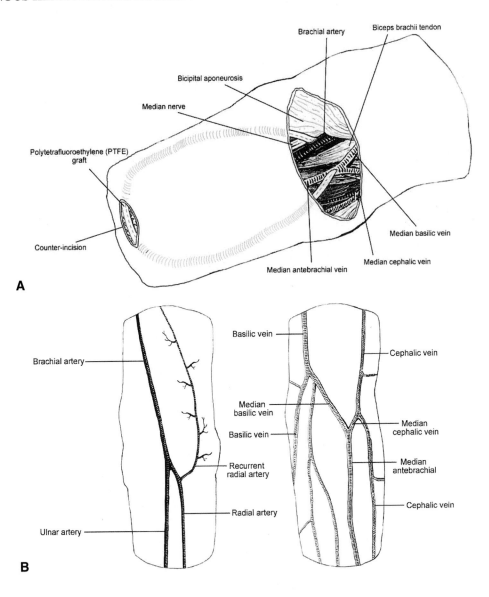

Brescia-Cimino Fistula (Side-To-End Anastomosis) (Fig. 32.3)

Technical and Anatomic Points

Spatulate the divided vein end to create a patulous anastomosis. Within the general guidelines of 6 to 10 mm, the actual length of the anastomosis is individually tailored. A vein 2.5 mm in diameter or greater is sufficiently large to promote successful fistula maturation. Avoid inserting dilators into the vein in order to minimize intimal injury. Carefully align the vein so that when it is distended with blood it will not be twisted or kinked because either may limit flow. Use a running 7-0 or 8-0 monofilament suture for the anastomosis. Sew the back wall from inside the lumen and the proximal suture line from outside the lumen.

Arteriovenous Hemodialysis Access with Prosthetic Graft (Fig. 32.4)

Technical Points

A graft of prosthetic material is used when the veins of the distal forearm are not adequate for creation of an arteriovenous fistula. Create a horizontal incision one fingerbreadth below the antecubital joint crease. Expose the brachial artery, median antebrachial vein, median basilic vein, and median cephalic vein (Fig. 32.4A). Expose the artery by retracting the bicipital aponeurosis, the fibrous expansion of the biceps brachii tendon, laterally. If necessary, divide a few of the aponeurosis fibers. Any of the veins may be used, depending on its position and quality. The veins in the antecubital region are relatively variable, but generally one of them is of sufficient caliber to serve as the venous outflow for the dialysis graft. Avoid dividing communicating venous branches because their patency will enhance graft venous outflow and graft patency.

Create a subcutaneous tunnel for the graft to lie in an ovoid or loop shape. The loop should be gently curved distally and about 10 to 12 cm long and 5 to 6 cm wide. A counterincision at the distal forearm will facilitate tunneling. Position a prestretched 6-mm, nonringed PTFE graft in the tunnel. Use care to avoid twisting or kinking of the graft especially at the distal forearm. The counterincision will aid in graft positioning. Systemically heparinize the patient. Perform the arterial anastomosis first. Minimally spatulate the arterial end of the PTFE graft. Anastomose it to an arteriotomy 7 to 8 mm long on the ventral side of the brachial artery using 6-0 monofilament suture.

Perform the venous anastomosis second. Carefully position the venotomy on the vein so that when the vein is distended with blood, it is neither twisted nor kinked. Spatulate the venous end of the graft so that an anastomosis of 7 to 10 mm is created. Use 6-0 or 7-0 monofilament suture for the anastomosis. Refrain from inserting dilators into the vein to avoid intimal injury.

Anatomic Points

There may be variability in the superficial veins of the forearm (Fig. 32.4B). In many instances, there is a median antebrachial vein that drains into the origins of the medial basilic and median cephalic veins. In other situations, it can drain into either. Recognizing anatomic variability is helpful so that a vein of appropriate quality and caliber can be identified for use.

Exposure of the median cephalic and median basilic veins should be done carefully to avoid injury to adjacent cutaneous nerves. Although these veins lie in the superficial fascia of the forearm, they are in close proximity to the medial and lateral antebrachial cutaneous nerves. These veins may cross superficially over these nerves. The median nerve enters the forearm medial to the brachial artery and should be carefully protected during arterial dissection.

REFERENCES

1. Bonalumi V, Civalleri D, Rovidas S, et al. Nine years' experience with end-to-end arteriovenous fistula at the anatomical snuffbox for maintenance hemodialysis. *Br J Surg* 1982;69:486. (Discusses most distal arteriovenous fistula.)
2. Brescia MJ, Cimino JE, Appel K, et al. Chronic hemodialysis using venipuncture and a surgically created arteriovenous fistula. *N Engl J Med* 1966;275:1089. (This is the original description of this technique.)
3. Butt KMH, Friedman EA, Kountz SL. Angioaccess. *Curr Probl Surg* 1976;13. (Provides good technical description of Scribner shunt and Brescio-Cimino fistula.)
4. Garcia-Rinaldi R, VonKoch L. The axillary artery to axillary vein bovine graft for circulatory access: surgical considerations. *Am J Surg* 1978;135:265. (Describes useful technique when more distal vessels are unsuitable.)
5. Humphries AL, Nesbit RR, Caruana RJ, et al. Thirty-six recommendations for vascular access operations: lessons learned from our first thousand operations. *Am Surg* 1981;47:145.
6. Koontz PG, Helling TS. Subcutaneous brachial vein arteriovenous fistula for chronic hemodialysis. *World J Surg* 1983;7:672. (Describes technique using autologous tissue.)
7. Matsumoto T, Simonian S, Kholoussy AM. *Manual of vascular access procedures.* Norwalk, CT: Appleton Century Crofts, 1987. (Provides concise, portable guide to a variety of access procedures for chronic renal failure and chemotherapy.)
8. McCormack LJ, Cauldwell EW, Anson BJ. Brachial and antebrachial arterial patterns: a study of 750 extremities. *Surg Gynecol Obstet* 1953;96:43.
9. Moosa HH, Peitzman AB, Thompson BR, et al. Salvage of exposed arteriovenous hemodialysis fistulas. *Surgery* 1985;2:610.
10. Morsy AH, Kulbaski M, Chen C, et al. Incidence and characteristics of patients with ischemia after hemodialysis access procedure. *J Surg Res* 1998;187:421–426.
11. Shemesh D, Mabjeesh NJ, Abramowitz HB. Management of dialysis access-associated steal syndrome: use of intraoperative duplex ultrasound scanning for optimal flow reduction. *J Vasc Surg* 1999;30:193–195.
12. So SKS. Arteriovenous communication: internal fistulas. Arteriovenous communication: bridge grafts. In: Simmons RL, Finch ME, Ascher NL, et al, eds. *Manual of vascular access, organ donation, and transplantation.* New York: Springer-Verlag, 1984;47:60.
13. Wixon CL, Hughes JD, Mills JL. Understanding strategies for the treatment of ischemic steal syndrome after hemodialysis access. *J Am Coll Surg* 2000;191:301–310.

CHAPTER 33

Tendon Repair

Preservation of mobility and function is a critical consideration in the repair of tendon injuries of the forearm and hand. In this chapter, the anatomy relating to the extensor and flexor tendons of the hand is explored, and the basic principles of tendon repair are described.

The flexor surface of the hand and wrist is divided into five zones, based on the anatomy (see the orientation figure). Zone I is distal to the insertion of the superficial flexor muscle of the fingers. Zone II extends from zone I to the proximal side of the A1 pulley, formerly termed *no-man's land* because the results of primary repair were poor. Zone III extends proximally from the A1 pulley to the flexor retinaculum. Zone IV is synonymous with the carpal tunnel, and zone V is proximal to the carpal tunnel.

The extensor aspect is also divided into zones, starting distally. These zones are defined as follows:

I—Dorsum of the distal interphalangeal joint
II—Dorsum of the middle phalanx
III—Dorsum of the proximal interphalangeal joint
IV—Dorsum of the proximal phalanx
V—Dorsum of the metacarpophalangeal joint
VI—Dorsum of the metacarpal bone
VII—Dorsum of the wrist
VIII—Dorsum of the distal forearm

The site of a skin laceration may not correspond directly to the site of tendon laceration, depending on the angle of the cutting instrument and the position of the hand (finger extension versus finger flexion) at the time of injury.

Surgical repair is only a small part of the treatment. Accurate diagnosis of all associated injuries, consideration of the timing of surgery (early versus delayed repair), careful splinting postoperatively, and rehabilitation are all critical factors in achieving a good result. The tendon must be able to glide smoothly within its sheath. Scar formation between the repaired tendon and the sheath will severely compromise mobility.

Incision (Fig. 33.1)

Technical Points

Surgery on the hand and forearm is generally performed using nerve-block anesthesia. Tourniquet ischemia is helpful to produce a bloodless field in which structures can be dissected accurately. Prepare the entire hand and all fingers and drape it free, allowing it to rest on an operating arm board.

Plan an incision that zigzags along the volar digital surface (Fig. 33.1A). This incision affords excellent exposure while minimizing problems secondary to wound contracture. It may be possible to make such an incision by extending the original laceration, after débriding the edges.

Anatomic Points

This incision provides excellent exposure and is not attended by problems associated with contracture. Laterally, however, care must be taken to avoid the palmar digital neurovascular bundles (the dorsal arteries are insignificant). These bundles lie along the sides of the digital flexor sheaths, not along

LIST OF STRUCTURES

Flexor muscles and tendons
Pronator teres
Pronator quadratus
Flexor carpi radialis
Flexor carpi ulnaris
Flexor digitorum superficialis
Flexor digitorum profundus
Flexor hallucis longus
Extensor muscles and tendons
Brachioradialis muscle
Extensor carpi radialis longus

Extensor carpi radialis brevis
Extensor carpi ulnaris
Abductor pollicis longus
Extensor pollicis brevis
Extensor pollicis longus
Extensor indicis
Extensor digiti minimi
Extensor digitorum
Other structures
Ulnar bursa
Radial bursa

Palmar aponeurosis
Superficial palmar arterial arch
Median nerve
Ulnar nerve
Carpal bones
Metacarpal bones
Phalanges
Carpal tunnel
Dorsal venous arch

ORIENTATION

Zones of the Hand

bone. Of the three components of the neurovascular bundle, the nerve is most palmar, and the vein is most dorsal.

The anterior (palmar) and medial aspects of the forearm, wrist, and hand include muscles and tendons involved with flexion of the extremity (Fig. 33.1B). One muscle, the palmaris longus, attaches to the palmar aponeurosis, and its tendon is superficial to the middle of the flexor retinaculum. Two muscles in the anterior compartment—the pronator teres and pronator quadratus muscles—are concerned solely with rotation of the radius relative to the ulna and, hence, do not extend into the wrist and hand region. Two other muscles—flexor carpi radialis and ulnaris—are powerful flexors that likewise do not flex into the hand and have no components that pass through the carpal tunnel. Three additional muscles are concerned with flexion of the digits, and all components of these muscles pass through the carpal tunnel. Two of these—flexor digitorum superficialis and profundus—each divide into four tendons that provide flexion of digits 2 through 5. The final function of the muscle, the long flexor muscle of the thumb, is solely flexion of the thumb (digit 1). Because flexor tendon injuries most often involve digital flexors, the following

anatomic description will be limited to these muscles and their relationships.

The digital flexors, including the flexor hallucis longus, all have fleshy origins from the medial epicondylar region and the anterior aspect of the radius, ulna, and interosseous membrane. In the distal third of the forearm, these muscles become tendinous, and all tendons pass through the carpal tunnel, an osteofibrous tunnel formed by the carpal bones and the flexor retinaculum. The latter structure forms the roof of the canal. Components of the carpal tunnel can be considered in three layers. The most superficial structure is the median nerve, which is just deep to the flexor retinaculum. This nerve has a tendency to be located toward the radial side of the canal. Deep to the median nerve are the four tendons of the flexor digitorum superficialis. The deepest layer includes the four tendons of the flexor digitorum profundus, plus the tendon of the flexor hallucis longus. All tendons of both the superficial and deep flexor muscles of the fingers are enclosed in a common synovial sheath, the ulnar bursa. This bursa extends proximally into the wrist and distally into the hand, where it continues as the synovial bursa for the fifth finger,

FIGURE 33.1
INCISION

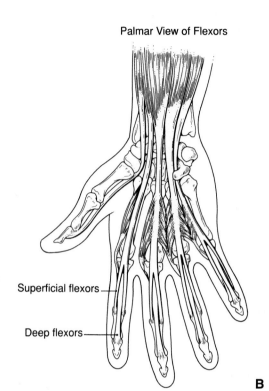

Palmar View of Flexors

Incision line

Superficial flexors

Deep flexors

A

B

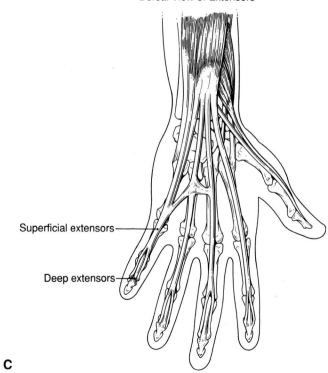

Dorsal View of Extensors

Superficial extensors

Deep extensors

C

extending essentially to the insertions of the extrinsic flexor tendons of this finger. The flexor hallucis longus is surrounded by its own synovial sheath, the radial bursa, which invests this tendon along its entire length.

After passing through the carpal tunnel, the flexor tendons fan out in the palm of the hand to pass to their respective digits. Superficial flexor tendons of the fingers are superficial to the deep tendons and immediately deep to the palmar aponeurosis, except where the superficial palmar arterial arch and its branches and the digital branches of the median and ulnar nerves intervene. Also in this region, the four lumbrical muscles originate from the deep tendons and pass to the radial side of their respective digit to insert into the extensor apparatus distal to the metacarpophalangeal joint.

When the flexor tendons enter the finger, they are invested in a strong osteofibrous canal, the ligamentous part of which is termed a *tendon sheath*. Each tendon sheath is lined by a synovial sheath or digital bursa, which is reflected on the contained tendons. Different regions of the fibrous sheath are thickened to form retinacula or "pulleys"; these so-called pulleys are named (annular or cruciate) according to the orientation of their component fibers and are numbered consecutively (A1 through A4, C1 through C3) from proximal to distal. Within the digital sheath, the superficial and deep tendons are tethered to the phalanges by expressions of the mesotendon termed *vincula brevia* and *longa*. In addition to tethering the tendons to bone, the vincula also carry a blood supply to the tendons.

The manner of insertion of the extrinsic flexor tendons is of crucial importance in the treatment of digital tendon injuries. At the level of the metacarpophalangeal joint, the tendons of the superficial flexor muscles of the fingers divide into two divergent slips, forming a chiasma through which the deep tendon passes. The two slips of each superficial flexor tendon spiral around and decussate dorsal to the deep tendon, finally inserting onto the sides of the midportion of the middle phalanx. The deep tendon continues through the chiasma to insert onto the base of the distal phalanx.

The muscles of the posterior (dorsal) and lateral aspects of the forearm, wrist, and hand are basically involved with extension and supination of the wrist and hand, although one muscle, the brachioradialis muscle, serves as a weak flexor of the elbow (Fig. 33.1C). Three muscles—extensor carpi radialis longus and brevis and extensor carpi ulnaris—function as extensors of the wrist. Three muscles function in thumb movements: the abductor pollicis longus, extensor pollicis brevis, and extensor pollicis longus. Two muscles—extensor indicis and extensor digiti minimi—control the extension of one digit only. One muscle, the extensor digitorum, is an extensor of digits 2 through 5. All of these tendons, with the exception of the brachioradialis tendon, pass through different osteofibrous compartments created by fusion of the extensor retinaculum with elevations of the dorsal surface of the radius and ulna. This fusion creates six extensor compartments. These compartments are numbered from radial to ulnar. The first compartment is occupied by tendons of the abductor pollicis longus and extensor pollicis brevis. The second

---

FIGURE 33.2
SUTURE OF TENDON

Tendon Repair Using the Bunnell Suture Technique

Tendon Repair

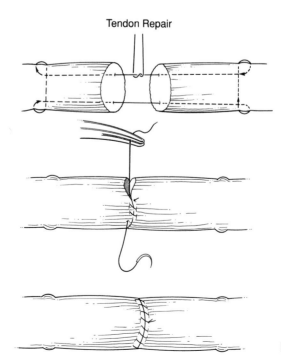

A

B

compartment contains the extensor carpi radialis longus and brevis. The extensor pollicis longus is the only tendon in the third compartment. Compartment four allows passage of the four tendons of the extensor digitorum and the extensor indicis. The tendon of the extensor digiti minimi passes through the fifth compartment, and the extensor carpi ulnaris occupies compartment six. It should be noted that, as the tendons pass through these osteofibrous compartments, they are invested in synovial bursa. With the exception of the bursa that is common to all tendons in the fourth compartment, each tendon has its own bursa.

On the back of the hand, the superficial fascia contains the dorsal venous arch, branches of the superficial branch of the radial nerve, and branches of the dorsal branch of the ulnar nerve. The superficial branch of the radial nerve is located in the fascia over the anatomic snuffbox and typically provides sensory innervation to the radial two thirds (approximately) of the dorsum of the hand and the dorsum of the radial three and one-half digits, about as far distally as the proximal interphalangeal joint. (Distal to this, sensory innervation is provided by digital branches of the median nerve.) The dorsal branch of the ulnar nerve supplies the rest of the ulnar one third (approximately) of the dorsum of the hand and the ulnar one and one-half digits.

Tendons of the extensor digitorum, located on the dorsum of the hand, are variably connected to each other by intertendinous connections. These connections, which possibly limit independent extension of the digits, are attached only to the extensor tendons of the fingers. Their recognition can be of value in surgical identification of tendons, especially of the extensor indicis and extensor digiti minimi.

At the level of the metacarpophalangeal joints, the extensor tendons become continuous with complicated aponeurotic extensor "hoods," to which are attached the extensor tendons, lumbrical muscles, and both dorsal and palmar interosseous muscles. This intricate mechanism involves all digital joints.

Suture of Tendon (Fig. 33.2)

Technical and Anatomic Points

Identify the cut ends of the tendon. It may be necessary to flex the wrist and digits sharply to bring the retracted tendon into the operative field. Handle the ends of the tendon as little as possible and perform as little débridement as possible. Do not strip the delicate areolar tissue from the tendon because this tissue contains small vessels and is especially critical in zones III and V.

The classic suture for tendon repair is the Bunnell suture (Fig. 33.2A). Unfortunately, this tends to accordion the tendon, and for this reason, many surgeons prefer the Kessler modification of the Maxon-Allen stitch (Fig. 33.2B). In either case, approximate the cut ends accurately and handle the tendon as little as possible. A 4-0 or 5-0 coated Dacron suture is useful for this.

Place a fine running suture of 6-0 nylon to approximate the epitenon securely. Place this suture in a slightly inverting fashion, so that the smooth epitenon completely encases the cut tendon, thereby producing a smooth-gliding surface.

REFERENCES

1. Ariyam S. *The hand book.* New York: McGraw-Hill, 1984. (Good basic reference with emphasis on emergency situations.)
2. Bruner JM. The zig-zag volar digital incision for flexor tendon surgery. *Plast Reconstr Surg* 1967;40:571.
3. Chase RA, Laub DR. The hand: therapeutic strategy for acute problems. *Curr Probl Surg* 1966. (Provides excellent review of emergency surgery of the hand.)
4. Idler RS. Anatomy and biomechanics of the digital flexor tendons. *Hand Clin* 1985;1:3.
5. Kessler I. The grasping technique for tendon repair. *Hand* 1973;5:253.
6. Kleinert HE, Schepel S, Gill T. Flexor tendon injuries. *Surg Clin North Am* 1981;61:267.
7. Lampe EW. Surgical anatomy of the hand. *CIBA-Geigy Clin Symp* 1988;40.
8. Lluch AL. Repair of the extensor tendon system. In Aston SJ, Beasley RW, Thorne CHM. eds. *Grabb and Smith's plastic surgery.* 5th ed. Philadelphia: Lippincott-Raven, 1997:883–888.
9. Taras JS, Schneider LH. *Atlas of the hand clinics: flexor tendon repair.* Vol. 1. Philadelphia: WB Saunders, 1996.
10. Zidel P. Tendon healing and flexor tendon surgery. In Aston SJ, Beasley RW, Thorne CHM. eds. *Grabb and Smith's plastic surgery.* 5th ed. Philadelphia: Lippincott-Raven, 1997:875–882.

CHAPTER 34

Carpal Tunnel Release

The median nerve passes through a narrow, rigid-walled canal (the carpal tunnel) as it enters the hand. Here, it is vulnerable to compression from trauma, anomalous muscles within the canal, poorly healed fractures (causing slight shifts in the dimensions of the canal), and swelling from adjacent tenosynovitis. In selected cases, release of the median nerve by surgical incision of the roof of the canal may be required. This procedure, termed *carpal tunnel release,* is discussed in this chapter as a means of illustrating the relevant anatomy of the volar surface of the wrist and hand.

Incision (Fig. 34.1)

Technical Points

Surgery on the hand is performed under nerve-block anesthesia at the level of the brachial plexus. Tourniquet-produced ischemia provides a dry operative field within which surgery can be performed with precision. Prepare the entire hand and drape it free. Place it comfortably on an operating armboard, with the volar surface of the wrist and hand turned upward.

Outline an incision that curves in the natural skin crease at the base of the thenar eminence, beginning about halfway from the wrist to the web space of the thumb. As the incision approaches the wrist crease, draw it longitudinally across this crease, and then angle the proximal extension of the incision toward the ulnar side of the wrist.

Anatomic Points

This incision is designed to accommodate the anatomic variations of the median nerve and to provide an adequate release for the carpal tunnel segment of this nerve. If the incision is kept wholly within the skin and superficial fascia, no motor nerves and no trunks of sensory nerves should be encountered. However, the potential for damage to the motor or recurrent median nerve always exists if one is not cognizant of its presence and its possible anatomic variations. Most frequently, the recurrent (motor) branch of the median nerve is given off the radial division or side of the median nerve distal to the flexor retinaculum and is recurrent (in about 50% of cases). The next most common variant is for the nerve to arise on the radial side of the median nerve in the carpal tunnel but to pass through the tunnel and take a recurrent course to innervate the thenar muscles (in about 33% of cases). The third most common variant (in about 20% of cases) is for the nerve to arise from the radial side of the median nerve in the carpal tunnel, then to pass through fibers of the flexor retinaculum to reach the thenar muscles; in this case, its course is not recurrent. In addition to these variants, in rare instances, the nerve arises from the ulnar side of the median nerve and takes a recurrent course to the thenar muscles. This can be further complicated by the recurrent branch lying on the superficial aspect of the flexor retinaculum. Further variants of note include a high division of the median nerve, so that two nerves lie in the carpal tunnel; accessory branches of the recurrent nerve to the thenar muscles; and instances in which the recurrent branch leaves the median nerve proximal to the carpal tunnel and passes through or superficial to the fibers of the flexor retinaculum. One additional anatomic variation of note is the occasional presence of a persistent median artery accompanying the median nerve through the carpal tunnel and, occasionally, an aberrant muscle in the tunnel.

LIST OF STRUCTURES

Median nerve
  Anterior interosseous branch
  Palmar cutaneous branch
  Recurrent (motor) branch
  Lateral ramus
  Medial ramus
Carpal tunnel
Thenar eminence
Flexor retinaculum

Median artery (persistent)
Antebrachial fascia
Transverse carpal ligament (flexor
  retinaculum)
Carpal bones
  Pisiform bone
  Hamate
  Scaphoid
  Trapezium

Tendons of the flexor digitorum
  superficialis
Tendons of the flexor digitorum
  profundus
Tendon flexor hallucis longus
Radial bursa
Ulnar bursa
Superficial palmar arterial arch
Deep palmar arterial arch

FIGURE 34.1
INCISION

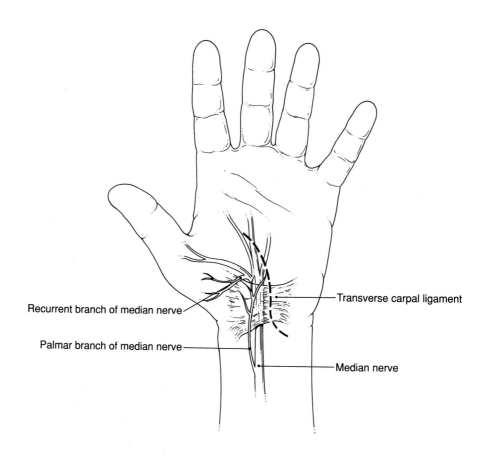

Recurrent branch of median nerve

Palmar branch of median nerve

Transverse carpal ligament

Median nerve

Exposure of the Carpal Tunnel (Fig. 34.2)

Technical Points

Identify the palmaris longus tendon and retract it radially. This should also retract and protect the palmar branch of the median nerve. Incise the palmar fascia to expose the transverse carpal ligament.

Anatomic Points

The median nerve at the wrist is almost entirely sensory. Proximal to the flexor retinaculum, it is immediately deep to the tendon of the long palmar muscle, which inserts on the palmar aponeurosis, with fibers adherent to the flexor retinaculum. Typically, in the distal forearm and hand, the nerve has the following branches:

FIGURE 34.2
EXPOSURE OF THE CARPAL TUNNEL

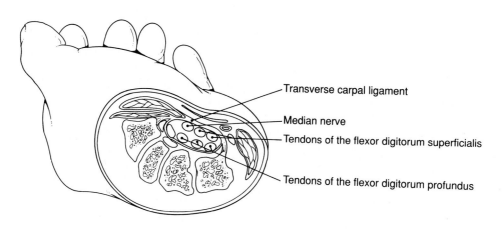

Transverse carpal ligament

Median nerve

Tendons of the flexor digitorum superficialis

Tendons of the flexor digitorum profundus

1. *Anterior interosseous.* This branch originates as the median nerve passes through the pronator teres muscle. It runs distally on the anterior surface of the interosseous membrane. Proximally, it supplies the radial half of the flexor digitorum profundus and flexor pollicis longus. Distally, it passes posterior to the pronator quadratus, which it supplies, and then provides innervation to joints of the wrist.
2. *Palmar cutaneous.* This branch typically starts just proximal to the flexor retinaculum, then pierces either the retinaculum or the distal deep fascia of the forearm. It then divides into lateral branches supplying the skin of the thenar eminence, some of which connect with the lateral cutaneous nerve (from the musculocutaneous nerve) of the forearm, and medial branches that supply the central palmar skin and connect with a palmar cutaneous branch from the ulnar nerve.
3. *Recurrent branch.* This branch typically arises from the radial side of the median nerve in the carpal tunnel, exiting the tunnel and taking a recurrent path to supply the flexor pollicis brevis, abductor pollicis brevis, opponens pollicis, and occasionally, the first dorsal interosseous muscle.
4. *Lateral ramus.* This branch arises in the carpal tunnel or distally. Through subsequent branching into the common and proper digital nerves, this branch provides sensory innervation to the thumb and the radial side of the index

finger. In addition, the proper digital branch to the radial side of the index finger also supplies the first lumbrical muscle. These digital branches are initially deep to the superficial palmar arch and its common digital branches.
5. *Medial ramus.* This branch, too, arises either in the carpal tunnel or distally. Through subsequent branching into the common and proper digital nerves, it provides sensory innervation to the ulnar side of the index finger, both sides of the middle finger, and the radial side of the ring finger. The common digital branch to the contiguous sides of the index and middle fingers supplies the second lumbrical muscle. Again, the common digital nerves are initially deep to the superficial palmar arterial arch and its common digital branches. Division of the common digital nerves into proper digital nerves occurs in the palm, much more proximally than the corresponding division of common digital arteries in the web spaces. In the distal palm, the common digital artery passes posteriorly between proper digital branches of the nerve, so that, in the fingers, the nerve is most posterior (dorsal).

Carpal Tunnel Release (Fig. 34.3)

Technical Points

Expose the median nerve in the distal forearm by incising the antebrachial fascia. Follow the median nerve into the carpal

FIGURE 34.3
CARPAL TUNNEL RELEASE

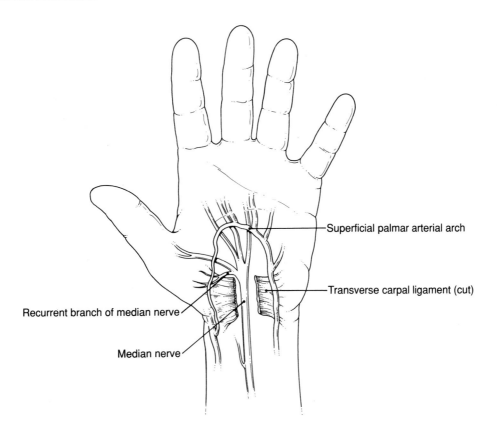

Superficial palmar arterial arch

Transverse carpal ligament (cut)

Recurrent branch of median nerve

Median nerve

tunnel, carefully incising the transverse carpal ligament with the median nerve in direct view. Avoid the palmar arterial arch, which is in close proximity to the distal end of the carpal tunnel. Identify and protect the recurrent nerve. Occasionally, it may be necessary to release this nerve from surrounding scar tissue.

Anatomic Points

The carpal tunnel is an osteofibrous canal formed by the carpal bones posteriorly and laterally, and by the transverse carpal ligament anteriorly. In the tunnel are four tendons of the flexor digitorum superficialis, four tendons of the flexor digitorum profundus, the tendon of the flexor pollicis longus, and the median nerve. The tendon of the latter is enveloped in an isolated (usually) synovial sheath, the radial bursa, whereas the other tendons are enveloped in a common synovial sheath, the ulnar bursa.

The transverse carpal ligament is attached medially to the pisiform bone and hook of the hamate bone, and laterally to the scaphoid and trapezium bones. It is 2.5 to 3 cm long transversely and has about the same dimensions longitudinally. It is important to note that the median nerve is immediately posterior to the ligament and either directly in the midline or somewhat to the radial side of the tunnel. Further, the surgeon should be aware that the ulnar nerve and artery do not pass through the carpal tunnel, but pass superficial to the medial attachment of the ligament. Posterior to the median nerve are the four tendons of the superficial flexor muscles of the fingers. Of these, the tendons to the third and fourth digits are immediately posterior to the median nerve, whereas those to the second and fifth digits are somewhat more posterior and further removed from the axis of the wrist and hand. Deep (posterior) to these are the tendons of the deep flexor muscles of the fingers. Unlike those of the superficial muscle, these four tendons lie side by side, on the same plane. In this plane, as well, is the tendon of the long flexor muscle of the thumb.

The relations of arteries to the flexor retinaculum and carpal tunnel are important. The superficial palmar arterial arch, which lies just deep to the palmar aponeurosis, is a continuation of the ulnar artery. It lies about 1 to 2 cm distal to the flexor retinaculum and should be avoided if at all possible. The deep palmar arterial arch, the continuation of the radial artery, enters the palm of the hand between the bases of the first two metacarpal bones. It then courses across the bases of the metacarpal bones to anastomose with the deep branch of the ulnar artery. It is more proximal than the superficial arch, lying approximately at the distal limit of the flexor retinaculum. It is seldom injured in lacerations of the wrist, either by lay people or by surgeons performing carpal tunnel releases, because it is so deeply situated.

REFERENCES

1. Amadio PC. Anatomic variations of the median nerve within the carpal tunnel. *Clin Anat* 1988;1:23.
2. Amadio PC. Bifid median nerve with a double compartment within the transverse carpal canal. *J Hand Surg [Am]* 1987;12:366–368.
3. Ariyan S, Watson HK. The palmar approach for the direct visualization and release of the carpal tunnel. *Plast Reconstr Surg* 1977;60:539.
4. Burton RI, Littler JW. Entrapment syndromes of the retinacular or restraining systems of the hand. *Curr Probl Surg* 1975;17. (Provides excellent brief description of technique.)
5. Graham WP. Variations of the motor branch of the median nerve at the wrist. *Plast Reconstr Surg* 1973;51:90.
6. Lanz U. Anatomical variations of the median nerve in the carpal tunnel. *J Hand Surg [Am]* 1977;2:44.
7. Netscher DT, Cohen V. Ulnar nerve entrapment at the wrist: cases from a hand surgery practice. *South Med J* 1998;91:451–456. (Describes a rare common compression syndrome.)
8. Propeck T, Quinn TJ, Jacobson JA, et al. Sonography and MR imaging of bifid median nerve with anatomic and histologic correlation. *AJR Am J Roentgenol* 2000;175:1721–1725.
9. Sennett BJ, Savoie FH. Surgery of the hand. In Greenfield LJ, et al, eds. *Surgery: scientific principles and practice.* 2nd ed. Philadelphia: Lippincott-Raven, 1999;2155–2156. (Presents nice illustration of endoscopic technique.)
10. Skandalakis JE, Colborn GL, Skandalakis PN, et al. The carpal tunnel syndrome: Parts I, II, and III. *Am Surg* 1992;58:72, 77, 158. (Provides excellent description of anatomy and surgical technique.)
11. Taleisnik J. The palmar cutaneous branch of the median nerve and the approach to the carpal tunnel: an anatomical study. *J Bone Joint Surg Am* 1973;55:1212.

SECTION IV

The Abdominal Region

This is the longest section of this book, reflecting the complexity and diversity of abdominal operative procedures commonly performed during training and by practicing general surgeons. It is divided into several parts.

The first part, *Basic Abdominal Procedures and the Abdomen in General* (Chapters 35 to 39), deals with the anatomy of the anterior abdominal wall and peritoneal recesses. The general layout of the peritoneal cavity is described.

The next part, *The Upper Gastrointestinal Tract and Structures of the Left Upper Quadrant* (Chapters 40 to 55), continues the anatomy first introduced in Chapters 28 and 29. The distal esophagus, stomach, duodenum, and spleen are described.

Next, the right upper quadrant is addressed in the part on *The Liver, Biliary Tract, and Pancreas* (Chapters 56 to 65), including a description of the operative procedures performed on the extrahepatic biliary tree and liver. The pancreas, which strictly speaking is a retroperitoneal structure, is included here because of tradition and because operations involving the pancreas and biliary tree often overlap.

The next part, devoted to *The Small and Large Intestine* (Chapters 66 to 74), continues the discussion of the alimentary tract, presenting the anatomy of the small and large intestine. Both operative and endoscopic procedures are discussed as a means of describing these organs. The anatomy of *The Pelvis* is described through the operations of abdominoperineal and low anterior resection of the rectum (Chapters 75 and 76) as well as total abdominal hysterectomy and oophorectomy (Chapters 77 and 78).

The next part, *The Retroperitoneum* (Chapters 79 to 85), explores renal and adrenal (suprarenal) surgery, aortic surgery, and the rarely performed operation of lumbar sympathectomy. Finally, the part entitled *The Inguinal Region* (Chapter 86 to 89) provides a transition to the next section of the text, **The Sacral Region and Perineum.**

BASIC ABDOMINAL PROCEDURES AND THE ABDOMEN IN GENERAL

The detailed anatomy of the muscles and fascial layers of the anterior abdominal wall is described in Chapters 35 to 37. Peritoneal lavage is the first procedure illustrated in this section because it is often the first "laparotomy" performed by the junior resident or student. The general topography of the abdominal cavity is introduced in Chapter 35. The relationships of the viscera and a method for systematic exploration of the abdominal cavity, with considerations for trauma laparotomy, are described in Chapter 36 and 37. Additional information on the lateral abdominal wall may be found in the chapters on colon resection (Chapter 73), cholecystectomy (Chapter 56), appendectomy (Chapter 68), and lumbar sympathectomy (Chapter 85), in which special abdominal incisions are described.

Weakness in the anterior abdominal wall may lead to hernia formation. Congenital weakness in the region of the umbilicus causes the formation of umbilical hernias, and imperfect healing of laparotomy incisions can result in incisional (ventral) hernia formation. The repair of these defects is described in Chapters 38 and 39. Other, less common, abdominal wall hernias and their repair are described in references at the end of these chapters.

CHAPTER 35

Peritoneal Lavage: Insertion of a Peritoneal Dialysis Catheter

Peritoneal lavage is a diagnostic maneuver in which a catheter is inserted into the peritoneal cavity and fluid is aspirated. The character of the fluid (presence of blood, bile, or food particles, and its odor) is noted. If no fluid is obtained, 1 L of Ringer's lactate solution is instilled, allowed to equilibrate with any fluid in the peritoneal cavity, and then aspirated. Although peritoneal lavage has largely been superseded by other diagnostic modalities such as FAST (focused abdominal ultrasound for trauma) or computed tomography scan, the procedure is still indicated under special circumstances.

A temporary or permanent peritoneal dialysis catheter is placed for peritoneal dialysis in patients with acute or chronic renal failure.

In this chapter, placement of a catheter for diagnostic peritoneal lavage is discussed first, followed by a description of the modifications necessary for placement of a permanent catheter. This procedure is used to introduce the anatomy of the anterior abdominal wall and the topography of the peritoneal recesses.

Diagnostic Peritoneal Lavage: Choice of Site (Fig. 35.1)

Technical Points

Note any scars from prior abdominal surgery. Because intraperitoneal adhesions form most densely on the underside of old scars, avoid such areas. In the absence of old scars or pelvic fractures, the preferred site is the lower midline, about 4 to 5 cm below the umbilicus. Alternative sites include the upper midline (for patients with pelvic fractures) and right lower quadrant. Ensure that the patient's bladder is empty by having the conscious, cooperative patient void or by placing

LIST OF STRUCTURES

Linea alba
Umbilicus
Rectovesical pouch
Rectouterine pouch (of Douglas)
Pyramidalis muscle
Rectus abdominis muscle
   Rectus sheath
Pubis

an indwelling Foley catheter. Shave, prepare, and infiltrate the area of the proposed skin incision. The use of lidocaine with epinephrine minimizes bleeding into the incision and may decrease the chance of a false-positive result. Careful hemostasis throughout the procedure is important.

Make an incision about 5 cm long in the midline. Place a self-retaining retractor and deepen the incision until the linea alba is seen.

Anatomic Points

The linea alba changes as one progresses from the pubic crest to the costal margin. Inferior to the umbilicus, it is quite thin, because the rectus abdominis muscles attach immediately adjacent to the pubic symphysis. Medial fibers of the recti can originate from the linea alba, or quite inferiorly, tendinous fibers of one side can interdigitate with fibers of the contralateral rectus. The pyramidalis muscles lie in the rectus sheath immediately anterior to the rectus. These paired muscles originate from the anterior surface of the pubis and from the pubic ligament and insert into the linea alba. Fibers of this muscle are attached to the linea alba midway between the umbilicus and pubis. Above the umbilicus, the rectus muscles widen (but become thinner), diverging from the midline to attach to the costal cartilages of the fifth through seventh ribs. Here, the linea alba is about 1.5 to 2 cm wide.

The topographic anatomy of the abdomen in the sagittal plane provides a rationale for making an incision 4 to 5 cm below the umbilicus. At this location, you should be directly anterior to the fifth lumbar vertebral body or L5 or S1 disk. Because the aorta bifurcates superiorly and the right common iliac artery crosses the midline superiorly, no major arteries are at risk for injury. The left common iliac vein, however, does cross the midline somewhat lower than the major arteries and thus can be susceptible to injury. If the bladder is empty, the only structures between the retroperitoneum and the anterior parietal peritoneum should be mesenteric (greater omentum) or suspended by mesentery (loops of small bowel or redundant transverse or sigmoid colon).

Placement of Catheter (Fig. 35.2)

Technical Points

If the tap is to be done completely open, make a longitudinal incision 1 to 2 cm in length in the linea alba. Infiltrate

ORIENTATION

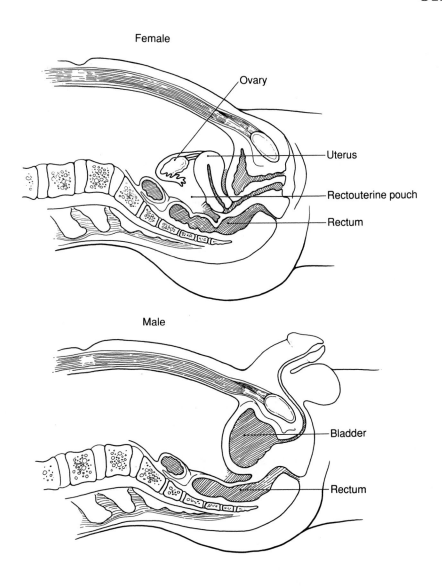

Female

Ovary

Uterus

Rectouterine pouch

Rectum

Male

Bladder

Rectum

FIGURE 35.1
DIAGNOSTIC PERITONEAL LAVAGE: CHOICE OF SITE

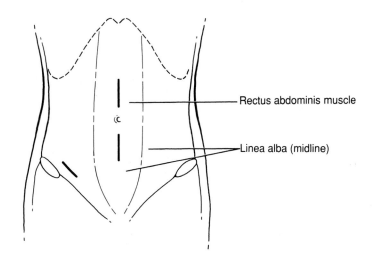

Rectus abdominis muscle

Linea alba (midline)

FIGURE 35.2
PLACEMENT OF CATHETER

the preperitoneal fat with local anesthetic. Spread the fatty preperitoneal tissues with a hemostat until the peritoneum is identified. Grasp it with two hemostats and incise between them with a knife. Place the catheter in the incision thus made and slide it in gently until all its holes are within the abdomen.

Perform a semiclosed tap (as shown in the figure) using a peritoneal dialysis catheter with a central trocar. Make a nick in the linea alba and pop the catheter-trocar assembly through the peritoneum and slide the catheter down into the pelvis. Withdraw the trocar.

The catheter should slip in easily, without resistance. Direct the catheter downward into the dependent recesses of the pelvis. Aspirate fluid. If blood, bile, or fecal material is obtained, the test is positive, and the procedure can be terminated at this point.

If no fluid is obtained, instill Ringer's lactate solution and proceed with a formal peritoneal lavage. Place a purse-string suture in the peritoneum around the catheter and tie it tightly. Place a gauze sponge in the wound both to decrease the chance of any blood from the incision contaminating the lavage and to cover the incision.

Connect the dialysis catheter to an intravenous infusion setup equipped with a macrodrip chamber. Instill 1 L of Ringer's lactate solution. It should flow in "wide open" by gravity alone. If the solution does not run in easily, the catheter may be in preperitoneal fat rather than in the peritoneal cavity. In this case, stop the infusion, cut the pursestring, and remove the catheter. Wash it clean of any blood. Check the incision into the peritoneum and confirm the location by visualizing omentum or bowel. Replace and resuture the catheter.

Allow the fluid to equilibrate for 5 minutes. Then place the bag of solution on the floor, allowing drainage from the peritoneum by gravity. If the intravenous infusion setup has a one-way valve in the tubing, it will not drain. In this case, cut the tubing and allow the lavage fluid to flow into a basin on the floor. Send the lavage fluid for amylase determination and cell count.

Close the incision in layers. If the lavage is clearly positive and laparotomy will be required, closure is not necessary.

Anatomic Points

The objective of catheter placement is to place the catheter in the lowest point possible in the peritoneal cavity. Ideally, this is the rectovesical pouch in the male, or the rectouterine pouch (of Douglas) in the female.

Insertion of a Tenckhoff Catheter for Dialysis in Patients with Chronic Renal Failure (Fig. 35.3)

Technical Points

When a permanent catheter is placed, special care must be taken (as with the implantation of any foreign device) to ensure asepsis. A paramedian incision is preferred by many surgeons because this approach permits better sealing of the tract.

The procedure may be done using local or general anesthesia.

The Tenckhoff chronic peritoneal dialysis catheter is designed for long-term peritoneal dialysis. It has two Dacron cuffs that encourage tissue ingrowth and provide a barrier against bacterial migration along the catheter. These cuffs must be positioned properly at the time of implantation. The deep cuff should lie just superficial to the peritoneum, whereas the superficial cuff should be located in the subcutaneous tissue below the skin.

Make a short paramedian incision (Fig. 35.3A) and place a 4-0 Dexon pursestring suture on the peritoneum. Guide the Tenckhoff catheter into the pelvis and the rectovesical pouch (in males) or the rectouterine pouch of Douglas (in females) using a guidewire if necessary. Position the first cuff just superficial to the fascia.

Instill fluid and confirm that there is no leakage of fluid when the pursestring suture is tied. If fluid leaks, place additional sutures to ensure a watertight closure. Close the fascia around the catheter and position the second cuff just superficial to the fascia in a subcutaneous position. Tunnel the exit site of the catheter a short distance from the surgical incision. Secure the catheter in place.

FIGURE 35.3
INSERTION OF A TENCKHOFF CATHETER FOR DIALYSIS IN PATIENTS WITH CHRONIC RENAL FAILURE

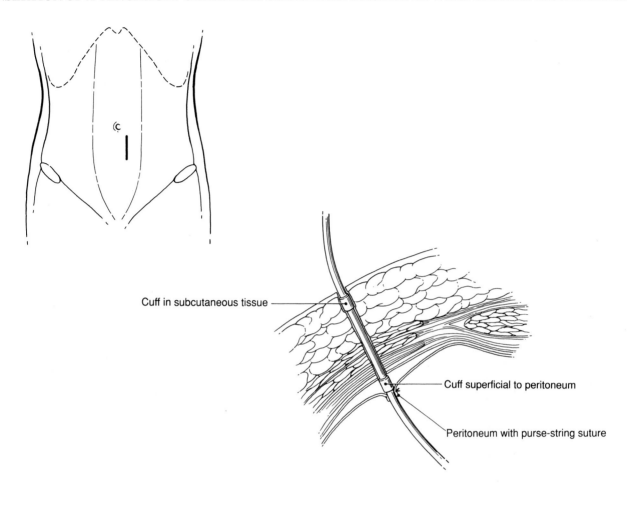

Cuff in subcutaneous tissue

Cuff superficial to peritoneum

Peritoneum with purse-string suture

REFERENCES

1. American College of Surgeons Committee on Trauma. Diagnostic peritoneal lavage. In: *Advanced trauma life support.* Chicago: American College of Surgeons, 1997:217–218. (Describes the currently accepted technique for trauma.)
2. Gokal R, Mallick NP. Peritoneal dialysis. *Lancet* 1999;353:823–828. (Presents a thorough review.)
3. Hodgson NF, Stewart TC, Girotti MJ. Open or closed diagnostic peritoneal lavage for abdominal trauma? A meta-analysis. *J Trauma* 2000;48:1091–1095. (Results show no difference between open and closed technique.)
4. Peritoneal dialysis. In: Matsumoto T, Simonian S, Kholoussy AM, eds. *Manual of vascular access procedures.* East Norwalk, CT: Appleton Century Crofts, 1984:47.
5. Payne WD. Peritoneal dialysis. In: Simmons RL, Finch ME, Ascher NL, et al, eds. *Manual of vascular access, organ donation, and transplantation.* New York: Springer-Verlag, 1984:88.
6. Rozycki GS, Ochsner MG, Schmidt JA, et al. A prospective study of surgeon-performed ultrasound as the primary adjuvant modality for injured patient assessment. *J Trauma* 1995;39:492. (Describes technique that has largely supplanted diagnostic peritoneal lavage in trauma management.)
7. Scott DF, Marshall VC. Insertion and complications of Tenckhoff catheters: surgical aspects. In: Adkins RC, Thomson NM, Farrell PC, eds. *Peritoneal dialysis.* Edinburgh, Scotland: Churchill Livingstone, 1981:61.
8. Tenckhoff H, Schechter H. A bacteriologically safe peritoneal access device. *Trans Am Soc Artif Intern Organs* 1968;14:181. (This is the original description of device that bears Tenckhoff's name.)
9. Velmahos GC, Demetriades D, Stewart M, et al. Open versus closed diagnostic peritoneal lavage: a comparison on safety, rapidity, efficacy. *J R Coll Surg Edinb* 1998;43:235–238.
10. Walsh RM, Popovich MJ, Hoadley J. Bedside diagnostic laparoscopy and peritoneal lavage in the intensive care unit. *Surg Endosc* 1998;12:1405–1409.

CHAPTER 36

Exploratory Laparotomy

The choice of incision for laparotomy is influenced by the operation planned, the location of the probable pathology, the body habitus of the patient, and the presence or absence of previous scars. Choose an incision that will provide good exposure, that can be extended if necessary, and that will heal well. The vertical midline incision is discussed here as the prototype for an abdominal incision. The McBurney and Rockey-Davis incisions, Kocher incision, paramedian incision, and transverse and oblique incisions are discussed in conjunction with the operative procedures for which they are most frequently used.

The vertical midline incision is rapidly made and affords equal access to all quadrants of the abdomen. Few vessels are encountered in the midline, and no nerves are sacrificed. It is the preferred incision in cases of traumatic injury, in situations in which access to multiple areas is required, and in any situation in which the nature of the pathology is in doubt. The potential disadvantages of the incision are that only one layer of fascia is present to be closed and that contraction of the abdominal wall muscles tends to pull the incision apart (in contrast to transverse or muscle-splitting incisions, in which the pull of the muscles does not act as a distracting force on the edges of the fascial incision). The vertical midline incision can be extended into the chest as a median sternotomy to improve exposure in the patient with traumatic injuries.

The Vertical Midline Incision (Fig. 36.1)

Technical Points

Cut cleanly through skin and subcutaneous tissue with a sharp knife, maintaining equal traction on both sides of the incision to ensure that the incision is straight. Make the incision

LIST OF STRUCTURES

External oblique muscle and aponeurosis
Internal oblique muscle and aponeurosis
Transversus abdominis muscle
Preperitoneal fat
Peritoneum
Linea alba
Median umbilical ligament (urachus)
Bladder

in the upper midline or the lower midline, or extend it from xiphoid to pubis, depending on the expected findings. Curve the incision around to the left of the umbilicus to avoid dividing the ligamentum teres hepatis. As the incision deepens, place laparotomy pads on the subcutaneous fat and use strong traction and countertraction to assist in exposure. In massively obese patients, "pull" the fat apart by strong traction and countertraction. This seemingly brutal maneuver helps to maintain orientation in the relatively avascular midline and leads directly to the linea alba.

Clean the linea alba of fat for a few millimeters on each side of the midline to help define the exact midline and to facilitate closure. Confirm the midline by the visible decussation of fibers at the linea alba. Check the wound for hemostasis and use electrocautery to coagulate any bleeding points.

Incise the linea alba for the length of the incision and pick up the peritoneum. (Often, a transparent area can be identified in the upper midline through which intraabdominal viscera can be seen.) The preperitoneal fat becomes thicker below the umbilicus and, as the pubic bone is reached, the urinary bladder may be encountered. Therefore, the abdomen should be entered in the upper midline, where the risk for injury to the bladder is eliminated, where preperitoneal fat is least prominent, and where the left lobe of the liver protects underlying hollow viscera from injury. Open the incision for its entire length using electrocautery. If the incision extends to the lower midline, incise fascia first, bluntly pushing preperitoneal fat and bladder away from the fascia. Once the fascia is opened, thin the preperitoneal fat by squeezing it between thumb and forefinger, feeling for the muscular wall of the bladder. If in doubt, feel for the balloon of the Foley catheter and pull it up to define the anterior extent of the bladder. Generally, the obliterated urachus will become visible as the fat is thinned out and a relatively free area lateral to the urachus can be identified.

Anatomic Points

Key dermatomes of the anterior abdominal wall include T-5 and T-6 (xiphoid), T-9 and T-l0 (umbilicus), and L-1 (pubis). Each dermatome receives supplemental innervation from the contiguous spinal nerves, both superiorly and inferiorly. Thus, an incision that results in a zone of denervated skin must section branches from at least two consecutive spinal nerves.

If a true midline incision is made, only minor nerves and arteries will be encountered. No named arteries or nerves

ORIENTATION

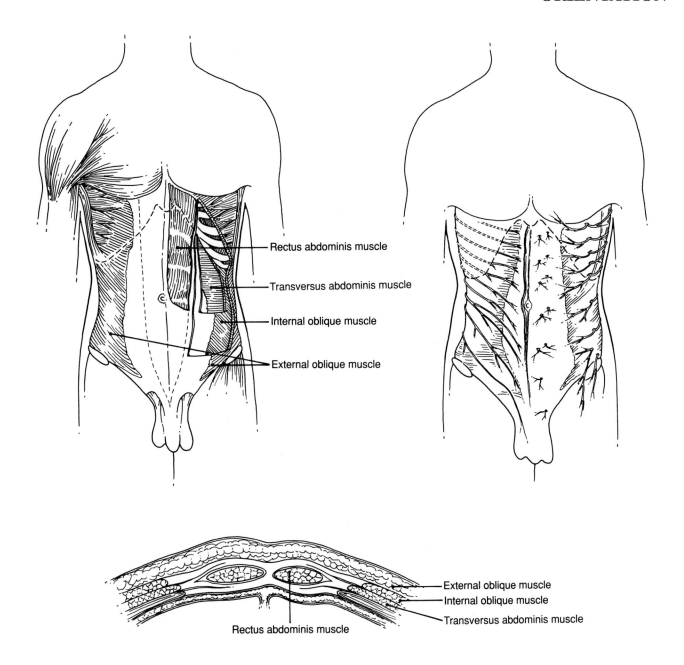

occupy the midline because they enter the anterior abdominal wall laterally (in the case of spinal nerves and the intersegmental arteries), or are lateral to the midline (as is true of the superior and inferior epigastric arteries). Superficial veins are minimal, although one should expect a greater number as the umbilicus is approached. As usual, these vessels can be ligated or cauterized with impunity.

Deep to the linea alba and attached to the anterior body wall are remnants of two embryologically important structures. Superior to the umbilicus, the *ligamentum teres hepatis,* or round ligament of the liver, which is the obliterated

left umbilical vein, passes in the free edge of the falciform ligament from the umbilicus to the fissure separating the left and right hepatic lobes. Because this fissure lies to the right of midline, the round ligament deviates to the right. The falciform ligament is attached along its base to the midline, but it lies to the right. Thus, its left surface is in contact with the left lobe of the liver and its right side is in contact with the abdominal wall. Inferior to the umbilicus, the median umbilical ligament—the obliterated *urachus*—passes from the umbilicus to the vertex of the bladder. The urachus is a narrow canal, originating from the vesicourethral portion

FIGURE 36.1
THE VERTICAL MIDLINE INCISION

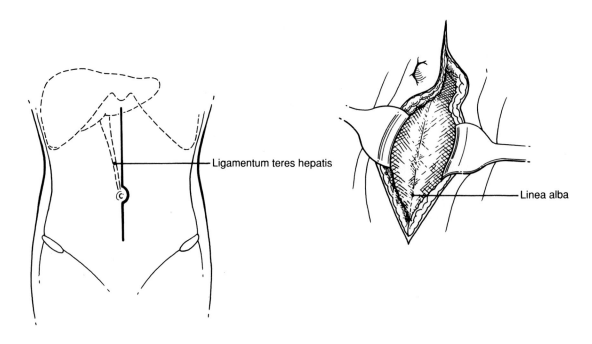

Ligamentum teres hepatis

Linea alba

of the hindgut, that connects developing urinary bladder to allantois. Distally, the urachus is continuous, through the umbilical cord, with the entirely extraembryonic allantois.

Finally, one should be aware of abdominopelvic organs just deep to the linea alba, from xiphoid to pubis. Most superiorly, and for a variable distance inferiorly, is the left lobe of the liver. Immediately inferior to the liver is the antrum of the stomach, to which is attached the thin gastrocolic ligament, through which the transverse colon is usually visible. From the inferior edge of the transverse colon (roughly midway between xiphoid and umbilicus, but quite variable in location), the greater omentum, which varies in both thickness and length, lies between the parietal peritoneum anteriorly and loops of small bowel, which should extend inferiorly to, or almost to, the pelvic brim. As the pelvic brim is approached, the extraperitoneal urinary bladder will be encountered. When the bladder is empty, its vertex typically is still superior to the pubis; thus, it may be encountered even if the urinary bladder is adequately drained.

Opening the Abdomen in the Case of Previous Abdominal Surgery (Fig. 36.2)

Technical and Anatomic Points

Adhesions are generally most prominent where there is foreign material (sutures, lint, talc) or at areas of injury or ischemia. Generally, there will be adhesions from any old incision to the underlying viscera or omentum. If possible, enter the abdomen through a virgin area, above or below the old incision. If this is not possible, it is generally advisable to enter the upper pole of the incision where the underlying left lobe of the liver, rather than the colon or small bowel, is likely to be encountered first.

Once you have made an opening into the peritoneal cavity, place Kocher clamps on the fascia and lift up. Use a laparotomy pad in your nondominant hand to pull down and provide countertraction. Lyse adhesions between loops of bowel or omentum and abdominal wall using Metzenbaum scissors or a knife. Do not cut fascia, dense fibrous adhesions, or old suture material with the Metzenbaum scissors; rather, reserve these scissors for cutting soft tissue to avoid dulling the blades. As you free up bowel and omentum from the underside of the incision, extend the peritoneal incision until more adhesions are encountered.

When you have opened the entire incision, place Kocher clamps on the fascia of one side and have your assistant pull up on the fascia. Apply downward countertraction with a laparotomy pad on bowel and omentum adherent to the underside of the abdominal wall. Sharply lyse adhesions; if necessary, take a small amount of peritoneum with a loop of bowel to avoid inadvertent injury. Generally, the adhesions will become less dense as you progress laterally away from the incision, and it may be possible to pass the fingers of the left hand behind adherent bowel to define the anatomy more clearly and to provide exposure. Adhesions are usually relatively avascular (in the absence of portal hypertension); bleeding from the serosal surface of the bowel can often be stopped with pressure from a laparotomy pad, and bleeding from the abdominal wall can be controlled with electrocautery.

Alternatives to the Vertical Midline Incision (Fig. 36.3)

Technical Points

Alternative incisions are discussed in detail with the operations for which they are most commonly used. The following

FIGURE 36.2
OPENING THE ABDOMEN IN THE CASE OF PREVIOUS ABDOMINAL SURGERY

is simply a list of commonly used incisions, along with the advantages and disadvantages of each. All share the potential advantage of creating an incision directly over the pathology to be dealt with and the potential disadvantage of accordingly limiting exposure of other areas.

Kocher Incision

The Kocher incision is an oblique right upper quadrant incision made about 4 cm below and parallel to the costal margin. It provides excellent exposure for surgery of the liver and biliary tract (see Chapter 56), and it can be extended partially or completely across the midline, as a chevron, and used for surgery of the pancreas (Fig. 36.3A).

Disadvantages of this incision include pain (because muscles are cut) and the potential for inducing muscular weakness of the abdominal wall if several segmental nerves are cut in a long Kocher incision.

A left-sided Kocher-type incision provides excellent exposure for elective splenectomy of the small or only moderately enlarged spleen (see Chapter 54).

McBurney and Rocky-Davis Incisions

These two closely related incisions are the standard incisions used for appendectomy (see Chapter 68). Extended, they afford adequate exposure for pelvic surgery and right colon resection, should this be required. These incisions heal very well, with minimal chance of hernia formation because each muscular or aponeurotic layer of the abdominal wall is split in the direction of its fibers; hence, muscle contraction tends to close further, rather than to pull apart, the incision. The only disadvantage is limited exposure, particularly

of the upper abdomen. Use these incisions only when the pathology is known to be localized to the right lower quadrant (Fig. 36.3B).

Transverse Incisions

Transverse incisions afford excellent exposure for right colon resections (see Chapter 73). They are of limited use in other abdominal procedures in the adult but are commonly employed in infants. A transverse incision generally heals well because the pull of the abdominal wall muscles tends to close the incision (Fig. 36.3C,D).

Lateral or Oblique Left Lower Quadrant Incisions

These incisions provide excellent exposure for left colon resections and may be preferred in obese patients or in instances in which surgery is performed with the patient in the lateral position (see Chapter 52). Exposure of the right upper quadrant is particularly poor; hence, these incisions are used only under very special circumstances (Fig. 36.3E,F).

Paramedian Incisions

Paramedian incisions are vertical incisions made parallel to the midline a few centimeters to the right or the left of the linea alba (Fig. 36.3G,H). The anterior rectus sheath is incised, and the rectus muscle is then retracted laterally to expose the posterior rectus sheath. The posterior sheath is then incised to enter the midline.

One of the advantages of a paramedian incision is that it is a vertical incision that is closed in two layers (rather than one, as is the case with a midline incision), affording perhaps

FIGURE 36.3
ALTERNATIVES TO THE VERTICAL MIDLINE INCISION

FIGURE 36.3 (Continued)

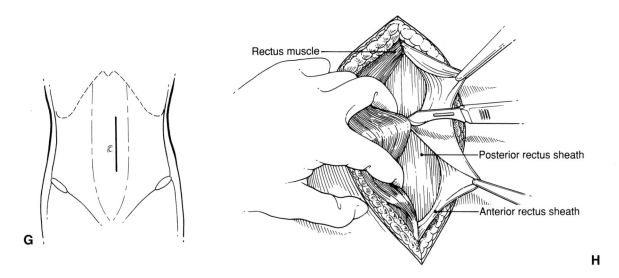

almost always will cut the eighth thoracic nerve, which continues inferomedially to a position just inferior to the ninth costal cartilage. This is of little consequence, however, owing to overlapping of the segmental innervation. If the larger ninth thoracic nerve is also severed, then part of the rectus is denervated, and muscle weakness can be expected. As these nerves are encountered, it must also be noted that they are one component of a neurovascular bundle, and it may be necessary to use electrocautery or ligatures to control bleeding.

McBurney and Rocky-Davis Incisions

Classically, these incisions are made over McBurney's point (junction of the middle and outer thirds of a line from the umbilicus to the anterosuperior iliac spine), which is the most probable location of the appendix. Because these are muscle- splitting rather than muscle-dividing incisions, it is necessary to remember the direction of muscle fibers at this location. The external oblique fibers run inferomedially, the internal oblique fibers run superomedially (almost at right angles to the external oblique fibers), and the transversus abdominis muscle fibers are approximately transverse; these usually can be split as a unit with the internal oblique muscle fibers because the direction of their fibers at this point is quite similar. Keep in mind that neurovascular bundles occupy the plane between the internal oblique and transversus abdominis muscles.

Transverse Incisions

Transverse incisions are usually somewhat oblique, so that the skin incision approximates the direction of Langer's lines, affording excellent cosmetic results. When muscle layers are encountered, they can be split in the direction of their fibers rather than divided, thus achieving the same goals as the McBurney incision. In addition, transverse incisions

some extra strength. Also, there may be a slight advantage, in terms of exposure of structures to the left or right of the midline, gained by moving the incision from the midline to the paramedian position. The left paramedian incision is used for left colon resections, for splenectomy, and for some gastric surgery. A high right paramedian incision may be used for biliary tract surgery in the patient with a narrow costal angle. Lower abdominal paramedian incisions heal poorly because the posterior rectus sheath is weak and, thus, are used relatively infrequently. A low right paramedian incision is used by some when the etiology of right lower quadrant pain is uncertain. The potential advantage of this approach is that the incision can be extended to gain exposure of the upper abdomen. Generally, this incision is not favored for appendectomy because it is associated with a high incidence of wound complications.

A major disadvantage of the paramedian incision is the increased time it takes to enter the abdomen. Closure is also slower than with other incisions because two layers must be sutured. Hence, it is not an appropriate choice for emergency situations. Long paramedian incisions limit the options for access when a second abdominal operation is performed; if a midline incision is chosen for the subsequent operation, the strip of abdominal wall between the old paramedian and new midline incisions may have inadequate blood supply for proper healing.

Anatomic Points

Kocher Incision

The Kocher incision divides the rectus abdominis muscle at about a right angle to its fibers. Fibers of the lateral abdominal wall muscles are also cut. The superior epigastric artery, which is typically located on or in the deep aspect of the muscle, and more medially than laterally, is divided. This incision

FIGURE 36.4
EXPLORATION OF THE ABDOMEN: ELECTIVE LAPAROTOMY

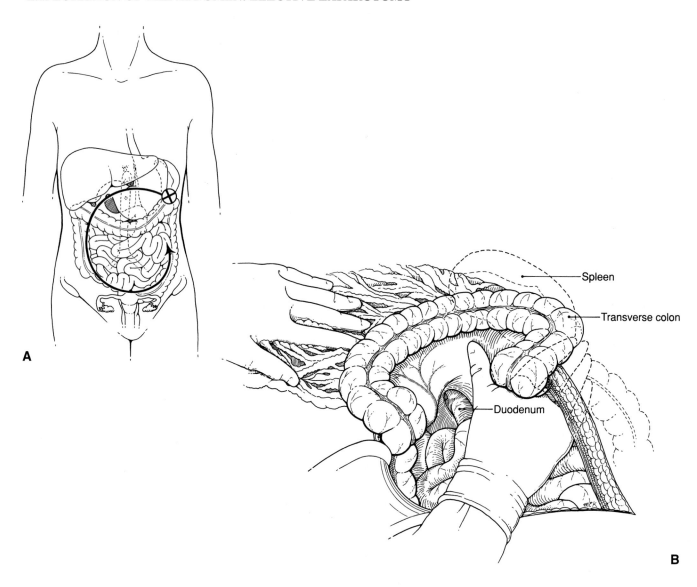

Spleen

Transverse colon

Duodenum

A

B

approximate the course of the neurovascular bundles, thus destroying fewer nerves and blood vessels.

Lateral or Oblique Left Lower Quadrant Incisions

These incisions also involve splitting the rectus sheath inferior to the arcuate line (of Douglas), where there is no posterior rectus sheath. The inferior epigastric vessels enter the rectus sheath from an inferolateral direction at this line and must be ligated and divided.

Paramedian Incisions

These vertical incisions are made in the same direction as the fibers of the rectus abdominis muscle. The tendinous inscriptions of the rectus muscle are attached to the anterior rectus sheath but not to the posterior sheath. Care should be taken to retract all of the rectus muscle laterally, especially

if the desired exposure is extensive, to prevent denervation to a median strip of the rectus muscle. Retraction of this muscle medially is not an accepted procedure because neurovascular bundles enter laterally and can be inadvertently disrupted.

Exploration of the Abdomen: Elective Laparotomy (Fig. 36.4)

Technical and Anatomic Points

Laparotomy provides the unique opportunity to observe and systematically palpate all of the infraabdominal viscera. A thorough, systematic exploration is the first step in laparotomy. Do not "zero-in" on known pathology before carefully checking the entire abdomen for unexpected findings.

Begin in the left upper quadrant. Place a Richardson retractor on the left upper abdominal wall and have an assistant retract it. Pass your dominant hand up under the left hemidiaphragm and feel the spleen, assessing it for size, mobility, and the presence of nodules. Note that the spleen is generally anchored to the diaphragm superiorly, the retroperitoneum posteriorly, and the stomach and colon medially and inferiorly. The spleen is a pulpy, blood-filled organ with a capsule of little tensile strength. It is easily damaged by vigorous retraction or palpation.

Next, pass the dominant hand under the left lobe of the liver, anterior to the stomach, and run the hand up toward the esophageal hiatus. Strong pulsations in the abdominal aorta (which should be assessed for size) assist in orientation. The esophagus lies anterior and slightly to the left of the aorta. An indwelling nasogastric tube, placed for most laparotomies, should be readily palpable and helps in the identification of the esophagus. The esophageal hiatus through which the esophagus passes should accept, at most, one finger. It may be dilated if the patient has a hiatal hernia; if so, make note of its approximate size by determining how many fingers it will admit easily. Next, feel the esophagogastric junction and stomach for masses, passing your hand down to the pylorus. Note any thickening or scarring that may be indicative of ulcer disease.

Feel the left lobe of the liver between the fingers of your dominant hand, assessing it for consistency and the presence of nodules or masses. Do not neglect to feel the underside of the diaphragm, a common site of metastases in patients with ovarian carcinoma.

Progress in a counterclockwise fashion to the right lobe of the liver. Place the retractor on the right upper abdominal wall and pass your dominant hand under the right hemidiaphragm as far as it will go. Normally, this potential space is clear, but sometimes adhesions from previous peritonitis limit access to this region; alternatively, a subphrenic abscess, by producing adhesions anteriorly between the right lobe of the liver and the diaphragm, may prevent palpation. The gallbladder should be felt and the presence or absence of stones noted. Passing a finger into the epiploic foramen (of Winslow) allows limited palpation of the common bile duct and hepatic artery. The head of the pancreas should also be felt for masses. (For systematic exploration of the entire pancreas, follow the procedure described in Chapter 63.) Next, feel the right kidney, noting its size and degree of mobility.

Progress down into the right lower quadrant and feel the terminal ileum, appendix, and cecum. Palpate the right colon up to the hepatic flexure. Lift the greater omentum out of the abdomen. Feel the omentum, assessing it for metastatic deposits or cysts. Note that the transverse colon runs on the undersurface of the greater omentum and hence must be approached from this surface. Assess the hepatic flexure both by feeling up the ascending colon and by coming across from the midtransverse colon along the underside of the omentum. Lesions in the hepatic and splenic flexure are easy to miss because the flexures pass higher and more laterally (becoming almost retroperitoneal) than one might expect.

Follow the transverse colon over to the left side of the abdomen and assess the splenic flexure, then palpate the descending and sigmoid colon. Feel the left kidney for size and mobility.

Follow the sigmoid colon into the pelvis and palpate the upper rectum. Assess the bladder and confirm the position of the balloon of the Foley catheter. In the female patient, assess the uterus, ovaries, and fallopian tubes. Feel for nodular metastatic deposits on the pelvic peritoneum.

Next, identify the duodenum at the ligament of Treitz. Then "run" the small bowel, with the aid of your first assistant, in the following manner: grasp a 10- to 15-cm length of small intestine in two hands and inspect it first on one side and then on the other. Then pass this section of bowel to your assistant, who then holds the loop as you grasp the next section. In this manner, your assistant helps you keep track of your progress, thereby avoiding missing segments or losing your point of reference as you pass distally. Check the entire small intestine to the ileocecal valve. Replace the omentum and small and large intestines into the abdomen in an orderly fashion.

Finally, feel the abdominal aorta and left and right common, internal, and external iliac arteries, assessing each for strength of pulsations, atherosclerotic plaque, and aneurysmal dilatation. Retroperitoneal lymphadenopathy (enlargement of paraaortic or iliac nodes) should be noted, if present.

Exploration of the Abdomen: Traumatic Injury (Fig. 36.5)

Technical and Anatomic Points

The first step in any laparotomy is a thorough and systematic exploration of the abdomen. Although it may be necessary to proceed expeditiously to identify and control active hemorrhage in patients with injuries, complete exploration is still mandatory before closure. A systematic approach helps to prevent the disastrous error of missed injuries.

First, note the character and distribution of blood or peritoneal fluid. Remove large quantities of blood, peritoneal fluid, or debris by suction or by scooping clots and semisolid material out into a basin. Identify and rapidly control any active bleeding or holes in hollow viscera to decrease contamination. Culture the peritoneal fluid if contamination by enteric contents has occurred. Then, irrigate the abdomen copiously and explore in a systematic fashion (Fig. 36.4), keeping in mind the additional considerations listed below.

Laparotomy in cases of trauma is performed with knowledge of the mechanism of injury. The probable course of the missile is known or suspected in cases of penetrating trauma. Be aware, however, that this is of limited predictive value. The relative positions of victim and assailant, the phase of respiration at the time of injury (and hence, the height of diaphragms), and the overall mobility of the intraabdominal viscera are all unknown factors. Search for clues, such as blood or bile staining or gas in the retroperitoneum, and investigate not only the intraabdominal organs but also retroperitoneal structures, such as the duodenum.

FIGURE 36.5
EXPLORATION OF THE ABDOMEN: TRAUMATIC INJURY

Mobilize viscera as needed to expose possible sites of injury. The anterior surface of the stomach is immediately visible; expose the posterior surface by widely opening the gastrocolic omentum between clamps and ties. This also exposes the body and tail of the pancreas.

Full exposure of the duodenum is obtained by mobilizing the right colon as for right hemicolectomy. Do this by cutting along the avascular line of Toldt just lateral to the colon. This line is the result of fusion of the embryologic visceral peritoneum of the antimesenteric and right surface of the colon with the parietal peritoneum. By recreating the embryonic condition, few, if any, significant vessels will be encountered. Sweep the colon and small bowel mesentery to the midline and superiorly (toward the

FIGURE 36.6
CLOSURE OF LAPAROTOMY

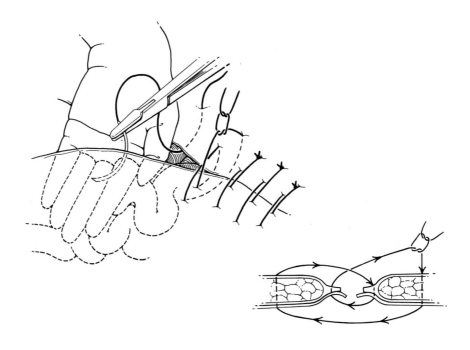

patient's left shoulder) to expose the entire duodenum. If colonic injury is a possibility, mobilize the involved segment of colon as for colon resection, so that all sides can be checked.

Approach retroperitoneal hematomas with respect. Contained hematomas secondary to pelvic fractures should be left alone. Obtain vascular control of the renal artery and vein before opening perinephric hematomas. Localized hematomas may be the only clue to retroperitoneal duodenal, pancreatic, or colonic injuries.

Always search for both entry and exit sites of the penetrating instrument in injuries to viscera. Be highly suspicious whenever you find an odd number of holes because you may have inadvertently missed one.

Closure of Laparotomy (Fig. 36.6)

Technical and Anatomic Points

Check carefully for hemostasis and make sure that no foreign bodies (e.g., laparotomy pads, clamps) have been left behind.

Pull the greater omentum down and interpose it between the viscera and the incision if possible.

Place Kocher clamps on the fascia. Interrupted Smead-Jones sutures can be used to close most incisions. Each suture is an asymmetric figure-of-eight and incorporates both "far bites" (which act as buried retention sutures) and "near bites" (which provide accurate fascial apposition). As your assistant retracts skin and subcutaneous fat to expose as much fascia as possible, take your first far bite from out to in; this bite should pass at least 2 cm back from the cut edge of the fascia. Then cross over and place a second far bite, from in to out, on the opposite side. Progress about 1 cm down the incision and place a near bite from out to in (about 1 cm back from the edge). Complete the stitch by passing another near bite from in to out on the opposite side.

A limited number of absorbable sutures may be placed in the subcutaneous tissues to obliterate dead space. Only do this to prevent a large cavity. The presence of foreign material (e.g., sutures) significantly reduces the inoculum of bacteria needed to cause infection.

REFERENCES

1. A-Malik R, Scott NA. Double near and far prolene suture closure: a technique for abdominal wall closure after laparostomy. *Br J Surg* 2001;88:146–147.
2. Ballinger WF, ed. Unexpected findings at laparotomy. *Probl Gen Surg* 1984;1:1. (The entire issue is devoted to the unforeseen and how to deal with it.)
3. Burch JM, Ortiz VB, Richardson RJ, et al. Abbreviated laparotomy and planned reoperation for critically injured patients. *Ann Surg* 1992;215:476–483.
4. Cattell RB, Braasch JW. The surgeon at work: technique for the exposure of the third and fourth portions of the duodenum. *Surg Gynecol Obstet* 1960;111:378. (Discusses wide exposure of the right retroperitoneum and entire duodenum.)
5. Cohn SM, Giannotti G, Ong AW, et al. Prospective randomized trial of two wound management strategies for dirty abdominal wounds. *Ann Surg* 2001;233:409–413. (Reaffirms value of delayed primary closure for dirty wounds.)
6. Feliciano D, Burch JM, Graham JM. Abdominal vascular trauma. In: Moore EE, Mattox KL, Feliciano DV, eds. *Trauma.* 2nd ed. East Norwalk, CT: Appleton & Lange, 1991:533.
7. Franchi M, Ghezzi F, Benedetti-Panici PL, et al. A multicentre collaborative study on the use of cold scalpel and electrocautery for midline abdominal incision. *Am J Surg* 2001;181:128–132. (Reports that the incidence of complications is similar.)
8. Greene MA, Mullins RJ, Malangoni MA, et al. Laparotomy wound closure with absorbable polyglycolic acid mesh. *Surg Gynecol Obstet* 1993;176:213–218. (Describes use of absorbable mesh when primary closure is not possible.)
9. Jones TE, Newell ET, Brubaker RE. The use of alloy steel wire in the closure of abdominal wounds. *Surg Gynecol Obstet* 1941;72:1056.
10. Matory WE Jr, O'Sullivan J, Fudem G, et al. Abdominal surgery in patients with severe morbid obesity. *Plastic Reconstr Surg* 1994;94:967–987. (Discusses techniques for manipulating a large pannus.)
11. McNeill PM, Surgerman HJ. Continuous absorbable vs. interrupted nonabsorbable fascial closure. *Arch Surg* 1986;121:821.
12. Morris JA Jr, Eddy VA, Blinman TA, et al. The staged celiotomy for trauma: issues in unpacking and reconstruction. *Ann Surg* 1993;217:576–584.
13. Shapiro MB, Jenkins DH, Schwab CW, et al. Damage control: collective review. *J Trauma* 2000;49:969–978.
14. Soteriou MC, Williams LF Jr. Unexpected findings in gastrointestinal tract surgery. *Surg Clin North Am* 1991;71:1283.
15. Spencer FC, Sharp ED, Jude JR. Experiences with wire closure of abdominal incisions in 293 selected patients. *Surg Gynecol Obstet* 1963;117:235.
16. Tejani FH, Zamora BO. The surgeon at work: placement of retention sutures. *Surg Gynecol Obstet* 1977;144:573.

CHAPTER 37

Laparoscopy: Principles of Access and Exposure

Laparoscopic surgery requires intense attention to the details of equipment used. Become familiar with the equipment used in your operating room. Ensure that it is in working order and that the supplies that you will need for the procedure are at hand or readily available. An equipment troubleshooting chart, such as that produced by Society of American Gastrointestinal Endoscopic Surgeons (SAGES) (referenced at the end), can be invaluable when problems arise.

Patient positioning and layout of equipment can facilitate a laparoscopic procedure or immensely complicate it. Locate the primary monitor directly opposite the surgeon in a straight line of sight. A secondary monitor may be located across from the first assistant, who will generally stand on the opposite side of the table. Part A of the orientation figure shows how this is accomplished for laparoscopic cholecystectomy. Arrange the insufflator, light source, cautery and other energy sources, suction irrigator, and so on, and the associated cords in such a fashion that you are free to move from one side of the table to the other if necessary.

For lower abdominal procedures, such as laparoscopic appendectomy (Chapter 69), it is best to tuck the arms at the side. This allows the surgeon and first assistant to move as far cephalad as needed without being cramped by the armboards (orientation figure part B). Gynecologic laparoscopists will generally place the patient in stirrups to allow manipulations from below, for example, elevating the cervix to enhance visualization of the pelvic organs (see Fig. 78.1A in Chapter 78).

Advanced laparoscopic procedures performed around the esophageal hiatus, such as laparoscopic fundoplication (Chapter 42) or esophagomyotomy (Chapter 43) are also best performed with the patient's legs spread to enable the surgeon to stand between the legs (orientation figure part C). This provides the straightest possible line of sight to the operative field and enables two assistants to stand comfortably, one on each side. Further information is given in the chapters for specific procedures. References at the end give additional information about equipment setup and troubleshooting.

Access to the Abdomen—Closed, with Veress Needle (Fig. 37.1)

Technical Points

The umbilicus is the usual site of initial entry. An infraumbilical "smile" or supraumbilical "frown" incision made in a natural skin crease is virtually invisible when healed (Fig. 37.1A). If conversion to open laparotomy is a strong possibility, a vertically oriented circumumbilical incision gives equally good access and is easily incorporated into a vertical midline incision.

Visualize the probable site of the pathology within the abdomen and consider the location of the umbilicus relative to this site. The level of the umbilicus varies considerably from individual to individual—do not hesitate to make the entry site slightly above or below the umbilicus if necessary. If the umbilicus is low on the abdomen and the target site is in the upper abdomen, an incision above the umbilicus may be necessary. Conversely, an incision below the umbilicus may provide the best visualization for laparoscopic cholecystectomy in a small patient. If all other things are equal, it is a bit easier to enter the abdomen through a smile incision because this avoids the falciform ligament. Make the incision a millimeter or two longer than the diameter of the trocar you plan to use. Deepen the incision through skin and subcutaneous tissue until the fascia at the base of the umbilicus is encountered. If the patient is obese, place a Kocher clamp on the underside of the umbilicus and pull up. Because skin is adherent to fascia at the umbilicus, this will elevate the fascia. Place Kocher clamps side by side on the fascia. Hold one in your nondominant hand and have your first assistant hold the other.

Test the Veress needle and confirm that the tip retracts easily (Fig. 37.1B). Introduce the Veress needle with steady controlled pressure, attentive to the popping sensations as it passes through the fascia and then the peritoneum (Fig. 37.1C). When the Veress needle is properly positioned, the tip should move freely from side to side as the hub is gently moved back and forth.

LIST OF STRUCTURES

Linea alba
Rectus abdominis muscle
Umbilicus
Urachus
Falciform ligament
Inferior epigastric artery and vein

ORIENTATION

A

B

Attach a syringe filled with saline. Aspirate, observing for gas, blood, or succus entericus. If the needle is properly positioned, a vacuum will be created. Inject saline; there should be no resistance to injection. Leave a meniscus of saline within the hub of the needle when you remove the syringe. Elevate both Kocher clamps while observing the meniscus. The saline should be drawn into the abdomen by the negative pressure thus created, confirming proper intraperitoneal positioning of the needle. Insufflate the abdomen. It is extremely important to take the time to ascertain proper placement to avoid visceral injury. On the other hand, if the Veress needle is not deep enough, the preperitoneal space can absorb an amazing amount of CO_2, making subsequent entry into the abdomen more difficult (Fig. 37.1D).

Anatomic Points

The umbilicus is an easy entry site because skin, fascia, and peritoneum lie in close apposition with minimal intervening fat, even in obese patients. Converging on the umbilicus are four structures, all remnants of fetal development (Fig. 37.1E).

Cephalad, the ligamentum teres hepatis, with its obliterated umbilical vein enters, potentially complicating supraumbilical access in two ways. First, the fat-laden ligamentum teres and falciform ligaments must be traversed. Difficulty increases as one moves slightly cephalad from the umbilicus. Second, dilated venous collaterals form in patients with portal hypertension, in whom the umbilical vein remains patent or recanalizes, acting as an outflow conduit by anastomosing with the systemic circulation (veins in the anterior abdominal wall). Profuse bleeding may accompany attempted supraumbilical (or even infraumbilical) access in these patients.

Inferiorly, the midline obliterated urachus and paired obliterated umbilical arteries converge but represent less of a mechanical problem.

If a vitelline duct remnant persists, it will be encountered in this region as well.

The proximity of the anterior abdominal wall to the underlying great vessels is accentuated by the manner in which the sacral promontory juts anteriorly (see the orientation figures that accompany Chapter 35). Directing the Veress needle toward the pelvis helps minimize the danger of vascular injury.

FIGURE 37.1
ACCESS TO THE ABDOMEN—CLOSED, WITH VERESS NEEDLE (A–C, from Soper NJ. Access to abdomen. In: Scott-Conner CEH, ed. *The SAGES manual.* New York: Springer Verlag, 1999, with permission; **D** Bailey RW. Complications of laparoscopic general surgery. In: Zucker KA, ed. *Surgical laparoscopy.* 1st ed. St. Louis: Quality Medical Publishing, 1991:311–342, with permission.)

FIGURE 37.1 (Continued)

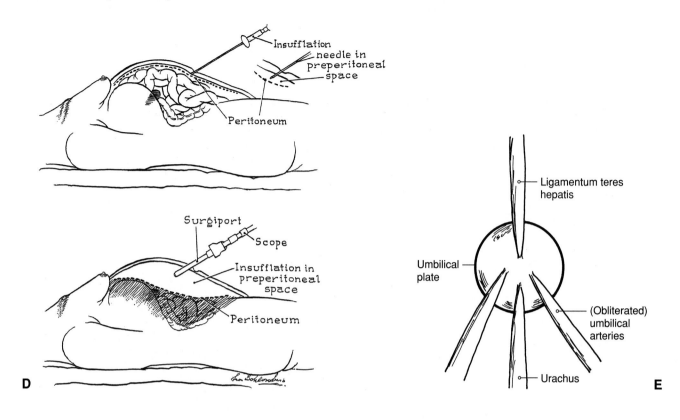

Open Entry with Hasson Cannula (Fig. 37.2)

Technical and Anatomic Points

A Hasson cannula allows open entry by minilaparotomy. Make a circumumbilical incision, as described previously. The skin incision should be several centimeters long, to allow easy exposure of the fascia. Make the fascial incision about two centimeters long. Attain careful hemostasis and place retractors (Fig. 37.2A). Elevate and incise the peritoneum (Fig. 37.2B). Confirm peritoneal entry by direct vision or by inserting your index finger. Place two figure-of-eight anchoring sutures, one on each side of the incision. These will be used to anchor the cannula during laparoscopy and will be tied when the cannula is removed, providing fascial closure.

Insert the cannula and push the tapered obturator into the fascia so that it is snugly engaged. Anchor the stay sutures by winding them into the retaining grooves on the obturator (Fig. 37.2C). This helps to minimize leakage of CO_2.

Alternative Puncture Sites (Fig. 37.3)

Technical Points

The left and right upper quadrants, where the costal margin elevates the anterior abdominal wall, may be used for alternative Veress needle puncture sites in cases in which the midline is inaccessible (Fig. 37.3A,B). Choose a site close to the costal margin and remote from old scars, ideally in the

midclavicular line. Make a transverse incision long enough to accommodate the planned trocar. Deepen the incision to fascia. Elevate the abdominal wall below the incision by grasping the full thickness of the abdominal wall with your nondominant hand. Insert the Veress needle as previously described and confirm intraperitoneal placement.

Anatomic Points

This method depends on the lower costal arch to provide counterpressure and resistance against which the Veress needle can be driven. Most often, the left upper quadrant site is employed because only stomach (decompressed with a nasogastric tube) should lie beneath the site. In the right upper quadrant, liver, gallbladder, or colon may be encountered. This entry site is commonly employed in morbidly obese patients because the pannus is generally thinner in the upper abdomen, or when surgery is being done in the lateral decubitus position.

Exploration of the Abdomen and Placement of Secondary Trocars (Fig. 37.4)

Technical Points

Insert the laparoscope and inspect the abdomen in a systematic fashion. Place secondary trocars as needed to palpate and manipulate loops of bowel. The optimum location of secondary trocars depends on the specific pathology anticipated or the procedure to be performed. Become familiar with the use of angled (30- and 45-degree) as well as straight (0-degree) laparoscopes. The angled scopes allow the surgeon to look at structures from several viewpoints (Fig. 37.4A). If the view you are obtaining with the straight scope is inadequate, try an angled scope. Alternatively, move the laparoscope to another location for a different point of view.

Conceptualize your working space within the abdomen as a triangle. The laparoscope forms the apex of the triangle and corresponds to your eyes. Working ports to left and right of the laparoscope, and generally closer to the surgical target than the port for the laparoscope, are at your left and right hands. If the ports are placed too close together, it will be difficult to manipulate instruments (Fig. 37.4B). Each laparoscopic chapter in this text describes the usual port locations. Sometimes, these locations must be modified according to individual anatomy.

Adjust the table and monitors so that a monitor is in the direct line of sight of both the surgeon and first assistant (Fig. 37.4C). Make sure the operating table is at a comfortable height; this will generally mean dropping it to a lower height than normal because of the length of the instruments.

FIGURE 37.2
OPEN ENTRY WITH HASSON CANNULA (A,B from Soper NJ. Access to abdomen. In: Scott-Conner CEH, ed. *The SAGES manual.* New York: Springer Verlag, 1999, with permission; **C** from Wind GG. *Special operative considerations.* Baltimore: Williams & Wilkins, 1997, with permission.)

A

B

FIGURE 37.2   (Continued)

C

FIGURE 37.3
ALTERNATIVE PUNCTURE SITES

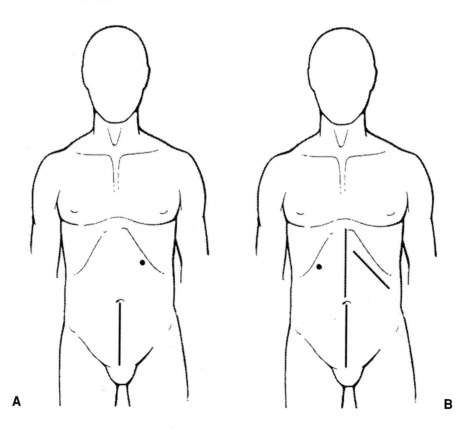

A   B

FIGURE 37.4

EXPLORATION OF THE ABDOMEN AND PLACEMENT OF SECONDARY TROCARS (**A** from Romanelli JR, Litwin DEM. Hand-assisted laparoscopic surgery. *Probl Gen Surg* 2001;18:45–51, with permission; **B** from Wind GG. *Special operative considerations*. Baltimore: Williams & Wilkins, 1997, with permission; **C** from Scott-Conner CEH. Choice of laparoscope: straight versus angled? In: Chassin's operative strategy in general surgery. 3rd ed. New York: Springer, 2002, with permission.)

FIGURE 37.4 (Continued)
(**D** from Scott-Conner CEH, Cuschieri A, Carter FJ. Anterior abdominal wall. In: *Minimal access surgical anatomy.*
Philadelphia: Lippincott Williams & Wilkins, 2000:1–5, with permission.)

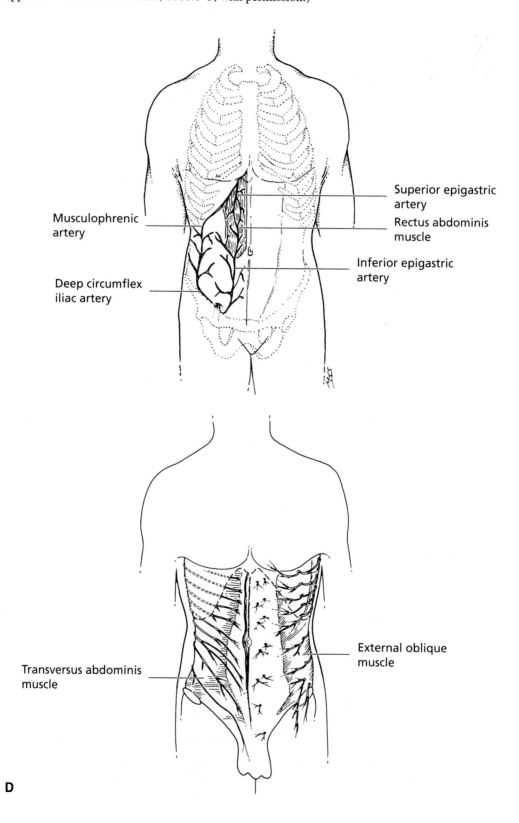

D

In the upper abdomen, ports can be placed essentially anywhere without significant risk for bleeding. Below the umbilicus, ports should either be placed in the midline or lateral to the rectus sheath in order to avoid the inferior epigastric vessels. Although injury to a patent urachus is a theoretical possibility in the lower midline, it does not appear to be a problem in practice. Injury to the bladder is best avoided by preoperative decompression by an indwelling catheter.

For exploration of the upper abdomen, place the table in steep reverse Trendelenburg position to allow gravity to retract the viscera caudad. Examine the diaphragm (a common site of metastatic deposits), liver, gallbladder, stomach, and spleen.

Turn the patient into a right-side-up position to examine the right colon, cecum, and appendix. The transverse colon can only be seen if the greater omentum is elevated.

The entire small bowel can be systematically run between two atraumatic graspers or Babcock clamps.

Turn the patient to a left-side-up position to examine the descending colon. Steep Trendelenburg positioning is crucial for adequate visualization of pelvic structures. The detailed normal laparoscopic anatomy of each region is shown in the specific chapters that follow.

Anatomic Points

The superior and inferior epigastric vessels run in the rectus sheath, posterior to the rectus abdominis muscles. Generally, only the inferior epigastric vessels are problematic.

Laterally, the musculophrenic arteries are noted (Fig. 37.4D), but these are rarely encountered during laparoscopic surgery.

REFERENCES

1. Blichert-Toft M, Koch F, Neilson OV. Anatomic variants of the urachus related to clinical appearance and surgical treatment of urachal lesions. *Surg Gynecol Obstet* 1973;137:51–54.
2. Bonjer HJ, Hazebroek EJ, Lange JF, et al. Open versus closed establishment of pneumoperitoneum in laparoscopic surgery. *Br J Surg* 1997;84:599–602.
3. Easter DW. Diagnostic laparoscopy for acute and chronic abdominal pain. In: Zucker KA, ed. *Surgical laparoscopy*. 2nd ed. Philadelphia: Lippincott Williams & Wilkins, 2001:97–102.
4. Green FL, Taylor NC. Operative room configuration: laparoscopic surgery. Philadelphia: WB Saunders, 1994:34–41.
5. Halpern NB. The difficult laparoscopy. *Surg Clin North Am* 1996;76:601–613.
6. MacVay CB, Anson BJ. Composition of the rectus sheath. *Anat Rec* 1940;77:213–217.
7. Milloy FJ, Anson BJ, McFee DK. The rectus abdominis muscle and the epigastric arteries. *Surg Gynecol Obstet* 1960;110:293–298.
8. Orda R, Nathan H. Surgical anatomy of the umbilical structures. *Int Surg* 1973;58:454–64.
9. Oshinsky GS, Smith AD. Laparoscopic needles and trocars: an overview of designs and complications. *J Laparoendosc Surg* 1992;2:117–125.
10. Riza ED, Deshmukh AS. An improved method of securing abdominal wall bleeders during laparoscopy. *J Laparoendosc Surg* 1995;5:37–40.
11. Romanelli JR, Litwin DEM. Hand-assisted laparoscopic surgery. *Probl Gen Surg* 2001;18:45–51.
12. SAGES Guidelines for the optimum placement and adjustment of the operating room table and the video monitor during laparoscopic surgery. Available online at: www.sages.org.
13. SAGES Laparoscopy Troubleshooting Guide. Available online at: www.sages.org.
14. Schafer M, Lauper M, Krahenbuhl L. A nation's experience of bleeding complications during laparoscopy. *Am J Surg* 2000;180:73–77. (Describes major vascular injuries.)
15. Scott-Conner CEH, Cuschieri A, Carter FJ. Anterior abdominal wall. In: *Minimal access surgical anatomy*. Philadelphia: Lippincott Williams & Wilkins, 2000:1–5.
16. Soper NJ, Halpin VJ, Meyers BF. Minimally invasive surgery: laparoscopic and thoracoscopic techniques. In: Baker RJ, Fischer JE, eds. *Mastery of surgery*. 4th ed. Philadelphia, Lippincott Williams & Wilkins, 2001:264–276.

CHAPTER 38

Repair of Ventral and Umbilical Hernias

Most ventral hernias occur through previous laparotomy incisions. Small defects may be closed by reopening the incision, clearing the fascia, and then closing as one would close a laparotomy incision. Frequently, multiple defects are present; thus, it is important to explore the entire incision. If closure cannot be accomplished without excessive tension, synthetic mesh may be used to bridge the gap. Two methods of incisional hernia repair using prosthetic mesh are detailed in this chapter. In addition, a variety of repair techniques using autogenous tissue are described and referenced at the end. Laparoscopic ventral hernia repair (Chapter 39) is an increasingly popular alternative to open herniorrhaphy in selected patients.

Umbilical hernias are a special category of ventral hernias. Repair can usually be accomplished by a primary fascial overlap (Figs. 38.4 to 38.6).

Ventral Hernia Repair

Exposure of Fascia and Definition of Defect (Fig. 38.1)

Technical and Anatomic Points

Excise the old scar and deepen the incision cautiously until you encounter the hernia sac. Often, the sac lies quite close to the skin surface. It may be adherent to the old scar. It will look somewhat like a large lipoma and, like a lipoma, is easily "shelled out" of the surrounding tissues. Dissect laterally around the sac and then deep to expose good fascia well past the edge of the defect. Define the defect on all sides, raising flaps of subcutaneous tissue and skin as the dissection progresses. In most cases, the entire length of the old incision should be exposed because multiple defects are quite common and may otherwise be overlooked. Lateral defects, which frequently occur at points where retention sutures have cut through the fascia or at old drain sites, must be sought as well. Expose good fascia on all sides of the old incision. If possible, dissect the sac away from the fascia and reduce it. You will then be able to perform the repair in a totally extraperitoneal fashion. It is critical to clean the underside of the fascia carefully so that gut is not caught in a stitch during the repair.

Generally, multiple adjacent defects should be made into one defect by excising intervening bridges of attenuated fascia. Débride all attenuated fascia, hernia sac, or scar tissue.

If the defect is small, close it with interrupted nonabsorbable sutures. Be careful to avoid excess tension. If tension is required to appose the fascial edges, the repair will fail. Remember that it is difficult to assess the tension on the repair under the conditions of muscle relaxation associated with general or spinal anesthesia. Therefore, if there is any tension, consider using prosthetic material to bridge the gap.

Usher Repair (Fig. 38.2)

Technical and Anatomic Points

Cut two strips of prosthetic mesh the length of the incision. Each strip should be at least 5 cm wide. Suture one strip of mesh to each fascial edge with a running nonabsorbable suture. The prosthetic mesh thus serves to lengthen and reinforce the fascia. Then suture the two edges of mesh together with a running stitch. Close the subcutaneous tissues and skin. If large flaps have been raised in the subcutaneous tissue, place closed-suction drains under the flaps.

Patch Technique (Fig. 38.3)

Technical and Anatomic Points

The patch technique, which is somewhat more complicated than the technique just described, is applicable to large defects, especially those that are more nearly circular than slit-like. Two prosthetic mesh patches are placed above and below the fascia.

First, cut two mesh patches to size. A piece of glove wrapping paper may be used to cut a pattern first, if desired. Make the patches about 2 to 3 cm larger than the hole in all dimensions.

Place the inner patch inside the fascial opening. The first four "quadrant" sutures are critical in terms of orientation and should be placed with extreme care. Place the first suture at the superior edge of the defect (at 12 o'clock). Place the other sutures at 3, 6, and 9 o'clock. Place each suture as a horizontal mattress suture in the following fashion, using a heavy nonabsorbable (preferably, monofilament) suture material. First, pass the suture from out to in on the upper patch, 1.5 to 2 cm from the cut edge. Then take a bite through the fascia, again 1.5 to 2 cm back from the edge, from out to in. The next bite can be taken as a horizontal bite from out to in, then from in to out on the mesh of the inner patch. Then simply pass from in to out on the fascia, progressing about 1 cm along the fascial edge from the first bite. Finally, pass from in to out on the outer patch. Cut the needle off and clamp the suture. All sutures will be tied at the end.

FIGURE 38.1
EXPOSURE OF FASCIA AND DEFINITION OF DEFECT

After the four quadrant sutures are placed, suture each quadrant using a "divide and conquer" strategy. Tie all sutures snugly, but not so tight as to cause fascial necrosis. To ensure that no viscera are caught under the inner patch, lift up on all sutures and pass a finger underneath.

If the patch is too loose, plicate it by running a suture down the anterior mesh patch to turn in part of the mesh. Generally, the large flaps produced by undermining to expose good fascia require that closed-suction drains be placed.

Umbilical Hernia Repair

Incision (Fig. 38.4)

Technical Points

Small umbilical hernias, particularly when they occur in young, slender patients, can be repaired through an incision placed within or just outside the umbilicus. The resulting scar will be indistinguishable from the other wrinkles in the

FIGURE 38.2
USHER REPAIR

FIGURE 38.3
PATCH TECHNIQUE

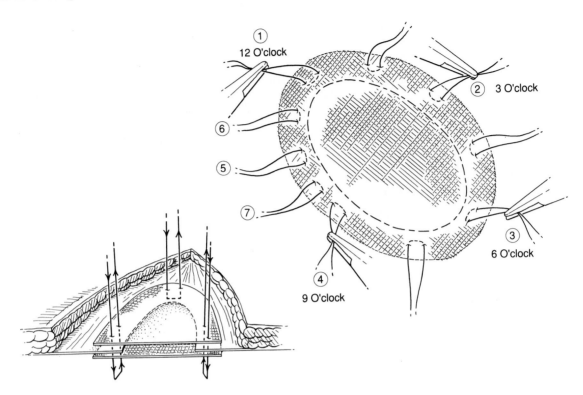

umbilical area. Large umbilical hernias or hernias in obese patients should be repaired through a large circumumbilical or modified transverse "smile" incision.

Anatomic Points

Remember that the periumbilical superficial fascia is more vascular than other regions of the anterior abdominal wall. Although this is primarily venous, almost a plexus, or rete, of small arteries is also present. These vessels must be ligated or cauterized.

Paraumbilical veins act as important portosystemic collaterals when portal venous hypertension is present. In patients so affected, multiple engorged vessels will be encountered.

Identification and Dissection of the Sac (Fig. 38.5)

Technical Points

Deepen the incision through the subcutaneous tissues until the hernia sac is identified. As dissection around the sac progresses superiorly, free up the underside of the umbilicus from the sac. Note that the umbilicus is the one place in the

FIGURE 38.4
INCISION

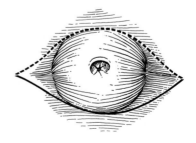

FIGURE 38.5
IDENTIFICATION AND DISSECTION OF THE SAC

anterior abdominal wall where the skin is adherent to fascia without intervening fat. Thus, in the case of a hernia, the skin is adherent to the hernia sac. It may be so densely adherent that sharp scalpel dissection is necessary for this step. Then dissect the rest of the sac free of subcutaneous tissue and carefully define the neck of the sac. Reduce the hernia, if possible. Enlarge the fascial defect, if necessary, by cutting laterally on one or both sides of the sac in order to reduce the hernia and to convert a round coinlike defect into a slit that can be closed more easily.

Anatomic Points

Congenital umbilical hernias are the result of a slightly enlarged umbilical ring. It is postulated that this is the result of the rectus abdominis muscles failing to approximate properly after reduction of the physiologic herniation of small bowel during development. Incomplete decussation of fibers forming the linea alba in this area then allows peritoneal structures (omentum or small intestine) to herniate. Congenital umbilical hernias are always within the umbilicus. Acquired umbilical hernias can present within the umbilical ring or, frequently, just superior or inferior to this cicatrix. It is postulated

FIGURE 38.6
CLOSURE OF THE FASCIAL DEFECT

that acquired umbilical hernias again relate to abnormalities in the decussation of linea alba fibers, which only fail after repeated stress, such as can occur with increasing age, multiple pregnancies, or ascites. Anatomically, there is little difference between congenital and acquired umbilical hernias, except that the latter need not be surrounded by the umbilical ring.

Two special kinds of umbilical defects are encountered in the neonate. *Omphaloceles* develop as a result of the failure of intestinal loops to reduce spontaneously following their physiologic herniation into the umbilical cord. These herniated loops of bowel are covered only by avascular amnion (extraembryonic coelom or "peritoneum"). At the apex of this amniotic sac is the umbilicus. By contrast, *gastroschisis* is a congenital muscular defect of the anterior abdominal wall. It is characterized by the following features: (a) the defect through which the abdominal contents herniate lies to the right of the umbilicus; (b) herniated structures always include thickened, adherent loops of small bowel; and (c) the herniated bowel is void of a covering. Clearly, gastroschisis must be treated immediately because the bowel has no covering. By comparison, the surgeon has more time in which to correct an omphalocele.

Closure of the Fascial Defect (Fig. 38.6)

Technical and Anatomic Points

Clean the fascial edges as described for ventral hernia repair (Fig. 38.1). Then close the defect with interrupted nonabsorbable sutures placed in a vest-over-pants fashion (Mayo repair).

First, place a suture from out to in on the upper flap (1 to 1.5 cm from the edge). Then pass the suture from out to in on the lower flap, then from in to out on the lower flap (about 1 cm from the previous stitch) and from in to out on the upper flap. Place a hemostat on each suture; do not tie until all sutures are placed.

When the sutures are tied down, the effect should be to pull the upper flap down over the lower flap. If you are uncertain whether you are placing sutures correctly, pull up on the sutures and observe how the flaps come together. Tie all sutures. Place a second row of interrupted sutures to tack down the free edge of the upper flap.

Tack the umbilicus to the fascia with an interrupted absorbable suture. Close subcutaneous tissue and skin and place a sponge in the umbilicus to obliterate the dead space and maintain an inverted contour as healing occurs.

REFERENCES

1. Bellon JM, Bujan J, Contreras LA, et al. Comparison of a new type of polytetrafluoroethylene patch (Mycro mesh) and polypropylene prosthesis (Marlex) for repair of abdominal wall defects. *J Am Coll Surg* 1996;183:11–18.
2. Bertelsen S. The surgical treatment of spigelian hernia. *Surg Gynecol Obstet* 1966;122:567.
3. Browse NL, Hurst P. Repair of long, large midline incisional hernias using reflected flaps of anterior rectus sheath reinforced with Marlex mesh. *Am J Surg* 1979;138:740. (Describes a relatively simple reinforced flap method.)
4. DeBord JR. The historical developments of prosthetics in hernia surgery. *Surg Clin North Am* 1998;78:973–1006. (Primarily concerned with inguinal hernia repair, but is an excellent overall review.)
5. DiBello JN Jr, Moore JH Jr. Sliding myofascial flap of the rectus abdominis muscles for the closure of recurrent ventral hernias. *Plastic Reconstr Surg* 1996;98:464–469. (Describes a complex flap closure for difficult, multiple recurrent hernias.)
6. Houlihan J. A review of spigelian hernias. *Am J Surg* 1976;131:734. (Provides a classic review of an uncommon hernia.)
7. Houston GC, Drew GS, Vazquez B, et al. The extended latissimus dorsi flap in repair of anterior abdominal wall defects. *Plastic Reconstr Surg* 1988;81:917–924. (Describes another flap method.)
8. Knolmayer TJ, Cornell KM, Bowyer MW, et al. Imbrication versus excision for fascial healing. *Am J Surg* 1996;172:506–511. (Reports on an animal study demonstrating that cut edges heal better.)
9. Larson GM, Harrower HW. Plastic mesh repair of incisional hernia. *Am J Surg* 1978;135:559. (Describes the "sandwich" technique.)
10. Luijendijk RW, Jop WCJ, Van Den Tol P, et al. A comparison of suture repair with mesh repair for incisional hernia. *N Engl J Med* 2000;343:392–398. (Multicenter trial demonstrating that mesh repair is better than simple suture repair for incisional hernias.)
11. Snesoz O, Arifoglu K, Kocer U, et al. A new approach for the treatment of recurrent large abdominal hernias: the overlap flap. *Plastic Reconstr Surg* 1997;99:2074–2078. (Describes a combination of abdominoplasty with flap closure.)
12. Singer JA, Mansberger AR. Spigelian hernia. *Arch Surg* 1973;107:515. (Provides a good description of an uncommon lateral abdominal wall hernia.)
13. Usher FC. A new technique for repairing large abdominal wall defects. *Arch Surg* 1961;82:108.
14. Usher FC. New technique for repairing incisional hernias with Marlex mesh. *Am J Surg* 1979;138:740.

CHAPTER 39

Laparoscopic Repair of Ventral Hernias

The theory behind laparoscopic ventral hernia repair is that because the problem is a defect in the fascia, an approach from inside the abdomen makes perfect sense. The role of this technique is still being defined. At present, it appears particularly appropriate for patients with relatively small defects who have not had previous mesh repair (hence no dense adhesions).

Initial Entry and Lysis of Adhesions (Fig. 39.1)

Technical and Anatomic Points

Choose an entry site remote from the defect and any old incision. This may require open entry with a Hasson cannula (see Fig. 37.2 in Chapter 37). Blind entry with a Veress needle in the left upper quadrant is an alternative in properly selected patients. This depends on the costal margin to provide resistance as the Veress needle is inserted and can only be used in patients in whom this area is free of old scars or probable adhesions from previous surgery in the region (eg, splenectomy).

To perform blind left upper quadrant entry, select a point at the left costal border (Fig. 39.1A) well away from the hernia sac. Elevate the abdominal wall below the proposed insertion site with a towel clip, and rely on counterpressure from the costal margin to elevate the cephalad portion. Make an incision and insert the Veress needle, checking for peritoneal entry in the usual fashion. Insert a laparoscope and explore the abdomen.

The hernia may contain omentum or bowel that is adherent to the sac. Place secondary ports and gently attempt to reduce the contents into the abdomen (Fig. 39.1B). Divide omental adhesions with cautery or ultrasonic scalpel. Often, the abdominal expansion caused by the pneumoperitoneum will have reduced the hernia. Inspect the undersurface of the anterior abdominal wall and identify all defects; frequently, multiple defects are present.

LIST OF STRUCTURES

Linea alba
Rectus abdominis muscle
Inferior epigastric vessels

Preparing and Securing the Patch (Fig. 39.2)

Technical and Anatomic Points

Take a small-gauge spinal needle and pass it through the abdominal wall at the approximate edge of the hernia defect to confirm that the skin location corresponds to the actual edge of the fascial defect. Mark this point on the skin with a skin marker. Repeat the procedure at several points around the circumference, producing a map on the skin surface of the underlying fascial defect. Repeat this procedure for any additional defects (Fig. 39.2A).

Cut a DualMesh patch large enough to cover all defects with an overlap of 2 cm on each side. Unless the shape is circular, mark the four corners as 1, 2, 3, and 4 with a skin marker. Mark the side that should face the peritoneal surface (and hence be visible to the laparoscope) as well. Mark the corresponding corners on the skin with the same numbers. Confirm that the mesh will be properly oriented, with the peritoneal surface facing the omentum and bowel and with the appropriate corners matched.

Place a horizontal mattress suture through each of four corners of the mesh. Mark the locations on the skin where these sutures should exit when the mesh is properly situated. Then roll the mesh up into a narrow cylinder and introduce it through a trocar. Unroll the mesh and orient it so that the numbers correspond and the proper side of the mesh faces the bowel. There will be a tendency for the mesh to obscure visualization, much like a sail. Work with the two corners closest to the laparoscope first.

Select the first corner. Make a skin incision about 1 cm in length over the site previously identified. Pass a needle passer through the incision and the fascia at one side of the incision. Maneuver one end of the suture into the needle passer and bring it out through the abdominal wall. Do the same thing with the second end, taking care to allow about 1 cm of fascia between the two entry sites (Fig. 39.2B). Tie the knot; it should bury itself in the subcutaneous fascia. Observe through the laparoscope as you snug the knot down; the patch should rise to the abdominal wall and lie comfortably against it. Complete the knot, securing the first corner of the patch.

Repeat the process with the remaining three corners. The patch should now be secured against the abdominal wall, completely covering the defect. The peritoneal side of the mesh should face the intraabdominal viscera.

FIGURE 39.1
INITIAL ENTRY AND LYSIS OF ADHESIONS (**A,B** from Larson GM. Laparoscopic repair of ventral hernia. In: Scott-Conner CEH, ed. *The SAGES manual.* New York: Springer Verlag, 1999:379–385, with permission.)

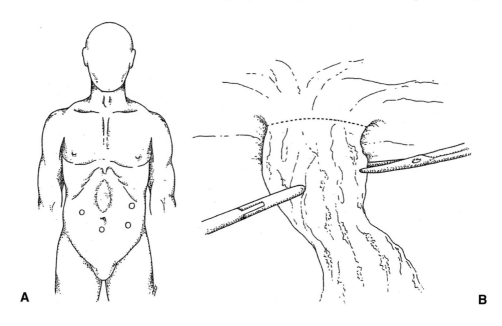

FIGURE 39.2
PREPARING AND SECURING THE PATCH (**A,B** from Larson GM. Laparoscopic repair of ventral hernia. In: Scott-Conner CEH, ed. *The SAGES manual.* New York: Springer Verlag, 1999:379–385, with permission.)

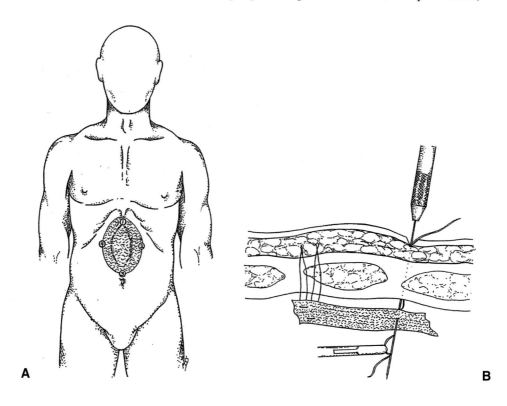

Use a hernia tacking device to place tacks or staples between the four sutures so that there are no gaps through which bowel could herniate.

Withdraw the laparoscope. Close the trocar sites and skin incisions.

REFERENCES

1. Felix EL, Michas C. Laparoscopic repair of spigelian hernias. *Surg Laparosc Endosc* 1994;4:308–310.
2. Holzman MD, Puret CM, Reintgen K. Laparoscopic ventral and incisional hernioplasty. *Surg Endosc* 1997;11:32–35.
3. Larson GM. Laparoscopic repair of ventral hernia. In: Scott-Conner CEH, ed. *The SAGES manual.* New York: Springer Verlag, 1999:379–385.
4. Larson GM, Vandertroll DJ. Approach to repair of ventral hernia and full-thickness losses of abdominal wall. *Surg Clin North Am* 1984;64:335–349.
5. MacFadyen BV, Arregui ME, Corbitt JD. Complications of laparoscopic herniorrhaphy. *Surg Endosc* 1993;7:155–158.
6. Park A, Gagner M, Pomp A. Laparoscopic repair of large incisional hernias. *Surg Laparosc Endosc* 1996;6:123–128.
7. Saiz AA, Willia IH, Paul DK. Laparoscopic ventral hernia repair: a community hospital experience. *Am Surg* 1996;62:336–338.
8. Temudom T, Siadati M, Sarr MG. Repair of complex giant or recurrent ventral hernias by using tension-free intraparietal prosthetic mesh (Stoppa technique): lessons learned from our initial experience (fifty patients). *Surgery* 1996;120:738–744.

THE UPPER GASTROINTESTINAL TRACT AND STRUCTURES OF THE LEFT UPPER QUADRANT

It is evident that if the abdomen is divided into quadrants, the left upper quadrant includes more than the upper gastrointestinal tract and spleen and the pylorus and duodenum pass out of this quadrant. Nevertheless, it is convenient to group these structures together. Perhaps because these are the structures palpated when this region of the abdomen is manually explored (see Chapter 36), along with the left lobe of the liver, these structures are commonly considered together by surgeons.

The region of the lower esophagus, including the esophageal hiatus, stomach, duodenum, vagus nerves, and spleen, is described in this section. First, the procedure of upper gastrointestinal endoscopy (Chapter 40) is described in order to present the general topography of the esophagus, stomach, and duodenum as well as a view from inside. Hiatal hernia repair (Chapters 41 and 42) introduces the anatomy in the region of the esophageal hiatus, the opening in the diaphragm through which the esophagus enters the abdomen. Chapter 43 describes laparoscopic esophagomyotomy, continuing the description of the distal esophagus. The discussion of this region is concluded in the chapter on vagotomies (Chapter 50).

The section on gastric surgery begins with the simplest procedure, feeding gastrostomy (Chapter 44 and 45). Surgical, laparoscopic, and endoscopic techniques are described, and a related procedure—feeding jejunostomy—is included for convenience. Chapters on plication of perforated ulcers introduce the anatomy of the pylorus and first portion of the duodenum as well as the subhepatic and subphrenic spaces from the traditional and laparoscopic approaches (Chapters 45 and 46). Gastric resections (Chapters 48 and 49), two operations performed for trauma—pyloric exclusion and duodenal diverticulization (Chapter 51) and gastric procedures for obesity (Chapters 52 and 53)—complete the discussion of anatomy and surgery of the stomach and duodenum (transduodenal sphincteroplasty and choledochoduodenostomy are included in the next part).

Finally, Chapters 54 and 55, open and laparoscopic splenectomy and splenorrhaphy (repair of injury), conclude the discussion of this region.

CHAPTER 40

Upper Gastrointestinal Endoscopy

Upper gastrointestinal endoscopy is performed for diagnostic and therapeutic purposes. In this chapter, the endoscopic anatomy and the technical maneuvers necessary for safe visualization of the upper gastrointestinal tract are described. For detailed information on endoscopic findings, indications, and technique of biopsy, as well as therapeutic endoscopy of the upper gastrointestinal tract, the reader is referred to several excellent texts listed in the references.

Position of the Patient and Initial Passage of the Endoscope (Fig. 40.1)

Technical Points

Thorough topical anesthesia of the pharynx is essential. This is best produced with the patient sitting facing the examiner and holding a basin.

The patient should then be placed in the left lateral decubitus position. Intravenous sedation is a useful adjunct and may be used at this point. In addition to the suction channel of the endoscope, a Yankauer suction apparatus should be available at the patient's head to avoid aspiration if the patient vomits.

Place a bite block over the endoscope. Check to make certain that the controls of the endoscope are not locked. Pass the endoscope into the posterior pharynx. Use the index and middle fingers of your nondominant hand to guide the endoscope and keep it in the midline. Ask the patient to swallow. Gently advance the endoscope as you feel the sphincter open as swallowing is initiated. Because this maneuver is done essentially blindly, it must be done gently. If the endoscope deviates from the midline, it will probably enter the left or right piriform sinus, a blind diverticulum. Forced attempts at passage may then result in perforation. Occasionally, the endoscope will enter the larynx; this generally results in coughing.

Anatomic Points

The pharynx, which is the vertical, tubular passage extending from the base of the skull to the beginning of the esophagus,

LIST OF STRUCTURES

Pharynx
    Nasopharynx
    Oropharynx
    Laryngopharynx

is in open communication with the nasal, oral, and laryngeal cavities. It is customarily considered to have three components: the nasopharynx (superior to the soft palate), the oropharynx (the area extending from the soft palate superiorly to the hyoid bone inferiorly), and the laryngopharynx (the region extending from the hyoid bone to the lower border of the cricoid cartilage).

The nasopharynx communicates with the auditory tubes (whose ostia open into its lateral wall) and with the nasal cavities (through the choanae). The pharyngeal tonsils (adenoids) are located on the posterior wall of the nasopharynx. The cavity of this portion of the pharynx is always patent and is the widest part of the pharynx.

The oropharynx, sometimes called the *posterior pharynx,* widely communicates anteriorly with the mouth, where the cavity faces the pharyngeal aspect of the tongue. The palatine tonsils are on the lateral wall, between the anterior palatoglossal arch and the posterior palatopharyngeal arch. These lymphoid tissue masses, in conjunction with the pharyngeal tonsil in the nasopharynx and with lymphoid tissue on the pharyngeal part of the tongue (lingual tonsil), form Waldeyer's ring. The oropharyngeal isthmus can be closed by approximation of the palatoglossal arches, accompanied by retraction of the tongue. This lingual movement also occludes the lumen of the oropharynx above the bolus during swallowing.

The laryngopharynx communicates anteriorly with the opening of the larynx. Lateral to the laryngeal aditus (inlet) on either side is an elongated fossa, the piriform recess. Inferiorly, the laryngopharynx is continuous with the esophagus. This junction is the narrowest part of the pharynx.

At the pharyngoesophageal junction, the pharyngeal musculature consists of the inferior pharyngeal constrictor, the thickest of the three pharyngeal constrictors. This muscle can be logically subdivided into a superior thyropharyngeus, whose fibers arise from the thyroid cartilage and are directed superomedially to insert on a posterior median raphe, and an inferior cricopharyngeus, whose fibers originate from the cricoid cartilage and pass horizontally to insert on the median raphe. During swallowing, contraction of the thyropharyngeus propels the bolus, while the cricopharyngeus acts as a sphincter. Failure of the cricopharyngeus to relax during swallowing can result in herniation of the mucosa between the two parts of the inferior constrictor (Zenker's diverticulum; see Chapter 12), or a predisposition to perforation of the esophagus with the endoscope.

FIGURE 40.1
POSITION OF THE PATIENT AND INITIAL PASSAGE OF THE ENDOSCOPE

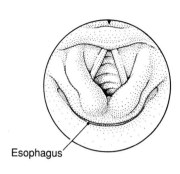

Esophagus

FIGURE 40.2
THE ESOPHAGUS

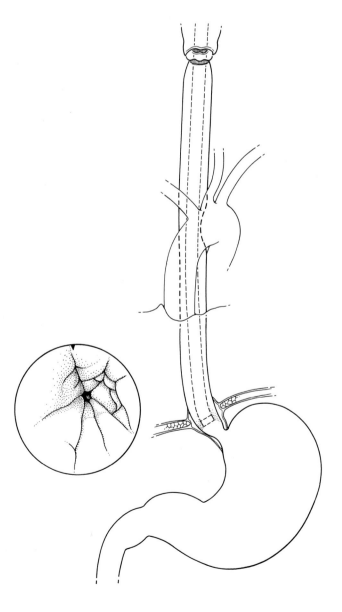

The Esophagus (Fig. 40.2)

Technical Points

Once the endoscope is within the esophagus, visualize the lumen and advance the endoscope to the cardioesophageal junction under direct vision. This is a fairly straight shot and should require minimal motion of the controls. Periodic light puffs of air keep the lumen open and assist in passage of the instrument. Recognize the cardioesophageal junction by the change in color at the squamocolumnar junction (the Z line). Generally, the cardioesophageal junction lies about 40 cm from the incisor teeth. The lower esophageal sphincter, a physiologic high-pressure zone without any consistent anatomic landmark, will generally be closed. Gentle pressure with the endoscope will allow the endoscope to pass into the stomach unless the distal esophagus is narrowed by a stricture or tumor.

Anatomic Points

The esophagus, which begins at the lower border of the cricoid cartilage, is about 25 cm long. It descends through the neck and thorax just anterior to the vertebral bodies. It passes through the diaphragm at about the level of the tenth thoracic vertebra, and ends by opening into the cardia of the stomach at about the level of the eleventh thoracic vertebra. It lies in the median plane at its origin but deviates slightly to the left until the root of the neck. At the root of the neck, it gradually deviates to the right so that, by the level of the fifth thoracic vertebra, it is once again midline. At the seventh thoracic vertebra, it again deviates to the left, and ultimately turns anteriorly to pass through the esophageal hiatus of the diaphragm. The thoracic esophagus also has anterior and posterior curves that follow the curvature of the vertebral column. The intraabdominal esophagus turns sharply to the left to become continuous with the stomach.

The anatomic relationships of the esophagus are important. In the neck, the esophagus is posterior to the trachea and anterior to the cervical vertebra and the prevertebral muscles.

Lateral to the cervical esophagus and trachea on both sides are the recurrent laryngeal nerve (in or near the tracheoesophageal groove), the common carotid artery, and the thyroid lobes. In the lower neck, the thoracic duct ascends to the left of the trachea. In the mediastinum, from superior to inferior, the esophagus has the following relationships:

Anterior: trachea, left main-stem bronchus, right pulmonary artery, left atrium within the pericardial sac, and diaphragm

Posterior: vertebral column and prevertebral muscles, right intercostal arteries of aortic origin, thoracic duct, azygos vein and the termination of the hemiazygos and accessory hemiazygos veins, and, as it approaches the diaphragm, the aorta

Right lateral: right parietal pleura and intervening arch of the azygos vein and the right vagus nerve, which will principally form the posterior esophageal plexus

Left lateral: left subclavian artery and thoracic duct, left recurrent laryngeal nerve, terminal portion of the aortic arch, left parietal pleura, left vagus nerve (which will principally form the anterior esophageal plexus), and the descending aorta

In the abdomen, the esophagus is anterior to the left crus of the diaphragm and the left inferior phrenic artery.

Four narrow areas of the esophagus are described. These are (a) the cricoesophageal junction (15 cm from the incisors); (b) the point at which the aortic arch crosses the esophagus (22 cm from the incisors); (c) the point at which the esophagus is crossed by the left main-stem bronchus (27 cm from the incisors); and (d) the point at which the esophagus traverses the diaphragm (40 cm from the incisors).

Although the distal esophageal sphincter cannot be identified anatomically, it can be demonstrated as a manometric high-pressure zone about 2 cm proximal to the gastroesophageal junction. Just distal to this physiologic sphincter, the gastroesophageal junction (ora serrata or Z line) can be recognized. The abrupt transition from esophageal squamous epithelium to gastric columnar epithelium is visualized endoscopically as a color change from gray-pink (esophageal mucosa) to yellow-orange (gastric mucosa).

The Stomach (Fig. 40.3)

Technical Points

First inflate the stomach by insufflating air, noting the mobility of the gastric walls as the stomach distends. Identify the gastric notch (incisura angularis) on the lesser curvature. Advance the scope to the notch. At this point, the scope may

FIGURE 40.3
THE STOMACH

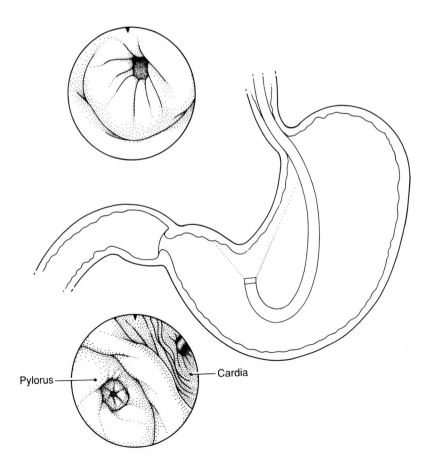

Pylorus

Cardia

be passed distally toward the pylorus, or retroflexed to visualize the cardioesophageal junction from below. It is helpful to think of a double-barreled configuration at this point. As you look at the incisure, one "barrel" is the view toward the pylorus, and the second barrel is the retroflexed view upward toward the cardia. Distention of the stomach with air pushes the greater curvature out and away from the incisure. The relatively fixed lesser curvature of the stomach looks like a septum, creating the double-barreled appearance. Slight changes in angulation of the tip of the endoscope will allow you either to proceed to the pylorus or to retroflex.

First retroflex the scope by entering the barrel leading back to the cardia. Push both control wheels away from you and pull back on the scope as you sharply angulate the tip. Look for the black tube of the endoscope as it emerges from the cardia. Twist and angulate the tip of the scope to visualize fully the cardia and fundus. Then return to the region of the incisure by advancing the scope and straightening the tip.

Identify the antrum by the relative paucity of folds. Advance the scope, hugging the lesser curvature, toward the pylorus and inspect the pylorus. Unless the pylorus is distorted by ulcer or tumor, it will open and close in a rhythmic fashion and will appear to be roughly circular. Advance the endoscope to visualize the pylorus face on. As the pylorus opens, gently push the scope through the pylorus. At this point, visualization of the lumen is generally lost as the scope enters the confines of the duodenal bulb. Note the numbers on the scope at the patient's incisor teeth. If a length of more than 60 cm of scope has been introduced, pull back on the scope gently to straighten the redundancy in the stomach.

Anatomic Points

The stomach is highly variable in its morphology and changes size and shape when full or empty. However, certain anatomic features can always, or almost always, be described. The greater curvature is directed to the left and inferiorly, whereas the lesser curvature is directed to the right and superiorly.

The esophagus opens into the stomach at the cardiac orifice. The immediate postesophageal part of the stomach is dilated in comparison to the esophagus and is referred to as the *cardiac antrum.* The left margin of the esophagus, at its junction with the stomach, makes an acute angle with the beginning of the greater curvature; this junction is the cardiac incisure. The fundus is that portion of the stomach that is superior to the cardiac incisure or cardiac notch. Along the lesser curvature, nearer to its distal end than to its proximal end, there is usually a distinct notch, the angular incisure. A line drawn from the angular incisure perpendicular to the axis of the stomach demarcates the proximal body from the distal, slightly dilated, pyloric antrum. The pyloric antrum is limited on the right by a slight groove, the sulcus terminalis. Immediately distal to the sulcus terminalis, the short segment of terminal stomach is termed the *pyloric canal.* The pyloric canal terminates at the pyloric sphincter, the restricted lumen of which is termed *pyloric channel.* The pyloric channel

is the terminal part of the stomach lumen and is continuous with the lumen of the duodenum.

Internally, the mucosa and submucosa of the stomach are characterized by thick folds and rugae. Along the lesser curvature and in the pyloric canal, the rugae are oriented longitudinally. It is the part of the lumen of the stomach that is referred to as the *gastric canal.* Elsewhere, the rugae assume a honeycomb pattern.

On endoscopic examination, the gastric notch can be identified as a crescentic fold projecting into the lumen from the lesser curvature. In passing the endoscope distally, the antrum is entered, identified on the basis that, here, as more distally, the relatively few rugae are aligned parallel to the longitudinal axis, rather than having a honeycomb appearance. The pylorus can be distinguished because the walls of the stomach converge at this point, severely restricting the diameter of the lumen, and a rhythmic opening and closing of the pyloric channel are noted. When the endoscope is retroflexed, the endoscope can be seen passing through the gastroesophageal sphincter, also characterized by a sudden reduction in luminal diameter as well as by the so-called cardiac rosette, which is a cluster of mucosal folds radiating from the gastroesophageal junction.

The Duodenum (Fig. 40.4)

Technical Points

Withdraw the endoscope slightly in order to advance the tip by straightening the scope in the stomach. Once the scope is straight, advance it gently while insufflating air; the circumferential folds of the duodenum should be visible. If the scope pops out of the pylorus and back into the stomach, traverse the pylorus again. Clear bile is generally visible in the duodenum. The normal ampulla of Vater, frequently covered by a fold of mucosa, is rarely seen with the end-viewing endoscope. Pass the scope down the duodenum as far as possible, keeping in mind that most pathologic processes are found in the first and second portions of the duodenum.

As the scope is withdrawn, carefully inspect the duodenal bulb. This arrowhead-shaped chamber lacks the circular folds seen in the remainder of the duodenum. Because this region is small and poorly distensible, it may be necessary to make several passes through the pylorus to visualize this region adequately.

As you withdraw the scope, inspect the stomach and esophagus again. Use the suction channel of the endoscope to decompress the stomach when visualization is complete.

Anatomic Points

The duodenum, which is the widest, shortest, and most fixed portion of the small intestine, is usually 20 to 25 cm long. Beginning at the pylorus, it passes posteriorly, superiorly, and to the right (the first or superior part) for about 5 cm. This portion is comparatively mobile and is the duodenal bulb of radiologists. In contrast to the stomach, where the mucosa is yellow-orange, the mucosa of the duodenum is

FIGURE 40.4
THE DUODENUM

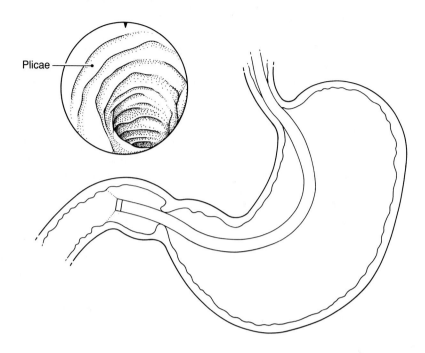

Plicae

yellow-gray. Proximally, mucosal folds are lacking, but as the second part is approached, the beginnings of the characteristic plicae circulares of the small intestine appear.

The duodenum then makes an abrupt curve inferiorly, forming the superior duodenal flexure, and passes to the right of the vertebral bodies and head of the pancreas for a distance of 8 to 10 cm. This part, the second or descending portion, receives the united common bile and pancreatic duct (ampulla of Vater or hepatopancreatic ampulla), which has an oblique intramural path on the medial aspect of the duodenum. The ampulla of Vater opens on the summit of the major duodenal papilla, about 10 cm from the pylorus and often protected by a mucosal hood. Distal to the papilla, a single or bifid longitudinal mucosal fold can frequently be seen. Elsewhere, typical plicae circulares should be noted. About 2 cm proximal to the major duodenal papilla, a minor duodenal papilla may frequently be noted; at its apex, the accessory pancreatic duct (duct of Santorini) empties into the duodenum.

The third or horizontal portion of the duodenum starts at the inferior duodenal angle (flexure), another sharp bend to the left and across the vertebral bodies. The third portion is about 10 cm long, containing plicae circulares and nothing else of endoscopic or anatomic significance.

The ascending or fourth part of the duodenum is short (about 2.5 cm in length). Just before its termination, it makes an abrupt turn anteriorly to end at the duodenojejunal flexure. The duodenojejunal flexure is held in position by the suspensory muscle or ligament of the duodenum, commonly termed the ligament of Treitz.

The Postgastrectomy Stomach (Fig. 40.5)

Technical and Anatomic Points

Gastric surgery alters the appearance of the stomach. Pyloroplasty and partial gastrectomy using the Billroth I reconstruction both result in a patulous or nonexistent pylorus. (The Billroth I and II reconstructions are described in Chapter 37; pyloroplasty is described in Chapter 38.) Endoscopy in such situations proceeds normally, with the scope traversing a surgically altered "pylorus" to enter the duodenum. Pay special attention to the appearance of the anastomosis (if it can be identified). Generally, only the first portion of the duodenum will have been altered surgically.

A Billroth II reconstruction can generally be recognized by a septum with two identifiable outlets (afferent and efferent limbs). Although it is often difficult to ascertain which limb is which, the afferent limb generally contains copious bile, whereas the efferent limb does not. Cannulate and inspect both limbs.

A simple gastrojejunostomy (with antrum and pylorus left *in situ*) has a similar endoscopic appearance, but frequently, the antrum and pylorus can also be identified.

Intraoperative Upper Gastrointestinal Endoscopy (Fig. 40.6)

Technical Points

Operative upper gastrointestinal endoscopy is performed when urgent laparotomy for upper gastrointestinal bleeding

FIGURE 40.5
THE POSTGASTRECTOMY STOMACH

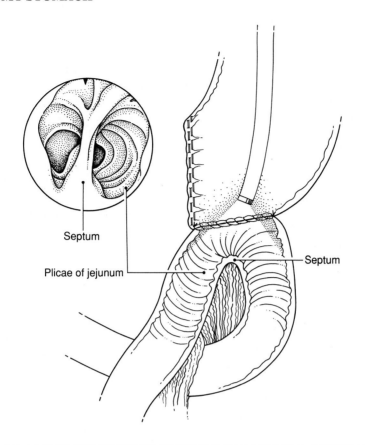

Septum

Plicae of jejunum

Septum

FIGURE 40.6
INTRAOPERATIVE UPPER GASTROINTESTINAL ENDOSCOPY

Bleeding site

Bleeding site

of unknown origin is necessary. It is particularly helpful for identifying bleeding sites within the small intestine.

Safe passage of the endoscope in an unconscious, intubated patient requires skill and a firm but gentle touch. The anesthesiologist must hold and guard the endotracheal tube against accidental dislodgment. Pass your nondominant hand deep into the posterior pharynx above the endotracheal tube and displace the endotracheal tube, mandible, and tongue anteriorly. Pass the scope into the posterior pharynx and guide it in the midline between the fingers of the nondominant hand. An indwelling esophageal stethoscope or nasogastric tube can sometimes be "followed" into the esophagus, but this is not always easy.

Traverse the upper esophageal sphincter by applying gentle pressure and pass the scope as previously described (Figs. 40.2 to 40.5). Remember that endoscopic relationships will be altered by the supine position of the patient. If the abdomen is open, the inflated stomach will rise up into the wound, further distorting the angle between stomach and duodenum; moreover, the pylorus will appear to lie much more posterior than usual.

An assistant within the sterile field of the abdomen should gently compress the proximal jejunum to limit passage of air into the small bowel. If the small bowel is allowed to become distended with air, closure of the abdomen will be difficult. If no source of bleeding is found proximal to the ligament of Treitz, endoscopy of the small intestine is often helpful. Often, the assistant can facilitate passage of the scope around the duodenum and into the proximal small intestine. A long scope, such as a colonoscope, can be passed by mouth and threaded through the small intestine to the ileocecal valve. The assistant should use both hands to "reef" the intestine over the scope as it is advanced. It is unnecessary and undesirable to distend the entire small intestine with air. Have your assistant maintain a sausage-shaped segment of air-filled intestine at the tip of the scope by occluding the bowel proximally and distally using gentle digital pressure. Look through the scope for fresh bleeding as the assistant inspects the transilluminated serosal surface of the intestine for prominent vessels or other abnormalities. Have your assistant mark any suspicious areas with silk sutures.

Anatomic Points

The predominant feature of the entire small bowel will be the plicae circulares. In addition, the diameter of the small bowel will be noted, both endoscopically and directly, to decrease progressively from the beginning of the jejunum to the ileocecal valve.

REFERENCES

1. Botet JF, Lightdale C. Endoscopic ultrasonography of the gastrointestinal tract. *Gastrointest Endosc Clin North Am* 1995;24:385–412. (Describes useful adjunct for staging gastric malignancies and assessing the pancreas.)
2. Cooper GS. Indications and contraindications for upper gastrointestinal endoscopy. *Gastrointest Endosc Clin North Am* 1994;4:439–454. (Provides excellent overall review.)
3. Demling K, Kloster K, Koch H, et al, eds. Endoscopy and biopsy of esophagus, stomach and duodenum. Philadelphia: WB Saunders, 1982. (Contains an atlas of typical findings.)
4. Jaffe PK. The use of endoscopic ultrasonography in the evaluation and diagnosis of gastric lesions. *Gastrointest Endosc Clin North Am* 1996;6:566–584.
5. Jane PK. Technique of upper gastrointestinal endoscopy. *Gastrointest Endosc Clin North Am* 1994;4:501–521.
6. Mellinger JD, Ponsky JL. Endoscopic evaluation of the postoperative stomach. *Gastrointest Endosc Clin North Am* 1996;6:621–639. (Gives specific pointers relevant to postsurgical anatomy.)
7. Pearl RK, ed. *Gastrointestinal endoscopy for surgeons.* Boston: Little, Brown, 1984:21.
8. Scott-Conner CEH, ed. *The SAGES manual. Section II: upper gastrointestinal endoscopy. Section III: small bowel enteroscopy.* New York: Springer-Verlag, 1999:422–484. (Contains information about therapeutic endoscopy.)
9. Sivak MV, ed. *Gastroenterologic endoscopy.* Philadelphia: WB Saunders, 1987:272.

CHAPTER 41

Hiatal Hernia Repair

The purpose of hiatal hernia repair is to generate a functional lower esophageal sphincter mechanism that will effectively prevent reflux of gastric contents into the esophagus but will allow swallowing, belching, and vomiting.

Increasingly, most hiatal hernia repairs are performed laparoscopically (see Chapter 42). Open repair is still necessary when the laparoscopic approach fails or is not feasible. The transabdominal Nissen procedure is presented in this chapter. For this repair, a 360-degree wrap of gastric fundus is placed around the distal esophagus, producing a functional valve. As intragastric pressure increases, the pressure in the wrap increases as well, closing off the distal esophagus. Other surgical techniques for hiatal hernia repair are detailed in the references.

Exposure of the Cardioesophageal Junction (Fig. 41.1)

Technical Points

The right-handed surgeon should stand on the right side of the patient. Make an upper midline laparotomy incision. Extend the incision up and to the left of the xiphoid for a little additional exposure. Clamp and ligate the small vessels that are frequently encountered in the angle between the xiphoid and costal margin. Do not divide the xiphoid: this adds little to the exposure and may stimulate heterotopic bone formation within the incision. Explore the abdomen and confirm the position of a nasogastric tube at the cardioesophageal junction. Place a fixed retractor (such as the Omni system) to provide strong cephalad retraction of the left costal margin, placing additional blades to hold the incision open in the midportion. If this type of retractor is not available, a satisfactory alternative is an "upper-hand" type of retractor in the left upper margin of the incision, and a Balfour retractor in the middle of the incision. Reverse Trendelenburg position assists as gravity pulls the upper abdominal viscera caudad into the field.

In most cases, adequate exposure can be obtained by placing a liver blade under the left lobe and retracting it upward. If exposure is not sufficient, mobilize the left lobe of the liver by incising the triangular ligament. Pass your left hand around the inferior edge of the left lobe of the liver, grasp it, and pull down. The triangular ligament will be seen as a thin, tough, membranous structure passing along the posterosuperior aspect of the liver. Divide the small vessel at the free edge between hemoclips. Use electrocautery to divide the triangular ligament. As you progress to the right, an anterior and posterior leaf of the triangular ligament will become apparent, with loose areolar tissue between. At this point, continue the dissection cautiously with Metzenbaum scissors until the left lobe of the liver can be folded down to expose the cardioesophageal junction. Place a moist laparotomy pad and Harrington retractor over the left lobe of the liver to hold it out of the way.

The inferior aspect of the diaphragm and the cardioesophageal junction should now be clearly visible. Confirm the location of the esophagus by palpating the nasogastric tube, which is anterior and a little to the left of the aorta at the esophageal hiatus. Incise the peritoneum overlying the cardioesophageal junction to expose the esophagus. Take care to avoid injury to the vagal nerve trunks.

Anatomic Points

Anteriorly, the diaphragm arises from the inner surface of the xiphoid process by two fleshy slips (sternal origin). Its costal

LIST OF STRUCTURES

Xiphoid	Thoracic duct	Short gastric arteries
Costal margin	Inferior vena cava	Left gastroepiploic artery
Diaphragm	Aorta	Superior epigastric artery
Median arcuate ligament	Left inferior phrenic artery	Liver
Esophageal hiatus	(and vein)	Left lobe
Mediastinum	Celiac artery	Left triangular ligament
Pericardium	Left gastric artery	Esophagus
Phrenic nerve	Splenic artery	Mesoesophagus
Left and right pleural sacs		

FIGURE 41.1
EXPOSURE OF THE CARDIOESOPHAGEAL JUNCTION

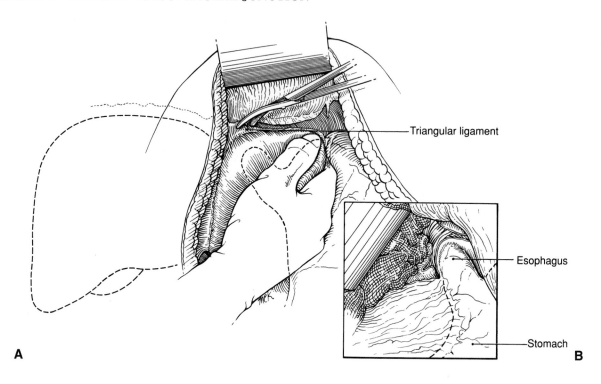

Triangular ligament

Esophagus

Stomach

A   B

origin is from the inner surfaces of the costal cartilages and adjacent bone of ribs 7 through 12. The costal cartilage of the seventh rib is the last to attach directly to the sternum at the xiphisternal articulation. The superior epigastric artery, a terminal branch of the internal thoracic (mammary) artery, enters the sheath of the rectus in the interval (termed the *foramen of Morgagni* or *space of Larrey*) between the sternal and costal origins of the diaphragm. This "defect" permits a retrosternal or parasternal hernia to occur. A paraxiphoid incision, then, will almost assuredly sever the superior epigastric artery or its branches. The artery anastomoses with the inferior epigastric artery in the substance of the rectus abdominis muscle and its division are of no consequence if bleeding is controlled.

Divide the free edge of the left triangular ligament between clamps. This ligament often contains vascular structures and may have both bile canaliculi (80%) and liver stroma (60%) present. Medially, the posterior layer of the left triangular ligament is continuous with the mesoesophagus, a more or less vertically disposed peritoneal reflection. Thus, careful division of the left triangular ligament should lead one to the esophagus.

Divide the peritoneum at the cardioesophageal junction, taking care to avoid the anterior and posterior vagal trunks. Typically (88% of the time), there are a single anterior vagal trunk and a single posterior vagal trunk at the esophageal hiatus. Both trunks lie to the right of the esophageal midline, with the anterior vagal trunk lying on the esophagus and the posterior vagal trunk lying either immediately posterior to the esophagus or up to 2 cm to the right of the esophagus;

thus, great care must be taken to avoid trauma to the vagi, especially the posterior vagal trunk.

Mobilization of the Esophagus (Fig. 41.2)

Technical Points

Mobilize the distal esophagus by blunt dissection in the mediastinum. Do not clear much of the lesser curvature of the stomach because tissue here will help to prevent the wrap from slipping. Encircle the mobilized esophagus and vagal trunks with a long Penrose drain to assist in subsequent dissection.

Anatomic Points

Dissection into the mediastinum requires some knowledge of the anatomy of the region of the esophageal hiatus, both on the abdominal and on the thoracic side of the diaphragm. The left inferior phrenic artery and vein lie on the left crus of the diaphragm and pass behind the esophagus. Occasionally, the left phrenic vein passes anterior to the esophageal hiatus, terminating in the inferior vena cava. The median arcuate ligament separates the aortic hiatus from the esophageal hiatus. The celiac artery arises from the aorta in the region of the arcuate ligament. The inferior vena cava lies on the right crus of the diaphragm. The thoracic duct lies in areolar and adipose tissue just to the right of the aorta.

Superior to the esophageal hiatus, the right and left pleurae are approximated between the esophagus and aorta, forming a mesoesophagus. This is a rather broad ligament, with an

FIGURE 41.2
MOBILIZATION OF THE ESOPHAGUS

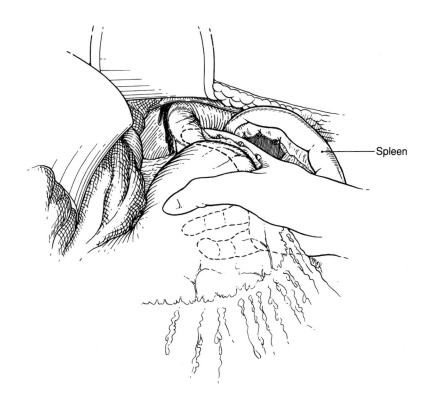

Spleen

abundance of areolar tissue between the left and right pleurae. If perforation occurs, it is usually the right pleural sac that is compromised because this is in contact with the lower esophagus, whereas the left is somewhat more removed. Only rarely are both pleural sacs perforated. The pericardial sac is immediately anterior to the esophagus at the level of the esophageal hiatus, and the left phrenic nerve is just to the left of the pericardium. Blunt dissection should not harm either of these structures; however, later, if the anterior margin of the hiatus is to be approximated, care must be taken not to include them in the suture.

Division of the Short Gastric Vessels (Fig. 41.3)

Technical Points

Three or four short gastric vessels that tether the greater curvature of the stomach to the spleen must be divided. Begin this dissection at the lowest short gastric vessel and progress toward the esophagus. Identify the point on the greater curvature where the right gastroepiploic artery terminates; then make a window into the lesser sac by dividing and ligating the pair of vessels above. Through this window, continue to progress up, serially clamping, dividing, and ligating vessels until the esophagus is reached. Take care not to tear the capsule of the spleen by excessive traction on the stomach. Mobilize the greater curvature fully to ensure that a good wrap can be performed. Elevate the stomach and esophagus to expose filmy gastropancreatic folds. Divide these sharply.

The wrap is generally performed over a calibrated bougie. There are two ways to accomplish this. One involves passing a 40-French esophageal dilator from above. Alternatively, a Hegar dilator may be placed next to the esophagus. If a Hurst-Maloney dilator is to be passed from above, it should be done at this time and its position within the esophagus confirmed by direct palpation. Generally, it will be necessary to remove the nasogastric tube.

Anatomic Points

The short gastric arteries are branches of the splenic artery or one of its terminal divisions. These arteries run through the gastrosplenic (lienogastric) ligament to supply the fundus; in the substance of the fundus, they anastomose with branches of the left gastric and gastroepiploic arteries. These arteries can be sacrificed within the substance of the gastrosplenic ligament but must not be pulled for fear of avulsing the delicate splenic capsule.

Construction of the Wrap (Fig. 41.4)

Technical and Anatomic Points

Pass a Babcock clamp posterior to the esophagus and grasp the greater curvature of the stomach, well down into the mobilized segment. Feed the mobilized greater curvature behind the esophagus, applying only gentle traction on the stomach with the Babcock clamp. Pull down and out on the Penrose

FIGURE 41.3
DIVISION OF THE SHORT GASTRIC VESSELS

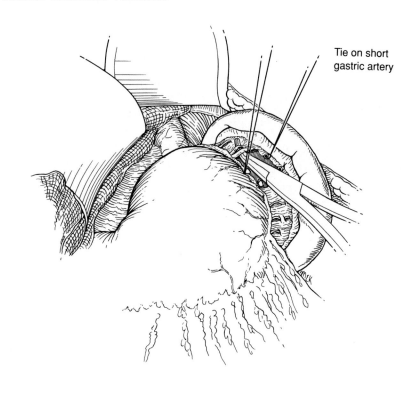

Tie on short gastric artery

FIGURE 41.4
CONSTRUCTION OF THE WRAP

A

B

drain, encircling the esophagus to facilitate passage of the wrap behind the esophagus and above the cardioesophageal junction. Do not hesitate to mobilize additional greater curvature if the stomach does not pass easily behind the esophagus.

If a Hurst-Maloney dilator has not been passed from above, place a 40-French Hegar dilator next to the esophagus (which should also contain a nasogastric tube).

Construct the wrap by suturing stomach on the left side to mobilized greater curvature on the right with four or five Lembert sutures of 0-0 or 2-0 silk. The lower two sutures may include bites of esophagus but should not enter the esophageal lumen. Tie the sutures, confirming that the wrap is patulous and not under tension. Remove the Hegar or Hurst-Maloney dilator. Reinsert the nasogastric tube, if it was removed earlier. Check hemostasis and close the abdomen.

REFERENCES

1. Baue AE, Belsey RH. The treatment of sliding hiatus hernia and reflux esophagitis by the Mark IV technique. *Surgery* 1967;62:396.
2. Donahue PE, Samelson S, Nyhus LM, et al. The floppy Nissen fundoplication: effective long-term control of pathologic reflux. *Arch Surg* 1985;120:663.
3. DeMeester TR, Stein JH. Minimizing the side effects of antireflux surgery. *World J Surg* 1992;16:335–336.
4. Deschamps C, Trastek VF, Allen MS, et al. Long-term results after reoperation for failed antireflux procedures. *J Thorac Cardiovasc Surg* 1997;113:545–550.
5. Gott JP, Polk HC. Repeat operation for failure of antireflux procedures. *Surg Clin North Am* 1991;71:13.
6. Gray SW, Rowe JS, Skandalakis JE. Surgical anatomy of the gastroesophageal junction. *Am Surg* 1979;45:575.
7. Hill LD. An effective operation for hiatal hernia: an eight year appraisal. *Ann Surg* 1967;166:681.
8. Horgan S, Pohl D, Bogetti D, et al. Failed antireflux surgery: what have we learned from reoperations? *Arch Surg* 1999;134:809–815.
9. Kauer WK, Peters JH, DeMeester TR, et al. A tailored approach to antireflux surgery. *J Thorac Cardiovasc Surg* 1995;110:141–146.
10. Luostarinen ME, Isolauri JO. Randomized trial to study the effect of fundic mobilization on long-term results of Nissen fundoplication. *Br J Surg* 1999;86:614–618.
11. Orringer MB, Skinner DB, Belsey RHR. Long-term results of the Mark IV operation for hiatal hernia and analyses of recurrences and their treatment. *J Thorac Cardiovasc Surg* 1972;63:25.
12. Peillon C, Manouvrier JL, Labreche J, et al. Should the vagus nerves be isolated from the fundoplication wrap? A prospective study. *Arch Surg* 1994;129:814–818.
13. Polk HC. Fundoplication for reflux esophagitis: misadventures with the operation of choice. *Ann Surg* 1976;183:645. (Provides excellent review of technical pitfalls.)
14. Richardson JD, Larson GM, Polk HC. Intrathoracic fundoplication for shortened esophagus: treacherous solution to a challenging problem. *Am J Surg* 1982;143:29.
15. Rieger NA, Jamieson GG, Britten-Jones R, et al. Reoperation after failed antireflux surgery. *Br J Surg* 1994;81:1159–1161.
16. Wald H, Polk HC. Anatomical variations in hiatal and upper gastric areas and their relationship to difficulties experienced in operations for reflux esophagitis. *Ann Surg* 1983;197:389.

CHAPTER 42

Laparoscopic Hiatal Hernia Repair

Isaac Samuel

Patients with gastroesophageal reflux disease (GERD) who have failed 8 to 12 weeks of medical therapy or have developed complications of GERD are candidates for antireflux surgery. Preoperative evaluation must include: (a) esophageal manometry to demonstrate a defective lower esophageal sphincter and to assess esophageal motility, and (b) esophagogastroduodenoscopy (EGD) to evaluate esophagitis, metaplasia, dysplasia, esophageal shortening, and stricture. A 24-hour pH study to confirm exposure of the lower esophageal sphincter to acid pH is essential only if EGD does not show esophagitis and if manometry is normal, but some surgeons perform this preoperative investigation routinely.

The laparoscopic Nissen fundoplication, described here, is a minimal access technique very similar to the open Nissen fundoplication (see Chapter 41), an operation that has proved highly successful and durable. An alternative laparoscopic fundoplication, the 270-degree Toupet, is described by McKernan and Champion (see references).

Hiatal Dissection and Crural Closure (Fig. 42.1)

Technical and Anatomic Points

Five ports are used (Fig. 42.1A). The size of these ports depends on the instruments used. Five 10-mm ports will accommodate all needed instruments; if 5-mm instruments are available (e.g., 5-mm liver retractor, ultrasonic shears), correspondingly smaller trocars may be substituted.

Place the midline port for the laparoscope well above the umbilicus. This is crucial for adequate visualization of the hiatus. Use a 45-degree angled laparoscope for hiatal dissection. Place a right subcostal port along the anterior axillary line for a liver retractor, and a left subcostal port along the anterior axillary line. This left subcostal port will be used by the assistant surgeon for retraction. The final two ports are inserted on either side of the camera port along the midclavicular line 3 inches below the costal margin. These allow the operating surgeon to work using both hands with good triangulation with the camera and operative field. Incline the patient into 35 to 45 degrees of reverse Trendelenburg position. Stand to the right side of the patient with the assistant to the left. Some surgeons prefer to stand in between the patient's legs with the patient in a modified lithotomy position.

Pass a liver retractor through the right anterior axillary line port and gently retract the left lobe of the liver up against the diaphragm. It is not necessary to divide the left triangular ligament. The stomach and undersurface of the diaphragm should come into view below the liver. A fat pad generally marks the gastroesophageal junction and obscures visualization of the esophagus.

The assistant surgeon should grasp the esophageal fat pad and retract it inferiorly to expose the phrenoesophageal membrane. When the hiatal defect is large, an opening into the chest will be seen. Divide the phrenoesophageal membrane to display the apex of the hiatus. Continue the dissection toward the right crus of the diaphragm, reducing any associated hiatus hernia (Fig. 42.1B). Focus attention on dissecting and defining the right crus of the diaphragm.

Divide the transparent part of the lesser omentum over the caudate lobe of the liver. Take care to avoid injury to the hepatic branch of the anterior vagus nerve. Because as many as one in four patients may have an aberrant left hepatic artery arising from the left gastric artery, exercise caution during this part of the dissection. With the stomach retracted inferiorly and to the left by the assistant surgeon, dissect the peritoneum off the abdominal surface and hiatal border of the right crus.

LIST OF STRUCTURES

Diaphragm	Stomach	Vagus nerves
Crura, right and left	Fundus	Liver
Hiatus	Mediastinum	Left lobe
Phrenoesophageal membrane	Left inferior phrenic artery (and vein)	Segments II and III
Gastrosplenic ligament	Short gastric arteries	Caudate lobe (segment I)
Gastrophrenic ligament	Esophagus	Left triangular ligament

FIGURE 42.1
HIATAL DISSECTION AND CRURAL CLOSURE (B and **D** from Scott-Conner C, Cushieri A, Carter FJ. Diaphragm, hiatus, and esophagus. In: *Minimal access surgical anatomy.* Philadelphia: Lippincott Williams & Wilkins, 2000, with permission; **C** and **E** from Wind GG. The stomach. In: *The applied laparoscopic anatomy: abdomen and pelvis.* Baltimore: Williams & Wilkins, 1997, with permission.)

FIGURE 42.1 (Continued)

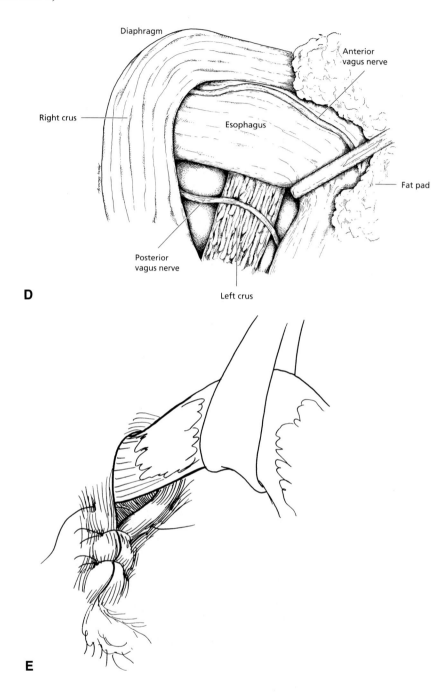

Gently dissect the loose connective tissue in the posterior mediastinum to visualize the distal esophagus. Next, gently displace the distal esophagus anteriorly and the right crus laterally to identify the right vagal nerve trunk. Use the shaft of an instrument to displace the esophagus gently forward; do not grasp it directly. Occult injury to the esophagus with peritonitis or mediastinitis is a potentially lethal complication. Similarly dissect and define the left crus of the diaphragm by working behind the esophagus from the right side, displacing the esophagus toward the anterior abdominal wall.

Retract the esophagus to the right to approach the left crus of the diaphragm from the left side. Retract the gastric fundus inferiorly and complete the circumferential dissection of the distal esophagus by dividing the peritoneum along the left crus of the diaphragm, the angle of His, and the gastric fundus. Retract the stomach carefully, by grasping the fundus very gently with atraumatic forceps; gastric perforations have occurred after vigorous retraction. Avoid injury to the phrenic vessels near the hiatus.

Pass a short segment of Penrose drain into the abdomen and use it to encircle the distal esophagus (Fig. 42.1C). Apply traction on this drain in such as way as to retract the esophagus anteriorly and to the left. Complete the hiatal dissection by cleaning away any loose connective tissue and defining the hiatal borders (Fig. 42.1D). To avoid pleural injury and resulting pneumothorax, do not transgress unnecessarily high into the posterior mediastinum.

Approximate the crura behind the esophagus with three to four interrupted nonabsorbable sutures, working from below upward (Fig. 42.1E). This step is generally omitted during open Nissen fundoplication. It is required during the laparoscopic procedure because extensive crural dissection and lack of adhesion formation combine to permit postoperative herniation through the hiatus.

FIGURE 42.2
FUNDIC MOBILIZATION AND NISSEN FUNDOPLICATION (A from Scott-Conner C, Cushieri A, Carter FJ. Stomach and duodenum. In: *Minimal access surgical anatomy.* Philadelphia: Lippincott Williams & Wilkins, 2000, with permission; **B–D** from Wind GG. The stomach. In: *The applied laparoscopic anatomy: abdomen and pelvis.* Baltimore: Williams & Wilkins 1997, with permission; **E** from Scott-Conner C, Cushieri A, Carter FJ. Diaphragm, hiatus, and esophagus. In: *Minimal access surgical anatomy.* Philadelphia: Lippincott Williams & Wilkins, 2000, with permission.)

FIGURE 42.2   (Continued)

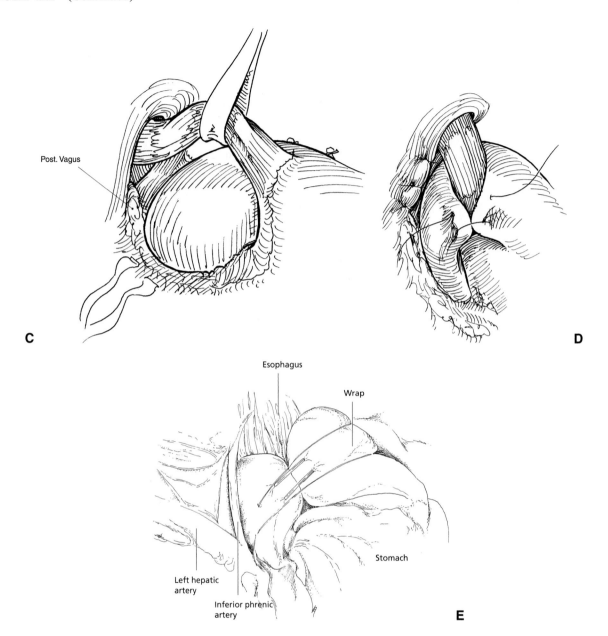

Fundic Mobilization and Nissen Fundoplication (Fig. 42.2)

Technical and Anatomic Points

It is essential to mobilize the gastric fundus completely in order to produce a tension-free Nissen fundoplication. This entails meticulous division of the short gastric vessels (Fig. 42.2A), the gastrosplenic ligament, and the gastrophrenic ligament.

Retract the gastric fundus inferiorly and to the right. Begin dividing the short gastric vessels in the upper third of the greater curvature of the stomach and progress superiorly (Fig. 42.2B). The ultrasonic dissecting shears are ideal for this purpose. Confirm that sufficient fundus has been mobilized by pulling it anteriorly across to the right side.

Pass a Babcock forceps behind the esophagus and grasp the mobile portion of the fundus (Fig. 42.2C). Bring the posterior wall of the fundus behind the esophagus and around to the patient's right side. Suture this to the anterior wall of the fundus in such a manner as to wrap the distal esophagus and gastroesophageal junction (Fig. 42.2D). Use nonabsorbable interrupted sutures. Include a bite of the esophagus with one stitch at the level of the gastroesophageal junction, and a second stitch placed 0.5 to 1 cm above it. Take care to avoid the left vagus nerve. Complete the wrap with an additional stitch above, and one below, these sutures (Fig. 42.2E). Do not include the esophagus in these latter two sutures.

The completed suture line should face to the right (9-o'clock position) and include both vagus trunks. Some surgeons leave the right (posterior) vagal trunk outside the wrap, but this tends to restrict the size of the posterior window.

Use a 60-French bougie to size the wrap, and do not create a wrap longer than 2 cm. If the wrap is too tight or too long, dysphagia may result. Avoid tension on the wrap by completely mobilizing the fundus. Ensure that the wrap is not twisted and that the posterior lip of the wrap has not been rendered ischemic by a narrow posterior window.

Remove the bougie and place a nasogastric tube. Suture the trocar sites closed.

REFERENCES

1. McKernan JB, Champion JK. Minimally invasive antireflux surgery. *Am J Surg* 1998;175:271–276.
2. Peters JH, DeMeester TR, Crookes P, et al. The treatment of gastroesophageal reflux disease with laparoscopic Nissen fundoplication: prospective evaluation of 100 patients with "typical" symptoms. *Ann Surg* 1998;228:40–50. (Provides detailed description of patient selection, preoperative evaluation, surgical technique, and assessment of postoperative physiologic alterations.)
3. Peters JH, DeMeester TR. Gastroesophageal reflux and hiatal hernia. In: Zinner MJ, Schwartz SI, Ellis H, eds. *Maingot's abdominal operations.* 10th ed. New York: McGraw Hill, 1997;787–842.
4. Peters JH, Heimbucher J, Kauer WKH, et al. Clinical and physiologic comparison of laparoscopic and open Nissen. *J Am Coll Surg* 1995; 180:385–393.
5. Scott-Conner C, Cushieri A, Carter FJ. Diaphragm, hiatus, and esophagus. In: *Minimal access surgical anatomy.* Philadelphia: Lippincott Williams & Wilkins, 2000. (Provides extensive illustration and description of regional laparoscopic anatomy.)

CHAPTER 43

Laparoscopic Esophagomyotomy

Laparoscopic esophagomyotomy uses the magnification and precise dissection associated with minimally invasive surgery to divide the hypertrophied distal esophagus associated with esophageal achalasia. This operation has largely supplanted the older transthoracic Heller myotomy, which required a left thoracotomy. References at the end of this chapter give details of the transthoracic myotomy (now generally performed thoracoscopically), which is still useful when a long-segment myotomy must be performed. Because achalasia is generally limited to the distal esophagus, the exposure attained at laparoscopy is usually ample.

Addition of a partial fundoplication is optional. The technique described here brings the fundus of the stomach anteriorly, where it may serve as a buttress for the myotomy. It is particularly useful if inadvertent entry into the esophagus has been made and repaired.

Exposure of Distal Esophagus and Proximal Stomach (Fig. 43.1)

Technical Points

Set up the room as described for laparoscopic fundoplication (see Chapter 42). The trocar sites and initial exposure are identical. Confine dissection of the esophageal hiatus to the anterior and lateral aspects of the esophagus; unless a partial fundoplication is planned, it is not necessary to dissect behind the esophagus (Fig. 43.1A,B). Visually confirm the thickened, narrowed segment of esophagus and mobilize the esophagus into the abdomen until dilated proximal esophagus is seen.

Excise Belsey's fat pad with electrocautery or ultrasonic shears (Fig. 43.1C,D). This allows unimpeded access to the gastroesophageal junction.

Anatomic Points

This dissection is confined to the anterior and lateral esophagus, in contrast to laparoscopic Nissen fundoplication, in which a more extensive dissection includes creation of a window behind the esophagus. As for Nissen fundoplication, dissection proceeds by outlining the crura of the diaphragm. These crura combine to form a muscular tunnel 2 to 3 cm long through which the esophagus and vagus nerves pass into the abdomen. There is considerable variability in the manner in which the fibrous and muscular parts of the hiatus form a sling around the esophagus; in actuality, dissection of the anterior and lateral parts of the hiatus rarely is affected by these variants. The median arcuate ligament crosses over the aorta just cephalad to the origin of the celiac axis and is not generally seen.

The left inferior phrenic artery runs along the left crus of the diaphragm and may give rise to an aberrant branch passing across the distal esophagus. The right inferior phrenic artery passes behind the inferior vena cava and is generally not encountered.

The phrenoesophageal ligament, more of a membrane than a ligament, covers the anterior surface of the hiatus and distal esophagus. It consists of a condensation of endoabdominal fascia and must be divided to expose the esophagus. Exposing the muscular fibers of the hiatus at its margins will automatically involve division of this structure, allowing exposure of the esophagus.

Belsey's (subhiatal) fat pad covers the gastroesophageal junction and contains Belsey's artery, a minor transversely

LIST OF STRUCTURES

Diaphragm
   Crura, right and left
   Hiatus
   Median arcuate ligament
Esophagus
Stomach
Belsey's fat pad
   Artery of Belsey
Phrenoesophageal membrane

Liver
   Segment I—caudate lobe
   Left lobe
      Segments II and III
   Coronary ligaments
   Left triangular ligament
   Ligamentum teres hepatis
      Falciform ligament
   Subphrenic space

Greater omentum
Lesser omentum
Colon
Pericardium
Phrenic nerves
Inferior phrenic artery and vein
Left gastric artery
Left and right vagus nerve

FIGURE 43.1
EXPOSURE OF DISTAL ESOPHAGUS AND PROXIMAL STOMACH (**A** and **B** from Wind GG. The stomach. In: *The applied laparoscopic anatomy: abdomen and pelvis.* Baltimore: Williams & Wilkins 1997, with permission; **C** and **D** from Pellegrini CA, Eubanks TR. Minimally invasive treatment of achalasia and other esophageal dysmotility. In: Baker, Fischer, eds. *Mastery of surgery.* 4th ed. Philadelphia: Lippincott Williams & Wilkins, 2001:803–812, with permission.)

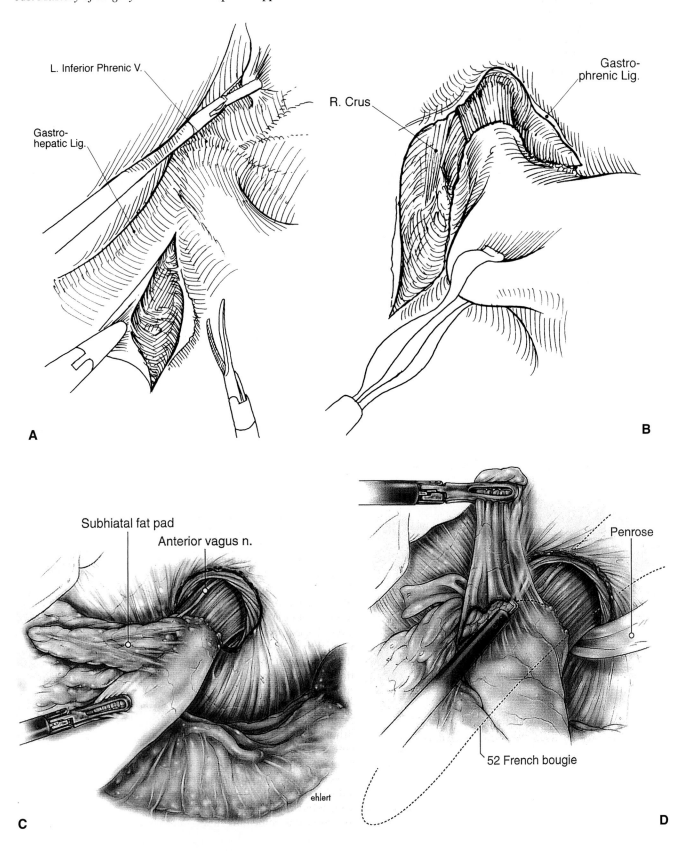

FIGURE 43.2
PERFORMANCE OF MYOTOMY (A, C, and **D** from Pellegrini CA, Eubanks TR. Minimally invasive treatment of achalasia and other esophageal dysmotility. In: Baker, Fischer, eds. *Mastery of surgery.* 4th ed. Philadelphia: Lippincott Williams & Wilkins, 2001:803–812, with permission; **B** from Scott-Conner C, Cushieri A, Carter FJ. Diaphragm, hiatus, and esophagus. In: *Minimal access surgical anatomy.* Philadelphia: Lippincott Williams & Wilkins, 2000, with permission.)

FIGURE 43.2   (Continued)

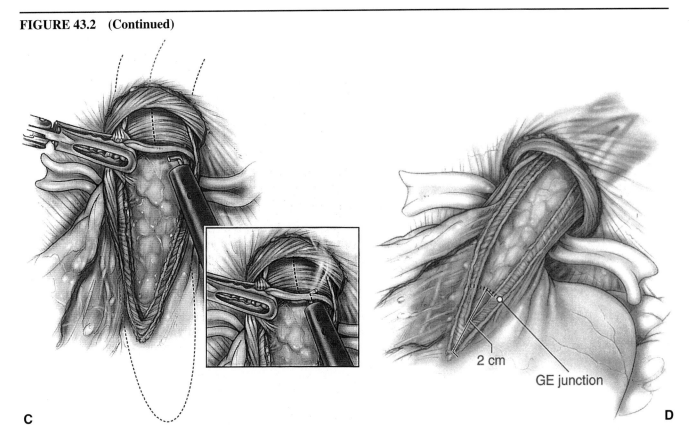

C   D

oriented collateral channel between the left gastric and left inferior phrenic arteries.

Performance of Myotomy (Fig. 43.2)

Technical Points

Begin the myotomy at a convenient point in the middle of the thickened, narrow segment of distal esophagus, taking care to avoid the vagus nerve. Using hook cautery to progress distally and laparoscopic scissors to progress proximally, create a line of incision on the anterior surface of the esophagus in a direction parallel to the longitudinal fibers. Placement of a Bougie in the esophagus may facilitate subsequent dissection by elevating and splaying out the layers of the esophagus and ensuring complete division. Use an atraumatic grasper to grasp the longitudinal fibers gently on each side of the myotomy and pull out and down (Fig. 43.2A).

Divide the thickened circular muscle in a similar fashion until the mucosal tube is seen (Fig. 43.2B). This is easily identified by its white color. Continue the myotomy proximal and distal until an ample myotomy has been created (Fig. 43.2C). This will generally require dissection 1.5 to 2 cm down on the stomach and extension proximal until the muscle layers thin out (Fig. 43.2D). If the myotomy extends too far down on the stomach, gastroesophageal reflux is more likely. There does not appear to be any adverse consequence if the myotomy extends too far proximally. If the myotomy is incomplete, relief of symptoms is likely to be inadequate. Confirm adequacy of the myotomy by passing an esophagogastroduodenoscope down and directly inspecting the distal esophagus.

Absence of blood confirms absence of gross injury, and the gastroesophageal junction should appear patulous. Pass the scope with great caution to avoid perforation. Do not shine the laparoscope at the distal esophagus during this maneuver because light from the laparoscope, transmitted through the thin esophageal mucosa, will complicate viewing from above.

Next, confirm absence of injury by insufflating air into the distal esophagus while observing under saline in the abdomen. Methylene blue may be of assistance in identifying small injuries. Repair any injury and perform a partial fundoplication (see later) to provide additional security. Do not hesitate to convert the procedure to an open operation if this appears to be the best way to manage an injury.

Irrigate the abdomen, ensure hemostasis, and close the trocar sites in the usual manner.

Anatomic Points

The esophagus is not covered by peritoneum. The outer layer consists of longitudinal muscle and rarely exceeds a millimeter in thickness at the distal esophagus. The distal esophageal sphincter is a physiologic rather than an anatomic structure, and normally there is no distinct thickening to the distal esophagus. The circular muscle layer in the normal esophagus is similarly generally about 1 mm. This layer is considerably thickened in achalasia. Beneath the circular muscle lies a submucosal layer containing a well-developed plexus of veins. The epithelial tube (squamous mucosa) is white and easily identified by three characteristics:

1. The white color, which contrasts with the pink-red of the muscle layers

FIGURE 43.3
OPTIONAL PARTIAL FUNDOPLICATION (**A–C** from Pellegrini CA, Eubanks TR. Minimally invasive treatment of achalasia and other esophageal dysmotility. In: Baker, Fischer, eds. *Mastery of surgery.* 4th ed. Philadelphia: Lippincott Williams & Wilkins, 2001:803–812, with permission.)

A   B

C

2. The tendency to "pout out" once the constricting circular muscle fibers are released
3. The overlying submucosal plexus of small veins

The vagus nerves coalesce into an anterior and a posterior trunk in the vicinity of the hiatus in most individuals. The anterior vagus nerve may be visible on the surface of the esophagus as a white band with a small vessel running on it; if seen, it is easily avoided. The posterior vagus is generally not seen and is not at risk.

Optional Partial Fundoplication (Fig. 43.3)

Technical and Anatomic Points

Proponents of this procedure believe that the partial fundoplication helps keep the muscle layers apart during healing, lessening the chances of recurrence. It also may provide some protection against gastroesophageal reflux. In addition, this form of fundoplication is useful as a buttress when an injury has been repaired. Minimal mobilization of the stomach is required, and it may be necessary to divide some short gastric vessels.

Ensure that the esophagus is circumferentially mobilized and that an adequate posterior window has been created. Divide short gastric vessels if necessary to generate sufficient mobility of the fundus (see Chapter 42). Pull the fundus of the stomach behind the esophagus and suture the fundus to the edges of the myotomy, rather than to each other (Fig. 43.3A). This provides a partial wrap and helps hold the edges of the myotomy apart. Take care during suturing not to lacerate the delicate epithelial layer (Fig. 43.3B).

Next, roll the floppy region of the anterior fundus over the myotomy and suture it to the right side of the wrap with several interrupted sutures (Fig. 43.3C). Do not place sutures in the epithelial tube—it is fragile and prone to laceration. Rather, suture the stomach to the muscular walls of the esophagus.

REFERENCES

1. Anselmino M, Perdikis G, Hinder RA, et al. Heller myotomy is superior to dilatation for the treatment of early achalasia. *Arch Surg* 1997; 132:233–240.
2. Oddsdottir M. Laparoscopic cardiomyotomy (Heller myotomy). In: Scott-Conner CEH, ed. *The SAGES manual:* Fundamentals of laparoscopy and GI endoscopy. New York: Springer-Verlag, 1999:213–220.
3. Patti MG, Pellegrini CA, Horgan S. et al. Minimally invasive surgery for achalasia: an 8-year experience with 168 patients. *Ann Surg* 1999;230: 587–594. (Compares thoracoscopic and laparoscopic approach, with notes on technique.)
4. Pellegrini CA, Eubanks TR. Minimally invasive treatment of achalasia and other esophageal dysmotility. In: Baker, Fischer, eds. *Mastery of surgery.* 4th ed. Philadelphia: Lippincott Williams & Wilkins, 2001: 803–812. (Presents excellent review of pathophysiology and surgical management.)
5. Rosati R, Fumagalli U, Bonavina L, et al. Laparoscopic approach to esophageal achalasia. *Am J Surg* 1995;169:424–427. (Describes use of dilated balloon to facilitate myotomy, with clear illustration of Dor fundoplication.)
6. Vogt D, Curet M, Pitcher D, et al. Successful treatment of esophageal achalasia with laparoscopic Heller myotomy and Toupet fundoplication. *Am J Surg* 1997;174:709–714. (Discusses use of Toupet fundoplication.)

CHAPTER 44

Gastrostomy and Jejunostomy

Gastrostomy may be performed for feeding or for decompression. The simplest open technique for creation of a gastrostomy is the Stamm procedure. Percutaneous endoscopic gastrostomy, an alternative to open gastrostomy, is briefly discussed in this chapter also. Laparoscopic gastrostomy is described in Chapter 45, and other techniques are included in the references.

Jejunostomy is sometimes preferred over gastrostomy in patients in whom free gastroesophageal reflux, mental obtundation, or abnormal upper gastrointestinal motility makes aspiration of gastric feedings likely. It has been difficult to prove conclusively any advantage for this procedure over gastrostomy.

Gastrostomy

The Incision (Fig. 44.1)

Technical and Anatomic Points

The patient is positioned supine, and an upper midline, short upper left paramedian, or left transverse incision is used. The choice of incision depends on the patient's body habitus. If an old midline scar is present, a left transverse incision provides good access through a space that is often free of adhesions.

General anesthesia is preferred; however, in the cachectic, weakened patient, local anesthesia may be safer. If the procedure is to be performed using local anesthesia, use a midline incision because it requires minimal muscle manipulation. Infiltrate the skin and subcutaneous tissues with local anesthesia. As dissection progresses, inject additional local anesthesia just under the fascia to numb the peritoneum.

Choice of Site on Stomach Wall and Placement of Sutures (Fig. 44.2)

Technical Points

Identify the stomach with certainty by observing its thick muscular wall, absence of haustral folds and taeniae, and the vessels entering on the greater and lesser curvature. Grasp the stomach with a Babcock clamp and pull it into the wound. Choose a site well proximal to the pylorus, on a mobile, accessible part of the anterior wall.

Place two concentric pursestring sutures of 2-0 silk, leaving the needles on. Begin and end one pursestring suture at the cephalad end of the incision and the other suture at the caudad end.

Anatomic Points

Remember the disposition of major organs in the upper abdomen, their attachments, and how to distinguish one from the other. On a surface projection, the stomach is located in the left hypochondriac and epigastric regions, with the pylorus just to the right of the vertebral column. The lesser curvature and adjacent part of the stomach lie deep to the left lobe of the liver. The body of the stomach lies just deep to the parietal peritoneum of the anterior body wall. The free edge of the left lobe of the liver typically lies about halfway between the umbilicus and the xiphoid in the midline and then angles upward and to the left to pass behind the eighth costal cartilage. The greater omentum is attached to the greater curvature of the stomach. It normally is draped over the transverse colon and the numerous loops of small intestine.

The transverse colon is attached to the greater curvature of the stomach by the gastrocolic ligament (developmentally, the anterior "root" of the great omentum) and to the posterior body wall by the transverse mesocolon. It can lie anywhere in the upper abdomen, depending on the degree of redundancy of this organ and the lengths of its peritoneal attachments. Although it is classically described to be immediately inferior to the stomach and superior to the small intestine, it may be interposed between stomach and body wall, or conversely, it may sag inferiorly into the pelvis. To visualize small bowel,

LIST OF STRUCTURES

Stomach	Duodenum	Liver
Fundus	Ligament of Treitz	Left lobe
Antrum	Jejunum	Greater omentum
Pylorus	Ileum	Transverse colon
Lesser curvature	Ileocecal junction	Gastrocolic ligament
Greater curvature		

FIGURE 44.1
THE INCISION

FIGURE 44.2
CHOICE OF SITE ON STOMACH WALL AND PLACEMENT OF SUTURES

Haustra

Taenia coli

Transverse colon

FIGURE 44.3
PLACEMENT OF TUBE

the greater omentum and often the transverse colon and transverse mesocolon must be reflected cranially.

Through the porthole of this small laparotomy incision, large bowel can be differentiated from other viscera by the presence of haustra, taenia coli, and fatty epiploic appendages. Small bowel can be differentiated from stomach by its narrow diameter, and from large bowel by the lack of the characteristics of large bowel just mentioned.

Unlike the colon, stomach lacks haustra and taeniae. Although the stomach is highly distensible and somewhat mobile, it should be remembered that it is attached along its lesser curvature to the liver by the hepatogastric ligament, along its greater curvature to the transverse colon by the gastrocolic ligament, to the esophagus proximally, and to the retroperi-

toneal duodenum distally. Because there are neurovascular structures in the ligaments and visceral continuity proximally and distally, care should be taken when delivering the anterior wall of the stomach into the wound to ensure that it is just the distensible anterior wall and that undue traction is not placed on the viscus wall or on accompanying neurovascular structures.

Placement of Tube (Fig. 44.3)

Technical and Anatomic Points

A large Malecot or mushroom catheter can be used. The holes in the catheter can be enlarged if desired. Choose an exit site for the catheter on the anterior abdominal wall and make

FIGURE 44.4
THE PULL TECHNIQUE

FIGURE 44.4 (Continued)

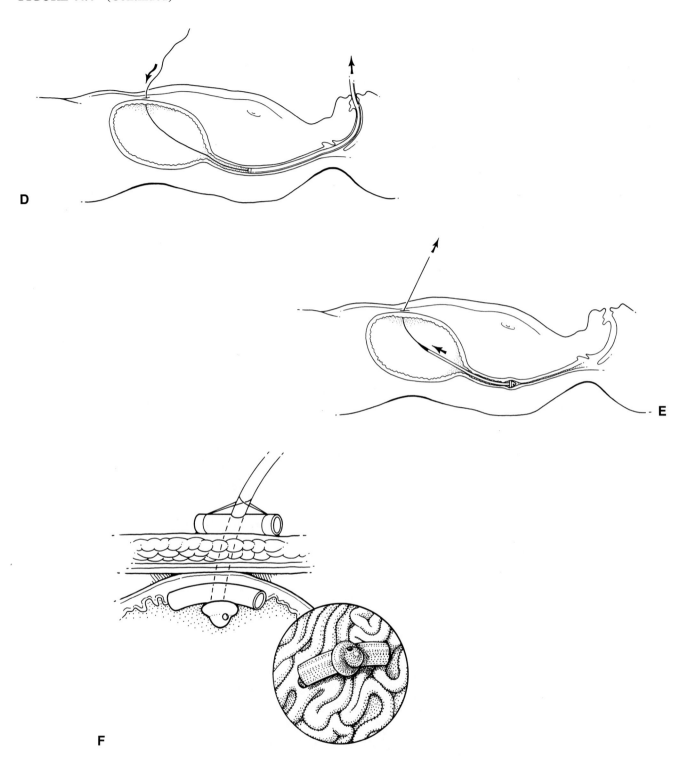

D

E

F

a small skin incision. Deepen the hole by poking a clamp through the abdominal wall. If local anesthesia is being used, remember to anesthetize this site also.

Pass the catheter through the abdominal wall. With electro-cautery, open the stomach in the center of the two pursestring sutures and enlarge the hole thus made with a hemostat.

Stretch and straighten the bulbous end of the catheter over a

Kelly clamp and push it into the hole. Confirm proper placement within the gastric lumen by irrigating and aspirating saline freely.

Tie the inner pursestring as an assistant dunks the hole in. Then tie the outer pursestring. Do not cut the needles off; these two sutures will be used to anchor the gastrostomy site to the undersurface of the anterior abdominal wall. Properly placed and tied, these two sutures should "inkwell" the stomach over the tube.

Place retractors to visualize the site where the catheter enters the peritoneal cavity. Place a 2-0 silk suture to approximate the far side of the stomach to the underside of the anterior abdominal wall beyond the catheter.

Then use the "top" and "bottom" pursestring sutures to tack the stomach above and below. Finally, place a suture anterior to the catheter entrance site and tie all sutures. Omentum, if available, can be packed around the gastrostomy and the incision can then be closed.

Percutaneous Endoscopic Gastrostomy

The Pull Technique (Fig. 44.4)

Technical and Anatomic Points

Percutaneous endoscopic gastrostomy (PEG) capitalizes on the fact that the distended stomach lies immediately under the anterior abdominal wall, displacing colon inferiorly, where it can be directly cannulated. Topical anesthesia of the oropharynx and local anesthesia of the gastrostomy site are all that is required. Sedation may be helpful.

FIGURE 44.5
INCISION AND IDENTIFICATION OF THE JEJUNOSTOMY SITE

Jejunum

Ileum

An assistant is positioned at the head of the table outside of the sterile field to perform the upper gastrointestinal endoscopy. The upper gastrointestinal endoscope is introduced into the stomach and a brief but thorough endoscopic examination is performed. The stomach is fully inflated with air, and the overhead lights are turned off. The endoscopist visualizes a point on the anterior gastric wall about two thirds of the distance from the cardioesophageal junction to the pylorus. The light of the endoscope should be easily visible through the abdominal wall of the patient at a point midway between the umbilicus and the left lateral costal margin. Touch the point of maximum light intensity, indenting the skin and anterior abdominal wall repeatedly. The endoscopist should see the wall of the stomach move in direct correspondence. This ensures that the gastric wall is up against the anterior abdominal wall without interposed viscera.

Turn the overhead lights back on and infiltrate the point that has just been identified with local anesthesia. Then introduce the needle supplied with the PEG kit into the stomach with a firm, straight, slightly screwing motion. Entry into the stomach is usually accompanied by a faint rush of air from the needle. The endoscopist then visualizes and confirms position of the needle in the stomach.

Use a number 11 blade to enlarge the skin hole and fascial opening adjacent to the needle. Pass a stout monofilament suture, supplied with the PEG kit, down through the needle into the stomach. The endoscopist must then grasp the end of the suture with biopsy forceps or snare it with a polypectomy snare and pull endoscope and suture out through the patient's mouth. The PEG tube is then tied securely to the suture by the endoscopist. Pull the suture slowly and firmly back through the abdominal wall until the PEG tube emerges and is snug against the stomach.

The endoscopist should pass the scope and visualize the PEG tube to confirm that the mushroom of the PEG tube is up against the anterior gastric wall, snug but not so tight as to produce pressure necrosis of the stomach. The PEG tube should be well secured in place because premature dislodgment (before a tract has formed) causes leakage of gastric juice and feedings into the peritoneal cavity and is often fatal.

Feeding Jejunostomy

The standard technique for creation of a Witzel jejunostomy is described here, followed by a derivation of the technique known as needle catheter jejunostomy.

Incision and Identification of the Jejunostomy Site (Fig. 44.5)

Technical Points

A feeding jejunostomy is frequently performed as an adjunct to complicated upper gastrointestinal surgery. When done as an isolated procedure, a midline or left paramedian incision may be used. The incision must be long enough to identify proximal jejunum with certainty by palpation of the ligament of Treitz. General anesthesia is usually required, although in exceptional circumstances, the procedure can be performed using local anesthesia.

Find the small bowel in the left upper quadrant by displacing the colon and omentum cephalad. Follow the small bowel up to the ligament of Treitz and identify a mobile segment of proximal jejunum, generally 40 to 60 cm from the ligament of Treitz.

Choose a site on the anterior abdominal wall that can easily and comfortably be reached by the jejunum without kinking,

FIGURE 44.6
CREATING A WITZEL TUNNEL AND ANCHORING THE JEJUNOSTOMY

FIGURE 44.7
NEEDLE CATHETER JEJUNOSTOMY

and pass a red rubber catheter or Broviac-type catheter through from the skin surface. Elevate the jejunal loop with a pair of Babcock clamps and place a single pursestring suture of 3-0 silk on the antimesenteric border at the point selected. Open the jejunum and introduce the catheter, taking care to pass it distally, in the direction of normal peristalsis. Confirm intraluminal passage rather than dissection in the submucosal plane by free injection and aspiration of air into the lumen of the jejunum. Tie the pursestring suture, leaving the needle in place.

Anatomic Points

Not only do physiologic functions of the small bowel differ in different locations along its length, but the anatomy changes as well. The diameter of the small bowel is largest at the ligament of Treitz and gradually tapers distally, so that it is narrowest at the ileocecal junction. The mesenteric attachment of the small bowel runs along a diagonal line from the ligament of Treitz (in the left upper quadrant) to the ileocecal junction (in the right lower quadrant). The feeding tube needs to be placed as far proximal as possible. This will ensure the maximum length of bowel downstream for absorption of nutrients. Fortuitously, it also allows placement of the tube at the point in the bowel that is of greatest caliber.

Creating a Witzel Tunnel and Anchoring the Jejunostomy (Fig. 44.6)

Technical and Anatomic Points

Construct a Witzel tunnel by placing multiple interrupted Lembert sutures in such a way as to pull the sides of the small bowel over and across the catheter, burying it from view. Tie these, leaving the needles on. Place several sutures past the entrance point of the catheter into the bowel. Take care that these sutures, tied over the catheter, do not unduly restrict the lumen of the jejunum.

Suture the jejunostomy to the underside of the abdominal wall by tacking the Witzel sutures sequentially. Place the sutures in the anterior abdominal wall in such a way that the bowel lies naturally and is not kinked. Anchor the bowel for 1.5 to 2 cm to minimize the risk for volvulus around a point.

Needle Catheter Jejunostomy (Fig. 44.7)

Technical and Anatomic Points

This rapidly performed technique is a useful adjunct to complicated upper gastrointestinal surgery when temporary nutritional support is required. Because the catheter is small (5 French), only elemental diets can be used. It is not a useful technique when prolonged nutritional support is likely to be needed.

Identify a loop of jejunum and place a pursestring suture (Fig. 44.5). Use the needle supplied with the catheter to pass the catheter through the abdominal wall, "floppy" guidewire first.

Take the second needle and pierce the seromuscular layers of the intestine in the center of the pursestring suture, passing the needle with its bevel down to decrease the risk for penetrating the lumen. Tunnel the needle for 2 to 3 cm in the submucosal plane, then pop it through into the lumen, first turning its bevel up.

Pass the catheter and guidewire through the needle into the lumen. Use the guidewire to facilitate passage of the tube into the small intestine and thread it 20 or 30 cm downstream.

Remove the guidewire and confirm intraluminal placement by injecting air. Suture the jejunum to the underside of the abdominal wall in several places to avoid volvulus. Secure the catheter to the skin using the device supplied by the manufacturer.

REFERENCES

1. Bergstrom LR, Larson DE, Zinsmeister AR, et al. Utilization and outcomes of surgical gastrostomies and jejunostomies in an era of percutaneous endoscopic gastrostomy: a population-based study. *Mayo Clin Proc* 1995;70:829–836.
2. Bradley RL. Feeding gastrostomy: a simplified technic. *Am J Surg* 1964;108:743. (Describes straightforward technique for Stamm gastrostomy performed with local anesthesia.)
3. Cohen OM, Donner Y, Berlatzky Y. Skin level permanent feeding gastrostomy. *Am J Surg* 1981;141:391.
4. Cosentini EP, Sautner T, Gnant M, et al. Outcomes of surgical, percutaneous endoscopic, and percutaneous radiologic gastrostomies. *Arch Surg* 1998;133:1076–1083.
5. Gauderer MW. Gastrostomy techniques and devices. *Surg Clin North Am* 1992;72:1285–1298. (Presents an excellent review.)
6. Heberer M, Bodoky A, Iwatschenko P, et al. Indications for needle catheter jejunostomy in elective abdominal surgery. *Am J Surg* 1987;153:545.
7. Joehl RJ. Gastrostomy. In: Ritchie WP Jr, ed. *Shackelford's surgery of the alimentary tract.* 3rd ed. Philadelphia: WB Saunders, 1991;121. (Provides good description of Janeway gastrostomy and other techniques for creating permanent, mucosa-lined tubes.)
8. McSherry CK. Interventional endoscopy. *Curr Probl Surg* 1985;22:1.
9. Ponsky JL, Gauderer MWL. Percutaneous endoscopic gastrostomy: indications, limitations, techniques, and results. *World J Surg* 1989; 13:165.
10. Ponsky JL, Gauderer MWL, Stellato TA, et al. Percutaneous approaches to enteral alimentation. *Am J Surg* 1985;149:102.
11. Preshaw RM. A percutaneous method for inserting a feeding gastrostomy tube. *Surg Gynecol Obstet* 1981;152:659.
12. Steichen FM, Ravitch MM. Stapling in surgery. Chicago: Year Book Medical Publishers, 1984:95. (Shows Janeway gastrostomy construction with GIA stapler.)
13. Zickler RW, Barbagiovanni JT, Swan KG. A simplified open gastrostomy under local anesthesia. *Am Surg* 2001;67:806–808.

CHAPTER 45

Laparoscopic Gastrostomy and Jejunostomy

These procedures are useful either as incidental procedures during other laparoscopic operations (eg, gastrostomy performed in association with laparoscopic repair of paraesophageal hernia) or when other methods of access fail. The stapled Janeway gastrostomy, shown here, can also be done as an open procedure when a permanent gastrostomy is desired. The mucosa-lined tube that is formed will remain patent without a catheter, and can be covered with a simple dressing when not in use.

Laparoscopic Simple Gastrostomy (Fig. 45.1)

Technical and Anatomic Points

Obtain access through an infraumbilical incision. Identify the stomach. Place a second trocar through a right upper quadrant site (Fig. 45.1A) and insert an atraumatic grasper. Grasp the stomach and manipulate it until a suitable site high on the fundus is located. Confirm that it will pass easily to the underside of the anterior abdominal wall at the chosen location.

Make an about 1-cm skin incision at the proposed site. Through the skin incision, insert a 14-gauge needle. Under direct visualization, puncture the stomach with the needle at the chosen location. Use the grasper to stabilize the stomach, facilitating puncture. Confirm that the needle is in the stomach by injecting and aspirating air or saline. Pass a guidewire into the stomach. Using a Seldinger technique, follow the guidewire with a dilator and finally a sheath through which an 18-French gastrostomy tube (commonly called a Foley catheter) can be inserted into the stomach. Withdraw the sheath and inflate the balloon. Snug the gastric wall up against the anterior abdominal wall by pulling back on the tube gently. It may be necessary to release some pneumoperitoneum to bring the anterior abdominal wall into closer apposition to the stomach.

LIST OF STRUCTURES

Stomach
Pylorus
Ligament of Treitz
Jejunum

T fasteners (shown, Fig. 45.1B) are a simple method to secure the stomach to the anterior abdominal wall. Place these by passing a needle through the anterior abdominal wall and stomach. Insert the closed T fastener through the needle and snug it up. Alternatively, use a couple of simple sutures of 3-0 silk to tack the stomach to the anterior abdominal wall. Either method helps minimize the chance of leakage and increases the safety of the procedure by giving additional assurance that the stomach will be maintained in close apposition to the anterior abdominal wall during the healing phase.

Pull omentum up into the upper abdomen to surround the area. Close the trocar sites.

Place the gastrostomy tube on straight drainage.

Laparoscopic Janeway Gastrostomy (Fig. 45.2)

Technical and Anatomic Points

Obtain access and visualize the stomach as previously described. Place a 12-mm trocar through the right upper quadrant and identify a suitable region of stomach with an atraumatic grasper. Identify the optimum location for the gastrostomy and make a skin incision. Place a 10-mm trocar through this site and elevate the chosen region of stomach with an endoscopic Babcock clamp.

Pass an endoscopic cutting linear stapler through the right upper quadrant port and use it to staple and divide a tongue of stomach (Fig. 45.2A) long enough to pass through the abdominal wall. Note that the tongue must be wide enough to accommodate a gastrostomy tube; therefore, place the stapler about 1 cm from the edge of the stomach. It may be necessary to fire the stapler more than once to obtain sufficient length.

Grasp the tip of the tongue of stomach with the endoscopic Babcock forceps and draw it up through the anterior abdominal wall, withdrawing the trocar as you do so. The stomach should be pulled comfortably against the anterior abdominal wall, without excessive tension. Be especially careful to avoid excessive tension on the crotch of the staple line, which may lead to leakage. If the tongue of stomach is not long enough to reach the skin without tension, return it to the abdomen, reinsert the trocar, and fire the stapler again to lengthen it.

Open the tongue of stomach and mature it to the skin with multiple interrupted sutures of 4-0 Vicryl or PDS (Fig. 45.2B).

FIGURE 45.1
LAPAROSCOPIC SIMPLE GASTROSTOMY

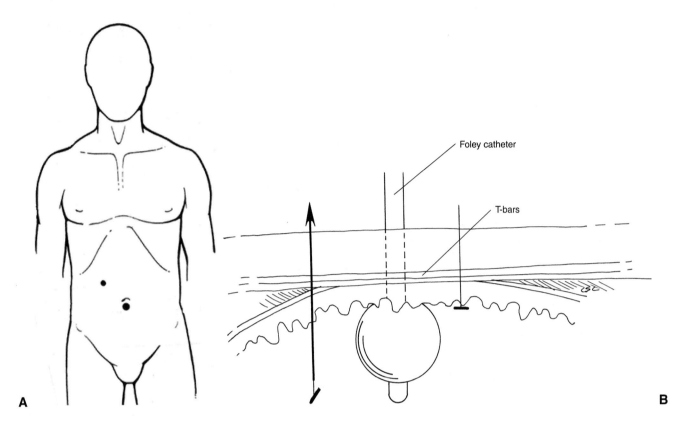

FIGURE 45.2
LAPAROSCOPIC JANEWAY GASTROSTOMY (**A** from Gadacz T. Laparoscopic gastrostomy.
In: Scott-Conner, CEH, ed. *The SAGES manual.* New York: Springer-Verlag, 1999:227–232, with permission.)

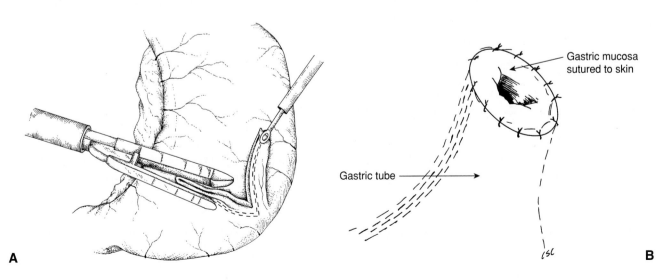

FIGURE 45.3

LAPAROSCOPIC JEJUNOSTOMY (B from Schirmer BD. Placement of jejunostomy tube. In: Scott-Conner, CEH, ed. *The SAGES manual.* New York: Springer-Verlag, 1999:267–274, with permission.)

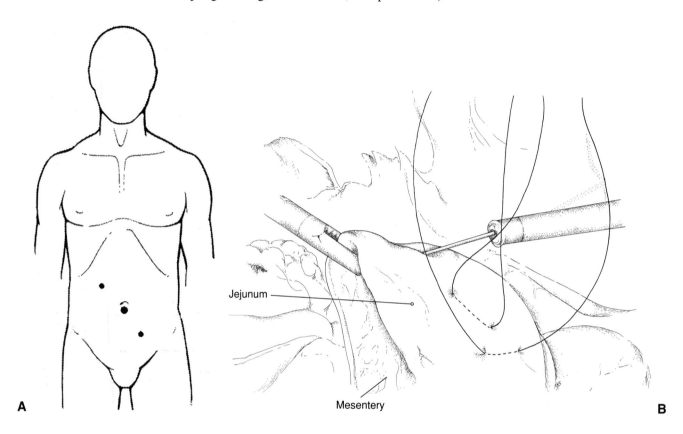

Laparoscopic Jejunostomy (Fig. 45.3)

Technical and Anatomic Points

Pass the laparoscope through an infraumbilical site and place additional trocars in the right upper quadrant and left lower quadrant (Fig. 45.3A). Select a loop of jejunum that is close to the ligament of Treitz yet sufficiently mobile to reach to the anterior abdominal wall at the tube site (usually left upper quadrant).

Place four quadrant sutures through the abdominal wall, arranged in a square around the tube site. These may be placed through small stab wounds using a straight (Keith) needle. First pass the Keith needle through the fascia, using the stab wound as a skin entry site. Grasp the Keith needle within the abdomen with a laparoscopic needle holder and take a seromuscular bite of jejunum. Then pass the Keith needle back through the abdominal wall, exiting the stab wound if possible (Fig. 45.3B).

Next use the needle from a needle-catheter jejunostomy kit to pierce the planned tube entry site, which is the center of the square formed by the four sutures on the anterior abdominal wall. Under laparoscopic guidance, pass this needle into the center of the square of sutures on the jejunum. Tunnel the needle through the bowel wall, if possible, and then pass it into the lumen. Dilate the tract and insert the catheter in the usual fashion (see Fig. 44.7 in Chapter 44).

Confirm passage into the lumen of the gut by free injection of saline and aspiration of bilious material. If there is any question about the position of the catheter, introduce water-soluble contrast material under fluoroscopy. Tie the four sutures.

Confirm that the loop of jejunum is not twisted but lies comfortably against the underside of the anterior abdominal wall. Place several additional sutures along the length of the jejunum to avoid potential torsion around a single fixed point. Secure the catheter, desufflate the abdomen, and close the trocar sites.

REFERENCES

1. Arnaud J-P, Casa C, Manunta A. Laparoscopic continent gastrostomy. *Am J Surg* 1995;169:629–630.
2. Duh QY, Senokozlieff-Englehart AL, Choe YS, et al. Laparoscopic

gastrostomy and jejunostomy: safety and cost with local vs general anesthesia. *Arch Surg* 1999;134:151–156. (Discusses use of local anesthesia for these procedures.)

3. Duh QY, Senokozlieff-Englehart AL, Siperstein AE, et al. Prospective evaluation of the safety and efficacy of laparoscopic jejunostomy. *West J Med* 1995;162:117–122.

4. Edelman DS, Unger SW. Laparoscopic gastrostomy. *Surg Gynecol Obstet* 173:401;1991.

5. Gadacz T. Laparoscopic gastrostomy. In: Scott-Conner, CEH, ed. *The SAGES manual.* New York: Springer-Verlag, 1999:227–232.

6. Murayama KM, Johnson TJ, Thompson JS. Laparoscopic gastrostomy and jejunostomy are safe and effective for obtaining enteral access. *Am J Surg* 1996;172:591–594.

7. Molloy M, Ose KJ, Bower RH. Laparoscopic Janeway gastrostomy: an alternative to celiotomy for the management of dislodged percutaneous gastrostomy. *J Am Coll Surg* 1997;185:187–189.

8. Schirmer BD. Placement of jejunostomy tube. In: Scott-Conner, CEH, ed. *The SAGES manual.* New York: Springer-Verlag, 1999:267–274.

CHAPTER 46

Plication of Perforated Duodenal Ulcer

Small anterior perforations of duodenal ulcers are treated by Graham patch plication, which may sometimes be performed laparoscopically (see Chapter 47). Larger perforations may require excision and closure by pyloroplasty or gastric resection for control.

In this chapter, the anatomy of the subhepatic space and its contents is introduced. The subphrenic spaces, frequent sites of associated abscess formation, are also demonstrated.

Identification of Perforation Site (Fig. 46.1)

Technical Points

Enter the abdomen through an upper midline or right paramedian incision (Fig. 46.1A) and thoroughly explore the abdomen. Culture the peritoneal fluid and remove as much contamination as possible by irrigation and suction. Place a Harrington retractor on the liver, lift it up, and expose the

LIST OF STRUCTURES

Liver
   Coronary ligament
   Triangular ligaments
   Falciform ligament
      Ligamentum teres
Left and right subphrenic spaces
Subhepatic space
Lesser sac
Duodenum
Greater omentum
Gastroepiploic vessels

FIGURE 46.1
IDENTIFICATION OF PERFORATION SITE

300

subhepatic space by applying gentle downward traction on the stomach and duodenum (Fig. 46.1B). Frequently, the left lobe of the liver will have "sealed" the perforation, which is typically located at the pylorus or first portion of the duodenum. This seal must be gently broken to expose the perforation. A flow of clear bile into the field usually results.

Anatomic Points

Topographically, the liver divides the upper abdominal region from the diaphragm superiorly to the transverse colon and mesocolon inferiorly into the smaller subphrenic space and subhepatic spaces. Each of these smaller spaces can be further subdivided, by peritoneal folds and reflections, into three spaces, each of which has clinical importance because abscesses can form in any of them. Immediately superior to the liver and anterior to the anterior layer of the coronary and triangular ligaments, the falciform ligament, with

its contained ligamentum teres, divides that space into a *left superior space* and a *right subphrenic space*. The *right subphrenic space* is limited by the anterior layer of the coronary ligament, the diaphragmatic surface of the liver, and the body wall.

The inferior aspect of the liver is divided by the ligamentum teres of the liver and the ligamentum venosum and associated mesenteric folds into a right and left side. To the right of these structures is a large *right subhepatic space*, bounded by the liver, transverse mesocolon and colon, and ligamentum teres. On the left side, a similar space lies between the liver and the anterior surface of the stomach and lesser omentum. The lesser sac *(lesser omental bursa)* is bounded superiorly by liver, anteriorly by stomach and lesser omentum, and posteriorly by parietal peritoneum over the parietes and structures in the retroperitoneal space. It is in this latter space that perigastric abscesses are most likely to form following perforation of a peptic ulcer. If the perforation

FIGURE 46.2
PLACEMENT OF SUTURES

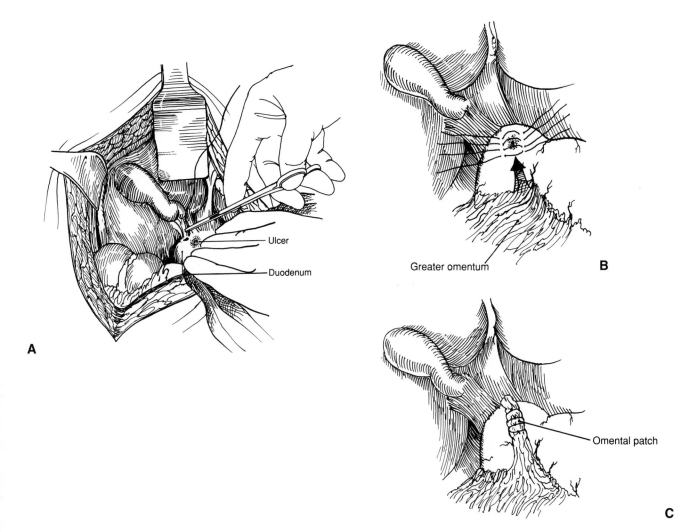

is through the anterior stomach or duodenum, abscess formation can occur in either or both of the other two subphrenic spaces.

Placement of Sutures (Fig. 46.2)

Technical Points

Typically, bile will flow continuously into the field from the perforation. Have an assistant maintain a clear field by suctioning the area. Select an appropriate piece of omentum from the free edge, mobilizing it if necessary to reach the site of perforation.

Place three or four interrupted 2-0 silk Lembert sutures across the perforation (Fig. 46.2A,B). Pass the tongue of the omentum under the silk sutures and tie the sutures over the omentum (Fig. 46.2C). Do not try to approximate the edges of the hole with the sutures because the tissue adjacent to the site of perforation is inflamed and edematous and the sutures may cut through.

If a highly selective vagotomy is to be performed, it may be done now. Recheck the patch after completing the highly selective vagotomy to ensure that the patch has not become dislodged during the course of the dissection.

Irrigate the abdomen again before closure and confirm that there is no leakage of bile from the patch. Place a closed-suction drain in the subhepatic space if a true abscess was found in association with the perforation.

Anatomic Points

The blood supply of the greater omentum is based on several rather long descending branches from the gastroepiploic arcade. Mobilization of a pedicle flap of omentum can be accomplished with little danger as long as continuity with the gastroepiploic arcade is maintained.

REFERENCES

1. Boyd DP. The subphrenic spaces and the emperor's new clothes. *N Engl J Med* 1966;275:911–917. (Provides classic description of spaces and techniques of surgical drainage.)
2. Donovan AJ, Berne TV, Donovan JA. Perforated duodenal ulcer: an alternative therapeutic plan. *Arch Surg* 1998;133:1166–1171. (Discusses role of therapy for *Helicobacter* species and other intensive medical therapy versus vagotomy.)
3. Graham RR. The treatment of perforated duodenal ulcers. *Surg Gynecol Obstet* 1937;64:235. (Presents original description of the technique that bears the author's name.)
4. Mouret P, Francois Y, Vignal J, et al. Laparoscopic treatment of perforated peptic ulcer. *Br J Surg* 1990;77:1006. (Presents clear description of a new technique.)
5. Ng EK, Lam YH, Sung JJ, et al. Eradication of *Helicobacter pylori* prevents recurrence of ulcer after simple closure of duodenal ulcer perforation: randomized controlled trial. *Ann Surg* 2000;231:153–158.
6. Sharma R, Organ CH Jr, Hirvela ER, et al. Clinical observation of the temporal association between crack cocaine and duodenal ulcer perforation. *Am J Surg* 1997;174:629–632.
7. Sirinek KR, Levine BA, Schwesinger WH, et al. Simple closure of perforated peptic ulcer. *Arch Surg* 1981;11:591.
8. Stabile BE. Redefining the role of surgery for perforated duodenal ulcer in the *Helicobacter pylori* era. *Ann Surg* 2000;231:159–160.
9. Svanes C, Lie RT, Svanes K, et al. Adverse effects of delayed treatment for perforated peptic ulcer. *Ann Surg* 1994;220:168–175.

CHAPTER 47

Laparoscopic Plication of Perforated Duodenal Ulcer

Laparoscopic plication is an easy way to manage a simple small anterior perforation of a duodenal ulcer.

Initial Exposure of the Right Upper Quadrant and Subhepatic Space (Fig. 47.1)

Technical Points

Set up the room as you would for laparoscopic cholecystectomy (see Fig. 57.1A in Chapter 57). Enter the abdomen through an infraumbilical puncture site and explore. Aspirate and irrigate all four quadrants of the abdomen. Frequently, the perforation is sealed by overlying liver. Leave this seal intact until you are finished irrigating and inspecting the rest of the abdomen. Be alert to the possibility of another etiology for the problem (eg, appendicitis, diverticulitis). If the appearance is consistent with a perforated duodenal ulcer, place secondary trocars as shown (Fig. 47.1A).

Gently elevate the liver to expose the perforation. An easy way to obtain initial exposure is to pass a grasper (closed) under the liver from the right lateral port and carefully lift up on liver and falciform ligament. Elevating the falciform ligament will lift the liver. Inspect the subhepatic space. Place a liver retractor to obtain a stable working field.

LIST OF STRUCTURES

Liver
    Falciform ligament
        Ligamentum teres
    Segment II
    Segment III
    Segment IV
Gallbladder
Left and right subphrenic spaces
Subhepatic space
Lesser sac
Duodenum
Prepyloric vein (of Mayo)
Greater omentum

Anatomic Points

The initial laparoscopic view of the left upper quadrant demonstrates the liver, falciform ligament, omentum, colon, and gallbladder (Fig. 47.1B). As the liver is elevated, stomach and duodenum come into view (Fig. 47.1C). The prepyloric vein of Mayo provides a convenient visual dividing point between stomach and duodenum. Branches of the supraduodenal artery are sometimes found in this region. As the laparoscope is brought closer, the manner in which gallbladder and segment IV of the liver overly the first and second portion of the duodenum becomes apparent (Fig. 47.1D).

The duodenum is conventionally divided into four parts. The first part of the duodenum extends from the pylorus to the point where the gallbladder overlies the duodenum. This is the portion that is easily accessible laparoscopically. Most simple anterior perforated duodenal ulcers are found in the first portion of the duodenum and are easily visualized when the liver is elevated. The second part of the duodenum extends from the gallbladder to approximately the right side of L3 or L4. It contains the ampulla of Vater. The third part of the duodenum runs from right to left, obliquely across to the left side of the aorta. The fourth part of the duodenum then ascends to the ligament of Treitz. To expose the duodenum fully, it is necessary to mobilize the right colon, as described in Chapter 66. A perforated duodenal ulcer that requires extensive mobilization is best managed by open surgery.

Gastric ulcers that perforate are frequently on the lesser curvature. Identify this situation by the location relative to the prepyloric vein. These are best managed by open surgery.

The relations of the various spaces of the upper abdomen, including the subhepatic space and lesser sac, are described in Chapter 46. Laparoscopic exposure of the lesser sac is described in Chapter 64.

Exposing the Perforation (Fig. 47.2)

Technical and Anatomic Points

Irrigate the anterior surface of the duodenum to expose the perforation (Fig. 47.2). Confirm that the entire circumference of the perforation is visualized by washing or picking away any fibrin debris from the edge. Be aware that, occasionally,

FIGURE 47.1
INITIAL EXPOSURE OF THE RIGHT UPPER QUADRANT AND SUBHEPATIC SPACE (B from Scott-Conner
CEH, Cushieri A, Carter FJ. Right upper quadrant: liver, gallbladder, and extrahepatic biliary tract. In: *Minimal access
surgical anatomy*. Philadelphia: Lippincott Williams & Wilkins, 2000:101–137, with permission; **C** from Scott-Conner CEH,
Cushieri A, Carter FJ. Stomach and duodenum. In: *Minimal access surgical anatomy*. Philadelphia: Lippincott Williams &
Wilkins, 2000:79–100, with permission.)

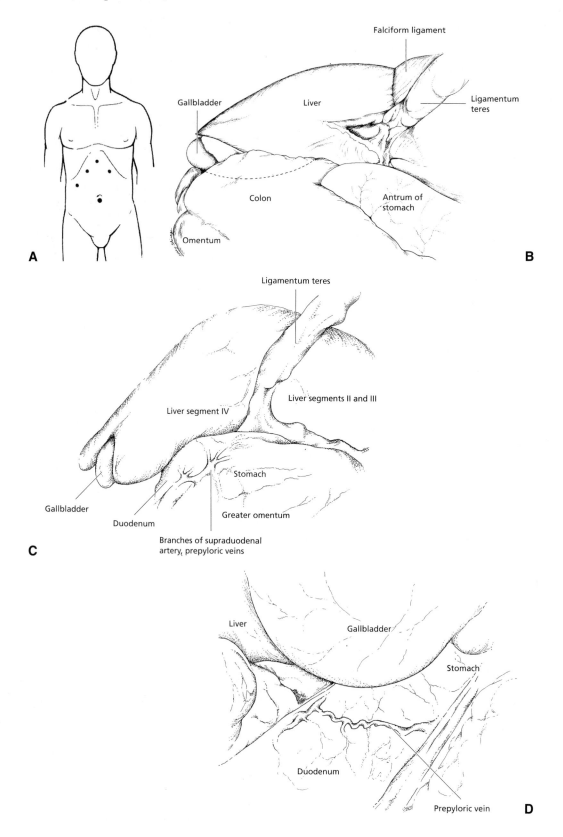

FIGURE 47.2

EXPOSING THE PERFORATION (From Thompson AR, Hall TJ, Anglin BA, et al. Laparoscopic plication of perforated ulcer: results of a selective approach. *South Med J* 1995;88:185–189, with permission.)

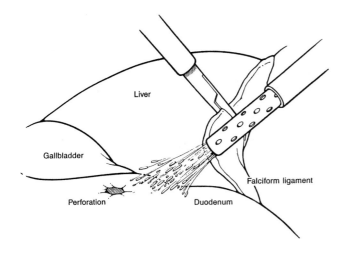

large perforations extend over the superior aspect of the duodenum into the retroperitoneum. In this situation, it is difficult to obtain secure closure. It is essential that the entire perforation be well visualized. Switch to a 30-degree angled laparoscope if necessary to view the anterior surface of the duodenum.

Omental Plication (Fig. 47.3)

Technical and Anatomic Points

Choose a mobile portion of omentum that reaches easily to the site of perforation. Generally, the omentum close to the ulcer will be inflamed and thickened; it is better to use omentum from the edge, distant from the perforation, because the texture is more pliable.

Suture Fixation of Patch

Suture the patch in place with three or four interrupted sutures of 2-0 or 3-0 silk, beginning with the apex (farthest from the scope) and progressing toward the scope (Fig. 47.3A). Place all the sutures first, then lay the omentum in place and tie the sutures.

Staple Fixation of Patch

A hernia stapler (not a helical tacker) can be used to secure the patch either as an adjunct to sutures or instead of sutures (Fig. 47.3B).

Completed Plication (Fig. 47.4)

Technical and Anatomic Points

Confirm adequacy of the patch by having the anesthesiologist instill air into the nasogastric tube while you watch for bubbles under saline. Reinforce the patch if necessary.

Irrigate and aspirate until returns are clear. Place a closed-suction drain in the subhepatic space and leave the nasogastric tube in place. Maintain nasogastric suction for 24 hours to allow the patch to seal.

FIGURE 47.3

OMENTAL PLICATION (**A** and **B** from Thompson AR, Hall TJ, Anglin BA, et al. Laparoscopic plication of perforated ulcer: results of a selective approach. *South Med J* 1995;88:185–189.)

A

B

FIGURE 47.4
COMPLETED PLICATION (From Gadacz TR. Laparoscopic plication of perforated ulcer. In: Scott-Conner CEH, ed. *The SAGES manual: fundamentals of laparoscopy and GI endoscopy.* New York: Springer-Verlag, 1999:233–235, with permission.)

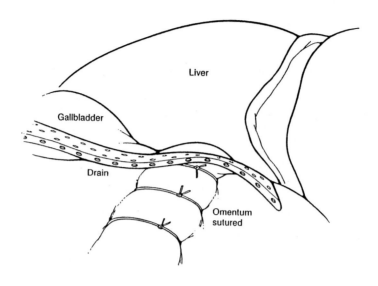

REFERENCES

1. Androulakis J, Colborn GL, Skandalakis PN, et al. Embryologic and anatomic basis of duodenal surgery. *Surg Clin North Am* 2000;80:171–199. (Provides excellent review of relevant anatomy.)
2. Gadacz TR. Laparoscopic plication of perforated ulcer. In: Scott-Conner CEH, ed. *The SAGES manual: fundamentals of laparoscopy and GI endoscopy.* New York: Springer-Verlag, 1999:233–235.
3. Mouret P, Francois Y, Vignal J, et al. Laparoscopic treatment of perforated peptic ulcer. *Br J Surg* 1990;77:1006. (Presents clear description of a new technique.)
4. Thompson AR, Hall TJ, Anglin BA, et al. Laparoscopic plication of perforated ulcer: results of a selective approach. *South Med J* 1995;88:185–189.
5. Scott-Conner CEH, Cushieri A, Carter FJ. Stomach and duodenum. In: *Minimal access surgical anatomy.* Philadelphia: Lippincott Williams & Wilkins, 2000:79–100. (Provides laparoscopic photographs and drawings illustrating regional anatomy.)

CHAPTER 48

Gastric Resection

Gastric resection, or gastrectomy, is performed mainly for treatment of gastric carcinoma. Benign ulcer disease, formerly a major indication, is now rarely treated by gastrectomy. Many modifications of the operation exist, differing in the extent of resection and the method of reconstruction of gastrointestinal continuity.

The extent of resection is determined by the pathology. An antrectomy (resection of the antrum of the stomach) is performed for peptic ulcer disease, usually with a concomitant truncal vagotomy. A subtotal gastrectomy involves resection of additional stomach and is generally quantitated according to the approximate amount removed (eg, a 60% gastrectomy). For radical subtotal gastrectomy, which is performed for carcinoma, resection of the omentum and regional lymph nodes is added. Total gastrectomy, also generally performed for carcinoma, entails removal of the entire stomach and the surrounding node-bearing tissue. The spleen is commonly also removed during operations for gastric cancer to resect regional lymph nodes in the splenic hilum.

The simplest method of reconstruction after partial gastrectomy is by direct anastomosis of the gastric remnant to the duodenum (Billroth I reconstruction). This creates what morphologically resembles a small stomach and is applicable when the gastric remnant and the duodenum can be brought together without tension. It is not used in operations for gastric carcinoma because the extent of resection generally precludes it and because recurrent disease can obstruct the new outlet.

The Billroth II reconstruction eliminates problems with tension after an extensive resection, as well as the potential for recurrent disease, by closing the duodenal stump and draining the gastric remnant by a gastrojejunal anastomosis. The two limbs of a Billroth II are termed the *afferent limb,* which drains the duodenal stump, and the *efferent limb,* through which food exits the stomach into the small intestine. Bile and pancreatic juice from the afferent limb continually pass the stoma and sometimes cause gastritis; the Roux-en-Y reconstruction is designed to surmount this.

In this chapter, partial or subtotal gastrectomy for benign disease is presented first with discussion of the Billroth I and Billroth II methods of reconstruction. Radical subtotal gastrectomy and total gastrectomy are then discussed, and the standard terminology used to describe the extent of resection is briefly explained. Less common procedures (rarely performed at present), such as proximal gastric resection, are discussed in the references at the end.

Subtotal Gastrectomy

Mobilization of the Greater Curvature (Fig. 48.1)

Technical Points

Enter the abdomen through an upper midline incision and explore it. Note the location of the pylorus by its landmark prepyloric veins of Mayo and determine the extent to

LIST OF STRUCTURES

Esophagus
Stomach
   Lesser curvature
   Greater curvature
   Antrum
   Cardioesophageal junction
Pylorus
Duodenum
   Ampulla of Vater
Ligament of Treitz
Spleen
Colon
   Epiploic appendices

Right gastric vein
   Prepyloric veins of Mayo
Transverse mesocolon
Greater omentum
Lesser omentum
   Hepatoduodenal ligament
Middle colic artery
   Marginal artery of Drummond
Pancreas
   Accessory pancreatic duct
Common bile duct
Celiac artery
   Common hepatic artery

Proper hepatic artery
   Gastroduodenal artery
     Right gastroepiploic artery
  Left gastric artery
Left gastroepiploic artery
Left gastric vein (coronary vein)
Portal vein
Liver
   Left lobe of liver
   Triangular ligament of liver
Splenorenal (lienorenal) ligament
Gastrosplenic ligament

ORIENTATION

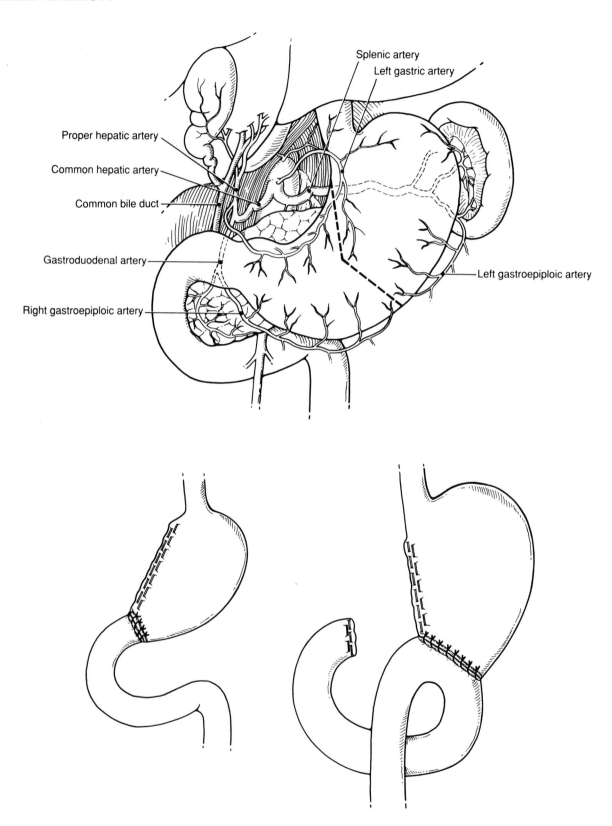

FIGURE 48.1
MOBILIZATION OF THE GREATER CURVATURE

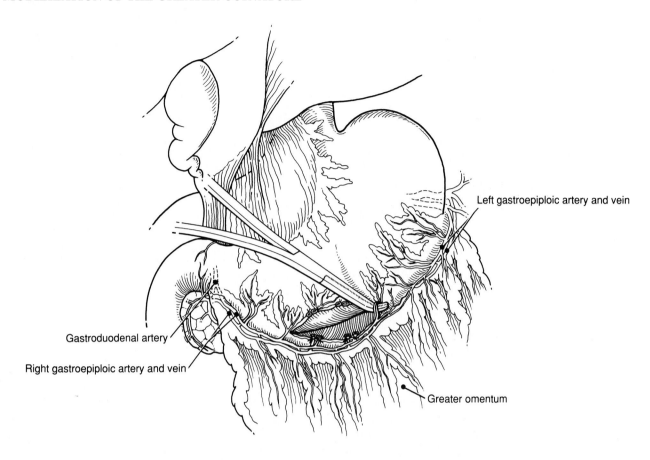

Left gastroepiploic artery and vein

Gastroduodenal artery

Right gastroepiploic artery and vein

Greater omentum

which scarring and old or active ulcer disease have altered the anatomy, particularly in the region of the pylorus and duodenum. Verify the position of the nasogastric tube. If a vagotomy is to be performed, do this first (see Fig. 38.1 in Chapter 38). Then commence mobilizing the stomach by serially dividing and ligating multiple branches of the right gastroepiploic artery and vein running to the greater curvature of the stomach. An opening into the free space of the lesser sac should become apparent. This free space is easier to enter to the left than to the right because multiple filmy layers of omentum can be difficult to separate from the antrum and transverse mesocolon.

Be aware of the close proximity of the transverse mesocolon (and middle colic artery) to gastrocolic omentum, and verify that you are in the correct plane by identifying the transverse mesocolon and pulling it inferiorly. Carry the dissection proximally on the greater curvature to the chosen point of transection of the stomach. The transition point between the left and right gastroepiploic arcades forms an easily recognizable landmark on the greater curvature, corresponding to about a 60% gastric resection.

Continue the dissection distally as far as it will go easily. As the pylorus is reached, chronic inflammation from ulcer disease may render the dissection more difficult. If so, it is best to delay this phase of the dissection until after the stomach is divided proximally. The added mobility will greatly facilitate dissection in the region of the pylorus and duodenum.

Place a Babcock clamp on the distal greater curvature and lift up. Divide multiple avascular adhesions between pancreas and posterior gastric wall with Metzenbaum scissors or electrocautery. A posterior gastric ulcer that is densely adherent to the pancreas is best managed by "buttonholing" the ulcer crater on the pancreas, rather than by attempting excision (which may result in injury to the pancreas).

Anatomic Points

Although the stomach is predominantly located in the upper left abdomen, the pylorus is inferior to the right seventh sternocostal articulation, typically at the level of the first lumbar vertebra. The prepyloric veins of Mayo are tributaries of the right gastric vein and aid in identification.

The right gastroepiploic artery is a terminal branch of the gastroduodenal artery that usually arises posterior to the first part of the duodenum and to the left of the common bile duct. The position of this artery varies from lying essentially in contact with the stomach to lying as much as 1 cm inferior; gastric branches pass to both anterior and posterior stomach.

FIGURE 48.2
MOBILIZATION OF THE LESSER CURVATURE

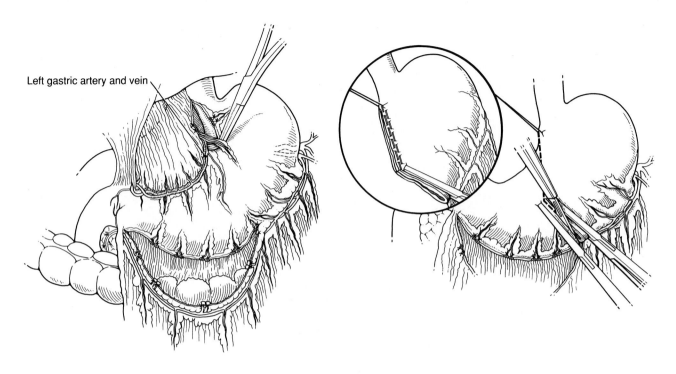

Left gastric artery and vein

A brief description of the development of the greater omentum enables an understanding of the relationship of this structure and of various peritoneal reflections in the upper abdomen. The greater omentum is derived from dorsal mesogastrium. The stomach rotates from its original sagittal orientation to its adult position and becomes more or less transversely disposed and rotated on its long axis. The original left side becomes anterior, and the original right side becomes posterior. The dorsal mesogastrium disproportionately increases in length and drapes anterior to the transverse colon. The portion of the dorsal mesogastrium that is in contact with the posterior parietal peritoneum fuses to it, and the apposed serosal layers degenerate. Dorsal mesogastrium in contact with transverse mesocolon and transverse colon then fuses to these serosal surfaces, and again, apposed serosal surfaces degenerate. Both the anterior and posterior inner serosa of the bursal recess contact each other, fuse, and as before, degenerate. Thus, the greater omentum typically has no cavity, but instead has a bloodless fusion plane between the original anterior and posterior leaves. This leaves the short gastrocolic ligament connecting the greater curvature of the stomach and the transverse mesocolon. Because of the close relationship of the greater curvature of the stomach to the transverse colon, and because the gastrocolic ligament (in which runs the gastroepiploic arcade) and one layer of the transverse mesocolon (in which runs the middle colic artery) are both developmentally related to dorsal mesogastrium, one can expect these arteries to be closely related. The middle colic artery generally passes into the mesocolon at the lower border of the neck of the pancreas, whereas the right gastroepiploic artery arises

just superior to the lower border of the first part of the duodenum, slightly to the right of midline. The spatial relationship of the middle colic and right gastroepiploic arteries may, in fact, be functional, because there can be a large anastomotic artery connecting the two.

Texts and atlases invariably depict a gastroepiploic arcade. However, a true anastomosis is absent in 10% of the cases. Typically, when no anastomosis occurs, there is no definitive left gastroepiploic artery; instead, there are several small branches that unite with similar-sized branches of the right gastroepiploic. In the other 90% of cases, the transition between left and right gastroepiploic supply is discerned by the change in angle of origin of the gastric branches.

Mobilization of the Lesser Curvature (Fig. 48.2)

Technical Points

Identify the descending branch of the left gastric artery in the lesser omentum. Pass a right-angle clamp under it and double-ligate and divide it. Clean the lesser curvature as high up as desired. Place a 2-0 silk Lembert suture at the upper end of the cleared lesser curvature for traction. Verify the position of the nasogastric tube, high in the gastric pouch and well above the line of proposed transection. Place two Kocher clamps across the greater curvature at the selected point of division and cut between the clamps with a knife. This will form the new outlet of the gastric remnant and should be sized accordingly (about 3 cm, or about the size of the duodenum, for a Billroth I reconstruction, and about 4 to 5 cm for a Billroth II procedure).

Construct a Hofmeister shelf by passing a linear stapling device (with 4.8-mm staples) into the opened crotch of the divided stomach, angling it as high up on the lesser curvature as possible. Use traction on the lesser curvature suture to define the upper extent of resection of the lesser curvature. Fire the stapler and divide the lesser curvature between the stapling device and a Kocher clamp. Check the staple line for bleeding points. Place a moist laparotomy pad over the proximal gastric remnant and allow it to retract into the left upper quadrant, out of the way.

Anatomic Points

The most important vascular structure in the lesser omentum is the left gastric artery. This, the smallest branch of the celiac artery, initially has a retroperitoneal course that runs superiorly and to the left. It then runs anteriorly to approach the gastroesophageal junction. Here, it gives rise to esophageal branches, turns inferiorly to follow the lesser curvature of the stomach, and terminates by anastomosing with the much smaller right gastric artery. Frequently (25% of the time), it gives rise to the left hepatic artery or to accessory left hepatic arteries, which course through the superior part of the lesser omentum. Even more commonly (42%), it divides into anterior and posterior branches.

The right gastric artery is usually a branch of the common or proper hepatic artery, although it frequently arises from the left hepatic or gastroduodenal artery. Like the left gastric artery, it frequently divides into anterior or posterior branches.

Gastric veins parallel the arteries and empty into the portal vein or its components at different levels, rather than as a single vessel. There are no functional valves in these veins, and because the left gastric vein (coronary vein) has free anastomoses with the caval system through the esophageal veins, it assumes great importance in portal hypertension.

Anterior and posterior vagal nerve components are also found within the lesser omentum. One or more hepatic branches from the anterior vagal trunk pass through the superior part of this ligament, from the level of the esophagus to the porta hepatis. Gastric branches from the anterior vagus either radiate from an origin at the cardioesophageal junction (in which case they are not found in the lesser omentum) or pass from the nerve of Latarjet (which accompanies the left gastric artery) to the stomach with the vessels. A posterior nerve of Latarjet also parallels the lesser curvature of the stomach, although its length as a discrete nerve is not as long as the anterior nerve. A major celiac branch (including more than half of the total nerve fibers) accompanies the left gastric artery to the celiac plexus. Gastric branches reach the stomach in a manner similar to the anterior gastric branches.

The extreme right part of the lesser omentum connects the duodenum and liver; hence, it is termed the *hepatoduodenal ligament.* This part of the lesser omentum forms the anterior wall of the epiploic foramen and contains the common bile duct, hepatic artery, and portal vein. The portal vein is posterior, the hepatic artery is anterior and somewhat to the left of the vein, and the common bile duct is anterior and somewhat to the right in the free edge of the ligament.

FIGURE 48.3
DISSECTION OF THE DISTAL ANTRUM AND DUODENAL STUMP

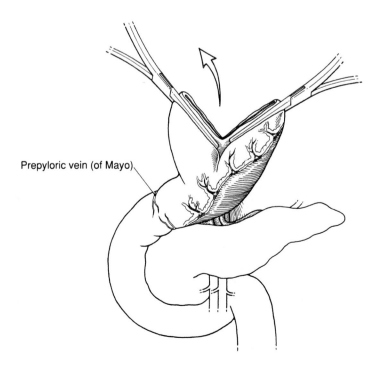

Prepyloric vein (of Mayo)

Dissection of the Distal Antrum and Duodenal Stump (Fig. 48.3)

Technical Points

Dissect circumferentially around the distal antrum and down the duodenum until soft, pliable tissue is encountered. Recognize the pylorus by direct palpation of the doughnut-shaped pyloric sphincter or by the overlying prepyloric veins of Mayo. If severe scarring from ulcer disease or previous surgery has distorted the anatomy, confirm that the duodenum has been reached by examining a frozen section of the resection margin. Brunner's glands are characteristic of the duodenum and are readily seen on histologic examination.

The gastroduodenal artery will be encountered if the dissection progresses more than about 1 cm down the duodenum. Dissection beyond this point should be done with extreme care lest the accessory pancreatic duct or common bile duct be damaged. Remove the stomach by transecting the duodenum.

Anatomic Points

Mobilization of the stomach, including the antrum, presents no further problems if none have been encountered with mobilization of the greater and lesser curvatures. This is not true with respect to the duodenum, which becomes a retroperitoneal organ shortly distal to the pyloric sphincter. Difficult anatomic relationships that can lead to complications also begin at this point. If the dissection proceeds from left to right and inferior tension is placed on the distal portion of the stomach, control of the right gastric vein superior to the pylorus will control bleeding from the prepyloric veins of Mayo. Further mobilization inferiorly and to the right should expose, posterior to the first part of the duodenum, the common hepatic artery and two of its branches, the proper hepatic and gastroduodenal arteries. Remember that the common bile duct should be located to the right of the common hepatic artery and anterior to the portal vein, both in the gastroduodenal ligament and immediately posterior to the duodenum, and that it is in the retroduodenal region that the common bile duct either becomes surrounded by pancreatic tissue or lies in the fascial plane between pancreas and duodenum. It, too, should be treated with utmost care.

If the second part of the duodenum is approached in this circumferential dissection, the surgeon should remember the significant features of pancreatic development. The superior part of the pancreatic head plus the neck and body of the pancreas develop from the dorsal pancreatic bud, initially a diverticulum of the original dorsal aspect of the duodenum. The elongated diverticulum forms the duct of Santorini. The ventral pancreatic bud begins as a diverticulum of the developing common bile duct. As a result of foregut rotation and differential growth, the ventral pancreatic bud migrates to a position immediately caudal to the dorsal pancreatic bud, where it develops into the uncinate process and lower part of the head of the pancreas. Its attachment (duct of Wirsung) to

the common bile duct is retained. Later, the duct systems fuse, and the definitive pancreatic duct is derived distally (neck, body, and tail) from the duct of Santorini and proximally (head and uncinate process) from the duct of Wirsung. In the adult, this main pancreatic duct opens into the duodenum, typically through the chamber (ampulla of Vater) that is common to the terminal common bile duct, at the major duodenal papilla, which is located somewhat posteriorly on the concave side of the duodenal lumen at about the level of the second lumbar vertebra. The proximal end of the duct of Santorini usually persists as the accessory pancreatic duct (in 70% of cases), opening into the duodenum somewhat more anteriorly than the major pancreatic duct and typically about 2 cm superior to the major duodenal papilla. In about 10% of cases, the accessory duct is the only grossly visible duct draining the pancreas.

This region is the site of many variations in the configuration and anatomic relationships of the biliary apparatus; blood supply to the liver, duodenum, and pancreas; and tributaries of the portal vein. A general rule that will help to prevent complications secondary to variant anatomy is to define carefully and identify accurately all tubular structures in this region before ligation and division.

Billroth I Reconstruction (Fig. 48.4)

Technical Points

Mobilize the duodenum by performing a Kocher maneuver (see Fig. 41.6 in Chapter 41). Place a posterior row of interrupted silk Lembert sutures to anastomose the duodenum to the gastric remnant. At the superior angle, where the Hofmeister shelf intersects the suture line, place a three-corner stitch, as shown in Fig. 48.7C. Visualize the three bites of this stitch as defining the sides of a triangle drawn around the "angle of sorrows." Place the inner suture line as a running lock-stitch of 3-0 absorbable suture, beginning at the midline of the back wall, and continue this anteriorly as a running Connell suture to achieve careful mucosal apposition. Then place an anterior row of interrupted Lembert sutures of 3-0 silk to complete the anastomosis.

Anatomic Points

The Kocher maneuver returns the duodenum and pancreas to their embryologic midline position. The duodenum originally is a midline segment of gut suspended by a dorsal mesoduodenum in which the dorsal bud of the pancreas (destined to become the upper part of the head plus the neck and body of the pancreas) develops. As a result of rotation of the upper gastrointestinal organs, the original right side of the duodenum and pancreas come to lie in contact with the dorsal parietal peritoneum. The apposing serosal surfaces then fuse and degenerate, leaving an avascular plane posterior to the now retroperitoneal duodenum and pancreas. In addition, on the original antimesenteric (convex) side of the duodenum, the parietal peritoneum and serosa of the original left side of the duodenum fuse.

FIGURE 48.4
BILLROTH I RECONSTRUCTION

Positional changes of the midgut loop (secondary to rotation, physiologic herniation and reduction, and fixation of those segments destined to become retroperitoneal) occur after fixation of the foregut-derived duodenum. Consequently, the root of the transverse mesocolon is frequently attached to the anterior surface of the second part of the duodenum and anterior surface of the pancreas. The hepatic flexure of the colon should be pulled inferiorly and medially to expose the superior part of the C loop of duodenum. At this point, one should identify the middle colic vessels because they frequently course immediately anterior to the second part of the duodenum. With these vessels identified, incision of the peritoneum along the lateral edge of the duodenum, followed by blunt finger dissection in the avascular fusion plane posterior to the duodenum and head of pancreas, should result

in adequate mobilization of these structures with little or no blood loss.

Billroth II Reconstruction: Closure of the Duodenal Stump (Fig. 48.5)

Technical and Anatomic Points

If Billroth II reconstruction is planned, first close the duodenal stump in two layers in the following manner. Start a Connell suture at the inferior end of the duodenal stump and run it superiorly. At the top, either terminate the suture line by tying the suture to itself, or turn the suture line back and invert again by running back to the point of origin as a running horizontal mattress suture. Then place an outer layer of interrupted 3-0 silk Lembert sutures. Alternatively, an easy duodenal

FIGURE 48.5
BILLROTH II RECONSTRUCTION: CLOSURE OF THE DUODENAL STUMP

FIGURE 48.6
BILLROTH II RECONSTRUCTION—GASTROJEJUNOSTOMY

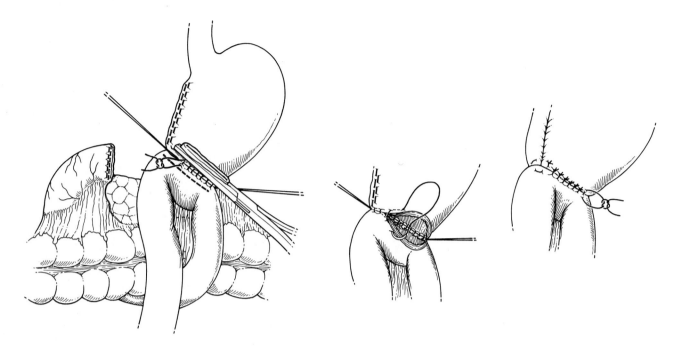

stump can be closed with a linear stapling device loaded with 3.5-mm staples.

The difficult duodenal stump, scarred by duodenal ulcer disease, can be closed by one of a variety of methods. Generally, pliable anterior duodenal wall is rolled down and over, with subsequent suturing to the pancreatic capsule if necessary. A tube duodenostomy can be placed through a separate stab wound and secured with an absorbable pursestring suture as an extra precaution. This creates a controlled fistula.

Pack omentum over the duodenal stump before closure. Place a closed-suction drain in the vicinity of the tube duodenostomy, if one was placed. Otherwise, do not drain the stump.

Billroth II Reconstruction—Gastrojejunostomy (Fig. 48.6)

Technical Points

The gastrojejunostomy may be performed in an antecolic or retrocolic fashion. Here, the basic antecolic gastrojejunostomy is described, with comments on the alternative retrocolic version.

Identify the proximal jejunum at the ligament of Treitz. Trace it down 20 to 30 cm and locate a loop of proximal jejunum that will reach to the gastric remnant without tension. The loop should be as close to the ligament of Treitz as possible. The jejunal loop will be routed to the left of the main bulk of the greater omentum, which will pass to the right and be used to pack off the duodenal stump and surround the gastrojejunostomy.

Suture the jejunal loop to the gastric remnant with a standard two-layer technique. Take special care to clamp

and ligate multiple small arterial branches in the gastric submucosa that can cause gastrointestinal bleeding in the postoperative period. Place a three-corner suture at the "angle of sorrows." The afferent limb should exit to the left, whereas the efferent limb should exit to the right. Allow the gastrojejunostomy to rise into the left upper quadrant, where it should lie comfortably without tension or kinking.

Anatomic Points

Technically, the antecolic anastomosis is the simpler of the two procedures. The gastrojejunal anastomosis is placed anterior to the colon, so that additional dissection is unnecessary. If a retrocolic anastomosis is to be performed, the transverse mesocolon must be incised. This should be done to the left of the middle colic artery and vein and to the right of the superior branch of the inferior mesenteric artery, taking care not to insult the marginal artery close to the mesenteric border of the colon. This area is essentially avascular.

Operations for Gastric Carcinoma

Radical Subtotal Gastrectomy (Fig. 48.7)

Technical Points

Radical subtotal gastrectomy is performed for carcinoma that is limited to the distal stomach. This resection differs from subtotal gastrectomy for benign disease in the following ways:

1. The gastrocolic omentum is resected in continuity with the greater curvature of the stomach.

FIGURE 48.7
RADICAL SUBTOTAL GASTRECTOMY

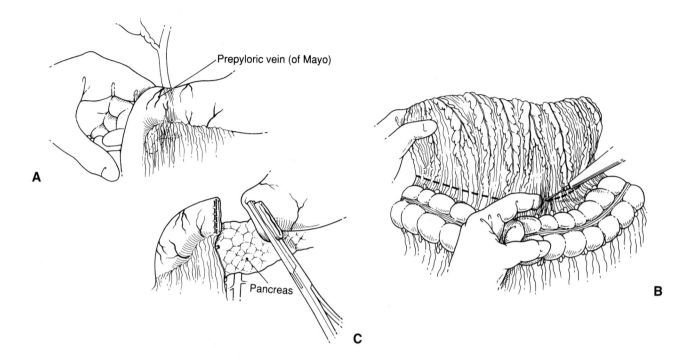

2. Lymph nodes along the left gastric and celiac arteries are resected with the lesser curvature.
3. The duodenal stump may need to be dissected a bit farther down to attain a clear tumor margin.
4. The spleen may be included with the resection to remove nodes in the splenic hilum (optional).

One standard terminology uses D1 to denote a resection with local (perigastric) nodes and D2 for a more extended resection with excision of nodes at the celiac axis and hepatoduodenal ligament. D3 adds the nodes in the retropancreatic space and along the vessels of the transverse mesocolon, and D4 adds the paraaortic lymph nodes from the aortic hiatus to its bifurcation. The value of these superradical dissections is still under discussion.

First, assess the tumor for resectability. Because resection offers the best chance for palliation, the presence of nonresectable metastatic disease does not preclude resection. The tumor commonly extends into adjacent structures. The tail of the pancreas is often involved in lesions of the body of the stomach. The mesentery of the transverse colon may be involved by tumors of the greater curvature. Resection of the tail of the pancreas or a segment of colon may be performed if necessary. Tumor tissue growing in the region of the lesser curvature may preclude resection because of the potential involvement of critical structures.

Radical subtotal gastrectomy is most easily performed by first dividing the duodenum, which usually has a normal consistency, and then progressing proximally. Identify a region of duodenum about 1 to 2 cm distal to the prepyloric vein or to any gross tumor (which generally stops at the pylorus).

Incise the peritoneum superiorly and inferiorly. Identify and confirm the position of the common bile duct in the hepatoduodenal ligament. The common bile duct should still lie deep to the region of dissection at this point. Develop a plane posterior to the duodenum by gentle blunt dissection using a peanut sponge. Close the duodenal stump with a linear stapling device using 3.5-mm staples; then place a Kocher clamp on the specimen side and divide it. Place a moist laparotomy pad over the duodenal stump and, lifting up on the proximal duodenum, divide the filmy adhesions that lie posterior, clamping any small vessels with mosquito hemostats.

Most of the gastrocolic omentum will be included with the specimen. Flip the gastrocolic omentum up and, while gently pulling down on the transverse colon, cut with Metzenbaum scissors in the normally avascular cleavage plane between the colon and omentum. Note that this plane lies about 1 cm from the bowel wall; multiple, small, fatty epiploic appendices should remain with the colon to avoid bleeding and the risk for perforating a small diverticulum.

Flip the specimen up and to the left, exposing the celiac axis by sweeping down lymph nodes along the lesser curvature. Identify the left gastric artery and ascertain that it does not give rise to an anomalous hepatic artery before dividing it at its origin. Choose the point of division of the stomach high on the lesser curvature and divide the gastrocolic omentum with clamps up to that point. Flip the stomach up and incise the avascular gastropancreatic folds until the stomach is fully mobilized. Divide the stomach (see Fig. 48.3).

Some surgeons include splenectomy as part of radical subtotal gastrectomy. This allows lymph nodes along the splenic hilum to be included with the specimen. By sacrificing the short gastric vessels, splenectomy may compromise the blood supply to the gastric remnant, particularly if the left gastric artery was ligated at its origin.

Proceed with reconstruction as for an antecolic Billroth II.

Anatomic Points

At this point, one should review the lymphatic drainage of the stomach. Remember that lymphatic vessels accompany arteries and basically drain lymph from areas supplied by the corresponding arteries. The lymphatic drainage of the stomach can be divided into four regions. One region includes the cardioesophageal junction, the right half of the fundus, and the lesser curvature half of the stomach to the approximate union of right and left gastric arteries—in essence, the area supplied by the left gastric artery. Regional lymph nodes serving this area include those along the left gastric artery, celiac nodes, and periesophageal nodes. The next largest region corresponds to the region supplied by the right gastroepiploic artery and includes about half of the greater curvature of the stomach, the antrum, and the pylorus. Regional lymph nodes for these lymphatics include nodes along the right gastroepiploic artery, pyloric nodes lying on the head of the pancreas, and celiac nodes. The gastroepiploic nodes, which can lie as much as 3 to 4 cm from the greater curvature in the greater omentum, also drain the greater omentum.

A third area includes the upper half of the greater curvature and fundus of the stomach—that is, that region that is supplied by the left gastroepiploic artery and short gastric arteries. Regional nodes are situated along the left gastroepiploic artery, short gastric arteries, and splenic artery. These also drain to celiac nodes. Finally, the fourth area includes the lymphatics draining that part of the stomach supplied by the right gastric artery. The region of the stomach drained by these lymphatics includes only the distal portion of the superior half of the pylorus. Regional lymph nodes include the right gastric nodes, nodes in the region of the portal triad, and finally, the celiac nodes. Remember that the transverse mesocolon, in part derived from the greater omentum and anatomically very close to the greater curvature of the stomach, may reasonably be suspected to be involved by tumor if the tumor is along the greater curvature. Further, because of the fact that carcinoma of the lesser curvature drains to nodes closely associated with the vital portal triad, tumors in this location may involve these structures and hence may be unresectable.

When skeletonizing the celiac axis, bear in mind that the celiac plexus, a plexus containing parasympathetic and sympathetic neurons, completely surrounds this artery. In addition, the artery is very closely related to the crura of the diaphragm, the left adrenal gland and its blood supply, and the left inferior phrenic arteries on the left diaphragmatic crus.

FIGURE 48.8
TOTAL GASTRECTOMY (RESECTION OF THE STOMACH)

Total Gastrectomy (Resection of the Stomach) (Fig. 48.8)

Technical Points

Assess the tumor for resectability and begin the resection at the distal margin, as described in Fig. 48.7. Take the gastrocolic omentum off the colon, progressing up the greater curvature. When the colon has been fully mobilized downward, mobilize the spleen by dividing the lateral peritoneal attachments. Elevate the spleen into the wound and ligate the splenic artery and splenic vein in the hilum. Sweep any lymph nodes along the splenic artery and vein into the specimen.

Divide the triangular ligament of the left lobe of the liver and reflect it to the right to improve exposure. Incise the peritoneum overlying the cardioesophageal junction and mobilize the distal esophagus (see Figs. 34.1 and 34.2 in Chapter 34).

Divide the posterior avascular attachments between the stomach and pancreas. Sweep down the node-bearing tissue along the lesser curvature and divide and ligate the left gastric artery at its origin.

The specimen now should be attached only by the esophagus. Place two stay sutures of 2-0 silk on the left and right distal esophagus and divide the esophagus at the cardioesophageal junction, above all gross tumor. One should obtain frozen-section confirmation of proximal and distal margins because submucosal tumor may extend several centimeters beyond grossly visible or palpable disease.

Anatomic Points

In this procedure, the peritoneal attachments of the spleen must be remembered. First, remember that the spleen is highly variable in position, as evidenced by the fact that its lower pole has been reported to range from L1 to L5. Typically, it is attached to the posterior body wall by the splenorenal (lienorenal) ligament (in which run the splenic vessels) and to the stomach by the gastrosplenic ligament (in which run the left gastroepiploic and short gastric vessels). These ligaments must be divided with care.

Reconstruction After Total Gastrectomy (Fig. 48.9)

Technical and Anatomic Points

The simplest reconstruction is to make a Roux-en-Y loop of jejunum. Several techniques for making reservoirs have been described and are referenced. Only the Roux-en-Y will be described here. This simple and serviceable reconstruction works remarkably well.

Identify the proximal jejunum and trace it to the ligament of Treitz. Measure down 30 to 40 cm distal to the ligament of Treitz and isolate a loop of jejunum. Hold the loop up and inspect its mesentery, looking for the pattern of the jejunal arcades. Plan to divide the jejunum at the midpoint of the arch of an arcade so that there is a good blood supply to both ends. Make a window through the mesentery and divide the mesentery for a total distance of about 10 cm, or until the

FIGURE 48.9
RECONSTRUCTION AFTER TOTAL GASTRECTOMY

root of the mesentery is reached. Divide the jejunum with a linear stapling device.

The Roux limb (distal limb) should pass comfortably up to the esophagus. The shortest path is retrocolic, through a small window in the transverse mesocolon. However, this may predispose the patient to obstruction if tumor recurs in the gastric bed. If possible, route the Roux limb in an antecolic path, passing it to the left of the transverse colon and major bulk of the omentum.

The esophagojejunal anastomosis may be sutured using a standard two-layer suture technique. Generally, it is preferable to sew the end of the stomach to the side of the jejunum along the antimesenteric border, several centimeters from the end of the loop. Complete the back wall, then have the anesthesiologist advance the nasogastric tube through the anastomosis and suture the front layer over the nasogastric tube.

Alternatively, a stapled anastomosis (end-esophagus to side-jejunum) may be fashioned using a circular stapling device. "Inkwell" the anastomosis by rolling jejunum up over it and securing it with a few interrupted Lembert sutures. Have the anesthesiologist advance the nasogastric tube slowly as you guide it through the anastomosis and down 10 to 15 cm into the jejunum.

Close the end of the loop with a linear stapling device using 3.5-mm staples.

Place two closed-suction drains, one on each side, in close proximity to the esophagojejunal anastomosis.

Finally, complete the Roux-en-Y reconstruction by suturing or stapling the proximal blind Roux loop (draining pancreatic and biliary secretions) 40 cm below the esophagojejunostomy. Close the mesenteric defect.

REFERENCES

1. Besson A. The Roux-Y loop in modern digestive tract surgery. *Am J Surg* 1985;149:656. (Describes the history and multiple applications of this technique.)
2. Bonenkamp JJ, Hermans J, Sasako M, et al. Extended lymph-node dissection for gastric. Dutch Gastric Cancer Group. *N Engl J Med* 1999;340:908–914. (Results are similar for D1 and D2 resections.)
3. Bozzetti F, Marubini E, Bonafanti G, et al. Subtotal versus total gastrectomy for gastric cancer: five-year survival rates in a multicenter randomized Italian trial. Italian Gastrointestinal Tumor Study Group. *Ann Surg* 1999;230:170–178. (Results show no benefit to total gastrectomy if negative margins attained with subtotal resection.)
4. Burch JM, Cox CL, Feliciano DV, et al. Management of the difficult duodenal stump. *Am J Surg* 1991;162:522–526. (Compares various techniques.)
5. Eagon JC, Miedema BW, Kelly KA. Postgastrectomy syndromes. *Surg Clin North Am* 1992;72:445. (Provides good review of problems that occur after gastric resection and their management.)
6. Gingrich GW. The use of the T-tube in difficult duodenal stump closures. *Am Surg* 1959;25:639. (Provides good description of tube duodenostomy.)
7. Harrower HW. Closure of the duodenal stump after gastrectomy for posterior ulcer. *Am J Surg* 1966;111:488.
8. Hermann RE. T-tube catheter drainage of the duodenal stump. *Am J Surg* 1973;125:364.
9. Herrington JL. Surgical management of duodenal ulcer and its complications. *Contemp Surg* 1986;29:13.
10. Hutson DG, Zeppa R, Levi JU, et al. An improved technique for total gastrectomy. *Surg Gynecol Obstet* 1977;145:249.
11. Maeta M, Yamashiro H, Saito H, et al. A prospective pilot study of extended (D3) and superextended para-aortic lymphadenectomy (D4) in patients with T3 or T4 gastric cancer managed by total gastrectomy. *Surgery* 1999;125:325–331.
12. Powers JC, Fitzgerald JF, McAlvanah MJ. The anatomic basis for the surgical detachment of the greater omentum from the transverse colon. *Surg Gynecol Obstet* 1976;143:105.
13. Roberts PL, Williamson WA, Sanders LB. Pitfalls in the use of staplers in gastrointestinal tract surgery. *Surg Clin North Am* 1991;71:1247.
14. Rodkey GV, Welch CE. Duodenal decompression in gastrectomy. Further experiences with duodenostomy. *N Engl J Med* 1960;262:498.
15. Scott HW, Gobbel WG, Law DH. Clinical experience with a jejunal pouch (Hunt-Lawrence) as a substitute stomach after total gastrectomy. *Surg Gynecol Obstet* 1965;121:1231.
16. Smith JW, Brennan MF. Surgical treatment of gastric cancer: proximal, mid, and distal stomach. *Surg Clin North Am* 1992;72:381.
17. Steichen FM, Ravitch MM. Operations on the stomach. In: *Stapling in surgery.* Chicago: Year Book Medical Publishers, 1984:173. (Describes a variety of procedures by pioneers in surgical stapling.)

CHAPTER 49

Laparoscopic Gastrojejunostomy

Laparoscopic gastrojejunostomy is a simple procedure that may be used when palliation of malignant upper gastrointestinal obstruction is required. It has the same drawbacks as the corresponding open procedure but may be of use when a nonresectable pancreatic cancer requires palliation of gastric outlet or duodenal obstruction.

Laparoscopic Gastrojejunostomy—Orientation and Setup (Fig. 49.1)

Technical and Anatomic Points

The usual trocar pattern (Fig. 49.1A) may be modified if both gastrojejunostomy and biliary bypass (see Chapter 59).

LIST OF STRUCTURES

Stomach
  Greater curvature
  Lesser curvature
Lesser omentum

Pancreas
Left gastric artery
Gastroepiploic artery
Prepyloric vein (of Mayo)

Jejunum
Duodenum
Pylorus
Ligament of Treitz

FIGURE 49.1
LAPAROSCOPIC GASTROJEJUNOSTOMY—ORIENTATION AND SETUP (**B** from Scott-Conner CEH, Cuschieri A, Carter FJ. Small intestine and appendix. In: *Minimal access surgical anatomy*. Philadelphia: Lippincott Williams & Wilkins, 2000:164–184, with permission; **C** from Scott-Conner CEH, Cuschieri A, Carter FJ. Stomach and duodenum. In: *Minimal access surgical anatomy*. Philadelphia: Lippincott Williams & Wilkins, 2000:79–100.)

A

B

Mesentery

Jejunum

Vasa recta

FIGURE 49.1 (Continued)

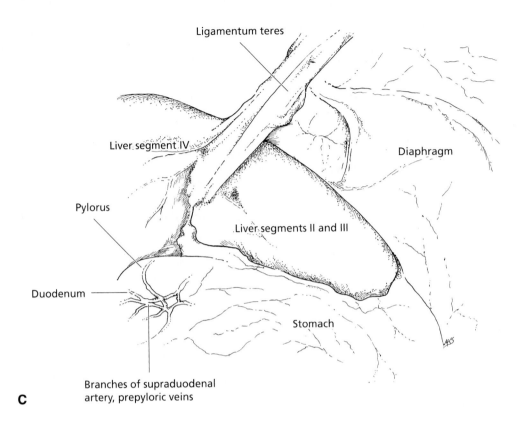

Ligamentum teres

Liver segment IV

Diaphragm

Pylorus

Liver segments II and III

Duodenum

Stomach

Branches of supraduodenal
artery, prepyloric veins

C

FIGURE 49.2
LAPAROSCOPIC GASTROJEJUNOSTOMY—STAPLING THE GASTROJEJUNOSTOMY (From Scott-Conner
CEH. Laparoscopic cholecystojejunostomy, laparoscopic gastrojejunostomy. In: Scott-Conner CEH, ed. *The SAGES manual:
fundamentals of laparoscopy and GI endoscopy.* New York: Springer-Verlag, 1999:314–325.)

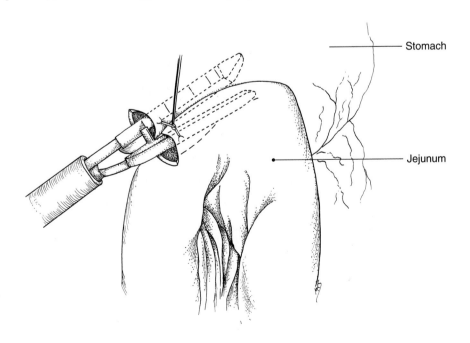

Stomach

Jejunum

Thoroughly explore the abdomen and determine the extent of disease. Choose a loop of proximal jejunum that will reach comfortably to the stomach without tension (Fig. 49.1B). Confirm that this is indeed proximal small intestine by tracing the loop to the ligament of Treitz.

Identify an appropriate point on the greater curvature of the stomach (Fig. 49.1C). If necessary, clear the omentum from part of the greater curvature, securing branches of the gastroepiploic vessels with the ultrasonic shears (see Fig. 64.1B in Chapter 64).

Laparoscopic Gastrojejunostomy—Stapling the Gastrojejunostomy (Fig. 49.2)

Technical and Anatomic Points

Create an opening in the stomach and pass one limb of the endoscopic stapler into the stomach. Gently close, but do not fire, the stomach. This will both partially close the gastrotomy, minimizing leakage, and stabilize the location of the gastrotomy relative to the stapler.

Similarly create an opening in the jejunum. Maneuver the jejunum close to the stomach and open the stapler. Pull the jejunum over the second limb of the stapler, manipulating both stomach and jejunum well up into the jaws of the stapler. Close and fire and stapler. Repeat if necessary to create a generous lumen.

Remove the stapler and use the suction irrigator to check hemostasis of the staple line.

Laparoscopic Gastrojejunostomy—Completing the Anastomosis (Fig. 49.3)

Technical and Anatomic Points

The two stab wounds will now have coalesced into a single anterior incision in stomach and jejunum. Close this by suturing or with the endoscopic linear stapler. Confirm that the anastomosis lies comfortably without tension. Trace the loops of small bowel to ensure that there are no kinks or twists. Attain hemostasis and close the port sites.

FIGURE 49.3
LAPAROSCOPIC GASTROJEJUNOSTOMY—COMPLETING THE ANASTOMOSIS (From Scott-Conner CEH. Laparoscopic cholecystojejunostomy, laparoscopic gastrojejunostomy. In: Scott-Conner CEH, ed. *The SAGES manual: fundamentals of laparoscopy and GI endoscopy.* New York: Springer-Verlag, 1999:314–325.)

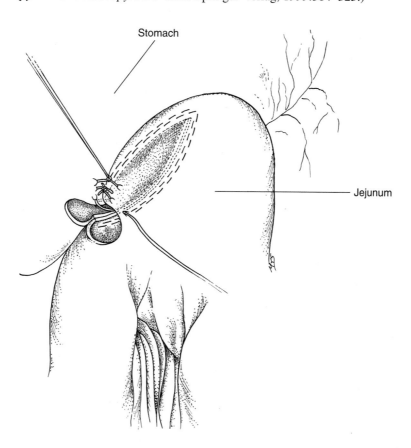

REFERENCES

1. Rhodes M, Nathanson L, Fielding G. Laparoscopic biliary and gastric bypass: a useful adjunct in the treatment of carcinoma of the pancreas. *Gut* 1995;36:778–780.

2. Scott-Conner CEH. Laparoscopic cholecystojejunostomy, laparoscopic gastrojejunostomy. In: Scott-Conner CEH, ed. *The SAGES manual: fundamentals of laparoscopy and GI endoscopy*. New York: Springer-Verlag, 1999:314–325.

3. Scott-Conner CEH, Cuschieri A, Carter FJ. Stomach and duodenum. In: *Minimal access surgical anatomy*. Philadelphia, Lippincott Williams & Wilkins, 2000:79–100.

4. Wind GG. Stomach. In: *Applied laparoscopic anatomy: abdomen and pelvis*. Baltimore: Williams & Wilkins, 1997:143–186.

CHAPTER 50

Laparoscopic Gastric Resection

Laparoscopically assisted gastric resection is used for benign disease or for palliation of malignancy. The laparoscopic portion may be limited to mobilization, with an extracorporeal anastomosis. Although totally intracorporeal anastomotic techniques are certainly feasible, difficulties with function and the need to create an incision to remove the specimen

LIST OF STRUCTURES

Esophagus	Duodenum	and vein
Stomach	Greater omentum	Short gastric vessels
Greater curvature	Lesser omentum	Spleen
Lesser curvature	Left gastric artery	Pancreas
Pylorus	Left and right gastroepiploic artery	Gastropancreatic folds

---

FIGURE 50.1

LAPAROSCOPIC GASTRIC RESECTION—MOBILIZING THE STOMACH (B from Scott-Conner CEH, Cuschieri A, Carter FJ. Stomach and duodenum. In: *Minimal access surgical anatomy.* Philadelphia: Lippincott Williams & Wilkins, 2000:79–100, with permission; **C** and **D** from Goh PMV, Cheah WK. Laparoscopic gastrectomy for cancer. In: Zucker KA, ed. *Surgical laparoscopy.* 2nd ed. Philadelphia: Lippincott Williams & Wilkins, 2001:531–541, with permission; **E** from Cuschieri A. Gastric resections. In: Scott-Conner CEH, ed. *The SAGES manual: fundamentals of laparoscopy and GI endoscopy.* New York: Springer-Verlag, 1999:314–325, with permission.)

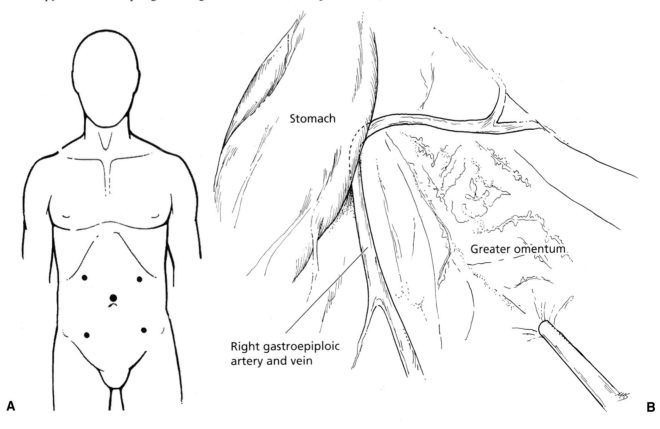

Stomach

Greater omentum

Right gastroepiploic
artery and vein

A

B

323

FIGURE 50.1   (Continued)

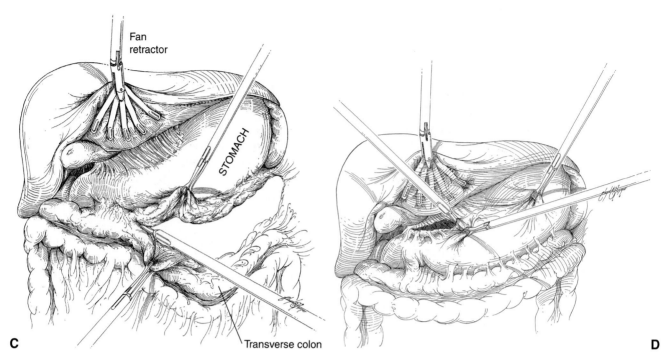

C

Fan retractor

STOMACH

Transverse colon

D

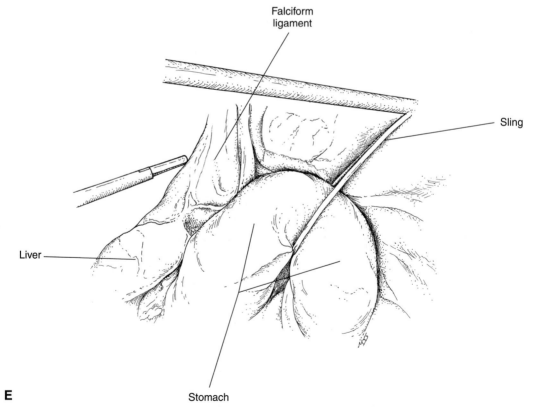

E

Falciform ligament

Sling

Liver

Stomach

FIGURE 50.2
SUBTOTAL GASTRECTOMY: VASCULAR DIVISION (**A** from Scott-Conner CEH, Cuschieri A, Carter FJ. Stomach and duodenum. In: *Minimal access surgical anatomy.* Philadelphia: Lippincott Williams & Wilkins, 2000:79–100, with permission; **B** from Wind GG. Stomach. In: *Applied laparoscopic anatomy: abdomen and pelvis.* Baltimore: Williams & Wilkins, 1997:143–186, with permission.)

A

B

FIGURE 50.3
LAPAROSCOPIC SUBTOTAL GASTRECTOMY—RESECTION (A and **B** from Goh PMV, Cheah WK. Laparoscopic gastrectomy for cancer. In: Zucker KA, ed. *Surgical laparoscopy.* 2nd ed. Philadelphia: Lippincott Williams & Wilkins, 2001:531–541, with permission.)

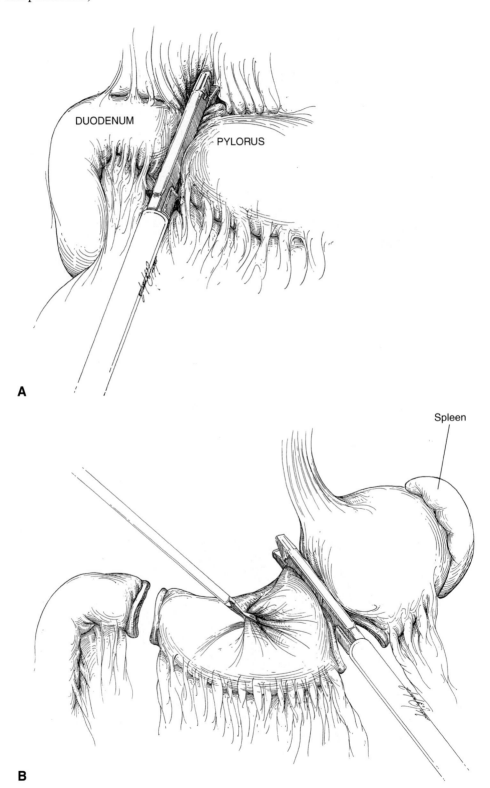

FIGURE 50.4
LAPAROSCOPIC TOTAL GASTRECTOMY (**A** and **B** from Wind GG. Stomach. In: *Applied laparoscopic anatomy: abdomen and pelvis.* Baltimore: Williams & Wilkins, 1997:143–186, with permission; **C** from Goh PMV, Cheah WK. Laparoscopic gastrectomy for cancer. In: Zucker KA, ed. *Surgical laparoscopy.* 2nd ed. Philadelphia: Lippincott Williams & Wilkins, 2001:531–541, with permission.)

FIGURE 50.4   (Continued)

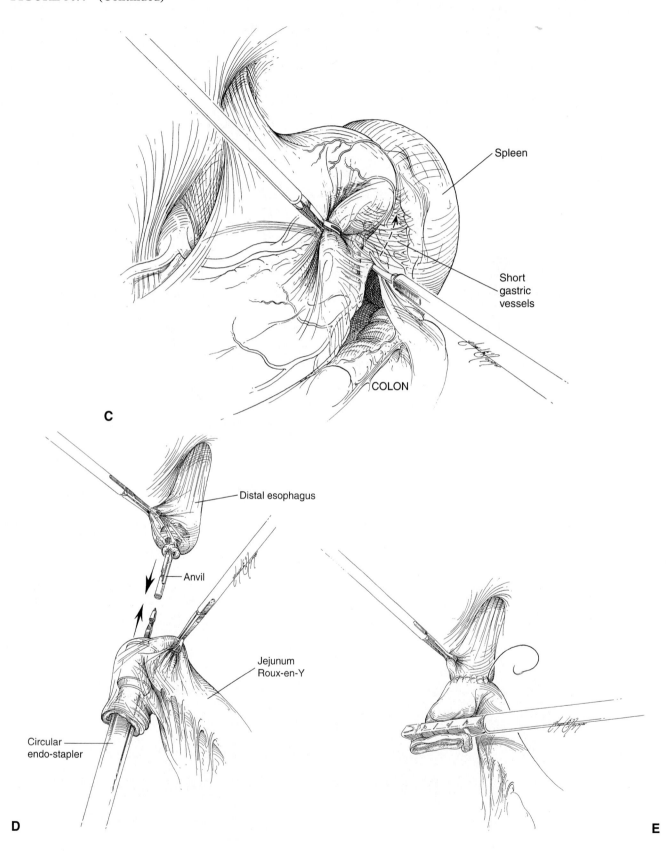

Spleen

Short
gastric
vessels

COLON

C

Distal esophagus

Anvil

Jejunum
Roux-en-Y

Circular
endo-stapler

D

E

have rendered these less desirable alternatives, particularly after subtotal resection. In this chapter, laparoscopic subtotal gastrectomy with standard (open) reconstruction and laparoscopic total gastrectomy with intracorporeal anastomosis are described. Considerations of extent of resection, whether or not to resect omentum with the stomach, and type of reconstruction should not be altered by the use of a laparoscopic technique. Laparoscopic node dissection has also been described, but the use of laparoscopic gastrectomy for cure of gastric cancer is as yet unproved.

References at the end give details of alternative approaches, including hand-assisted techniques and totally intracorporeal anastomoses.

Laparoscopic Gastric Resection—Mobilizing the Stomach (Fig. 50.1)

Technical and Anatomic Points

The extent of resection will determine the amount of mobilization required. Trocar sites are shown in Fig. 50.1A.

Begin by mobilizing the greater curvature. Elevate the stomach with an atraumatic grasper and divide branches of the gastroepiploic vessels along the greater curvature to create a window into the lesser sac (Fig. 50.1B; see also Fig. 64.1B in Chapter 64). Enlarge this window proximally and distally to mobilize fully the greater curvature of the stomach (Fig. 50.1C). Elevate the stomach and sharply divide the avascular gastropancreatic folds.

Open the avascular portion of the lesser omentum (Fig. 50.1D). Pass a short segment of Penrose drain into the abdomen. Pass it through the windows in the greater and lesser omentum, behind the stomach, and use this as a sling to elevate and retract the stomach atraumatically (Fig. 50.1E).

Subtotal Gastrectomy: Vascular Division (Fig. 50.2)

Technical and Anatomic Points

Dissection may then progress proximally and distally as far as needed. First divide any additional branches of the gastroepiploic arcade that remain. At the conclusion of this phase, the stomach should be completely elevated from underlying structures, including pancreas (Fig. 50.2A). The left gastric artery and vein should be visible. Depending on the extent of planned resection, divide these at the origin (total gastrectomy) or identify and divide the descending branch of the left gastric artery (subtotal resection). Secure these sizable vessels with ties or clips (Fig. 50.2B).

At the conclusion of this phase, the stomach should be completely elevated from underlying structures, including the pancreas. Use the prepyloric vein of Mayo and branches of the supraduodenal artery as visual landmarks to locate the pylorus (see Fig. 47.1C in Chapter 47 and Fig. 49.1C in Chapter 49).

Laparoscopic Subtotal Gastrectomy—Resection (Fig. 50.3)

Technical and Anatomic Points

Circumferentially mobilize the pylorus by blunt dissection to create a window large enough to pass an endoscopic linear stapler. Divide the duodenum just beyond the pylorus with the stapler (Fig. 50.3A).

Similarly divide the stomach proximally with an endoscopic linear stapler (Fig. 50.3B), firing it several times if necessary to complete the transection.

Make a short midline or left paramedian incision to deliver the specimen and complete the reconstruction (Billroth I, Billroth II, or Roux-en-Y) in the standard open fashion, as described in Chapter 48.

Laparoscopic Total Gastrectomy (Fig. 50.4)

Technical and Anatomic Points

In the region of the esophageal hiatus, mobilization of the esophagus may be achieved by techniques described in Chapters 42 and 43. Carefully and completely divide the gastropancreatic folds (Fig. 50.4A) and short gastric vessels (Fig. 50.4B), rolling the stomach posteriorly as needed. The short gastric vessels can also be divided from an anterior approach as shown in Fig. 50.4C and in Fig. 42.2 in Chapter 42. Elevate the stomach to display the left gastric artery for ligation, if not previously performed.

The stomach should now be completely free. Divide the stomach at the pylorus and at the esophagogastric junction. Create a small incision to remove the specimen. Reconstruction may be done in the usual fashion with a circular stapler and endoscopic linear cutting stapler (Fig. 50.4D,E) in an intracorporeal or extracorporeal fashion as desired.

REFERENCES

1. Cuschieri A. Gastric resections. In: Scott-Conner, CEH ed. *The SAGES manual: fundamentals of laparoscopy and GI endoscopy.* New York: Springer-Verlag, 1999:314–325.
2. Goh PMV, Cheah WK. Laparoscopic gastrectomy for cancer. In: Zucker KA, ed. *Surgical laparoscopy.* 2nd ed. Philadelphia: Lippincott Williams & Wilkins, 2001:531–541.
3. Goh PMV, Kum CK. Gastrectomy. In: MacFadyen BV, Ponsky JL, eds. *Operative laparoscopy and thoracoscopy.* Philadelphia: Lippincott-Raven, 1996:523–534.

CHAPTER 51

Truncal Vagotomy and Pyloroplasty and Highly Selective Vagotomy

Vagotomy is performed to decrease the stimulus to acid output by the parietal cells. Most peptic ulcers respond to eradication of *Helicobacter* species and acid-suppressive medication. The remaining role of vagotomy is still being clarified. Three types of vagotomy have been described: truncal vagotomy, selective vagotomy, and highly selective (or parietal cell) vagotomy.

Truncal vagotomy is a total abdominal vagotomy in which both vagal trunks are divided at the esophageal hiatus. The procedure can be performed through the chest (transthoracic vagotomy), which is occasionally done when recurrent ulceration follows gastrectomy and it is known with certainty that a complete vagotomy was not done at the time of the original operation.

Selective vagotomy is a total gastric vagotomy, with preservation of the hepatic branch (innervating the biliary tract) and the celiac branch (innervating the small intestine). Highly selective (or parietal cell) vagotomy divides only the fibers to the parietal cells of the stomach, preserving innervation to the gastric antrum.

Because truncal vagotomy and selective vagotomy denervate the antrum, a drainage procedure, such as pyloroplasty, must be performed. No drainage procedure is needed after highly selective vagotomy because antral innervation is preserved.

In this chapter, truncal vagotomy and pyloroplasty (including a brief section on management of the bleeding duodenal ulcer), as well as highly selective vagotomy, are presented. References describing the less commonly performed selective vagotomy, transthoracic vagotomy, and laparoscopic techniques for vagotomy are listed at the end.

Truncal Vagotomy and Pyloroplasty

Vagotomy (Fig. 51.1)

Technical Points

Position the patient supine on the operating table. Make an upper midline incision. An indwelling nasogastric tube is important to facilitate identification of the esophagus and its mobilization.

Expose the esophageal hiatus and mobilize the esophagus (see Figs. 34.1 and 34.2), encircling it with a Penrose drain. Place the fingers of your nondominant hand behind the esophagus and elevate it, maintaining gentle traction on it.

The main vagal trunks feel like banjo strings. One large trunk lies on the left anterior surface and a slightly smaller one lies to the right and posterior. The anterior vagal trunk is often visible on the surface of the esophagus. Because it is easiest to find, it is generally taken first. Pass a right-angled clamp under the vagal trunk and mobilize it for a total length of 1.5 to 2 cm. Clamp the vagal trunk in the middle of the mobilized segment and place a medium hemoclip at the lower end of the trunk. Cut just above the clip. Lift up on the right-angled clamp to pull the mobilized segment away from the esophagus and clip this segment at the upper end; then cut below, excising a short segment of nerve.

Next identify the posterior vagal trunk. It is often palpable when gentle tension is placed on the esophagus and the back of the esophagus is felt. Roll the esophagus and posterior vagal trunk one way or the other to bring the vagal trunk into view. If you cannot feel the vagal trunk, search the posterior tissue between the esophagus and aorta. This nerve

LIST OF STRUCTURES

Esophagus	Stomach	Hepatic division
Esophageal hiatus	Lesser curvature	Anterior nerve of Latarjet
Left lobe of liver	Pylorus	Posterior esophageal plexus
Left triangular ligament	Greater curvature	Celiac division
Diaphragm	Vagus nerves	Posterior nerve of Latarjet
Inferior phrenic artery and vein	Anterior esophageal plexus	"Criminal nerve" of Grassi

ORIENTATION

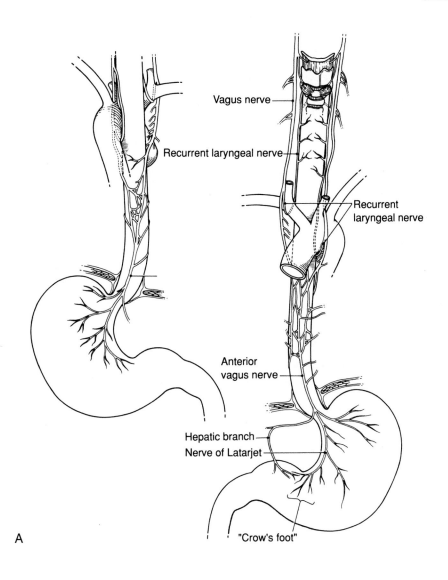

Vagus nerve

Recurrent laryngeal nerve

Recurrent laryngeal nerve

Anterior vagus nerve

Hepatic branch
Nerve of Latarjet

"Crow's foot"

A

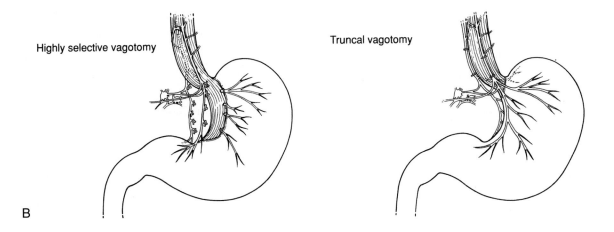

Highly selective vagotomy

Truncal vagotomy

B

FIGURE 51.1
VAGOTOMY

is frequently left behind when the esophagus is mobilized and encircled by the Penrose drain at the beginning of the dissection.

Vagal tissue cuts with a very slight crunching sensation that can be distinguished, with practice, from the sensation felt when cutting small blood vessels or muscle fibers. Nevertheless, submit the vagal fibers for frozen-section confirmation; two good segments of peripheral nerve should be obtained.

Search for other fibers. Carefully feel the entire esophagus, rolling it between your fingers. Divide any suspicious bands running longitudinally on the esophagus.

Check the area for hemostasis and place a moist laparotomy pad there while commencing the drainage procedure. Do not wait for frozen-section confirmation; if two trunks are not identified on frozen-section analysis, return to the esophageal hiatus after completing the drainage procedure.

Anatomic Points

The left lobe of the liver initially obscures visualization of this region. To mobilize the left lobe, cut the left triangular ligament. This ligament attaches the liver to the abdominal side of the diaphragm. Divide it close to the liver (to avoid injury to the inferior phrenic vessels) and between clamps because the ligament can contain bile duct radicals, vessels, and nerves. Divide the peritoneum at the esophageal hiatus with care because the left inferior phrenic vessels can pass immediately anterior to the esophageal hiatus.

When exposure is adequate, one will begin to see certain structures passing through the hiatus—namely, the esophagus, various arrangements of the vagal nerve trunks, and esophageal veins and arteries. The left and right vagus nerves form the anterior and posterior esophageal plexuses in the upper to middle thorax. Each plexus is predominantly derived from left or right vagus nerves. However, each receives contributions from its contralateral counterpart. Differential growth of the greater curvature of the stomach during development causes an apparent rotation. The left vagus nerve comes anterior and becomes the anterior vagal trunk, whereas the right vagus nerve becomes the posterior vagal trunk. Distally, both anterior and posterior esophageal plexuses typically reunite above the esophageal hiatus to form anterior (predominantly left vagus) and posterior (predominantly right vagus) trunks. Thus, in about 90% of cases, only two vagal structures pass through the hiatus. Typically, both of these structures are to the right of the esophageal midline. The anterior trunk should be located on the anterior surface of the esophagus. The posterior vagus is typically closer to the right margin of the esophagus than is the anterior trunk. It can be located as much as 2 cm from the esophagus and spatially is closer to the aorta than to the esophagus.

Soon after passing through the hiatus, the anterior vagal trunk divides into a hepatic division, which runs to the porta hepatis in the gastrohepatic ligament, and a principal anterior nerve of the lesser curvature of the stomach (anterior nerve of Latarjet), which accompanies the left gastric artery and gives off branches to the anterior stomach. Similarly, the posterior vagal trunk divides into a large celiac division, which accompanies the proximal left gastric artery to the celiac gan-

glion, and a principal posterior nerve of the lesser curvature of the stomach (posterior nerve of Latarjet), which gives off branches to the posterior stomach.

Variations in the number of vagal structures passing through the esophageal hiatus occur in about 10% of cases and depend on the distal extent of the esophageal plexuses. If the plexus terminates at a point more proximal than usual, the trunks can divide in the esophageal hiatus, so that four vagal structures can pass through the hiatus. More than four vagal structures may pass through the hiatus if additional gastric branches pass through independently, or if the esophageal plexuses extend into the abdomen and then later form the two principal trunks. Fortunately, variations involving the posterior vagal trunk are less common than those of the anterior trunk. However, because it is more difficult to visualize the posterior vagal elements than the anterior ones, a posterior gastric branch is probably more likely to be missed. The notorious "criminal nerve" of Grassi refers to the most

---

FIGURE 51.2
PYLOROPLASTY

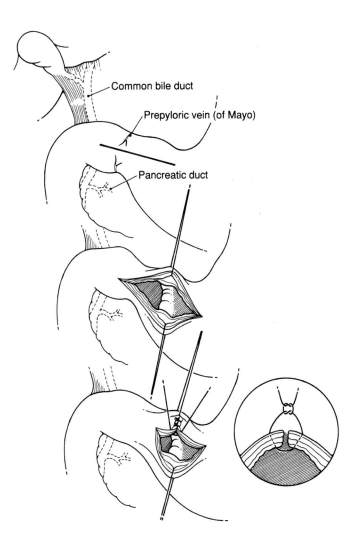

Common bile duct

Prepyloric vein (of Mayo)

Pancreatic duct

proximal posterior gastric branch that arises at, or above, the celiac division.

In short, because of the variation of the vagus nerves at the esophageal hiatus, it is absolutely necessary to skeletonize the distal esophagus and divide all nerve structures that pass through this opening.

Pyloroplasty (Fig. 51.2)

Technical and Anatomic Points

Although pyloroplasty is illustrated here, truncal vagotomy may be performed in conjunction with either antrectomy (see Chapter 48) or simple gastrojejunostomy.

Place a Harrington retractor over a moist laparotomy pad and retract the liver to expose the pylorus, which is identifiable by the two prepyloric veins of Mayo. Assess the pylorus for size, mobility, and the presence of thickening or edema from old or active ulcer disease.

The simplest and most commonly employed pyloroplasty is the Heineke-Mikulicz procedure, as described here. Several alternative techniques, which may be easier or safer to perform when severe scarring or active ulcer disease involves the pylorus, are described in the references at the end.

Place two traction sutures of 2-0 silk at the pylorus and lift up. Incise the pylorus by cutting longitudinally for a distance of 2 to 3 cm. Digitally explore the pyloric channel, confirming

division of the pylorus and the absence of obstruction from severe scarring.

Close the pyloroplasty incision transversely, using a single layer of interrupted 2-0 silk sutures. It is easiest to place all of the sutures first and then pull up and tie them at the end. Place each suture as a simple suture, taking a bite that is widest at the top in order to ensure accurate apposition of the layers with slight inversion. Place omentum over the pyloroplasty.

Management of the Bleeding Duodenal Ulcer (Fig. 51.3)

Technical Points

The first step is to confirm the site of bleeding. Perform a brief but thorough exploration of the abdomen, with particular attention to the liver (cirrhosis, metastatic disease), spleen (splenomegaly from splenic vein thrombosis), stomach, distal esophagus, duodenum, and proximal small bowel. In the absence of unexpected findings, make a generous longitudinal gastroduodenotomy beginning on the proximal antrum and continuing down across the pylorus into the first portion of the duodenum (Fig. 51.3A). Aspirate and remove clot. Irrigate proximally and distally and place small packs. The ulcer should be visible on the posterior wall of the duodenum, just beyond the pylorus.

In the classic situation, bleeding comes from a branch of the gastroduodenal artery. Remove any adherent clot and seek

FIGURE 51.3
MANAGEMENT OF THE BLEEDING DUODENAL ULCER

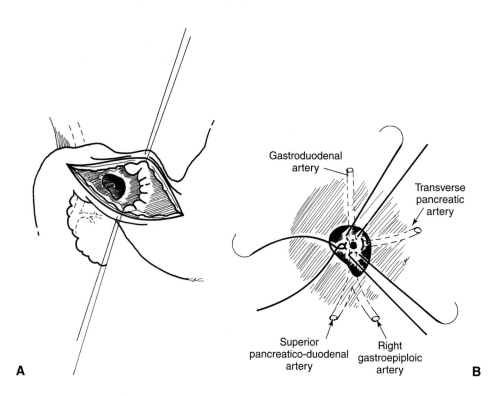

FIGURE 51.4
BEGINNING OF DISSECTION

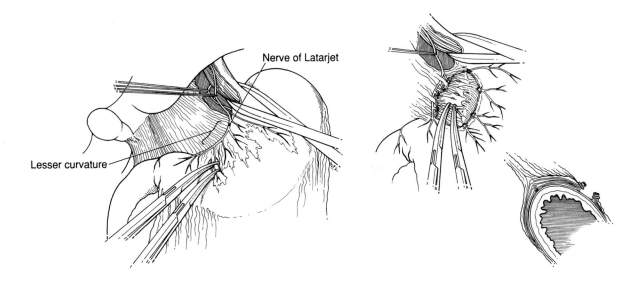

active bleeding. Place 2-0 silk sutures to control the artery above and below the bleeding site. Place a third suture on the pancreatic side of the site to control the transverse pancreatic artery, which may join at this site (Fig. 51.3B). Confirm that the bleeding has completely stopped. Place a pack over the site and proceed with truncal vagotomy. After performing a vagotomy, return your attention to the duodenum. Appearance of fresh bile from the duodenum below the operative site confirms patency of the distal common bile duct. Absence of fresh blood confirms adequate hemostasis. Always keep in mind that there may be more than one ulcer. Close the pyloroplasty when satisfied that bleeding is completely controlled.

Anatomic Points

The gastroduodenal artery arises from the common hepatic artery and passes behind the superior part of the duodenum and superficial to the pancreas. It divides into the right gastroepiploic and superior pancreaticoduodenal arteries and frequently gives rise to small pancreatic tributaries, including the transverse pancreatic artery. The location of this bifurcation and subsequent divergence of tributaries is highly variable and may occur in the region where posterior duodenal ulcers are most commonly located. If ulcer perforates into the region of a bifurcation or trifurcation, sutures must be placed in such a manner as to occlude all potential branches. The recommendation that three bites be placed—one above, one below, and one to the pancreatic side of the bleeding point—is intended to accomplish this objective.

The common duct passes deep to the gastroduodenal artery, and the exact relationship of the duct to the gastroduodenal artery varies. In the most common situation, the gastroduo-

denal artery passes to the left of the common bile duct. Sutures should be placed just deep enough to control the artery. Blind placement of deep sutures in this region may damage the common duct or pancreatic duct.

Highly Selective Vagotomy

Beginning of Dissection (Fig. 51.4)

Technical Points

Expose the hiatus as described in Fig. 51.1. Incise the peritoneum overlying the gastroesophageal junction. Encircle the esophagus with a Penrose drain and retract it to the right. Identify the anterior and posterior vagus trunks. Gently dissect these from the esophagus and surrounding soft tissues. Place a right-angled clamp under each and pass a Silastic loop around each vagus. Gently retract both vagal trunks to the left.

Next, turn your attention to the pylorus. Identify the prepyloric veins of Mayo. Look for the so-called crow's foot, the terminal branches of the nerves of Latarjet innervating the distal antrum. Using the pylorus as a landmark, measure 5 to 7 cm up the lesser curvature. Confirm that this will preserve the terminal three divisions of the crow's foot. Place a Babcock clamp on the greater curvature of the stomach and have your assistant provide downward traction to the left. Commencing just above the branch that extends to the crow's foot, begin dividing the upper leaf of the lesser omentum between long, fine-tipped hemostats. Work from the antrum up toward the gastroesophageal junction to skeletonize the lesser curvature.

Think of the lesser omentum as being wrapped around the lesser curvature and as being attached to it along a broad surface rather than in a narrow line. Do not attempt to divide the omentum entirely in one pass. Generally, three passes through the tissue will completely divide the omentum while preserving the nerves of Latarjet. On the first pass, divide the omentum from just above the crow's foot to the peritoneal incision of the gastroesophageal junction. Pull the lesser curvature down and then start on the middle portion of the dissection.

Anatomic Points

Because the objective of a highly selective vagotomy is to denervate the acid-producing parietal cells while preserving gastric motility, it is first necessary to understand the distribution of these cells in the stomach. The distribution of parietal cells is somewhat variable but is generally most dense in the midbody region, tapering somewhat both proximally and distally. Parietal cells are rarely present, if at all, in the distal antrum. Thus, the optimal highly selective vagotomy will denervate the proximal two thirds of the stomach while preserving innervation to the distal one third. This is possible because of the distribution of vagal nerve fibers to the stomach.

The anterior gastric division (anterior nerve of Latarjet) usually can be traced along the lesser curvature to the angular notch of the stomach, although occasionally, it can be traced distally as far as the pylorus or first part of the duodenum. As it passes along the lesser curvature, from 2 to 12 gastric branches supply the stomach. Ligate and divide all of these gastric branches except the last one. This is best accomplished by starting the denervation 5 to 7 cm proximal to the pylorus and proceeding proximally, taking care to identify all gastric branches, even those that may pass through the esophageal hiatus independently. The anterior nerve of Latarjet may be doubled; alternatively, there may be no true nerve of Latarjet, but rather a "spray" of vagal nerve fibers at the gastroesophageal junction. It is not uncommon to find that the hepatic division of the anterior trunk supplies the pyloric canal and pylorus, so that even if all of the gastric fibers of the nerve of Latarjet were severed, pyloric sphincter tone would be preserved. The variations of this distribution mandate meticulous dissection to identify and divide all fibers to the parietal cell mass of the stomach.

Completion of the Dissection of the Lesser Curvature (Fig. 51.5)

Technical Points

As the dissection becomes difficult in the region of the cardioesophageal junction, go back toward the region of the crow's foot. When a window has been made that extends completely through the lesser omentum, you will be able to pass your nondominant hand behind the stomach and pull down. This will facilitate the dissection and improve exposure. You or an assistant can then pull down on the stomach

FIGURE 51.5
COMPLETION OF THE DISSECTION OF THE LESSER CURVATURE

with the thumb and forefinger of your nondominant hand, elevating the lesser omentum with the spread third and fourth fingers and dividing it. Completely divide the lesser omentum from just above the crow's foot to the peritoneal incision at the cardioesophageal junction.

Anatomic Points

The gastric division of the posterior vagal trunk usually forms a principal posterior gastric nerve (posterior nerve of Latarjet) that parallels the anterior nerve. Compared with the anterior nerve, the posterior nerve terminates somewhat more proximally and has fewer gastric branches. In addition, frequently, the gastric branches of the posterior nerve are divided into superior and inferior groups. Because the inferior group typically supplies all of the stomach from the distal body to the pylorus, it is still necessary to divide gastric branches from a point 5 to 7 cm proximal to the pyloric sphincter proximally. In about 20% of cases, there is no true posterior nerve of Latarjet; rather, gastric branches emanate from the celiac division and recurve to innervate the stomach.

Dissection of the Distal Esophagus (Fig. 51.6)

Technical Points

Use the Penrose drain encircling the esophagus to elevate the esophagus, pulling it to the left to expose the posterior aspect of the stomach. Some filmy adhesions of the gastropancreatic folds will need to be divided to allow the back of the esophagus to be exposed and skeletonized. Do not divide the short gastric vessels connecting the greater curvature to the spleen. Take care that these are not inadvertently cut as the esophagus is pulled up and skeletonized. Maintain gentle right and upward traction on the Silastic loops on both vagal trunks and

FIGURE 51.6
DISSECTION OF THE DISTAL ESOPHAGUS

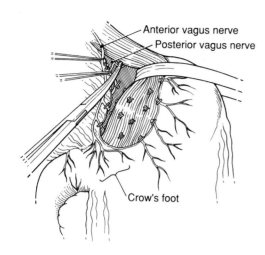

careful, steady traction on the esophagus to the left. This will facilitate dissection of the vagal trunks from the esophagus.

As the dissection progresses, the lower esophagus is pulled down out of the mediastinum into the abdomen. Clean the esophagus circumferentially for a total distance of 10 cm and divide any small nerve twigs that connect the vagal trunks with the esophagus. At the conclusion of the dissection, the distal esophagus should be completely skeletonized circumferentially for 10 cm, and the lesser curvature should

be completely free down to the crow's foot. Check the area for hemostasis.

Anatomic Points

The most superoposterior gastric branch—the so-called criminal nerve of Grassi—can arise at or cranial to the origin of the celiac division. As with division of the anterior gastric branches, a meticulous dissection is necessary to ensure that all desired gastric nerves are severed.

Reperitonealization of the Lesser Curvature (Fig. 51.7)

Technical Points

Reperitonealize the lesser curvature by placing multiple interrupted Lembert sutures of 3-0 silk from the serosal surface of the anterior wall of the lesser curvature to the serosal surface of the posterior wall of the lesser curvature. This will turn in the raw area, ensuring that any areas that may have been inadvertently traumatized or devitalized do not progress to perforation. At the completion of this part of the operation, the lesser curvature should be completely reperitonealized. Check the area again for hemostasis and close the abdomen without drainage.

Anatomic Points

It is technically impossible to separate the gastric branches of either the anterior or posterior gastric division from the vascular structures accompanying them to the lesser curvature.

FIGURE 51.7
REPERITONEALIZATION OF THE LESSER CURVATURE

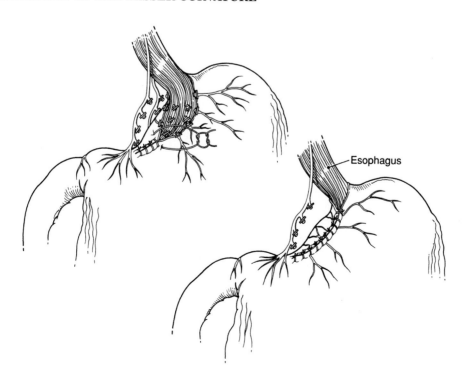

Thus, ligation and division of the neurovascular bundles supplying the lesser curvature is the rule. Division of the arteries is possible because of the rich intramural anastomoses of arteries derived from both gastric arteries, both gastroepiploic arteries, and the short gastric arteries. However, one of the recognized potential complications of highly selective vagotomy is devascularization, with subsequent necrosis, of the lesser curvature of the stomach. This complication results from variant arterial anatomy and so cannot be predicted, at least at the present time.

REFERENCES

1. Berne CJ, Rosoff L. Peptic ulcer perforation of the gastroduodenal artery complex: clinical features and operative control. *Ann Surg* 1969;169:141–144. (Provides classic description of trifurcation and three-stitch control.)
2. Branicki FJ, Coleman SY, Pritchett CJ, et al. Emergency surgical treatment for nonvariceal bleeding of the upper part of the gastrointestinal tract. *Surg Gynecol Obstet* 1991;172:113–120.
3. Cooperman AM, Hoerr SO. Pyloroplasty. *Surg Clin North Am* 1975;55: 1019.
4. Croft RJ. Reperitonealization and invagination of the lesser curvature of the stomach following proximal gastric vagotomy. *Arch Surg* 1978;113:206.
5. Dallemagne B, Weerts JM, Jehaes C, et al. Laparoscopic highly selective vagotomy. *Br J Surg* 1994;81:554–556.
6. Demos NJ. The elusive posterior vagus: its identification by palpation. *Am Surg* 1966;32:317.
7. Donahue PE. Ulcer surgery and highly selective vagotomy—Y2K. *Arch Surg* 1999;134:1373–1377.
8. Foster JH. Pyloroplasty, vagotomy, and suture ligation for bleeding duodenal ulcer. In: Nyhus LM, Baker RJ, Fischer JE, eds. *Mastery of surgery*. 3rd ed. Philadelphia: Little, Brown, 1997:911–915.
9. Gadacz TR. Laparoscopic vagotomy. In: Scott-Conner CEH, ed. *The SAGES manual*. New York: Springer-Verlag, 1999:227–232.
10. Goligher JC. A technique for highly selective (parietal cell or proximal gastric) vagotomy for duodenal ulcer. *Br J Surg* 1974;61:337.
11. Grassi G, Orecchia C. A comparison of intraoperative tests of completeness of vagal section. *Surgery* 1974;75:155.
12. Jordan PH Jr, Thornby J. Parietal cell vagotomy performed with fundoplication for esophageal reflux. *Am J Surg* 1997;173:264–269. (Emphasizes need for concomitant posterior gastropexy to avoid wrap slippage with this combination.)
13. Poon R, Chow L, Lim B, et al. Thoracoscopic vagotomy for recurrent ulcer after previous gastric operation. *Aust N Z J Surg* 1997;67:177–180.
14. Roberts JP, Debas HT. A simplified technique for rapid truncal vagotomy. *Surg Gynecol Obstet* 1989;168:539–541.
15. Skandalakis G. The history and surgical anatomy of the vagus nerve. *Surg Gynecol Obstet* 1986;162:75.
16. Skandalakis JE, Rowe JS, Gray SW, et al. Identification of vagal structures at the esophageal hiatus. *Surgery* 1974;75:233.
17. Taylor TV, Lythgoe P, McFarland JB, et al. Anterior lesser curve seromyotomy and posterior truncal vagotomy versus truncal vagotomy and pyloroplasty in the treatment of chronic duodenal ulcer. *Br J Surg* 1990;77:1007.
18. Wangensteen SL, Kelly JM. Gastric mobilization prior to vagotomy to lessen splenic trauma. *Surg Gynecol Obstet* 1968;127:603.
19. Wilkinson JM, Hosie KB, Johnson AG. Long-term results of highly selective vagotomy: a prospective study with implications for future laparoscopic surgery. *Br J Surg* 1994;81:1469–1471.

CHAPTER 52

Pyloric Exclusion and Duodenal Diverticulization

Injuries of the duodenum can be difficult to manage. In this chapter, exposure of the duodenum from the pylorus to the ligament of Treitz and two useful maneuvers for managing complex injuries to the duodenum are covered.

Duodenal injuries are rarely isolated. Careful assessment of the adjacent pancreas, common bile duct, colon, and neighboring vascular structures is an essential component of management.

Exposure of the Duodenum (Fig. 52.1)

Technical Points

First, mobilize the hepatic flexure of the colon by incising the lateral peritoneal attachments at the hepatic flexure. Make a small window in the peritoneum with Metzenbaum scissors, then pass the fingers of the nondominant hand behind the colon, sweeping the peritoneum up and thinning it out. Divide it with electrocautery. Often, there are filmy adhesions extending to the gallbladder; divide these by sharp dissection.

If you anticipate the need to expose the entire duodenum, pass your nondominant hand down behind the right colon and divide the lateral peritoneal reflection all the way down past the cecum. Lift the right colon with its mesentery, sharply dividing any filmy adhesions between the colon and retroperitoneum. The third portion of the duodenum will be visible as the colon is swept medially. Elevate the right colon and the mesentery of the small intestine (carefully preserving the superior mesenteric vessels) and swing them toward the left shoulder of the patient. The anterior surface of the duodenum from the pylorus to the ligament of Treitz should now be visible.

Mobilize the duodenum and head of the pancreas using a wide Kocher maneuver to gain access to the lateral and posterior surfaces of the duodenum in these regions. The fourth portion of the duodenum may be similarly mobilized by incising the antimesenteric border.

Anatomic Points

This procedure is made necessary, as well as technically possible, by the embryologic rotation of the gut. A knowledge of this developmental process enables a rational approach to the procedure.

The gut can be divided into foregut, midgut, and hindgut. For the purposes of the general surgeon operating on the abdomen, these divisions can be defined as follows: the foregut is that portion of the gut supplied by the celiac artery, the midgut is that portion supplied by the superior mesenteric artery, and the hindgut is that portion supplied by the inferior mesenteric artery. Foregut derivatives in the abdomen include the distal esophagus, the stomach, and the duodenum to just distal to the major duodenal papilla. The liver and biliary apparatus arise as the hepatic diverticulum from the terminal foregut, whereas the pancreas arises from a diverticulum of the hepatic diverticulum and from a separate dorsal pancreatic bud. Midgut derivatives include the rest of the duodenum, all of the small intestine, the appendix, the cecum, the ascending colon, and the proximal two-thirds of the transverse colon. Hindgut derivatives include the distal one-third of the transverse colon, the descending colon, the sigmoid colon, the rectum, and the anal canal to the anal valves.

The development of the abdominal gastrointestinal tract can be understood as a consequence of two phenomena. One of these is differential growth of the gut components

LIST OF STRUCTURES

Stomach	Pancreas	Hepatic flexure
Pylorus	Head of pancreas	Cecum
Duodenum	Ligament of Treitz	Transverse colon
First portion (duodenal bulb)	Gallbladder	**Embryologic terms**
Second portion	Common bile duct	Foregut
Third portion	Colon	Midgut
Fourth portion	Right (ascending) colon	Hindgut

ORIENTATION

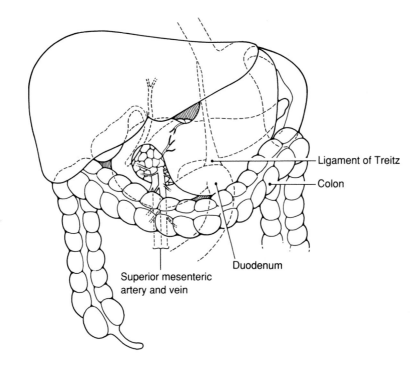

Ligament of Treitz

Colon

Duodenum

Superior mesenteric
artery and vein

in comparison to each other and to the developing peritoneal cavity. The other is the fusion and later degeneration, of apposed serosal surfaces. What follows is a conceptual description of some of the surgically relevant facets of the development of the infradiaphragmatic gastrointestinal system.

Initially, the gut is a midline intraperitoneal tube suspended from the dorsal body wall along its entire length by the dorsal mesentery. A ventral mesentery attaches the foregut to the anterior body wall from the umbilicus to the diaphragm, carrying the left umbilical vein from the umbilicus to its ultimate union with the caval system. As the fusiform dilatation destined to become stomach begins to develop by rapid elongation, the duodenum assumes the form of a C-shaped loop, with its convexity directed ventrally. Soon after these structures begin to be recognizable, the stomach changes its position by rotating 90 degrees to the right about its longitudinal axis. The end result of this rotation is that the right side of the stomach becomes the definitive posterior side and the left side becomes the definitive anterior side. Moreover, the original dorsal border becomes the greater curvature and the ventral border becomes the lesser curvature. As a result of the positional changes of the stomach, the C-loop of the duodenum rotates about a longitudinal axis so that the convex border becomes its definitive right border. This causes the right side of the duodenum and the right leaf of the mesoduodenum to be in apposition to the dorsal parietal peritoneum. The apposed serosal surfaces soon fuse and then degenerate, placing the bulk of the duodenum and pancreas, which develops primarily within the mesoduodenum, in a retroperitoneal position.

While foregut changes are occurring, the midgut rapidly lengthens, especially in comparison to the vertebral column. The midgut forms a ventrally directed loop that is suspended by the dorsal mesentery containing the superior mesenteric artery and vein. The proximal limb of the loop is cranial to the superior mesenteric artery, whereas the distal loop is caudal. Because the developing liver and urogenital system occupy most of the abdominal space, the midgut loop rotates 90 degrees counterclockwise around the superior mesenteric artery axis (as viewed anteriorly) and herniates into the umbilical cord. While herniated, the gut diverticulum destined to become vermiform appendix and cecum becomes recognizable, and the proximal limb, which elongates more than the distal limb, is thrown into numerous coils. At the same time, the abdominal cavity expands, resulting in a peritoneal cavity with sufficient room for the "herniated " midgut. The "herniation" is then reduced in an orderly fashion, and rotation (ultimately through a total of 270 degrees) of the midgut loop continues.

When the midgut returns to the abdominal cavity, the pattern of return progresses in a craniocaudal sequence, with the most cranial portions passing to the left upper quadrant and the rest of the midgut following obliquely toward the right lower quadrant. As the midgut returns into the peritoneal cavity, it forces the intraperitoneal hindgut (descending and sigmoid colon) to the left. As a consequence of this pattern of return, the left side of the descending colon and the left leaf of its mesentery come to lie in contact with the parietal peritoneum, and the inevitable fusion and degeneration of apposed serosal surfaces occur. The end result of this is that the descending

FIGURE 52.1
EXPOSURE OF THE DUODENUM

A

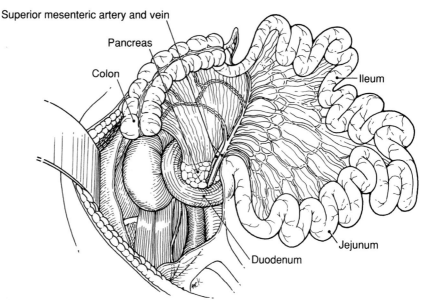

B

colon and its blood supply, contained in the mesentery, become retroperitoneal to a greater or lesser degree. The sigmoid colon retains its mesentery because midgut loops have entered the left upper quadrant (not the left lower quadrant), and consequently, the apposition of serosal surfaces necessary to allow fusion and degeneration is not achieved.

The last part of the midgut loop to return is the ascending and transverse colon. The ascending colon and its mesentery, similar to the descending colon, are fixed to the parietal peritoneum, and subsequent fusion and degeneration of apposed serosal surfaces again occur. Because the transverse colon is the last to return, it must pass anterior to the midgut loops that entered earlier; hence, it retains its mesentery. Later, a leaf of greater omentum, derived from dorsal mesogastrium, fuses with the cranial leaf of the original transverse mesocolon, so that the definitive transverse mesocolon develops from the original transverse mesocolon plus the original dorsal mesogastrium.

The procedure for exposure of the duodenum just described simply recreates the earlier developmental stage when the gut was an intraperitoneal structure. Fusion and degeneration of apposed serosal surfaces result in relatively avascular planes that allow massive mobilization with minimal blood loss.

Inspection of the dorsal side of the duodenum and head of the pancreas allows visualization of the terminal common bile duct, as this duct passes posterior to the duodenum and, in its "intrapancreatic" course, is more posterior than anterior with respect to pancreatic tissue. The same is true of the pancreatic duct; although embedded in pancreatic tissue, it is more posterior than anterior. In addition, the beginning of the portal vein, formed by the confluence of the superior mesenteric vein and splenic vein, should be visible.

FIGURE 52.2
DUODENAL DIVERTICULIZATION AS A MEANS OF "DEFUNCTIONALIZING" THE DUODENUM AND CONVERTING A LEAK INTO AN END-DUODENAL FISTULA

The third portion of the duodenum lies in the angle between the root of the superior mesenteric artery (and its accompanying vein) and the aorta. The leftward mobilization of duodenum and pancreas is thus limited by the superior mesenteric artery.

Duodenal Diverticulization as a Means of "Defunctionalizing" the Duodenum and Converting a Leak into an End-Duodenal Fistula (Fig. 52.2)

Technical and Anatomic Points

First, debride and repair the injury. Because enteric contents will bypass the duodenum, a considerable amount of narrowing can be tolerated, if necessary, to achieve a secure repair. A standard two-layered suture technique is preferred. Confirm the integrity of the biliary and pancreatic ducts and cannulate them, performing contrast studies if necessary.

Next, "defunctionalize" or diverticulize the duodenum by performing a limited gastric resection using the Billroth II reconstruction. Perform a truncal vagotomy. Place omentum over the duodenal suture line and duodenal stump closure. If closure of the duodenal stump has been difficult, a tube duodenostomy is a prudent additional step. Place drains in the region of the duodenal suture line.

Note that duodenal diverticulization is, in essence, gastric resection with vagotomy. This is a lengthy operation that

FIGURE 52.3
PYLORIC EXCLUSION

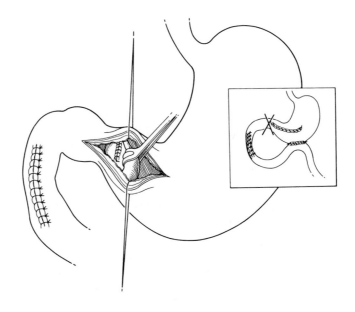

results in permanent anatomic changes. Pyloric exclusion (Fig. 52.3) accomplishes the same objective but is a much shorter procedure and results in only temporary diversion. In many patients, pyloric exclusion is the preferred alternative.

Pyloric Exclusion (Fig. 52.3)

Technical and Anatomic Points

Repair the duodenal injury as described in Fig. 52.2. Then, create a low anterior gastrotomy. Pass Babcock clamps into the stomach and grasp the pylorus, everting it through the gastrotomy. Close the pylorus firmly with a running suture of 2-0 synthetic absorbable suture. Take large bites through the pyloric ring.

Construct an anterior gastrojejunostomy by bringing up a loop of jejunum and suturing it at the site of the gastrotomy.

Place omentum over the duodenal suture line and place drains in close proximity to it. The pylorus will generally remain closed for only a few weeks. Even if a nonabsorbable suture is used, the pylorus will reopen spontaneously in most cases. If it does not, the suture can be cut endoscopically after the duodenal suture line has healed satisfactorily.

Severe combined duodenal and pancreatic injuries, particularly when accompanied by profuse bleeding, may require pancreaticoduodenectomy.

REFERENCES

1. Androulakis J, Colborn GL, Skandalakis PN, et al. Embryologic and anatomic basis of duodenal surgery. *Surg Clin North Am* 2000;80:171–199. (Provides excellent review of anatomy and embryology.)
2. Asensio JA, Demetriades D, Berne JD, et al. A unified approach to the surgical exposure of pancreatic and duodenal injuries. *Am J Surg* 1997;174:54–60. (Presents comprehensive review of management options.)
3. Cattell RB, Braasch JW. A technique for the exposure of the third and fourth portions of the duodenum. *Surg Gynecol Obstet* 1960;111:379. (Describes wide exposure of entire duodenum.)
4. Donohue JH, Crass RA, Trunkey DD. The management of duodenal and other small intestinal trauma. *World J Surg* 1985;9:904.
5. Martin TD, Feleciano DV, Mattox KL, et al. Severe duodenal injuries: treatment with pyloric exclusion and gastrojejunostomy. *Arch Surg* 1983;118:631.
6. Nauta RJ. Duodenojejunostomy as an alternative to anastomosis of the small intestine at the ligament of Treitz. *Surg Gynecol Obstet* 1990; 170:172–174.
7. Snyder WH, Weigelt JA, Watkins WL, et al. The surgical management of duodenal trauma: precepts based on a review of 247 cases. *Arch Surg* 1980;115:422.
8. Walley BD, Goco I. Duodenal patch grafting. *Am J Surg* 1980;140: 706.

CHAPTER 53

Laparoscopic Roux-en-Y Gastric Bypass

James W. Maher

Laparoscopic Roux-en-Y gastric bypass, one of the most technically demanding laparoscopic procedures, is emerging as the preferred method for treating morbid obesity when nonsurgical therapy has failed.

Patient Position and Trocar Position (Fig. 53.1)

Technical and Anatomic Points

A Foley catheter is inserted into the bladder. The patient is positioned supine on the table with the right arm tucked to the side. The left arm is positioned on an arm board. A foot board is applied to the end of the table to facilitate placement of the patient in reversed Trendelenburg position to aid exposure in the upper abdomen.

The surgeon stands on the patients right, the assistant and scope holder on the patients left. Elevate the umbilical plate with two Allis clamps and insert a Veress needle into the abdomen approximately 15 cm below the xiphoid and 2-3 cm to the left of the midline. Do not use the umbilicus as a landmark because it is displaced inferiorly in many morbidly obese patients. Insufflate the abdomen with a high flow insufflator to an intraabdominal pressure of 15 cm water. Next insert a five mm trocar in the left upper quadrant and place a 5 mm 30 degree scope to guide insertion of the other trocars. The next trocar is a 5 mm trocar inserted in the right upper quadrant laterally to allow liver retraction. Insert a 10 mm trocar into the midepigastrium to the patients left. Its position should generally be just below the level at which the ligamentum teres begins. This trocar will be used for the 10 mm 45 degree scope throughout the procedure. Insert a 12 mm port at the same level in the right epigastrium; this will serve as one of the surgeons' operating ports. Take care not to place this port too inferior since this may compromise the ability of the instruments to reach the operating area. Next place the liver retractor. Retract the liver superiorly and fix the retractor to the table with a retractor holder to provide stable exposure. Insert another 5 mm trocar into the right upper quadrant as the second operating port. Take care to place this port below the liver retractor and free of the round ligament. Inserting a long needle through the abdominal wall in the proposed trocar site may help prevent misplacement of this trocar. Finally, place a fourth 5 mm trocar in the left upper quadrant as a second port for the assistant.

Exposure of the Angle of His (Fig. 53.2)

Technical Points

Place the patient in reversed Trendelenburg position. The assistant retracts the omentum as well as the fundus inferiorly. A fat pad known as the gastroesophageal fat pad, or Belsey's fat pad, overlies and in many cases obscures the gastroesophageal junction and the angle of His. Excise this pad with an ultrasonic shears to expose the angle of His (Fig. 53.2A). Incise the peritoneum in this area with the ultrasonic shears and gently dissect the area behind the angle of His with an articulating angled dissector (Fig. 53.2B).

Anatomic Points

Recall that a small artery, termed Belsey's artery, frequently runs transversely across the gastroesophageal junction in the associated fat pad. Division of this pad must be performed with an instrument capable of achieving hemostasis such as the ultrasonic shears.

LIST OF STRUCTURES

Umbilicus	Greater curvature	Lesser (gastrohepatic) omentum
Stomach	Lesser curvature	Jejunum
Fundus	Esophagogastric junction	Ligament of Treitz
Incisura	Esophagus	Transverse colon
Angle of His	Belsey's fat pad	Mesocolon
	Greater omentum	

FIGURE 53.1
PATIENT POSITION AND TROCAR POSITION

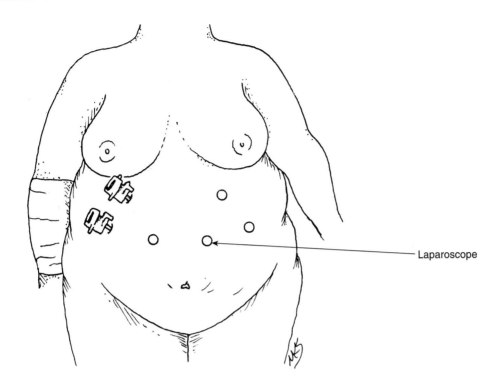

Laparoscope

Determining Pouch Size and Dissection of the
Lesser Curve (Fig. 53.3)

Technical and Anatomic Points

A Baker tube is inserted perorally into the stomach by the anesthetist. Have the balloon inflated with 15 cc of air and the tube then gently withdrawn until the balloon is stopped by the esophagogastric junction and resistance is felt. This balloon is used to estimate where the stomach should be divided to produce a 15 cc pouch. Mark this point on the serosa of the cardia with cautery. Next, the lesser curvature vessels below this must be divided with the ultrasonic shears on the

FIGURE 53.2
EXPOSURE OF THE ANGLE OF HIS

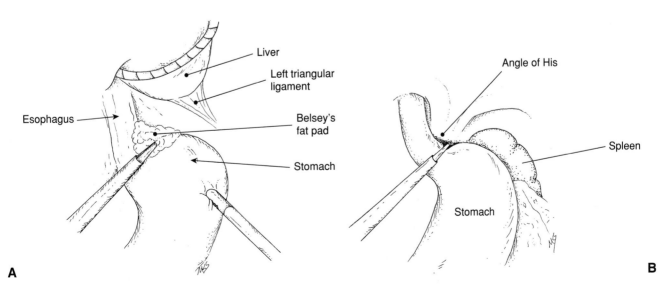

Liver

Left triangular ligament

Esophagus

Belsey's fat pad

Stomach

Angle of His

Spleen

Stomach

A

B

stomach wall to allow access to the lesser sac (Fig. 53.3A). The assistant should grasp the lesser curvature at the level of the marked spot with forceps and attempt to roll the lesser curvature laterally as the dissection progresses. With the other hand, the assistant may use a laparoscopic suction device to place traction distally near the incisura. Grasp the gastrohepatic omentum to give medial traction with the left hand while using the ultrasonic shears in the right. Work through the fatty lesser omentum until, eventually, the lesser sac is entered.

Enlarge this opening to allow dissection near the angle of His from behind connecting the two areas, lesser and greater sac (Fig. 53.3B). An articulating dissector may be helpful in this regard. Do not carry the dissection proximally on the lesser curve above the marked spot to avoid the risk of devascularizing the proximal gastric pouch.

Anatomic Points

Recall that the blood supply to the proximal stomach is derived from the left gastric artery, which is the smallest branch of the celiac artery (see also part A of the orientation figure that accompanies Chapter 48). Potential collateral circulation

---

FIGURE 53.3
DETERMINING POUCH SIZE AND DISSECTION OF THE LESSER CURVE

A

B

FIGURE 53.3   (Continued)

Esophagus

Grasper emerging
at angle of His

C

coming from the short gastric vessels will be divided in the course of developing the pouch.

Dividing the Stomach (Fig. 53.4)

Technical Points

Have the Baker tube and any other devices that may have been inserted into the stomach withdrawn. Use an endoscopic linear cutting stapler to transect the stomach. Orient the first stapler load transversely, then direct subsequent loads toward the angle of His until division of the stomach is complete. Obtain hemostasis with electrocautery or suture ligatures as needed.

Next, have the assistant elevate the distal stomach to allow the surgeon to clear the lesser sac of any adhesions that might later interfere with passage of the Roux limb. Insert a white Penrose drain inferiorly into the lesser sac. This drain will later be sutured to the Roux limb to assist in passing it into the upper abdomen. It is also an aid in identifying the lesser sac when making the mesocolic incision into the sac from below the colon.

FIGURE 53.4
DIVIDING THE STOMACH

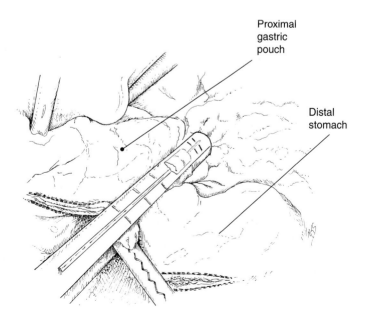

Proximal
gastric
pouch

Distal
stomach

FIGURE 53.5
OPENING THE MESOCOLON AND DIVIDING THE JEJUNUM

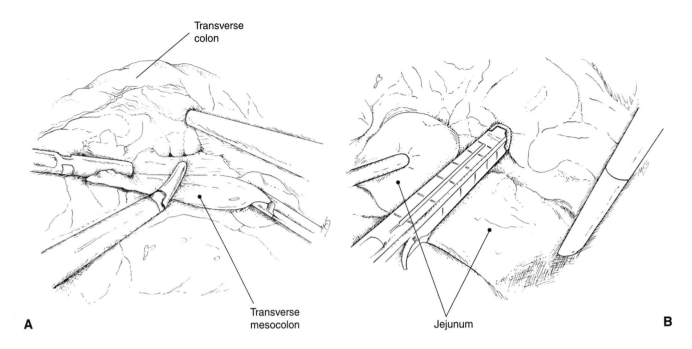

A

B

Opening the Mesocolon and Dividing the Jejunum (Fig. 53.5)

Technical Points

Have the table taken out of reversed Trendelenburg position. The scope holder moves temporarily to the patient's left. Retract omentum and transverse colon superiorly into the upper abdomen where it is held by the assistant.

Identify the ligament of Treitz and grasp the mesocolon two centimeters above and two centimeters to the patient's left of the ligament of Treitz. Use the ultrasonic shears to incise the mesocolon until the lesser sac is identified (Fig. 53.5A). In some patients the mesocolon is quite thick. When the sac is entered it should be possible to identify the white Penrose drain and draw the drain down into the opening.

Next, trace the jejunum 30 cm distal to the ligament of Treitz and divide it with a linear cutting stapler (Fig. 53.5B). Use a second firing of the linear stapler to divide small bowel mesentery if necessary. Mark the distal bowel with a stitch to avoid confusion with the proximal end of the bowel.

Fashioning the Enteroenterostomy (Fig. 53.6)

Technical Points

Measure the jejunum 75 cm distal to the point of transection. Approximate this point on its antimesenteric border to the antimesenteric border of the proximal bowel with a single stitch. The assistant holds up on this stitch and enterotomies are made with the harmonic scalpel. Insert a linear cutting

stapler and fire it to fashion the side to side stapled anastomosis (Fig. 53.6A).

Approximate the two edges of the staple line with another stitch (Fig. 53.6B). With the assistant holding up on this stitch, close the enterotomies with a second firing of the stapler, taking care not to compromise the lumen of the in-continuity bowel (Fig. 53.6C). Place sutures at the distal end of the enteroenterostomy staple line to take tension off the anastomosis and between the proximal jejunum and the in-continuity jejunum (the so-called "anti-obstruction" stitch). Close the mesenteric defect with a running suture.

Passage of the Distal Jejunum Through the Mesocolic Defect into the Lesser Sac (Fig. 53.7)

Technical Points

Suture the distal jejunum (with its marking stitch attached) to the Penrose drain. Grasp the drain with an articulating Babcock type clamp and pass it through the mesocolon into the upper abdomen with the articulation oriented anteriorly.

Again have the table placed in steep reversed Trendelenburg position and allow the colon and omentum to fall into the lower abdomen. Grasp the drain and use it to draw the attached jejunum into the appropriate position in the upper abdomen. Take care that the jejunum is not twisted on its mesentery. One helpful way to avoid this is to note the orientation of the drain and mesentery of the jejunum prior to passing it.

Attach the jejunum to the proximal gastric staple line at the angle of His with a single stitch.

FIGURE 53.6
FASHIONING THE ENTEROENTEROSTOMY

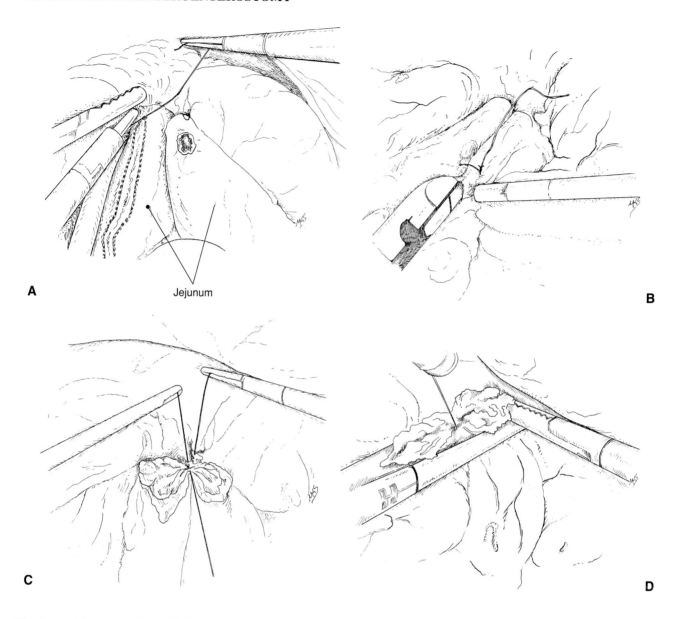

A

Jejunum

B

C

D

The Gastrojejunostomy (Fig. 53.8)

Technical and Anatomic Points

Attach the jejunum to the posterior aspect of the proximal gastric pouch using a running suture that begins at the angle of His and ends at the lesser curvature.

Next choose a suitable site for the gastrotomy and jejunotomy and make these with the harmonic scalpel. Insert a linear stapler into the two openings and pass it to the 2.5 cm mark (Fig. 53.8A). Fire the stapler, creating a 2.5 cm side to side anastomosis.

Next, go to the patient's head and pass the upper GI endoscope through the mouth and into the proximal stomach. The standard scope is 30 French in diameter. Pass this through the anastomosis, with the aid of the assistant, and into the proximal jejunum. The scope helps to prevent narrowing of

the anastomosis during closure of the enterotomies and will later be used to test the anastomosis.

Close the enterotomy with a running full-thickness stitch. Cover the gastric staple line from lesser to greater curve with a second running layer of Lembert sutures (Fig. 53.8B). Clamp the bowel distal to the anastomosis with a bowel clamp and use the irrigator to fill the left upper quadrant with fluid.

Again go to the patient's head and slowly withdraws the scope while insufflating air to test the anastamosis (Fig. 53.8C). The assistant carefully looks for any bubbling which might indicate a leak. If none is found, aspirate the insufflated air and remove the bowel clamp.

Insert a Jackson-Pratt drain and place it behind the gastrojejunostomy. Bring this drain out through the trocar site used for the liver retractor. The drain will remain in place for 10 days to detect any possible leaks.

FIGURE 53.7
PASSAGE OF THE DISTAL JEJUNUM THROUGH THE MESOCOLIC DEFECT INTO THE LESSER SAC

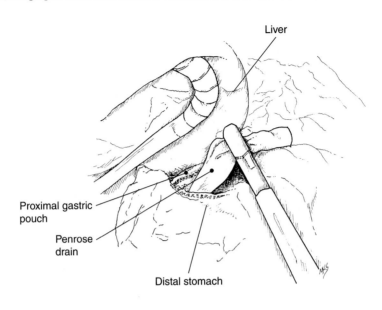

Liver

Proximal gastric pouch

Penrose drain

Distal stomach

FIGURE 53.8
THE GASTROJEJUNOSTOMY

A

B

C

D

FIGURE 53.9
CLOSING THE MESOCOLIC DEFECT AND PETERSON'S DEFECT

Closing the Mesocolic Defect and Peterson's Defect (Fig. 53.9)

Technical Points

Place the table flat and reestablish exposure of the mesocolon. Reduce any redundant jejunum into the lower abdomen and suture the mesocolon to the jejunum with several interrupted sutures.

Close Peterson's defect, that space between the jejunal mesentery and the mesocolon, with a few sutures as the assistant holds the jejunum towards the left.

Close the fascia of the large ports (10 mm and 12 mm). Inspect all port sites for secure hemostasis before removing the trocars. Close the skin in the usual fashion.

REFERENCE

1. Schauer PR, Ikramuddin S. Laparoscopic surgery for morbid obesity. *Surg Clin North Am* 2001;81:1145–1179.

CHAPTER 54

Splenectomy and Splenorrhaphy

Total splenectomy is performed for hematologic indications and for traumatic injury. Special techniques for repairing the injured spleen are discussed in Figs. 54.8 and 54.9. A staging laparotomy procedure for Hodgkin's disease is discussed in Fig. 54.10. Laparoscopic splenectomy an increasingly attractive alternative for elective splenectomy, is described in Chapter 55.

Splenic Exploration and Assessment of Mobility (Fig. 54.1)

Technical Points

Position the patient supine on the operating table. If the spleen is small, place a folded sheet under the left costal margin to elevate the operative field. A left subcostal incision (Fig. 54.1A) provides the best exposure for a small or normal-sized spleen. However, this incision divides muscles and may result in wound hematoma in patients with profound thrombocytopenia. As the spleen enlarges, it descends from the left upper quadrant, displacing the hilar vascular structures medially. Thus, in a patient with an enlarged spleen, use a midline or left paramedian incision for splenic exposure (Fig. 54.1B).

Explore the abdomen. Pass your nondominant hand up over the spleen and assess its mobility and size, as well as the nature and location of the attachments to the diaphragm and retroperitoneum.

At this point, decide whether or not to proceed with preliminary ligation of the splenic artery in the lesser sac. This maneuver decreases splenic blood flow and should be considered in the patient with a large spleen, particularly when difficulty in mobilization is anticipated.

Anatomic Points

The spleen develops embryologically in the dorsal mesogastrium. As the stomach rotates, the greater omentum develops as an elongation and subsequent redundancy of the dorsal mesogastrium. The pancreas (also initially within the dorsal mesogastrium) becomes retroduodenal. The spleen comes to lie in the left hypochondriac region, interposed between the diaphragm and left kidney posteriorly and the fundus of the stomach anteriorly. Unlike the pancreas, it does not become retroperitoneal, but instead retains its intraperitoneal status, at the left extremity of the lesser sacromental bursa.

Short bilaminar peritoneal folds attach the spleen to the fundus of the stomach (gastrosplenic or gastrolienal ligament) and to the left kidney and diaphragm (splenorenal or phrenicosplenic ligament) (Fig. 54.1C). The gastrosplenic ligament is really the left extremity of the gastrocolic ligament; thus, there is also a splenocolic ligament. The splenorenal ligament is the left extremity of the transverse mesocolon. The attachments of spleen to colon are avascular.

The sides of these ligaments (gastrosplenic and splenorenal) that contribute to the walls of the lesser sac are continuous at the hilum, whereas the sides that are part of the boundary of the general peritoneal cavity are separated by the visceral peritoneal investment of the spleen. In other words, the spleen is invested with the general peritoneal layer of the embryologic dorsal mesogastrium. Both gastrosplenic and splenorenal ligaments are vascular. The splenorenal ligament supports the splenic artery and vein (and their splenic ramifications), whereas the gastrosplenic ligament supports those branches of the splenic artery (and the accompanying veins)—namely, the left gastroepiploic artery and short gastric arteries—that supply the greater curvature and fundus of the stomach.

The left gastroepiploic artery may originate from one of the splenic branches, rather than from the splenic artery proper. The short gastric arteries, of which there are typically four to six, can arise from the left gastroepiploic artery, the splenic artery proper, the splenic branches of the splenic artery, or any combination thereof.

LIST OF STRUCTURES

Spleen	Transverse mesocolon	Pancreas
Splenic artery	Celiac nodes	Gastrosplenic ligament
Splenic vein	Hepatoduodenal nodes	Gastrocolic ligament
Stomach	Paraaortic nodes	Splenorenal ligament
Short gastric vessels	Iliac nodes	Lesser sac (omental bursa)
Left gastroepiploic artery	Mesenteric nodes	

FIGURE 54.1
SPLENIC EXPLORATION AND ASSESSMENT OF MOBILITY

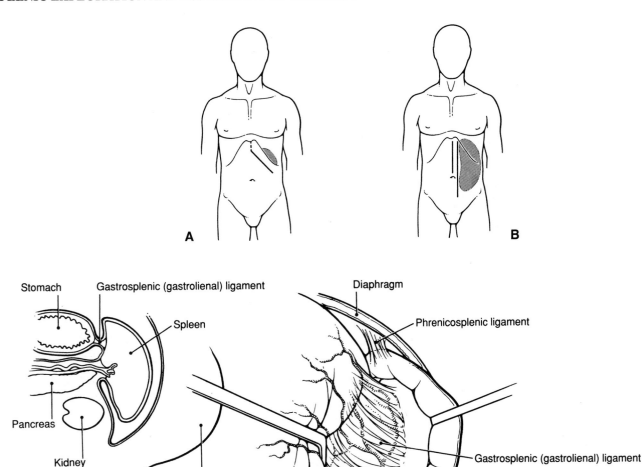

Stomach

Gastrosplenic (gastrolienal) ligament

Spleen

Pancreas

Kidney

Lesser curvature of the stomach

Diaphragm

Phrenicosplenic ligament

Gastrosplenic (gastrolienal) ligament

Splenocolic ligament

Gastrocolic ligament

A

B

C

Ligation of the Splenic Artery in the Lesser Sac (Fig. 54.2)

Technical Points

Enter the lesser sac by dividing the gastrocolic omentum. Serially clamp and ligate multiple branches of the gastroepiploic artery and vein until you have created a window in the gastrocolic omentum that is of sufficient size to admit retractors. Elevate the stomach, dividing the filmy avascular gastropancreatic folds as necessary to expose the pancreas. Identify the splenic artery where it loops along the upper border of the pancreas and pass a right-angle clamp under it. Ligate the splenic artery with a heavy silk tie.

FIGURE 54.2
LIGATION OF THE SPLENIC ARTERY IN THE LESSER SAC

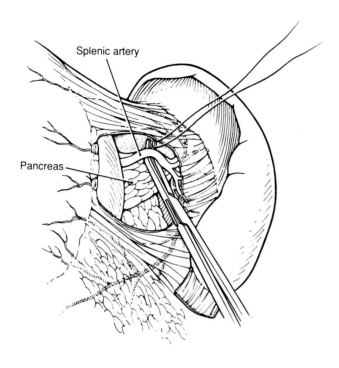

Anatomic Points

Make the gastrocolic window either between the stomach and gastroepiploic arcade or between the gastroepiploic arcade and colon. Nothing will be devascularized in either case owing to the free and abundant anastomoses in this area. After entering the lesser sac (omental bursa), observe the pancreas through the parietal peritoneum of the posterior wall of the lesser sac. The characteristic corkscrew course of the large splenic artery (which is about 5 mm in diameter) along the superior border of the pancreas is related to age. The tortuosity is maximal in the elderly, minimal in the young, and absent in infants and children. This tortuosity lifts the splenic artery up out of the retroperitoneum behind the pancreas. In a child, it may be necessary to incise the peritoneum carefully and elevate the superior border of the pancreas to find the splenic artery. The splenic vein is not invested in a common sheath with the artery. Instead, it is somewhat inferior, always retropancreatic, and never tortuous.

Mobilization of the Spleen (Fig. 54.3)

Technical Points

Place retractors on the left costal margin. Pass your nondominant hand up over the spleen and hook the posterior edge, pulling the spleen down strongly and rolling it medially. Use a laparotomy pad over the spleen to improve traction. By strong compression of the spleen and steady traction, coupled with good retraction up on the costal margin, one can create a space in which to work.

FIGURE 54.3
MOBILIZATION OF THE SPLEEN

A

B

Incise the peritoneum lateral to the spleen (Fig. 54.3A). Pass your nondominant hand under the medial leaf of the peritoneum and develop the plane deep to the spleen, the splenic vessels, and the tail of the pancreas. Mobilize the splenic flexure of the colon with the lower pole of the spleen. Mobilization of the spleen into the operative field will then be limited by the short gastric vessels and splenocolic ligaments (Fig. 54.3B).

Check the retroperitoneum and bed of the spleen for bleeding. Pack two laparotomy pads into the bed of the spleen.

Anatomic Points

Mobilization of the spleen should not exceed the limits imposed by the gastrosplenic ligament, as it is possible to avulse the short gastric blood vessels running in this ligament. The maneuver described partially recreates the embryonic midline position of the spleen in the dorsal mesogastrium. Incision of the peritoneum lateral to the spleen allows access to the relatively avascular fusion plane formed by fusion and subsequent degeneration of the original left leaf of dorsal mesogastrium with posterior parietal peritoneum. As the spleen, splenic vessels, and pancreas all begin their development in the dorsal mesogastrium, this fusion plane is posterior to these structures. The splenic flexure of the colon is mobilized with the spleen because of the variable presence of small vessels in this ligament. Placing traction on the short splenocolic ligament can tear the delicate splenic capsule. Although the spleen is to be removed, capsular damage at this point can result in a bloody operative field.

Division of the Short Gastric Vessels (Fig. 54.4)

Technical Points

Typically, three to four short gastric arteries (with accompanying veins) connect the spleen to the greater curvature of the stomach high up near the cardioesophageal junction. The highest of these is generally the shortest, and the gastric wall closely approximates the upper pole of the spleen. With the spleen mobilized into the operative field, pass a right-angle clamp behind the highest short gastric vessels and doubly ligate and divide them. Be careful not to include the wall of the stomach in the tie. Then, sequentially ligate and divide the remaining short gastric vessels. Inspect the ties on the greater curvature of the stomach. If the gastric wall has been injured or included in a tie, the area should be imbricated with a 3-0 silk Lembert suture.

Anatomic Points

As discussed earlier (Fig. 54.1C), the origin of the short gastric arteries is variable. As can be expected, the number of short gastric vessels is also variable. There may be as few as 2 or as many as 10. Often, these can be divided into a superior group and an inferior group. The superior group is shorter than the inferior one, and downward traction of the spleen, without concomitant movement of the gastric fundus, can result in troublesome bleeding at the time of operation. It is best to ligate and divide the most superior short gastric vessels first, working in an inferior direction. Because of the variability in the origin of the arteries, it is easier to ligate and divide them as close to the stomach as possible, rather than trying to ligate and divide them at their origin.

FIGURE 54.4
DIVISION OF THE SHORT GASTRIC VESSELS

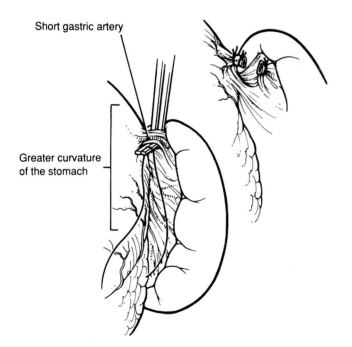

Short gastric artery

Greater curvature
of the stomach

FIGURE 54.5
DIVISION OF THE GASTROCOLIC LIGAMENT

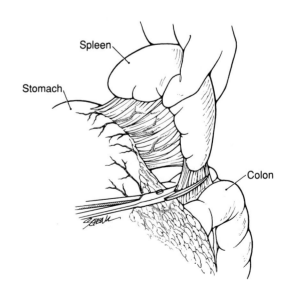

Spleen

Stomach

Colon

FIGURE 54.6
LIGATION OF THE HILAR VESSELS

Pancreas

A

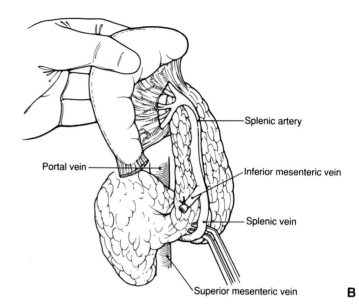

Splenic artery

Portal vein

Inferior mesenteric vein

Splenic vein

Superior mesenteric vein

B

Division of the Gastrocolic Ligament (Fig. 54.5)

Technical Points

The gastrocolic ligament commonly contains small, unnamed vessels that may cause troublesome bleeding. Thus, even if no vessels are visible in the fatty tissue connecting the lower pole of the spleen with the splenic flexure of the colon, divide this tissue with clamps and ties.

Anatomic Points

The gastrocolic ligament, when present, is the left continuation of the transverse mesocolon. It can have small vessels supplying the fat and other mesenteric structures, but there should be no anastomoses between vessels derived from the spleen and those derived from mesenteric structures. In all probability, the vessels will originate from the inferior proper splenic divisions of the splenic artery.

Ligation of the Hilar Vessels (Fig. 54.6)

Technical Points

The hilar vessels are best approached from the posterior aspect, with the spleen well-mobilized into the field. The tail of the pancreas extends for a variable extent into the region of the splenic hilum and may be difficult to differentiate from fatty and nodal tissue in the hilum. Individually ligate the terminal branches of the splenic artery and splenic vein close to the spleen. Suture-ligate the large branches.

Some surgeons prefer to ligate the splenic vein close to its juncture with the superior mesenteric vein, especially in cases of massive splenomegaly. This has the theoretical advantage of preventing thrombus within the stump of the splenic vein from propagating into the portal or superior mesenteric vein. To perform a more proximal ligation of the splenic vein, trace

the vein along the back of the mobilized tail of the pancreas and pass a right-angle clamp behind the vein at the desired point. Ligate the vein with a heavy silk tie.

Anatomic Points

Ligate the hilar vessels as close as possible to the spleen because the tail of the pancreas is frequently supplied by a recurrent branch from one of the segmental divisions of the splenic artery, usually an inferior segmental division. Although this recurrent artery, a caudal pancreatic artery, is frequently illustrated as anastomosing with pancreatic arteries that are more medial, the fact that necrosis of the tail of the pancreas is a recognized complication of splenectomy suggests that the anastomosis is either variable or potential.

With respect to ligation of the splenic vein, it is advisable, on the basis of anatomic arrangements, to locate the termination of the inferior mesenteric vein and ligate distal to this. As expected, this termination is variable. It can terminate by draining into the superior mesenteric vein, confluence of the superior mesenteric and splenic veins, or into the splenic vein. Regardless of where this termination occurs, it is always retropancreatic.

Searching for Accessory Spleens and Subsequent
Closure (Fig. 54.7)

Technical Points

Because many patients who undergo elective splenectomy have coagulation defects, hemostasis must be especially meticulous. The time spent double-checking for bleeding can also be used to conduct a search for accessory spleens which, if not found and removed, may cause a recurrence of the symptoms for which elective splenectomy was initially recommended.

FIGURE 54.7
SEARCHING FOR ACCESSORY SPLEENS AND SUBSEQUENT CLOSURE

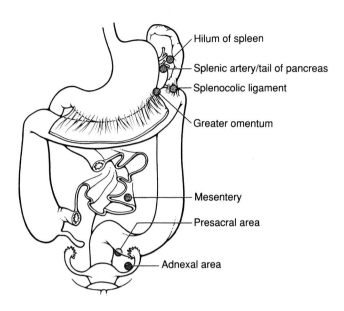

Hilum of spleen
Splenic artery/tail of pancreas
Splenocolic ligament
Greater omentum
Mesentery
Presacral area
Adnexal area

Check the sites of ligation of the hilar vessels and the region of the tail of the pancreas for bleeding. Remove the laparotomy pads that were placed in the bed of the spleen. Suture-ligate any persistent bleeding points in the retroperitoneum. If bleeding from the cut edges of the peritoneal reflection is a problem, oversew these edges with a running lock-stitch.

Search for accessory splenic tissue in the hilum of the spleen, in the gastrocolic omentum, around the tail of the pancreas, in the mesentery of the bowel, and in the pelvis. Most accessory spleens are found close to the spleen.

Anatomic Points

Accessory splenic tissue has been reported to be present in the abdominal cavity of 10% to 35% of individuals. Rarely, it has been reported found in the liver, scrotum, and pancreas. If an accessory spleen is present, there is typically only one; however, multiple accessory spleens have been reported. As stated earlier, most accessory spleens are located in the region of the spleen proper. The retroperitoneal region around the tail of the pancreas should be examined with great care, as this is an area in which accessory splenic tissue is often overlooked. The splenic tissue is usually less than 3 cm in diameter. In addition, a careful examination of the left ovary and uterine tube in the female, and the scrotum in males, is warranted because the spleen develops in close contact with the genital ridge.

Splenorrhaphy (Fig. 54.8)

Technical and Anatomic Points

Repair of the damaged spleen is often possible and should be attempted in patients who can tolerate the somewhat longer operative time required and the greater blood loss associated with it as compared with total splenectomy.

First, mobilize the spleen up into the operative field. Use the same procedure that is used for elective splenectomy. Ligate the short gastric vessels, if necessary, to mobilize the spleen fully. Use extreme care not to damage the spleen further. Obtain temporary control of any bleeding by applying direct pressure to the bleeding site using a laparotomy pad. It may be necessary to occlude the splenic vessels in the hilum with an atraumatic vascular clamp.

Capsular avulsion injuries occur when traction on the colon or stomach stretches the splenic capsule. These are common iatrogenic injuries. In such cases, apply direct pressure to the injury for 5 minutes. Then apply a piece of microfibrillar collagen sponge and again apply direct pressure. Do not use electrocautery; episodes of rebleeding are common. The argon beam coagulator is an ideal thermal hemostatic device for this situation.

Large capsular avulsion injuries or simple capsular lacerations (Fig. 54.8A) may require suturing. Choose a monofilament suture, such as 4-0 chromic catgut, and a fine taper-point needle. This particular suture is good because it is very soft when wet and hence is less likely than other monofilaments to saw through the capsule. Place a series of horizontal mattress sutures in such a way as to close the defect (Fig. 54.8B). As the capsule of the spleen is thin and flimsy, place sutures with precision and pull each suture through gently to avoid damaging the capsule. These sutures may be tied over pledgets, if desired, to decrease the chance of the suture's cutting through the capsule of the spleen (Fig. 54.8C). Tie the sutures gently. Use omentum to buttress the repair, if necessary (Fig. 54.8D).

If there is considerable damage to the spleen but the hilar vessels are intact, it may be possible to salvage the spleen by wrapping it in absorbable mesh (Fig. 54.8E,F). Debride the injured parenchyma and cut a piece of mesh large enough to enclose the spleen completely. Place a purse-string suture around the edge to create a bag. Tighten the purse-string around the hilum. Take care not to compromise venous return from the spleen. Make the wrap a little loose initially, then place a running suture on the outer aspect to tighten it. As the wrap works by compression, it must be snug and work to pull lacerated edges together in order to be effective. Check the completed wrap for hemostasis.

Partial Splenectomy (Fig. 54.9)

Technical Points

Extensive damage to one pole of the spleen, or damage to one of the hilar vessels, can be managed by partial splenectomy (Fig. 54.9A). Ligate the splenic artery branch or branches supplying the injured segment. The bleeding should stop or slow significantly. The spleen should turn dark and develop a line of demarcation. Cut through the spleen along this line of demarcation (Fig. 54.9B). Suture-ligate occasional bleeding points. If necessary, close the transected edge with a series of horizontal mattress sutures to ensure hemostasis (Fig. 54.9C,D).

FIGURE 54.8
SPLENORRHAPHY

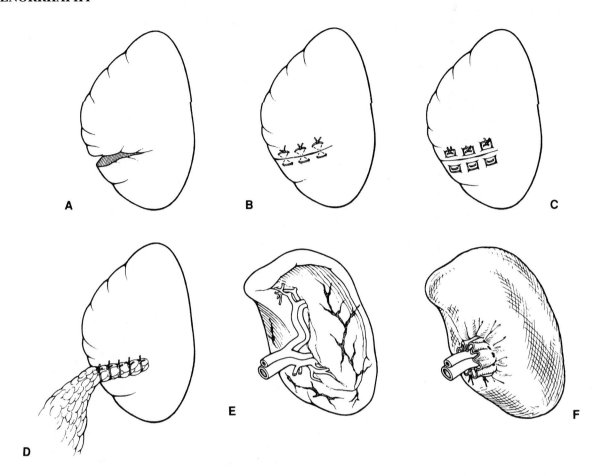

Anatomic Points

As the portal venous system lacks functional valves, it is necessary to ligate splenic segmental tributaries of the splenic vein, as well. These segmental tributaries drain segments supplied by corresponding arteries and are not intersegmental, as is the case in some other segmental organs.

Staging Laparotomy for Hodgkin's Disease (Fig. 54.10)

Technical Points

A staging laparotomy for Hodgkin's disease consists of splenectomy, liver biopsy, and biopsy of multiple intra-abdominal node groups; in addition, it may include biopsy of the iliac crest bone and oophoropexy (in the female). Use a long midline incision, as all four quadrants of the abdomen must be explored.

Liver Biopsy

Perform a liver biopsy first to minimize changes in liver histology caused by operative trauma. Obtain a biopsy specimen from any suspicious nodules. Take a wedge biopsy specimen from one lobe and a deep core biopsy specimen (using a liver biopsy needle) from the other lobe.

Splenectomy

Next, proceed with splenectomy. Include the splenic hilar lymph nodes with the specimen. Send the spleen in the fresh state to the pathologist. If the spleen shows obvious involvement by Hodgkin's disease, the tedious search for and biopsy of intra-abdominal node groups can be curtailed. Mark the hilum of the spleen with a hemoclip.

Next, systematically expose and palpate the para-aortic, celiac, hepatoduodenal, mesenteric, and iliac lymph nodes. Obtain biopsy specimens from representative nodes from each group, as well as from any suspicious masses.

Celiac Nodes

Expose the celiac (or upper para-aortic) nodes by opening a window through the lesser omentum along the lesser curvature of the stomach. This can usually be done through an avascular region, which can easily be identified in thin patients. Palpate the region of the celiac axis and excise or obtain

FIGURE 54.9
PARTIAL SPLENECTOMY

biopsy specimens from any enlarged nodes, or take a representative sample. Be careful not to damage the celiac artery or its branches.

Hepatoduodenal Nodes

Palpate the region of the hepatoduodenal ligament. Divide the filmy adhesions between the gallbladder and omentum or colon, if necessary, to expose the region. Nodes are commonly found in the region of the cystic duct and porta hepatis.

Paraaortic Nodes

Expose the abdominal aorta by lifting the omentum and transverse colon. Reflect the small bowel to the right, eviscerating the intestines, if necessary, to improve exposure. Palpate the abdominal aorta for the presence of enlarged nodes. Incise the peritoneum from just below the ligament of Treitz to the region just above the inferior mesenteric artery. If nodes are palpable behind the fourth portion of the duodenum at the ligament of Treitz, mobilize the fourth portion of the

duodenum by incising the peritoneum lateral to the duodenum, then reflect the duodenum upward to expose the nodes.

If no nodes are palpable, explore the region to the left and deep in the groove adjacent to the abdominal aorta, excising fatty tissue from this area. Avoid the nearby sympathetic trunk.

Iliac Nodes

Incise the peritoneum overlying the iliac vessels. Identify the ureter as it crosses the common iliac artery at the bifurcation of the iliac vessels. Iliac nodes lie lateral and deep to the iliac vessels, just past the bifurcation of the iliac artery.

Mesenteric Nodes

Nodes are commonly palpable in the mesentery of the terminal ileum and elsewhere along the mesentery of the small intestine. Incise the peritoneum overlying the largest of these nodes and carefully shell out a node or two for biopsy. In addition, remove any enlarged or suspicious node, regardless of its location.

FIGURE 54.10
STAGING LAPAROTOMY FOR HODGKIN'S DISEASE

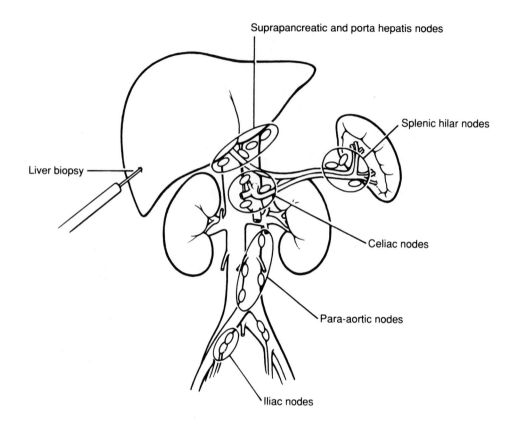

Biopsy of the Iliac Crest Bone

Expose the anterior iliac crest. Use a periosteal elevator to strip the periosteum. Use a small electric saw to remove a segment of the iliac crest that includes bone marrow.

Oophoropexy

Mobilize the tubes and ovaries gently by incising their lateral peritoneal attachments. Tack the ovaries to the posterior surface of the uterus with nonabsorbable suture. The ovaries and tubes should lie comfortably in the pouch of Douglas. Mark the lateral border of each ovary with a metal clip.

Anatomic Points

Celiac Nodes

The celiac nodes are the last in a chain of preaortic nodes that drain the gastrointestinal system. The para-aortic nodes in approximately the same location are terminal nodes in a chain that drain the lower extremities, parietes, and paired retroperitoneal and genitourinary organs.

Hepatoduodenal Nodes

The hepatoduodenal nodes are in the hepatoduodenal ligament, near the free right edge of the lesser omentum in close proximity to the hepatic artery. These nodes drain those structures supplied by the hepatic artery, and send efferents to the celiac nodes.

Paraaortic Nodes

Nodes in the para-aortic region (as described earlier in the section on technical points) are part of the chain draining the lower extremities, parietes, and genitourinary organs. They are close to the abdominal sympathetic chain, and care should be taken not to confuse them with these ganglia. Gentle palpation and attention to their size and their more "peritoneal" than "parietal" location should allow one to distinguish them.

Iliac Nodes

Nodes along the common and external iliac artery drain the extremities, parietes, and skin of the lower trunk. Nodes along the internal iliac artery are responsible for drainage of pelvic viscera.

Mesenteric Nodes

The mesenteric nodes drain the portion of bowel supplied by the intestinal artery (e.g., specific jejunal or ileal) with which they are associated.

Oophoropexy

The neurovascular supply to the ovaries and distal part of the uterine tubes runs through the suspensory ligament, that portion of the broad ligament extending from the pelvic wall to the uterine tube and ovary. Consequently, when these ligaments are incised, care must be taken to permit medial mobilization of the ovaries and uterine tubes.

REFERENCES

1. Cahill CJ, Wastell C. Splenic conservation. *Surg Annu* 1990;22:379. (Describes multiple techniques for splenic salvage.)
2. Cannon WB, Kaplan HS, Dorfman RF, et al. Staging laparotomy with splenectomy in Hodgkin's disease. *Surg Annu* 1975;7:103.
3. Cioffiro W, Schein CJ, Gliedman ML. Splenic injury during abdominal surgery. *Arch Surg* 1976;111:167. (Discusses mechanisms of iatrogenic splenic injury based on attachments of the spleen and mechanical forces exerted during surgery.)
4. Dawson DL, Molina ME, Scott-Conner CEH. Venous segmentation of the human spleen: a corrosion case study. *Am Surg* 1986;52:253. (Venous segmentation is similar to arterial segmentation.)
5. Dixon JA, Miller F, McCloskey D, et al. Anatomy and techniques in segmental splenectomy. *Surg Gynecol Obstet* 1980;150:516.
6. Douglas BE, Baggenstoss AH, Hollinshead WH. The anatomy of the portal vein and its tributaries. *Surg Gynecol Obstet* 1950;91:562.
7. Dunham CM, Cornwell EE III, Militello P. The role of the argon beam coagulator in splenic salvage. *Surg Gynecol Obstet* 1991;173:179.
8. Fingerhut A, Oberlin P, Cotte JL. Splenic salvage using an absorbable mesh: feasibility, reliability and safety. *Br J Surg* 1992;79:325.
9. Garcia-Porrero JA, Lemes A. Arterial segmentation and subsegmentation in the human spleen. *Acta Anat* 1988;131:276.
10. Gayet B, Fekete F. Splenorrhaphy by perisplenic prosthesis: a new method that is simple, reliable, and safe. *Contemp Surg* 1987;30:52.
11. Grieco MB, Cade B. Staging laparotomy in Hodgkin's disease. *Surg Clin North Am* 1980;60:369.
12. Hoppe RT, Castellino RA. The staging of Hodgkin's disease. *PPO Updates* 1990;4:4.
13. Lange DA, Zaret P, Merlotti GL, et al. The use of absorbable mesh in splenic trauma. *J Trauma* 1988;28:269.
14. Michels NA. The variational anatomy of the spleen and the splenic artery. *Am J Anat* 1942;70:21.
15. Millikan JS, Moore EE, Moore GE, et al. Alternatives to splenectomy in adults after trauma: repair, partial resection, and reimplantation of splenic tissue. *Am J Surg* 1982;144:711.
16. Mitchell RI, Peters MV. Lymph node biopsy during laparotomy for the staging of Hodgkin's disease. *Ann Surg* 1973;178:698.
17. Morgenstern L. Technique of partial splenectomy. *Probl Gen Surg* 1990;7:103.
18. Pemberton LB, Skandalakis LJ. Indications for and technique of total splenectomy. *Probl Gen Surg* 1990;7:85.
19. Trooskin SZ, Flancbaum K, Boyarsky AH, et al. A simplified approach to techniques of splenic salvage. *Surg Gynecol Obstet* 1989;168:546. (Provides excellent description of partial splenectomy.)
20. Uranus S, Kronberger L, Kraft-Kine J. Partial splenic resection using the TA-stapler. *Am J Surg* 1994;168:49. (Describes useful technique for small soft spleens.)
21. Waizer A, Baniel J, Zin Y, et al. Clinical implications of anatomic variations of the splenic artery. *Surg Gynecol Obstet* 1989;168:57.

CHAPTER 55

Laparoscopic Splenectomy

Laparoscopic splenectomy is easiest for small spleens (for example, the normal sized spleen associated with ITP). Techniques have been developed for moderate to large sized spleens, but in general, the larger the spleen the more difficult the surgery. The first laparoscopic splenectomies were performed with the patient supine, in a manner similar to that used during open splenectomy. The technique described here, in which the patient is placed in the lateral position and the peritoneal attachments of the spleen are used to suspend it in place is sometimes termed the "hanging spleen" technique. References at the end give details of other techniques and modifications for large spleens, as well as techniques for partial splenectomy and excision of splenic cysts.

Initial Exposure (Fig. 55.1)

Technical Points

Place the patient in the full lateral decubitus position, with the left side up. The general trocar pattern is shown in Fig. 55.1A. A 30 or 45 degree laparoscope gives optimum visualization. Place the laparoscope through an umbilical port. Operating trocars need to be large enough (generally 12 mm) to accommodate the endoscopic linear cutting stapler, if that is planned. Reverse Trendelenburg positioning allows gravity to assist in retraction.

Use the ultrasonic scalpel to mobilize and detach the splenic flexure of the colon from the spleen by first dividing the peritoneal reflection of the descending colon. Start inferiorly at a convenient point and progress cephalad (Fig. 55.1B). Fully divide the phrenicocolic ligament, and then the splenocolic ligament (Fig. 55.1C). Leave the splenophrenic ligament intact, to allow the spleen to "hang" from this ligament during subsequent dissection.

Rotate the colon medially and inferiorly out of the field. Then sequentially divide the anterior peritoneal folds and short gastric vessels (see Fig. 42.2A,B in Chapter 42). This creates an opening into the lesser sac through which the splenic hilum should be visible. Mobilize and rotate the stomach medially out of the field.

Anatomic Points

The peritoneal attachments and topographic relations of the spleen were discussed in Chapter 54. The shape of the spleen gives the laparoscopic surgeon a clue as to the pattern of vessels in the hilum. The rounded shape shown in Fig. 55.1A–C) correlates with late branching (within one or two centimeters of the hilum) of the splenic artery and vein. This implies a single well-defined vascular pedicle that is easy to identify and control. This magistral splenic artery pattern occurs in only approximately 30% of individuals.

In the remainder, the splenic artery and vein divide into branches at a distance from the hilum and multiple vessels must be identified and controlled, often in close proximity to the tail of the pancreas. The sharply notched border of the spleen shown in Fig. 55.1D correlates with early branching of the splenic vessels. A superior polar splenic artery is found in 13%, an inferior polar artery in 31%, and both are identified in 16% of normal individuals.

Division of Hilar Vessels (Fig. 55.2)

Technical and Anatomic Points

Ideally, identify the splenic artery near the hilum of the spleen but before it branches. Look for the tip of the pancreas and find a site on the splenic artery that is beyond the tip of the pancreas. Seek the splenic vein deep to splenic artery and pancreas, and generally a little inferior to the splenic artery (Fig. 55.2A). Multiple vessels associated with a notched splenic border are best individually ligated or clipped (Fig. 55.2A,B).

If the hilar vessels form a neat packet hear the splenic hilum, use an endoscopic linear stapler to secure them (Fig. 55.2C). It may be necessary to place a fan retractor and

LIST OF STRUCTURES

Spleen	Colon	Phrenicocolic ligament
Splenic artery	Descending colon	Splenophrenic ligament
Superior polar artery	Splenic flexure	Lesser sac
Inferior polar artery	Greater omentum	Stomach
	Splenocolic ligament	Short gastric vessels

FIGURE 55.1

INITIAL EXPOSURE (**B** and **C** from Wind GG. The spleen. In: *Applied laparoscopic anatomy: abdomen and pelvis.* Baltimore: Williams & Wilkins, 1997:187–216, with permission; **D** from Scott-Conner CEH, Cuschieri A, Carter FJ. Spleen and pancreas. In: *Minimal access surgical anatomy.* Philadelphia: Lippincott Williams & Wilkins, 2000:139–163, with permission.)

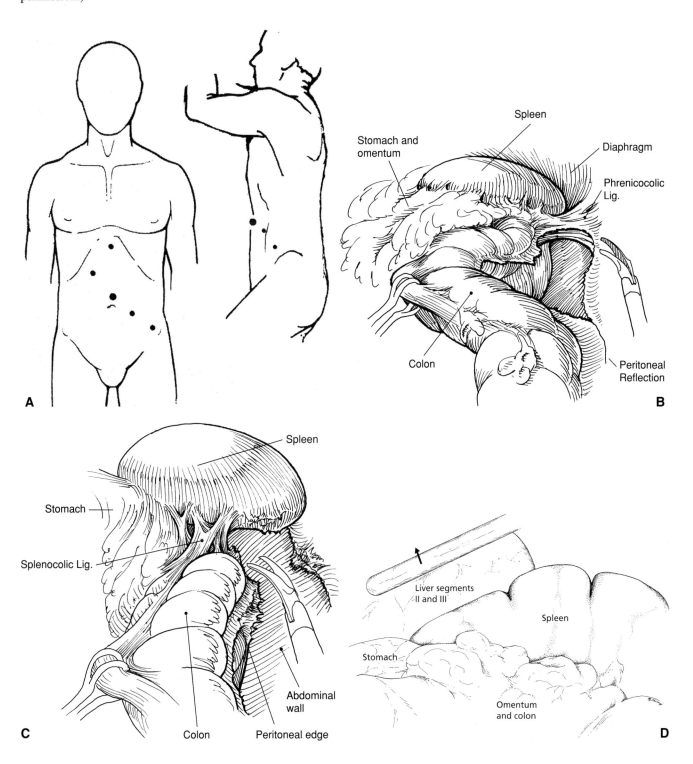

gently elevate the spleen to secure adequate visualization of the hilum. Manipulate the spleen with extreme gentleness to avoid bleeding; even a small amount of bleeding can obscure visualization.

Develop the plane above and below the hilar vessels. The vessels may be taken in a single firing of the stapler if located close to each other. Avoid superimposing one vessel on the other because postoperative arteriovenous fistula may complicate mass ligation or stapling. Gently insert the endoscopic cutting linear stapler (vascular cartridge) and manipulate splenic artery and vein within the jaws. Fire and remove the stapler.

Divide the remaining peritoneal attachments with an ultrasonic scalpel (Fig. 55.2D).

FIGURE 55.2

DIVISION OF HILAR VESSELS (**A** and **B** from Scott-Conner CEH, Cuschieri A, Carter FJ. Spleen and pancreas. In: *Minimal access surgical anatomy.* Philadelphia: Lippincott Williams & Wilkins, 2000:139–163, with permission; **C** and **D** from Wind GG. The spleen. In: *Applied laparoscopic anatomy: abdomen and pelvis.* Baltimore: Williams & Wilkins, 1997:187–216, with permission.)

FIGURE 55.2   (Continued)

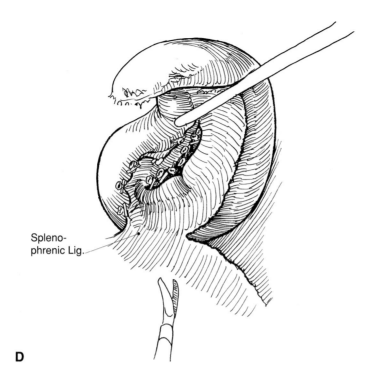

Spleno-
phrenic Lig.

D

FIGURE 55.3
REMOVAL OF SPLEEN AND SEARCH FOR ACCESSORY SPLEENS (**A** from Rege RV. Laparoscopic splenectomy.
In: Scott-Conner CEH, ed. *The SAGES manual.* New York: Springer-Verlag, 1999, with permission; **B** from Wind GG. The
spleen. In: *Applied laparoscopic anatomy: abdomen and pelvis.* Baltimore: Williams & Wilkins, 1997:187–216, with
permission.)

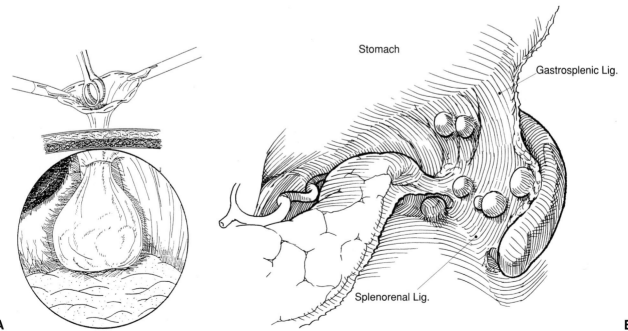

Stomach

Gastrosplenic Lig.

Splenorenal Lig.

A

B

Removal of Spleen and Search for Accessory Spleens (Fig. 55.3)

Technical Points

Place the spleen in a strong endoscopic retrieval bag. Withdraw the open mouth of the bag through the abdominal wall. Use a ring forceps, your fingers, a suction irrigator, or specially designed morcellator to fragment and suck out the spleen (Fig. 55.3A). Remove the bag.

Search for accessory spleens in the usual locations before desufflating the abdomen and closing the trocar sites.

Anatomic Points

There has been a suggestion that accessory spleens are more difficult to find during laparoscopic splenectomy. The most common location is in the splenic hilum, as previous discussed (see Fig. 54.7). Throughout the dissection, remain alert to the possibility of accessory spleens, particularly when the splenic hilum is first exposed, as shown in Figure 55.3B.

REFERENCES

1. MacFadyen BV, Litwin D, Park A, et al. Laparoscopic splenectomy. II. Technical considerations. *Contemp Surg* 2000;56:398–407.
2. Rescorla FJ, Breitfeld PP, West KW, et al. A case controlled comparison of open and laparoscopic splenectomy in children. *Surgery* 1998;124:670–676.
3. Silvestri F, Russo D, Fanin R, et al. Laparoscopic splenectomy in the management of hematological diseases. *Haematologica* 1995;80:47–49.
4. Terrosu G, Donini A, Silvestri F, et al. Laparoscopic splenectomy in the management of hematological diseases: surgical technique and outcome of 17 patients. *Surg Endosc* 1996;441–445.
5. Wind GG. The spleen. In: *Applied laparoscopic anatomy: abdomen and pelvis.* Baltimore: Williams & Wilkins, 1997:187–216. (Provides an excellent description of embryology and anatomy from the laparoscopist's viewpoint.)

THE LIVER, BILIARY TRACT, AND PANCREAS

This section is organized into two parts: the extrahepatic biliary tract (and liver) and the pancreas. Within each part, simple procedures are described first, followed by a discussion of more complex procedures. The extrahepatic biliary tract is introduced in Chapters 56 and 57, which are devoted to cholecystectomy, common bile duct exploration, and liver biopsy. Both open and laparoscopic cholecystectomy are described. Operations to bypass an obstructed bile duct by direct anastomosis to the gut, either by anastomosis to the duodenum (choledochoduodenostomy) or to a defunctionalized loop of jejunum (choledochojejunostomy) are then detailed (Chapters 58 and 59). A related procedure-transduodenal sphincteroplasty (Chapter 60)-illustrates the anatomy of the ampulla of Vater. More complex procedures that demonstrate the anatomy of the portal venous system (Chapter 61) and liver (Chapter 62) are then presented.

Pancreatic resections are described in Chapters 63 and 64, continuing the discussion of portal venous anatomy, celiac artery anatomy, the spleen, and the anatomy of the duodenum begun in earlier sections. Finally, a chapter on operations for drainage of pancreatic pseudocysts (Chapter 65) concludes this section. More complex hepatobiliary and pancreatic procedures are detailed in the references at the end of each chapter.

CHAPTER 56

Cholecystectomy, Common Bile Duct Exploration, and Liver Biopsy

Cholecystectomy can be performed by removing the gallbladder from the top down, reserving dissection in the region of the common bile duct until the last step, or it may be performed in a retrograde fashion, with the cystic duct being divided early and the gallbladder being removed subsequently. In this chapter, the former approach to cholecystectomy is described, as this method provides the greatest degree of safety in terms of avoiding inadvertent injury to the common bile duct or hepatic arteries. Laparoscopic cholecystectomy (see Chapter 57) is performed in a retrograde fashion.

Incision and Exposure of the Gallbladder (Fig. 56.1)

Technical Points

In most patients, a right-sided subcostal (Kocher) incision provides the best exposure. If the subcostal angle is very acute, a right paramedian incision may be chosen instead, especially in a slender patient.

Make the incision two fingerbreadths below the right costal margin and parallel to it. Divide the anterior rectus sheath sharply. Pass a long Kelly hemostat under the rectus abdominis muscle and divide it with electrocautery. Occasional small arteries may require suture ligation. Pick up and incise the posterior rectus sheath and preperitoneal fat to enter the abdomen. Medially, the ligamentum teres hepatis may need to be divided, particularly if exposure is difficult and surgery on the common bile duct is anticipated.

Explore the abdomen. Pass a hand over the right lobe of the liver and pull down, allowing air to enter the subphrenic space and providing increased exposure of the subhepatic region. Filmy adhesions between the gallbladder and gastrocolic omentum or transverse colon may need to be cut.

If the gallbladder is tense and acutely inflamed, preliminary decompression with a trocar will decrease the chance of uncontrolled spillage of infected bile during dissection. Place a pursestring suture of 3-0 silk on the top of the gallbladder, in an easily accessible location. Support the gallbladder with the left hand and insert a trocar through the center of the pursestring. Aspirate bile and calculus material from the gallbladder. Withdraw the trocar, taking care not to spill bile, and tie the pursestring suture to close the hole. Obtain a culture of the bile.

If the gallbladder is not tense, place a Kelly clamp on the fundus of the gallbladder and pull down and out. Use the clamp to gain traction and expose Calot's triangle. Place packs to depress the colon and to hold the stomach and duodenum medially out of the field.

Anatomic Points

A short Kocher incision does not cause any functional deficit of the rectus abdominis muscle. However, a very long Kocher incision may result in weakness of the rectus, especially if several segmental nerves are divided. The superior epigastric artery and vein lie posterior to the rectus abdominis muscle, about halfway (at this level) between the linea alba and the costal margin. These vessels are generally small and are either divided with electrocautery or ligated and divided.

The falciform ligament (and its contained ligamentum teres hepatis, in the free edge of the falciform ligament) runs from the umbilicus to the fissure separating the right and left lobes. This lies to the right of the midline, so the falciform ligament is oriented with its left surface in contact with liver and its right in contact with the anterior parietal peritoneum. If the falciform and round ligaments must be divided, this should be done between clamps. The reasons for this are twofold. First, the round ligament, which is the obliterated left umbilical vein, may retain a patent lumen. Second, paralleling the round ligament are a variable number of paraumbilical veins, which provide a potential collateral circuit between the portal vein and the caval system via the superficial veins of the abdomen.

LIST OF STRUCTURES

Liver
Gallbladder
  Hartmann's pouch
Cystic duct
Common hepatic duct
Common bile duct
Ligamentum teres hepatis
Right and left hepatic arteries
Cystic artery
Cholecystoduodenal ligament
Calot's triangle

FIGURE 56.1
INCISION AND EXPOSURE OF THE GALLBLADDER

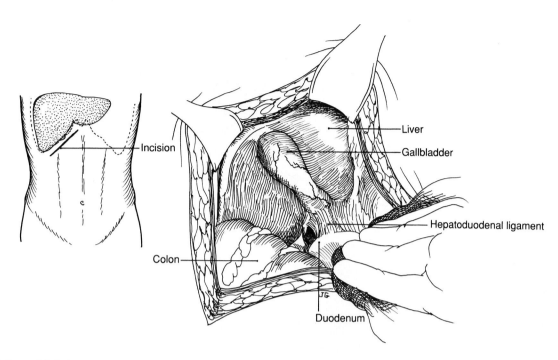

The right and left hepatic ducts leave their corresponding liver lobes and unite close to the porta hepatis to form the common hepatic duct, typically the most anterior tubular structure in this region. The cystic duct, which drains the gallbladder, joins the common hepatic duct at a variable distance from the porta hepatis and at a variable angle. This union forms the common bile duct.

The gallbladder is a diverticulum of the extrahepatic biliary tree. From the cystic duct, the gallbladder is divided into a narrow neck (in which spirally arranged folds of mucosa form the so-called valve of Heister), a tapering body, and an expanded fundus that extends beyond the inferior border of the liver. Frequently, an asymmetric bulging of the right side of the neck may occur. This bulge, known as Hartmann's pouch, may be bound down toward the first part of the duodenum by a cholecystoduodenal ligament, the right edge of the lesser omentum. This ligament must be divided and Hartmann's pouch mobilized to clearly identify the cystic duct.

Identification of the Cystic Artery and Cystic Duct (Fig. 56.2)

Technical Points

Divide any filmy adhesions that remain between the gallbladder and colon or omentum. Place a second Kelly clamp farther down on the gallbladder; be careful to clamp the gallbladder and not the cystic or common bile duct. Incise the peritoneum overlying Calot's triangle and dissect bluntly with a Kitner dissector. Push fatty and areolar tissues away from the gallbladder to expose the common bile duct, cystic duct, and cystic artery.

Identify the cystic duct passing from the gallbladder to the common bile duct. Clean the duct gently and pass a right-angle clamp behind it. Double-loop the duct with a 2-0 silk suture to provide temporary but atraumatic occlusion of the duct. This helps to prevent small stones from being forced down into the common bile duct during the dissection, and facilitates the performance of a cholangiogram of the cystic duct.

Next, identify the cystic artery, which typically passes superior to the cystic duct and runs along the anterior surface of the gallbladder. Clean the cystic artery and divide it, securing the ends with 3-0 silk ligatures. Anomalies are common in this area; an unusually large cystic artery should raise the suspicion that the vessel may, in fact, be an anomalous right hepatic artery. Dissect along the course of the vessel to see whether it terminates on the gallbladder or loops back up into the liver.

Anatomic Points

Calot's triangle, according to current usage, is synonymous with the cholecystohepatic triangle. Its boundaries are the cystic duct inferiorly, the common hepatic duct medially, and the right lobe of the liver superiorly. It contains the right hepatic duct and right hepatic artery (usually posterior to the duct) in the superior part of the triangle, and the cystic artery more inferiorly. Anomalous vessels and bile ducts are common. The right hepatic artery can lie anterior to the right hepatic duct, or it may be up to 1 cm distant from the duct. As its course briefly parallels the cystic artery, it can be mistaken for the latter vessel. The cystic artery, typically a branch of the

FIGURE 56.2
IDENTIFICATION OF THE CYSTIC ARTERY AND CYSTIC DUCT

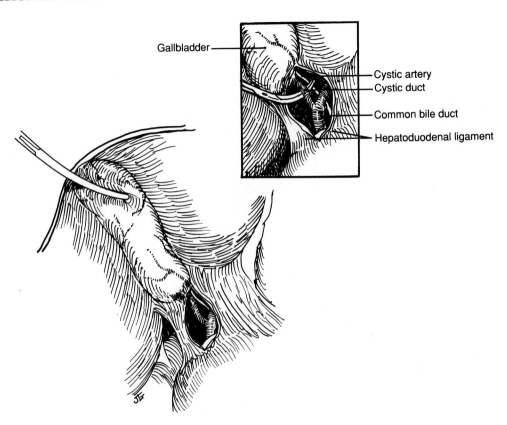

right hepatic artery, can arise from any artery in the vicinity (eg, the left hepatic, common hepatic, gastroduodenal, superior mesenteric, etc.). However, regardless of its origin, it usually passes through Calot's triangle.

Skeletonization of the cystic duct from the neck of the gallbladder to the bile duct is necessary, as it allows the surgeon to verify its identity. Variations in the biliary apparatus are also common. There can be accessory hepatic ducts (usually from the right), which can be mistaken for the cystic duct; bifurcated cystic ducts; multiple cystic ducts; and even absence of a cystic duct.

Removal of the Gallbladder (Fig. 56.3)

Technical Points

With the cystic artery and cystic duct controlled, dissection now progresses from the fundus of the gallbladder down. Incise the peritoneum overlying the gallbladder until the blue submucosal plane, which is superficial to a network of small vessels, is identified. Dissection in this plane will allow removal of the gallbladder without injury to the liver and with a minimum of blood loss. Carry the peritoneal incisions laterally as far as exposure will allow. Once the correct plane has been identified, use electrocautery to incise the peritoneum over a right-angle clamp.

Hold the Kelly clamp and the gallbladder with your nondominant hand, moving the gallbladder from side to side as

required to expose the attachments between the gallbladder and liver. Cut these attachments sharply, remaining as much as possible in the submucosal plane.

As the dissection progresses, connect the peritoneal incision over the gallbladder with that made previously over Calot's triangle. Hold the gallbladder in your nondominant hand and work on the edge of the gallbladder.

Lift the gallbladder and incise the posterior peritoneum. Push fatty and areolar tissue overlying the gallbladder downward with a Kitner dissector. Although most of the dissection in the critical region close to the common bile duct is done from the front, mobility gained by clearing peritoneum posteriorly will greatly facilitate the remaining phase of dissection. Ideally, the common bile duct should be visualized and the common duct/cystic duct juncture clearly identified.

Occasionally, severe inflammation or the presence of hepatic cirrhosis renders dissection of the back wall of the gallbladder from the liver difficult, hazardous, or almost impossible. In this case, leave the back wall of the gallbladder in place where it attaches to the liver. Remove the gallbladder by cutting through the full thickness of the wall as shown for the peritoneal incision. As you extend the dissection downward, attempt to reenter the wall of the gallbladder and dissect within the wall for the terminal 1 to 2 cm. This maneuver facilitates identification and ligation of the cystic duct. If inflammation is so severe that dissection within the wall of the gallbladder cannot be attempted, then remove the gallbladder

FIGURE 56.3
REMOVAL OF THE GALLBLADDER

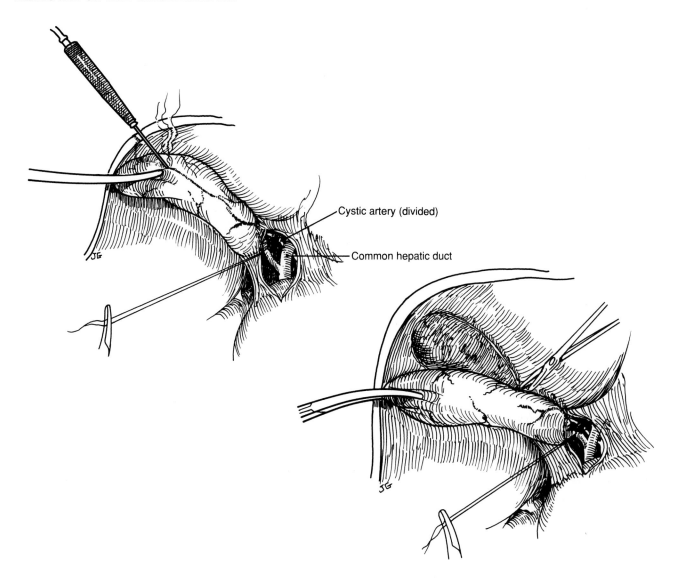

Cystic artery (divided)

Common hepatic duct

and suture-ligate the cystic duct orifice from within. Thoroughly obliterate the mucosa of the gallbladder remnant with electrocautery and pack the area with omentum. Drain the subhepatic space with a closed suction drain.

Anatomic Points

Do not remove the gallbladder until you have clearly identified all ancillary structures, components of the biliary apparatus, and associated vasculature. As you dissect the gallbladder from the liver bed, stay as close as possible to the gallbladder rather than to the liver surface. This avoids injury to subvesicular bile ducts (which are blind ducts, present in as many as 35% of gallbladder fossae, that do not communicate with the gallbladder but that can be a source of bile leakage) or to the intrahepatic anterior segmental branch of the right hepatic artery, which is very close to the subvesicular surface of the liver. Occasionally, there can be small accessory

cystohepatic ducts in the gallbladder fossa or in the vicinity that must be controlled to prevent bile leakage. Moreover, the right, left, or both hepatic ducts can empty directly into the gallbladder.

Operative Cholangiogram (Fig. 56.4)

Technical and Anatomic Points

At this point, the gallbladder should be attached only by the cystic duct, which has a 2-0 silk double-looped around it. Place a hemostatic clip on the gallbladder to prevent spillage of bile when the cystic duct is opened. Choose a catheter appropriate to the size of the cystic duct. Soft Silastic pediatric feeding tubes are safe, atraumatic, and available in several sizes. An 8 French feeding tube is a good catheter to use when the cystic duct is large. An 5 French feeding tube can generally be placed in even the smallest cystic duct.

FIGURE 56.4
OPERATIVE CHOLANGIOGRAM

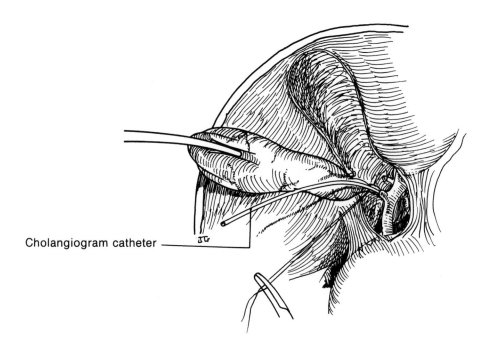

Cholangiogram catheter

Commercially available kits with stiffer catheters are convenient, but one must be very careful not to injure the common bile duct when a stiff catheter is used.

Flush the catheter and connecting tubes with sterile saline and remove any bubbles. While maintaining slight traction on the cystic duct, make a small incision in the upper surface with a No. 11 blade. A small drop of bile should appear at the site of incision, confirming entry into the biliary tree. Pass the catheter gently into the cystic duct and tie the silk suture around it. Confirm that bile can be aspirated and that saline can be injected easily, without extravasation.

Exchange the syringe of saline for one containing dilute water-soluble contrast medium. Generally, the contrast material should be diluted 1:1 or 1:2 so that small stones will not be hidden in a dense column of contrast medium. Check to make sure that no air bubbles have been introduced. Remove all packs and retractors, taking care not to dislodge the catheter. Obtain two exposures, one after a small amount of contrast medium has been instilled and the second after a larger amount. For a small common duct, 8 mL to 12 mL of contrast material are appropriate. If the common duct appears to be large, use correspondingly larger amounts. The common duct and intrahepatic biliary tree should be able to be well visualized, with good definition of the distal common duct. If too much contrast material is used initially, spillage of contrast into the duodenum may obscure visualization of the terminal common duct. On the second film, contrast material should be seen to flow into the duodenum.

After checking the cholangiograms, remove the gallbladder in the following fashion. Cut the suture holding the cholangiogram catheter in the cystic duct. Then pull the catheter out while an assistant clamps the cystic duct close to its juncture with the common bile duct. Suture-ligate the cystic duct with 3-0 silk. Check the field for hemostasis.

Common Bile Duct Exploration (Kocher Maneuver) (Fig. 56.5)

Technical and Anatomic Points

A recent, good-quality cholangiogram is critical; preferably, this should be obtained on the operating table, either as part of the preliminary cholecystectomy or by direct puncture of the common duct with a small-caliber butterfly needle. The cholangiogram guides the subsequent exploration by showing the regional anatomy and the approximate number and location of stones. Even if a recent preoperative cholangiogram is available, consideration should be given to obtaining a preliminary operative radiograph, as the number and location of the stones may have changed.

Ascertain that the incision is long enough to allow adequate exposure of the common bile duct. Because the gallbladder mobilizes upward in the course of the dissection, cholecystectomy can be done through a relatively short incision under favorable circumstances. Safe and thorough exploration of the common bile duct requires generous exposure.

Divide the ligamentum teres hepatis by doubly clamping and ligating the obliterated umbilical vessel in the free edge. Use electrocautery to divide the rest of this ligament.

Mobilize the hepatic flexure of the colon to expose the duodenum. Incise the peritoneum lateral to the duodenum. After creating an initial window large enough to admit a

FIGURE 56.5
COMMON BILE DUCT EXPLORATION (KOCHER MANEUVER)

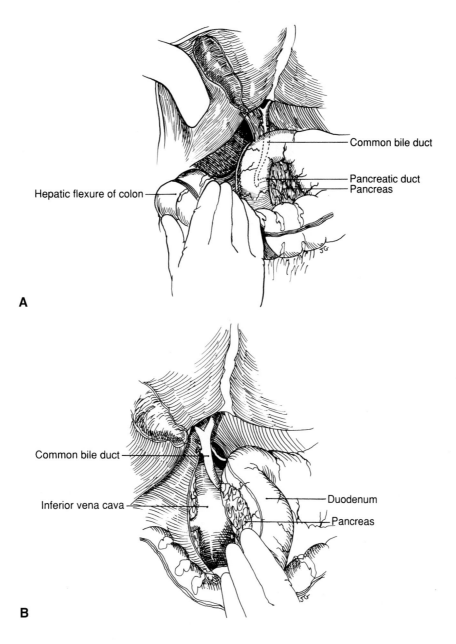

finger, pass the index finger of your nondominant hand into the retroperitoneum and elevate the remaining peritoneum, dividing it with electrocautery when it is thin enough to see through. Place traction on the duodenum with a laparotomy pad and incise the filmy, avascular adhesions between the duodenum and retroperitoneum using Metzenbaum scissors. As the dissection progresses, elevate the duodenum and head of the pancreas and rotate them medially. Continue mobilization until you can pass your nondominant hand comfortably behind the head of the pancreas and can feel the terminal common bile duct and ampulla. Palpate the hepatoduodenal ligament and terminal duct for stones and the pancreas for masses. Place a laparotomy pad behind the duodenum to elevate it into the field.

Common Bile Duct Exploration (Fig. 56.6)

Technical Points

Clean the upper surface of the common bile duct. Choose a site for choledochotomy. If a choledochoduodenostomy (see Figs. 59.1 and 59.2 in Chapter 59) is planned, make the choledochotomy low, just above the duodenum. Otherwise, a choledochotomy at about the level of the cystic duct stump is convenient.

FIGURE 56.6
COMMON BILE DUCT EXPLORATION

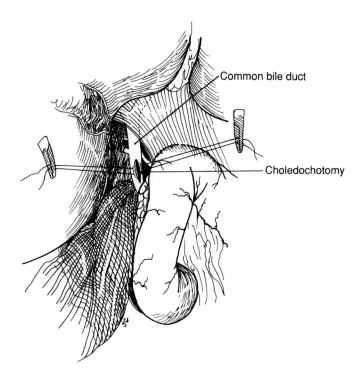

Common bile duct

Choledochotomy

Place two traction sutures of 4-0 silk through the superficial layers of the common bile duct, avoiding entering the lumen, if possible. Bile is a detergent and will pass through small holes; hence, even a needle hole can be the site of postoperative leakage of bile. Elevate the common duct with these sutures and make a 2- to 3-mm longitudinal slit in the common duct with a No. 11 blade. Entry into the common duct must be made cleanly, but with care taken to avoid penetrating the back wall. Extend the choledochotomy with Pott's scissors until it is about 1 cm in length.

Exploration of the common duct is traditionally performed as a blind procedure. As the choledochoscope allows direct visualization and manipulation under direct vision, its use has superceded many of the maneuvers described here. Nevertheless, these approaches are still useful and will be described briefly.

Often, a stone or two can be palpated in the duct and felt to be mobile. In this situation, one must be careful not to displace the stone into the intrahepatic tree, where retrieval can be difficult. Instead, it may be possible to gently push the stone up into the choledochotomy using gentle digital pressure. Stones retrieved from the duct should be saved and counted and their number and size compared to the estimates obtained from the preliminary cholangiogram. Stones in the common duct frequently acquire layers of muddy, easily dislodged sediment. Handle the stones gently to avoid fragmenting them. If the stones become fragmented, it is more difficult to ascertain whether all stones have been removed, and any debris left

behind in the common duct may act as a nidus for further stone formation.

Because most stones settle in the distal duct just above the ampulla, this part of the duct is generally explored first. Take care throughout not to dislodge stones from the lower part of the duct, where they are relatively easy to retrieve, into the intrahepatic biliary tree, where they may become impacted. When passing instruments into the distal common bile duct, place your nondominant hand behind the duodenum and head of pancreas and pull down to straighten the terminal duct and palpate the ampulla. The nondominant hand will help you judge the direction and course of the terminal common duct and you will probably be able to feel instruments as they are being passed into the region above the ampulla. When you explore the upper duct, bend the malleable handle of the instruments to allow both the left and right intrahepatic ducts to be entered. Allow the instrument to find its own path into the duct; you will have a sensation that the instrument is following a tract when it is passing into the intrahepatic tree.

Scoops of various sizes on malleable handles are passed proximal and distal to lift up and retrieve stones. Pass the scoop along the back wall of the duct and concentrate on the sensation of stone against steel that indicates the presence of a stone. Try to pass the scoop under the stone and lift up, pulling the scoop and stone back into the choledochotomy. An assistant should hold a medicine glass of saline ready for you to wash the stone after each passage. Typically, mucus and debris will also be obtained; stones should be visible in the bottom of the glass.

A large stone in a large duct may be retrieved using a stone forceps. Such forceps are available with several degrees of curvature. To grasp a stone in the lower duct, choose a stone forceps that is relatively straight. Pass the forceps with the jaws open as widely as the common duct will allow; then, gently close the forceps periodically as the instrument is advanced. If successful, you will feel the forceps grip the stone. Pull stone and forceps back and out the choledochotomy.

Biliary Fogarty catheters may be passed proximal and distal with the balloon deflated; then they may be inflated and pulled back to drag out stones and debris. Particularly in the intrahepatic biliary tree, it is important not to inflate the balloon too much as it is easy to rupture small intrahepatic radicles. Adjacent branches of the portal vein may be injured, resulting in troublesome bleeding. Inflate the balloon with just enough saline to feel a slight resistance when the catheter is withdrawn. Vary the amount of saline in the balloon in response to the feel of the catheter as the Fogarty catheter is pulled back. Additional saline may be introduced as the catheter enters the larger common bile duct. If the Fogarty catheter is passed through the ampulla, the balloon will catch on the ampulla as the catheter is withdrawn. It is then necessary to deflate the balloon, pull the catheter back through the ampulla, and reinflate the balloon.

Bakes dilators, which are calibrated dilators on malleable handles, are passed through the ampulla. Start with a small Bakes dilator (a No. 3 is usually the smallest available). Be extremely careful to feel the ampulla as the Bakes dilator is passed and to pass the dilator atraumatically. It is possible, and undesirable, to create a false passage with the use of these dilators. When the Bakes dilator passes into the duodenum, you will feel it pop through the ampulla, at which point you should be able to see the steel tip shining through the lateral wall of the duodenum if you stretch the duodenal wall over the dilator. Passage of successively larger Bakes dilators stretches and will ultimately tear the ampulla. There is a general lack of agreement as to what extent the ampulla should be dilated. Record the size of the largest Bakes dilator that is successfully passed. If it is not possible to pass even the No. 3 Bakes dilator, there is probably a stone lodged at the ampulla.

Finally, a large red rubber catheter can be passed proximally and distally to flush the duct out with saline. Observe the effluent and continue flushing until no stones or debris are obtained.

Anatomic Points

Proximal to the site of entrance of the biliary duct, the extrahepatic biliary apparatus consists of right and left hepatic ducts; these unite to form the common hepatic duct. This union is between 0.25 and 2.5 cm from the liver surface. Within the liver parenchyma, the right and left hepatic ducts are formed by the union of appropriate segmental ducts. As

would be expected, there are several possible variations in this pattern. Accessory hepatic ducts, usually with a diameter that is about half that of the main pancreatic ducts, may be present. These are really normal segmental ducts that join the biliary tract extrahepatically, rather than intrahepatically.

From its formation in the hepatoduodenal ligament, the common bile duct passes posterior to the first part of the duodenum, then passes posterior to or through the head of the pancreas, unites with the terminal pancreatic duct, and finally pierces the wall of the second part of the duodenum to open upon the summit of the major duodenal papilla. The pancreatic part of the common bile duct lies at a variable distance from the duodenum and may be entirely retroduodenal; alternatively and more commonly, it may be covered posteriorly by a small tongue or bridge of pancreatic tissue. In most cases, there is a fusion cleft to the right of the duct that permits exposure of this terminal duct. Rarely, the duct lies anterior to the pancreas rather than posterior to it.

As the bile duct approaches the duodenum, it is posterior and somewhat superior to the pancreatic duct. These ducts typically join extramurally, then follow an oblique course through the wall of the duodenum.

As the bile duct enters the wall of the duodenum, it narrows significantly (from about 10 mm to about 5 mm), sometimes resulting in the formation of an intraluminal ridge or step. This ridge can present problems during intraluminal procedures, and is an anatomic reason for the settling of common duct stones just proximal to the ampulla of Vater. The intramural part of its course can be as narrow as 2 mm. Here, the wall of the bile duct and pancreatic duct fuse, forming the ampulla of Vater, and both the biliary system and the exocrine pancreatic system open by the single ostium at the apex of the major duodenal papilla. The length of the common channel within the ampulla of Vater is variable. Typically, a variable septum separates the intra-ampullary bile duct from the pancreatic duct; this septum may be complete so that both ducts open independently on the apex of the papilla. The major duodenal papilla is normally on the posteromedial wall of the second part of the duodenum, approximately 7 to 10 cm distal to the pylorus.

Operative Choledochoscopy and Closure of Choledochotomy (Fig. 56.7)

Technical and Anatomic Points

Both rigid and flexible fiberoptic scopes are available and may be used for choledochoscopy. The rigid scope provides excellent optics but demands that the duodenum be fully kocherized so that the duct can be straightened and the scope passed. The fiberoptic scope is considerably easier to pass. Its use is described here.

Pass the scope distally first. Use the controls of the scope to introduce a slight bend in the tip and pass it from above down through the choledochotomy. Cross the traction sutures over the scope to "close" the duct over the instrument and allow it to fill with saline. Allow saline to run freely into

FIGURE 56.7
OPERATIVE CHOLEDOCHOSCOPY AND CLOSURE OF CHOLEDOCHOTOMY

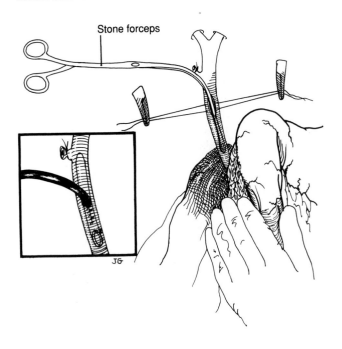

Stone forceps

direct vision. As the scope is pulled back, the common duct should be inspected.

The choledochoscope should then be passed into the right and left hepatic ducts. Several branches of the intrahepatic biliary tree may be visible. Retrieve any stones seen. Pull back the scope and inspect the common duct. It is easy to overlook stones in the region of the common duct adjacent to the choledochotomy unless you are especially careful.

Choose a T tube of appropriate size. If the duct is large and multiple stones have been obtained, use at least a No. 14 French T tube. A large tube will facilitate subsequent manipulation if stones are left behind at operation. If the duct is small, a smaller tube is appropriate. Cut the crossbars of the T short, and either cut out the back wall or cut a V into the back wall so that the crossarms bend easily when the tube is pulled. Confirm patency of both limbs by injecting saline. Place the T tube in the common duct and push it to the upper margin of the choledochotomy. Once in the common duct, it should slide freely, indicating that the crossbar of the T is not kinked within the lumen of the duct. Push the T tube to the upper limit of the choledochotomy so that closure can proceed from below, where visualization is easiest.

Start a running lock-stitch of 4-0 Vicryl at the inferior margin of the choledochotomy and proceed up to the T tube. Take full-thickness bites of the duct, but be careful not to narrow the lumen (especially if the duct is small). At the T tube, close the choledochotomy snugly around the tube, taking care not to catch the rubber tube within a suture. Run the suture back as a simple running stitch and tie it to itself. Inject saline to check for leaks.

Perform a completion cholangiogram by injecting dye into the T tube to confirm that all stones have been removed and that the duct has not been narrowed. Place omentum and a closed suction drain in the subhepatic space.

the duct through the instrument. The duct should become distended with saline, allowing the lumen to become visible. The ampulla will be visible as a sphincter at the terminal duct. The central lumen of the ampulla may be visualized. Generally, it is not possible to pass the scope into the ampulla and duodenum. If a stone is seen, pass the biliary Fogarty catheter next to the scope and, under direct vision, attempt to engage the stone. A stone basket can also be used under

FIGURE 56.8
WEDGE AND NEEDLE BIOPSY OF THE LIVER

Liver

Biopsy needle

Wedge and Needle Biopsy of the Liver (Fig. 56.8)

Technical and Anatomic Points

Liver biopsy is most easily performed at the free edge of the left or right lobe. If any obvious abnormalities are present, however, a biopsy specimen should be obtained from the affected area. If there are no visible or palpable masses, the free edge of the right lobe, away from any areas that may have been damaged in the course of dissection or by placement of retractors, should be selected.

Wedge Biopsy

The wedge biopsy technique provides a generous amount of tissue, but is limited in depth. To perform this procedure, place two sutures of 2-0 chromic in such a way as to outline a triangle. Tie the sutures and leave long ends. Cut a wedge of tissue from the inside of the triangle. Check the cut surface for hemostasis. Use electrocautery to control any small bleeding points. Persistent bleeding from the apex of the V-shaped defect may be controlled with a horizontal mattress suture placed above the apex. The long ends of the two lateral sutures may be tied together to close the defect. This should only be done after hemostasis has been achieved, as hidden bleeding may persist.

Needle Biopsy

Stabilize the liver with your nondominant hand and stick the liver on the free edge, using a disposable, core-cutting needle. Pass the needle as deeply as desired and cut a core of tissue. Remove the needle, using your nondominant hand to compress the edge of the liver for hemostasis, and inspect the core. Cut several cores through the same entry point by inserting the needle at several different angles. If bleeding persists from the puncture site, close the hole with a single 3-0 chromic suture placed across the hole in a figure-of-eight pattern.

REFERENCES

1. Benson EA, Page RE. A practical reappraisal of the anatomy of the extrahepatic bile ducts and arteries. *Br J Surg* 1976;63:853.
2. Browne EZ. Variations in origin and course of the hepatic artery and its branches: importance from surgical viewpoint. *Surgery* 1940;8:424.
3. Gross RE. Congenital anomalies of the gallbladder: a review of 148 cases, with report of a double gallbladder. *Arch Surg* 1936;32:131.
4. Johnston EV, Anson BJ. Variations in the formation and vascular relationships of the bile ducts. *Surg Gynecol Obstet* 1952;94:669.
5. Linder HH, Green RB. Embryology and surgical anatomy of the extrahepatic biliary tree. *Surg Clin North Am* 1963;44:1273.
6. Michels NA. The hepatic, cystic, and retroduodenal arteries and their relations to the biliary ducts with samples of the entire celiacal blood supply. *Ann Surg* 1951;133:503.
7. Michels NA. Variational anatomy of the hepatic, cystic, and retroduodenal arteries: a statistical analysis of their origin, distribution, and relations to the biliary ducts in two hundred bodies. *Arch Surg* 1953;66:20.
8. Moosman DA. Where and how to find the cystic artery during cholecystectomy. *Surg Gynecol Obstet* 1975;133:769.
9. Sutton JP, Sachatella CR. The confluence stone: a hazardous complication of biliary tract disease. *Am J Surg* 1967;113:719.

CHAPTER 57

Laparoscopic Cholecystectomy, Common Bile Duct Exploration, and Liver Biopsy

Laparoscopic cholecystectomy introduced operative laparoscopy to most general surgeons, and is often the first laparoscopic procedure performed by surgical residents. Although the anatomy is identical to that described in Chapter 56, the significance of some biliary anomalies is greater for the laparoscopic procedure. Accordingly, this chapter stresses not only surgical technique but also ways in which specific anatomic pitfalls can be avoided. It should be read in conjunction with Chapter 56.

Initial Exposure (Fig. 57.1)

Technical Points

Introduce the laparoscope through an umbilical portal. Place a 10-mm port in the epigastric region and two 5-mm ports in the right midclavicular line and right anterior axillary line (Fig. 57.1A). Explore the abdomen. Cautiously lyse any adhesions of gallbladder to colon, omentum, or duodenum (Fig. 57.1B). Pass a grasping forceps through the anterior axillary line port and grasp the fundus of the gallbladder, pulling it up and over the liver. This will expose the subhepatic space (Fig. 57.1C). If the stomach and duodenum are distended, have suction placed on an orogastric or nasogastric tube. Reverse Trendelenburg positioning and tilting the operating table right-side-up will help increase the working space by allowing the viscera to move caudad and to the left.

Place a second grasping forceps through the midclavicular line port and grasp Hartmann's pouch. Pull out, away from the liver. This maneuver will open Calot's triangle and create a safe working space (Fig. 57.1D).

Take a moment to orient yourself. Frequently, there is an obvious color difference between the pale blue or green of the gallbladder (unless severely diseased) and the yellow fat of Calot's triangle. This blue-yellow junction is a good place to begin dissection. A few filmy adhesions of omentum, transverse colon, or duodenum may need to be cautiously lysed to provide optimum visualization of the region. Calot's node, often enlarged in acute or resolving acute cholecystitis, nestles in Calot's triangle (Fig. 57.1E).

Another good landmark is the hepatic artery, which should be visible as a large pulsating vessel well to the left of the surgical field. This is a marker for the common duct, which generally lies just to the right.

Anatomic Points

The cystic artery arises from the right hepatic artery in Calot's triangle and ascends on the left side of the gallbladder in approximately 80% of individuals. A fatty stripe or slight tenting of the peritoneum overlying the gallbladder may serve as a clue to its probable location. In a significant minority of individuals, the cystic artery arises directly from the hepatic artery. Other anomalies of the cystic artery of laparoscopic significance are described in Fig. 57.2.

Calot's node is one of two fairly constant nodes in this region. The second node, termed the node of the anterior border of the epiploic foramen, lies along the upper part of the bile duct. Thus, simply noting the presence of a node in

LIST OF STRUCTURES

Liver
    Left lobe
        Segments I, II, III, and IV
    Right lobe
        Segments V, VI, VII, and VIII
    Falciform ligament
        Ligamentum teres

Common duct
    Common bile duct
    Right and left hepatic ducts
    Cystic duct
Left and right subphrenic spaces
Subhepatic space
Lesser sac

Duodenum
Greater omentum
Hepatic artery
Cystic artery

(**A** and **B** from Cullen JJ, Scott-Conner CEH. Surgical anatomy of laparoscopic common duct exploration. In: Berci G, Cuschieri A, eds. Bile ducts and bile duct stones. Philadelphia: WB Saunders, 1997:20–25, with permission.)

ORIENTATION

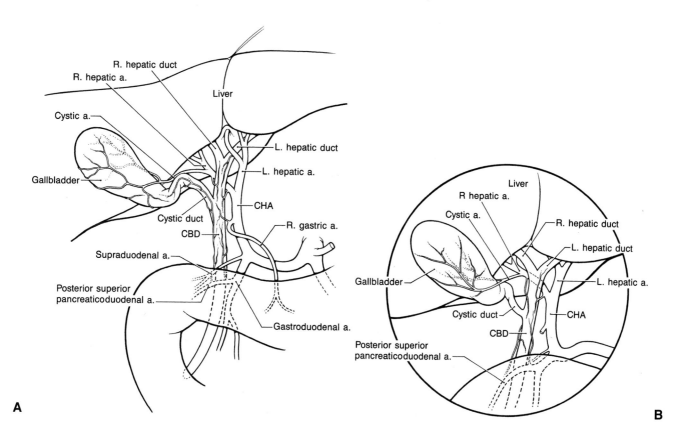

A

B

proximity to the bile duct does not guarantee a safe working distance from the common duct.

Initial Dissection (Fig. 57.2)

Technical Points

Incise the peritoneum overlying the blue-yellow junction (Fig. 57.2A). The cystic duct should become evident as a tubular structure which runs into the gallbladder. It is generally the closest structure to the laparoscope, and hence the first structure which is encountered. Develop a window behind the gallbladder by incising the gallbladder peritoneum on the left and right sides and blunt-dissecting behind cystic duct and gallbladder (Fig. 57.2B). The cystic artery should be visible to the left of the cystic duct (Fig. 57.2C).

Anatomic Points

The normal laparoscopic appearance is shown in Fig. 57.2D. As previously mentioned, this textbook pattern is present in approximately 80% of individuals. In 6 to 16% of normal individuals, the right hepatic artery passes close to the gall-

bladder (Fig. 57.2E). In such cases, the artery may assume a tortuous or "caterpillar hump," this redundancy, combined with small arterial twigs to the gallbladder rather than a single cystic artery, renders the right hepatic artery susceptible to injury. The artery may be mistaken for the cystic artery and ligated, or may be damaged when these small twigs are controlled. Suspect this abnormality when the "cystic artery" appears larger than normal. In up to 8% of normals, an accessory right hepatic artery may arise from the superior mesenteric artery or another vessel in the region, pass in close proximity to Hartmann's pouch as it ascends to the liver. More commonly, the cystic artery arises from the gastroduodenal artery or superior mesenteric artery and ascends to the gallbladder. This "low-lying" cystic artery will be encountered closer to the laparoscope than the cystic duct and may be mistaken for it.

In 25% of individuals, the superficial and deep branches of the cystic artery have separate origins, and thus, there appear to be paired or double cystic arteries. In this situation, one cystic artery may be identified in the normal position and the second may be a "low-lying" cystic artery encountered before the cystic duct.

FIGURE 57.1

INITIAL EXPOSURE (**A** from Scott-Conner CEH and Brunson CD. Surgery and anesthesia. In: Embury SH and Hebbel RP eds. Sickle cell disease-basic principles and clinical practice. New York: Raven, 1994:809–827, with permission; **B** from Wind GG. The biliary system. In: *Applied laparoscopic anatomy: abdomen and pelvis.* Baltimore: Williams & Wilkins, 1997:13–83, with permission; **C–E** from Scott-Conner CEH, Cushieri A, Carter F. Right upper quadrant: liver, gallbladder, and extrahepatic biliary tract. In: *Minimal access surgical anatomy.* Philadelphia: Lippincott Williams & Wilkins, 2000:101–138, with permission.)

FIGURE 57.1 (Continued)

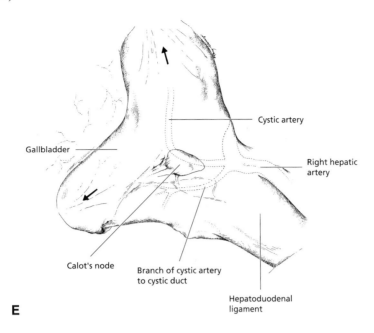

E

Cystic artery

Right hepatic artery

Gallbladder

Calot's node

Branch of cystic artery to cystic duct

Hepatoduodenal ligament

FIGURE 57.2

INITIAL DISSECTION (Scott-Conner CEH and Brunson CD. Surgery and anesthesia. In: Embury SH and Hebbel RP eds. Sickle cell disease: basic principles and clinical practice. New York: Raven, 1994:809–827; **D** and **E** from Scott-Conner CEH, Hall TJ. Variant arterial anatomy in laparoscopic cholecystectomy. *Am J Surg* 1992;163:590, with permission; **F** from Cullen JJ, Scott-Conner CEH. Surgical anatomy of laparoscopic common duct exploration. In: Berci G, Cuschieri A, eds. *Bile ducts and bile duct stones*. Philadelphia: WB Saunders, 1997:20–25, with permission.)

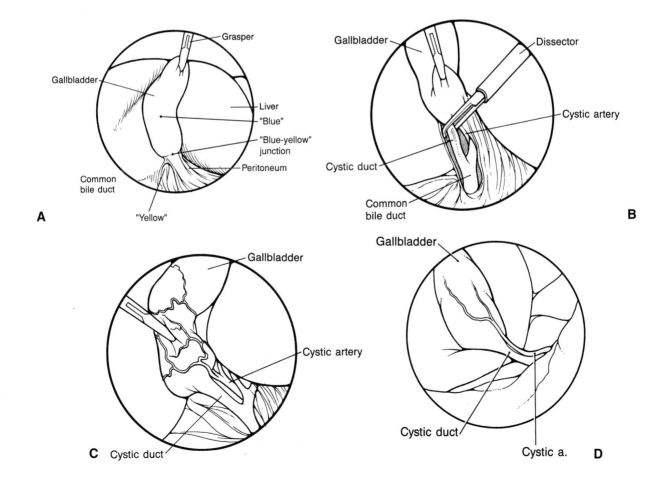

A
Grasper
Gallbladder
Liver
"Blue"
"Blue-yellow" junction
Peritoneum
Common bile duct
"Yellow"

B
Gallbladder
Dissector
Cystic artery
Cystic duct
Common bile duct

C
Gallbladder
Cystic artery
Cystic duct

D
Gallbladder
Cystic duct
Cystic a.

FIGURE 57.2   (Continued)

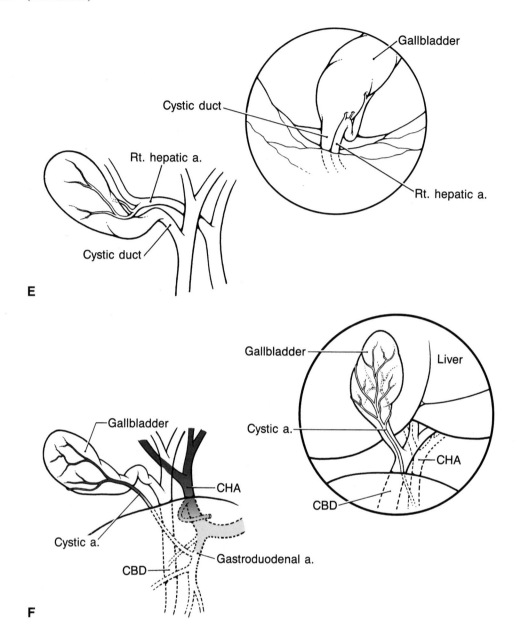

Division of Cystic Duct and Cystic Artery,
Cholangiogram (Fig. 57.3)

Technical Points

Skeletonize the cystic duct by blunt dissection. Place a clip proximal on the cystic duct, high on the gallbladder. It is generally easiest to use the midclavicular port for the cholangiogram. Place a grasper in the sub-xiphoid port and grasp the gallbladder to release the midclavicular port. Pass scissors through the midclavicular port and incise the cystic duct. Bile should flow freely when an adequate ductotomy has been made. Gently use the shaft of the scissors to milk any stones from the distal cystic duct by pressing from below upward toward the ductotomy. Place a cholangiogram catheter through the midclavicular aport and manipulate it into the cystic duct (Fig. 57.3A). Perform a cholangiogram in the usual fashion.

It is fairly common to see small filling defects, presumed to be bubbles of carbon dioxide; for this reason fluorocholangiography (rather than taking films and waiting for them to be developed) and the capability to flush the duct with copious amounts of saline are advisable. Generally bubbles and small stones can easily be flushed through the ampulla and a clean cholangiogram obtained.

If the cholangiogram confirms both normal anatomy and the absence of stones in the common bile duct, remove the cholangiogram catheter and clip the cystic duct with two clips proximally. Divide the cystic duct. The cystic artery will lie posterior and cephalad. Doubly clip and divide it.

Anatomic Points

In the normal situation, there is an adequate length of

FIGURE 57.3

DIVISION OF CYSTIC DUCT AND CYSTIC ARTERY, CHOLANGIOGRAM Scott-Conner CEH and Brunson CD. Surgery and anesthesia. In: Embury SH and Hebbel RP eds. Sickle cell disease: basic principles and clinical practice. New York; Raven, 1994:809–827.

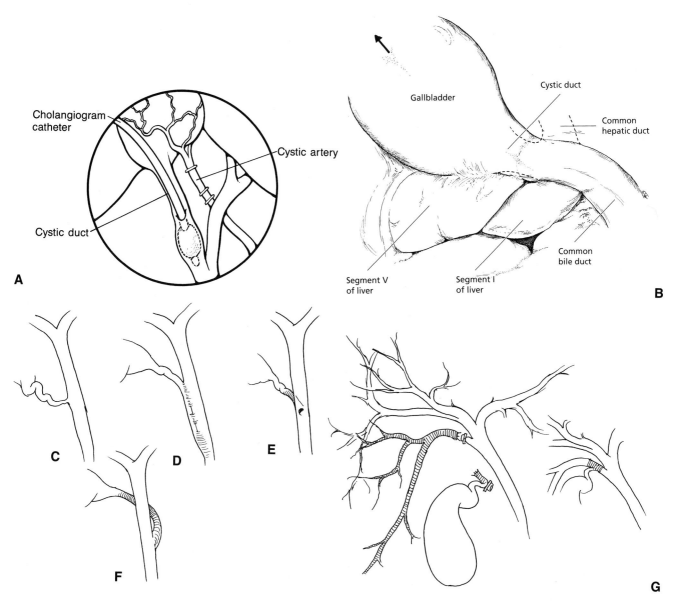

cystic duct available for cannulation and ligation. The cystic duct may be abnormally short, either as a result of chronic inflammation or as an anomaly. In such cases, it is often abnormally thick as well (Fig. 57.3B). There are several anatomic pitfalls here. First, it is very easy to assume that the common bile duct, which may appear as a visual continuation of the cystic duct and which may be similar in caliber, is the cystic duct. Traction on the gallbladder accentuates this tendency as shown. Second, it may be difficult or impossible to simply clip the cystic duct. Always confirm the anatomy by cholangiography in such situations and then secure the cystic duct by an alternative means—such as by stapler transection or by suturing the stump closed. The final anatomic pitfall may occur if this is encountered as a normal variant. The relatively large caliber and short cystic duct allows easy egress of stones

into the common duct; thus, an increased incidence of choledocholithiasis may be anticipated. This is another reason to perform cholangiography in these cases.

Most of the variants of the cystic duct that are stressed during open cholecystectomy are of little significance for the laparoscopic surgeon, provided the dissection is confined to the region of the gallbladder infundibulum. Although the normal situation in which a good length of cystic duct terminates obliquely but directly into the common duct (Fig. 57.3C), occurs in only 60% to 75% of individuals, the other common variants (Fig. 57.3D–F) are generally associated with an adequate length of cystic duct near the gallbladder. Hence, in all of these cases, the cystic duct can be safely dissected and ligated or clipped if the laparoscopic surgeon works close to the gallbladder.

FIGURE 57.4
DISSECTION OF GALLBLADDER FROM LIVER; REMOVAL OF GALLBLADDER

As laparoscopic surgeons have become more cognizant of the ways in which common duct injury can occur, a lesser known variant has emerged as a major source of ductal injuries. When the cystic duct terminates onto the right hepatic duct rather than the common duct, or when the right hepatic duct, the posterior or anterior segmental duct, or an accessory duct terminates onto the cystic duct, it is possible to clip or excise this part of the ductal system (Fig. 57.3GH). Only careful dissection and liberal use of cholangiography can provide secure guidance in this region.

Dissection of Gallbladder from Liver; Removal of Gallbladder (Fig. 57.4)

Technical Points

Apply upward traction on the gallbladder and separate it from its bed by sharp and blunt dissection. The hook cautery is the instrument most commonly used (Fig. 57.4A). Be extremely careful in the initial phase of this dissection because of the proximity of the gallbladder to the right hepatic duct and right hepatic artery. As the dissection progresses, obtain better access to the dissection plane by flipping the gallbladder up and over the liver (Fig. 57.4B). Remove the gallbladder from the bottom up, obtaining hemostasis in the gallbladder bed with electrocautery as the dissection progresses (Fig. 57.4C).

Move the laparoscope to the epigastric portal and pass grasping forceps through the umbilical portal. Pull the neck of the gallbladder up into the portal, engaging it firmly. Then pull both the portal and gallbladder out together. As the gallbladder neck appears in the incision, grasp it with Kelly clamps. Incise the gallbladder and decompress it with a suction, removing stones if necessary. It may be necessary to gently dilate the trocar site by introducing a ring forceps and opening it, taking care not to perforate the gallbladder (Fig. 57.4D).

Do not hesitate to use a retrieval pouch if difficulties are anticipated due to inflammation or large stones. Secure all stab wounds with interrupted 2-0 Vicryl sutures in the fascia and subcuticular sutures on the skin.

Anatomic Points

Small bile ducts are occasionally encountered in the gallbladder fossa. Normally, vascular structures will be found in the peritoneal reflections, thus any small tubular structure should be assumed to be a bile duct. Many of these ducts are actually running parallel to the gallbladder fossa and can be left alone by careful dissection. These are simply small segmental ducts draining parts of the liver into the right hepatic ductal system. Other ductal structures drain directly into the gallbladder (Fig. 57.4E). Most of these can be clipped or ligated. If a large ductal structure is encountered, attempt cholangiography to confirm that the segment of liver drained by the duct has other, more central, drainage into the biliary tree. If these ducts are not recognized and are simply divided with cautery, significant leakage of bile may result.

Laparoscopic Common Duct Exploration—Transcystic Exploration (Fig. 57.5)

Technical Points

There are two basic ways to explore the common duct laparoscopically. The simplest, termed transcystic common duct exploration, is by passing catheters through the cystic duct into the common duct. Success depends upon the size of the stones and the angle formed between the cystic duct and common duct. This method works best with small stones and a cystic duct that enters the common duct relatively high. Generally, it is only possible to explore the duct below the cystic-duct entry point, as it is not feasible to steer the catheter up into

---

FIGURE 57.5
LAPAROSCOPIC COMMON DUCT EXPLORATION—TRANSCYSTIC EXPLORATION

A   B

the proximal ductal system. In the second method, a chole-dochotomy is created through which the duct is explored. Fluoroscopy and a flexible choledochoscope are essential for both.

Pass a dilating balloon into the cystic duct and gently dilate it. Through the dilated duct, pass a choledochoscope and retrieve stones under direct vision ("picture in picture" video technology helps) using wire baskets or balloons (Fig. 57.5A,B). Alternatively, perform the manipulations under fluoroscopic control. It may be necessary to fragment stones using a lithotriptor and retrieve the fragments or flush them out through the ampulla. Obtain a completion cholangiogram and clip the duct at the conclusion. If it is not possible to completely clear the duct, consider threading a guidewire through the ampulla to facilitate subsequent ERCP cannulation.

FIGURE 57.6
LAPAROSCOPIC CHOLEDOCHOTOMY

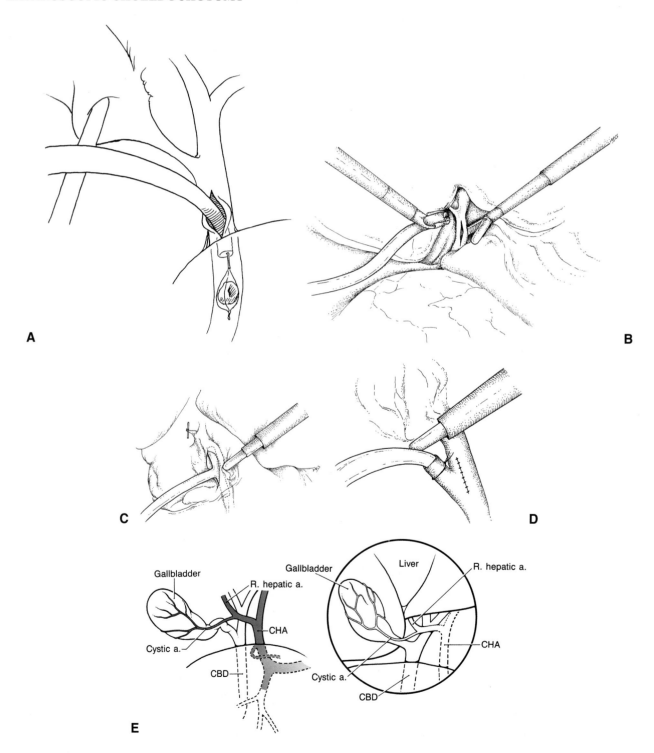

Anatomic Points

The success of this depends upon ease of dilatation and cannulation of the cystic duct, and the extent of common duct that can be explored depends upon how distal the cystic duct enters the common duct. In a situation such as that shown in Fig. 57.3D, where the cystic duct enters relatively low on the common duct, only the most distal segment of common duct is accessible for transcystic exploration.

Laparoscopic Choledochotomy (Fig. 57.6)

Technical Points

A 30 degree laparoscope works better than a straight (zero degree) scope for this operation, as it allows the surgeon to look "down" on the hepatoduodenal ligament.

Identify the common duct immediately to the left of the hepatic artery. Clear the surface to expose 1-2 cm. Place two stay sutures and incise the anterior surface for approximately .5 to 1 cm (Fig. 57.6A). Pass balloon catheters and baskets proximal and distal to retrieve stones. A flexible choledochoscope can be used to inspect the duct. At the conclusion of the procedure, tailor a small T-tube to fit and place it in the choledochotomy. Secure it in place with two or three interrupted sutures of 3-0 or 4-0 Vicryl (Fig. 57.6B,C). Alternatively, some surgeons close the choledochotomy and drain the biliary tree with a catheter secured into the cystic duct stump (Fig. 57.6D). Obtain a completion cholangiogram. Place a

FIGURE 57.7
LAPAROSCOPIC LIVER BIOPSY

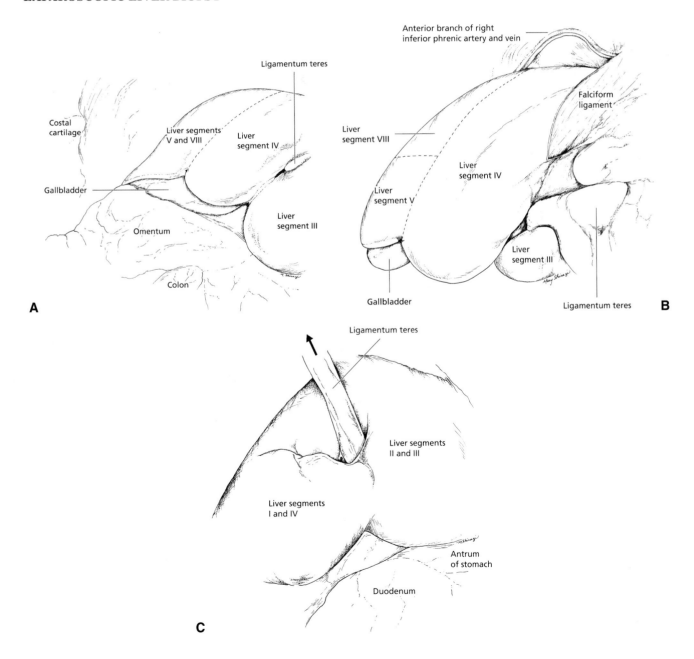

closed suction drain in proximity to the choledochotomy and bring omentum up to lie within the subhepatic space.

Anatomic Points

When the right hepatic artery crosses anterior (rather than posterior) to the common hepatic duct (Fig. 57.6E), it may be injured during the cephalad aspect of choledochotomy. Avoid this pitfall by carefully observing the field for pulsations before making any incision, and by limiting the incision to the distal duct, after incising the peritoneum and clearly exposing the anterior surface of the duct.

Laparoscopic Liver Biopsy (Fig. 57.7)

Technical Points

Perform needle biopsy by passing a cutting biopsy needle directly through the abdominal wall and puncturing the liver under direct vision. Wedge biopsy is best performed using the ultrasonic scalpel to divide a small portion of liver and secure hemostasis.

Anatomic Points

The most obvious laparoscopic landmarks are the ligamentum teres with its associated falciform ligament, which divides segments II and III of the left lobe from the rest of the liver (Fig. 57.7A). A line drawn through the gallbladder fossa indicates the demarcation of segment IV of the left lobe from the right lobe. As the laparoscope is passed higher into the abdomen, segment VIII, which is more posterior, comes into view (Fig. 57.7B). There is no visual landmark to demarcate segment V from segment VIII. Laparoscopic ultrasound may be of some assistance. Elevation of the ligamentum teres exposes segment I (Fig. 57.7C), which may also be seen through the transparent part of the lesser omentum during dissection along the lesser curvature.

REFERENCES

1. Davidoff AM, Pappas TN, Murray EA, et al. Mechanisms of major biliary injury during laparoscopic cholecystectomy. *Ann Surg* 1992;215:196. (Reviews 12 cases of major duct injury and discusses causes and management of these complications.)
2. Dubois F, Icard P, Berthelot G, et al. Coelioscopic cholecystectomy: preliminary report of 36 cases. *Ann Surg* 1990;211:60.
3. Fine A. The cystic vein: the significance of a forgotten anatomic landmark. *JSLS* 1997;1:263–266.
4. Franklin ME Jr. Laparoscopic choledochotomy for management of common bile duct stones and other common bile duct diseases. In: Arregui, M, Fitzqibbons, R, Katkhouda, N, McKernan, B, and Reich, R. (eds). *Principles of laparoscopic surgery: basic and advanced techniques.* New York: Springer-Verlag, 1995: pp. 197–204.
5. Huang S-M, Wu C-W, Chau G-Y, et al. An alternative approach of choledocholithotomy via laparoscopic choledochotomy. *Arch Surg* 1996;131:407–411.
6. Kitano S, Iso Y, Moriyama M, et al. A rapid and simple technique for insertion of a T-tube into the minimally incised common bile duct at laparoscopic surgery. *Surg Endosc* 1993;7:104–105.
7. Martin IG, Curley P, McMahon MJ. Minimally invasive treatment for common bile duct stones. *Br J Surg* 1993;80:103–106.
8. Phillips EH, Berci G, Carroll B, et al. The importance of intraoperative cholangiography during laparoscopic cholecystectomy. *Am Surg* 1990;56:792.
9. Reddick EJ, Olsen DO. Laparoscopic laser cholecystectomy: a comparison with mini-lap cholecystectomy. *Surg Endosc* 1989;3:131.
10. Rhodes M, Nathansom L, O'Rourke N, et al. Laparoscopic exploration of the common bile duct: lessons learned from 129 consecutive cases. *Br J Surg* 1995;82:666–668.
11. Robinson G, Hollinshead J, Falk G, et al. Technique and results of laparoscopic choledochotomy for the management of bile duct calculi. *Aust N Z J Surg* 1995;65:347–349.
12. Scott-Conner CEH, Hall TJ. Variant arterial anatomy in laparoscopic cholecystectomy. *Am J Surg* 1992;163:590.
13. Scott-Conner CEH, Cushieri A, Carter F. Right upper quadrant: liver, gallbladder, and extrahepatic biliary tract. In: *Minimal access surgical anatomy.* Philadelphia: Lippincott Williams & Wilkins, 2000:101–138.
14. Wind GG. The biliary system. In: *Applied laparoscopic anatomy: abdomen and pelvis.* Baltimore: Williams & Wilkins, 1997:13–83.

CHAPTER 58

Choledochoduodenostomy and Other Biliary Bypass Procedures

Choledochoduodenostomy is performed when multiple stones have been found in the common duct at exploration and when it appears unlikely that complete removal of all stones has been achieved. It is a simple side-to-side bypass procedure.

Choledochojejunostomy and cholecystojejunostomy are palliative procedures performed for advanced malignant disease involving the periampullary region. In choledochojejunostomy, an anastomosis of the common bile duct to a loop of jejunum is performed. Cholecystojejunostomy consists of anastomosis of the gallbladder to a jejunal loop.

Hepaticojejunostomy and choledochojejunostomy are also performed for reconstruction after bile duct injuries. Finally, resection of tumors of the hepatic duct bifurcation (Klatskin tumors) necessitates high reconstruction. References at the end of the chapter detail these applications.

Choledochoduodenostomy

Choledochotomy and Duodenotomy (Fig. 58.1)

Technical Points

Expose and prepare the common bile duct for exploration, as detailed in Chapter 56. Place two stay sutures and make a longitudinal incision in the lower third of the common duct. Make the incision approximately 2 cm in length and just above the appearance of the common duct over the superior aspect of the duodenum. Place the incision lower than you normally would for common duct exploration so as to facil-

LIST OF STRUCTURES

Common bile duct
Gallbladder
  Cystic duct
Pancreas
Duodenum
Jejunum
Transverse colon
Superior mesenteric artery
Jejunal branches
Middle colic artery

itate construction of the choledochoduodenal anastomosis. Explore the common duct thoroughly.

Anatomic Points

The close proximity of the distal common bile duct and duodenum make this anastomosis possible. Extra mobility of the duodenum may be obtained by performing a Kocher maneuver.

Anastomosis (Fig. 58.2)

Technical and Anatomic Points

Place stay sutures on the anterior duodenal wall just below the entry of the common bile duct into the duodenum. Center a longitudinal duodenotomy above the choledochotomy on the anterior superior surface of the duodenum. Make this incision approximately the same length as the incision in the common bile duct.

The two incisions will be perpendicular to each other and will produce a diamond-shaped opening when sutured together. Place a posterior interrupted row of 4-0 silk Lembert sutures, beginning at the apex of the choledochotomy and continuing laterally in both directions. This will form the back wall of the anastomosis. Interrupted mucosal sutures of 4-0 Vicryl can be placed if desired. Next, suture the anterior row with interrupted sutures of 4-0 Vicryl on the inner layer and interrupted 4-0 silk on the outer layer. Alternatively, a single layer of interrupted 4-0 PDS sutures may be used.

Do not stent the anastomosis or place a T tube or other drainage device in the common duct. A lumen should be palpable to the tip of the finger at the conclusion of the procedure. Place omentum around the choledochoduodenal anastomosis and then place two closed suction drains (generally, one on each side) in the vicinity of the anastomosis.

Choledochojejunostomy

Choledochotomy and Construction of a Roux-en-Y Anastomosis (Fig. 58.3)

Technical Points

When performed for malignant disease of the distal common duct or pancreas, the anastomosis should be made high enough to avoid tumor encroachment as the tumor enlarges.

FIGURE 58.1
CHOLEDOCHOTOMY AND DUODENOTOMY

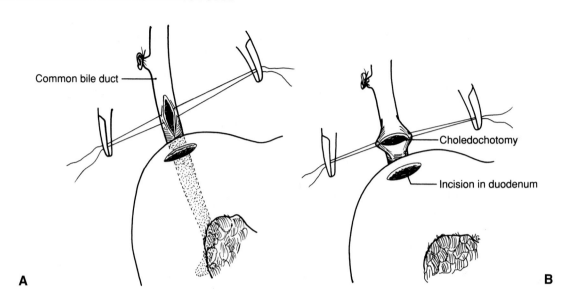

When benign biliary stricture is the indication for surgery, the anastomosis must be made to clean, healthy, unscarred duct. This may necessitate hepaticojejunostomy (see references at the end).

Identify the common duct and trace it proximally. Either a side-to-side duct-to-jejunum or an end-to-side anastomosis may be performed. Side-to-side anastomosis is usually reserved for patients in whom extensive tumor renders circumferential dissection of the duct hazardous.

Side-to-Side Anastomosis

Place stay sutures on the common duct and make a longitudinal choledochotomy approximately 2 cm in length. Explore the duct.

End-to-Side Anastomosis

Place stay sutures on the common duct. Gently dissect on both sides of the duct with a right angle clamp until it is possible to come behind it. Divide the duct, ligating the distal segment.

Then construct a Roux-en-Y loop of the jejunum. Bring the blind end of the Roux loop up to the choledochotomy. Construct a two-layer, side-to-side anastomosis between the loop of jejunum and the common duct using a single layer of interrupted 4-0 PDS sutures. Construct the back wall of the anastomosis and then roll the jejunum up and complete the front row of the anastomosis. Reinforce the anastomosis by inkwelling the jejunum up and tacking it to tissues surrounding the proximal duct or the capsule of the liver with three or

FIGURE 58.2
ANASTOMOSIS

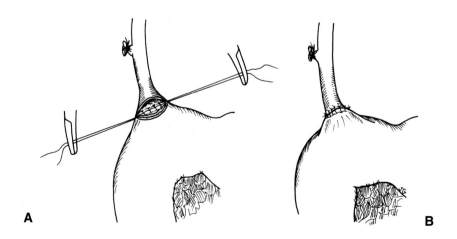

FIGURE 58.3
CHOLEDOCHOTOMY AND CONSTRUCTION OF A ROUX-EN-Y ANASTOMOSIS

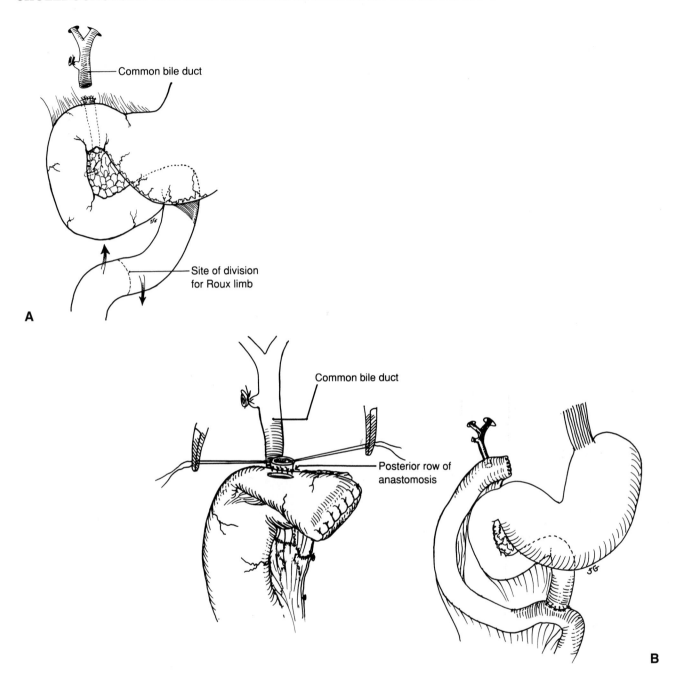

four sutures of 4-0 silk or Vicryl, taking care not to encroach on the lumen of the common duct.

Finish the Roux-en-Y by creating an anastomosis between the end of the proximal jejunum and the side of the distal segment (see Fig. 48.9 in Chapter 48).

As an alternative to the Roux-en-Y loop, the omega loop is simply a loop of jejunum (remaining in continuity) that is sewn in a side-to-side fashion to the common duct. An enteroenterostomy is constructed approximately 20 to 30 cm from the anastomosis to partially bypass the anastomosis. In some patients, an omega loop may be quicker or easier to construct than a Roux-en-Y, and it serves the same function. This procedure is generally reserved for patients with limited lifespans due to extensive disease.

Anatomic Points

Ligate and divide the jejunal branches of the superior mesenteric artery to mobilize the jejunum close to the superior mesenteric artery. The arterial arcades, which are relatively simple in the proximal bowel, provide a collateral route of blood supply for the Roux loop. This anastomosis is generally performed antecolic. This direct route is easier and less hazardous than a retrocolic route, because it avoids the transverse mesocolon and its contained vasculature. Occasionally, a retrocolic approach may be necessary. In such cases, identify the middle colic vessels and take care not to damage them or the marginal arteries. The best place to pierce the transverse mesocolon is to the right of the middle colic artery, taking care to control all mesenteric vessels before dividing them. If you pass to the left of the middle colic artery, you will enter the lesser omental bursa, necessitating a circuitous route to bring the loop of jejunum up to the bile duct. This route is used only when a concomitant pancreatic bypass is performed.

Cholecystojejunostomy

Construction of the Anastomosis (Fig. 58.4)

Technical and Anatomic Points

Cholecystojejunostomy is performed for palliation of advanced carcinoma of the head of the pancreas. It should only

FIGURE 58.4
CONSTRUCTION OF THE ANASTOMOSIS

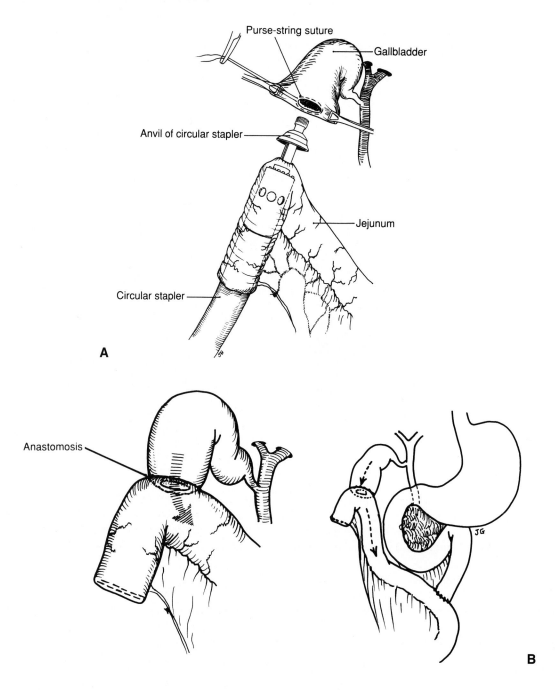

be elected when the cystic duct is known to be patent or when a grossly enlarged (Courvoisier) gallbladder is found. If the cystic duct is not patent, this anastomotic procedure will not adequately decompress the obstructed biliary tree and should not be attempted.

Place a pursestring suture of 4-0 silk on the apex of the distended gallbladder. Place this suture in the form of a small square measuring approximately 1 cm on each side. Introduce a gallbladder trocar through the pursestring, using the suture to control leakage. Decompress the distended gallbladder fully. Obtain a culture of the bile. Remove the trocar, taking care not to spill any bile as the trocar is removed. Place Babcock clamps on the gallbladder to maintain it in a high position within the operative field. Construct a Roux-en-Y loop of jejunum that will comfortably reach to the fundus of the gallbladder.

Sutured Anastomosis

Construct a two-layer anastomosis between the side of the Roux-en-Y loop of jejunum and the previously made opening in the gallbladder, using 4-0 silk for the outer layer and running 4-0 Vicryl for the inner layer. Interrupted single layer 3-0 PDS is an alternative preferred by some surgeons. Confirm that the anastomosis is patent and cover it with omentum at the conclusion of the surgical procedure. Place drains in proximity to any biliary enteric anastomosis.

Stapled Anastomosis

Pass a small EEA stapler (the largest that will fit within the lumen of the Roux loop) through the open end of the jejunum and then spike it out through the antimesenteric border at the proposed site of anastomosis. Create a pursestring suture of 3-0 prolene around the opening in the gallbladder made at the time of trocar decompression and introduce the anvil. Tie the pursestring, connect the anvil to the EEA and fire the stapler. Confirm patency of the anastomosis by palpation and inspect the donuts. Reinforce the anastomosis with a few interrupted 4-0 silk sutures. Close the open end of jejunum with a TA-55 stapler and complete the Roux-en-Y as previously described.

Consider performing a gastroenterostomy if the tumor is encroaching on the duodenum or if preoperative gastric outlet obstruction is suspected.

REFERENCES

1. Andersen JR, Sorensen SM, Kruse A, et al. Randomized trial of endoscopic endoprosthesis versus operative bypass in malignant obstructive jaundice. *Gut* 1989;30:1132–1135.
2. Bogt DP, Hermann RE. Choledochoduodenostomy, choledochojejunostomy or sphincteroplasty for biliary and pancreatic disease. *Ann Surg* 1981;193:161.
3. Gerhards MF, van Gulik TM, Bosma A, et al. Long-term survival after resection of proximal bile duct carcinoma (Klatskin tumors). *World J Surg* 1999;23:91–96.
4. Iwatsuki S, Todo S, Marsh JW, et al. Treatment of hilar cholangiocarcinoma (Klatskin tumors) with hepatic resection or transplantation. *J Am Coll Surg* 1998;187:358–364.
5. Jarnagin WR, Burke E, Powers C, et al. Intrahepatic biliary enteric bypass provides effective palliation in selected patients with malignant obstruction at the hepatic duct confluence. *Am J Surg* 1998;175: 453–460.
6. Launois B, Terblanche J, Lakehal M, et al. Proximal bile duct cancer: high resectability rate and 5-year survival. *Ann Surg* 1999;230: 266–275.
7. Lillemoe KD. Current status of surgery for Klatskin tumors. *Curr Opin Gen Surg* 1994;161–167.
8. Schein CJ, Gliedman ML. Choledochoduodenostomy as an adjunct to choledocholithotomy. *Surg Gynecol Obstet* 1981;152:797.
9. Stoker J, Lameris JS, Jeekel J. Percutaneously placed Wallstent endoprosthesis in patients with malignant distal biliary obstruction. *Br J Surg* 1993;80:1185–1187.
10. Taschieri AM, Elli M, Danelli PG, et al. Third-segment cholangiojejunostomy in the treatment of unresectable klatskin tumors. *Hepatogastroenterology* 1995;42:597–600. (Describes alternative technique that is useful when tumor precludes access to ducts in the hilum.)
11. Tocchi A, Mazzoni G, Liotta G, et al. Management of benign biliary strictures: biliary enteric anastomosis vs endoscopic stenting. *Arch Surg* 2000;135:153–157.
12. van den Bosch RP, van der Schelling GP, Klinkenbijl JHG, et al. Guidelines for the application of surgery and endoprostheses in the palliation of obstructive jaundice in advanced cancer of the pancreas. *Ann Surg* 1994;219:18–24. (Advocates use of surgical biliary bypass for patients with anticipated survival time longer than 6 months.)

CHAPTER 59

Laparoscopic Biliary Bypass

Laparoscopic cholecystojejunostomy is a simple procedure which is described in this chapter. Other, more complex forms of biliary diversion have also been performed laparoscopically and are referenced at the end.

LIST OF STRUCTURES

Liver
Gallbladder
   Cystic duct
Common bile duct

Initial Orientation and Setup for Anastomosis (Fig. 59.1)

Technical and Anatomic Points

Set up the room as for a laparoscopic cholecystectomy. Introduce the laparoscope through an infraumbilical portal and explore the abdomen. Cholecystojejunostomy will provide adequate decompression of the obstructed common duct only if the cystic duct is patent. If this is true, the gallbladder will appear tensely distended. Place secondary trocars as shown in Fig. 59.1A. The right lower quadrant trocar site will be used for a laparoscopic linear stapling device; current devices

FIGURE 59.1
INITIAL ORIENTATION AND SETUP FOR ANASTOMOSIS

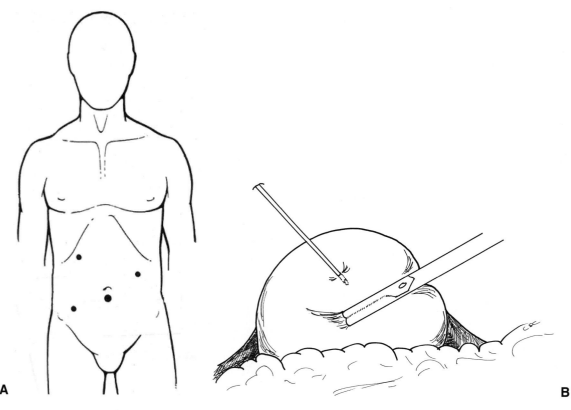

A   B

FIGURE 59.2
CONSTRUCTION OF ANASTOMOSIS (A and **B** from Bogen GL, Mancino AT, Scott-Conner CEH. Laparoscopy for staging and palliation of gastrointestinal malignancy. *Surg Clin North Am* 1996;76:557–569, with permission.)

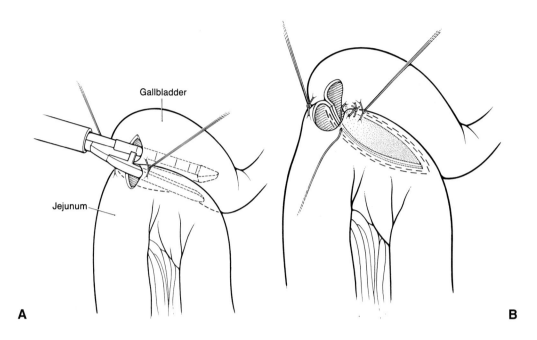

A   B

require a 12 mm port. The other two ports should accommodate graspers and needle holders. For most situations, two 5 mm ports will suffice.

Insert a Veress needle directly through the abdominal wall and puncture the gallbladder at a site suitable for anastomosis. Use an atraumatic grasper to stabilize the gallbladder during puncture (Fig. 59.1B).

Confirm patency of the cystic duct by cholangiography (if not previously obtained) and the aspiration of yellow bile from the gallbladder. Aspirate the bile to decompress the gallbladder. If the aspirated bile is white rather than yellow, suspect cystic duct obstruction with hydrops of the gallbladder.

Identify a loop of proximal jejunum that reaches comfortably to the gallbladder. Confirm that it is suitably proximal by tracing the bowel to the ligament of Treitz.

Place stay sutures to approximate the gallbladder and jejunum.

Construction of Anastomosis (Fig. 59.2)

Technical and Anatomic Points

Enlarge the puncture site in the gallbladder until it is sufficiently large (approximately 1 cm) to accommodate the endoscopic stapler. Create a second stab wound in the jejunum. Place the stapler through the 12 mm port and introduce one jaw into the gallbladder, and the other jaw into the jejunum. Use the stay sutures and atraumatic graspers to manipulate gallbladder and jejunum well up into the jaws of the stapler (Fig. 59.2A). Close and fire the device. Leave the stapler closed for one or two minutes to encourage hemostasis, then remove it.

Inspect the staple line for bleeding by irrigating within the lumen of the cholecystojejunostomy, looking for blood in the suction return. Close the anterior stab wounds by suturing jejunum to gallbladder (Fig. 59.2B). Alternatively, the endoscopic stapler may be introduced from a left-sided port and used to close the stab wounds by triangulation.

REFERENCES

1. Bogen GL, Mancino AT, Scott-Conner CEH. Laparoscopy for staging and palliation of gastrointestinal malignancy. *Surg Clin North Am* 1996;76:557–569. (Describes both cholecystojejunostomy and gastrojejunostomy and their applications.)
2. Fletcher DR, Jones RM. Laparoscopic cholecystojejunostomy as palliation for obstructive jaundice in inoperable carcinoma of pancreas. *Surg Endosc* 1992;6:147–149.
3. Rhodes M, Nathanson L, Fielding G. Laparoscopic biliary and gastric bypass: a useful adjunct in the treatment of carcinoma of the pancreas. *Gut* 1995;36:778–780.
4. Scott-Conner CEH. Laparoscopic cholecystojejunostomy, laparoscopic gastrojejunostomy. In: Scott-Conner CEH, ed. *The SAGES manual.* New York: Springer-Verlag, 1999.

CHAPTER 60

Transduodenal Sphincteroplasty

Sphincteroplasty is a useful adjunct to common duct exploration for calculous biliary tract disease. It produces a wide opening of the distal common duct, allowing impacted stones to be removed from the ampulla of Vater. The ampullary sphincter is enlarged, and any stones that are left behind in the upper ductal system should be able to pass naturally into the duodenum. It is only performed when there is reason to believe that stones may have been left behind, or when there are impacted stones in the distal ampulla. It has been termed an internal choledochoduodenostomy.

Occasionally, sphincteroplasty is performed for treatment of recurrent pancreatitis. Sphincteroplasty of the terminal pancreatic duct is included as part of that procedure (see references).

Visualization of the Ampulla (Fig. 60.1)

Technical Points

Generally, cholecystectomy and common duct exploration will have been performed immediately prior to sphincteroplasty. Open the common duct and place a probe through it to aid in subsequent dissection. This should be done even if the common duct is not explored prior to sphincteroplasty.

Place a No. 3 Bakes dilator into the choledochotomy and pass it through the ampulla. Confirm that the dilator is in the duodenum by visualizing the "single steel" sign. This refers to the manner in which the shiny stainless *steel* tip of the Bakes dilator is easily seen through a *single* layer of tissue (the duodenal wall). Fully mobilize the duodenum by performing a wide Kocher maneuver. Place stay sutures of 3-0 silk on the lateral aspect of the second portion of the duodenum in the approximate area where the ampulla is palpable over the Bakes dilator. Make a longitudinal duodenotomy approximately 4 cm in length and deliver the Bakes dilator into the duodeno-

LIST OF STRUCTURES

Gallbladder
Common bile duct
   Intramural portion
Ampulla of Vater
Major duodenal papilla
Pancreatic duct (of Wirsung)
Duodenum

tomy. The ampulla should be visible in the incision. Extend the incision along the duodenum proximally, or distally if necessary, to achieve good visualization of the ampulla.

Have ready in the operating room an ampule of secretin and instruct the anesthesiologist to administer this intravenously (IV) as you begin the sphincteroplasty. This will increase the flow of pancreatic juice and facilitate visualization of the pancreatic duct. Place stay sutures of 4-0 silk on the lateral aspect of the ampulla. Lifting up on these, insert the tip of Potts scissors into the ampulla and make a cut with the scissors approximately 2 mm in length, directing it between 10 o'clock and 11 o'clock on the ampulla. Place through-and-through sutures of 4-0 Vicryl, one on each side of the incision. Leave the sutures long and pull up gently on them, elevating the edges of the incision in the ampulla. Again, place the tip of the Potts scissors into the incision in the ampulla and extend it proximally another 2 mm or so. Place additional sutures of Vicryl to suture the duodenal mucosa securely to the mucosa of the ampulla and to provide hemostasis as the incision is widened. Extend the incision proximally until the muscular sphincter of the ampulla is divided and the common duct is entered. At this point, the opening in the sphincteroplasty should be large enough to admit a large Bakes dilator. Remove any stones that are impacted in the distal duct.

Anatomic Points

The clockface orientations given above refer to a mobilized duodenum rotated so that the convex side of the duodenal C loop is facing anteriorly, with a longitudinal duodenotomy on the convex, or antimesenteric, side of the duodenum. The major duodenal papilla should be visible on the posteromedial wall of the second part of the duodenum, usually 7 to 10 cm distal to the pylorus. Rarely, it may be as close as 1.5 cm, or as far distal as the third part of the duodenum.

The ampulla of Vater is the common channel of the terminal bile duct and the pancreatic duct (of Wirsung). Developmentally, this common channel extends throughout the entire intramural part of these ducts. As growth proceeds, the site of luminal union of the two ducts comes to lie progressively nearer the tip of the major duodenal papilla. Because of this developmental sequence, it is not surprising that the extent to which the two ducts are separated within the duodenal wall is quite variable. They can open separately into the duodenum, usually via independent ostia on the major duodenal papilla, and are reported to do so in up to 29% of the cases. Further,

ORIENTATION

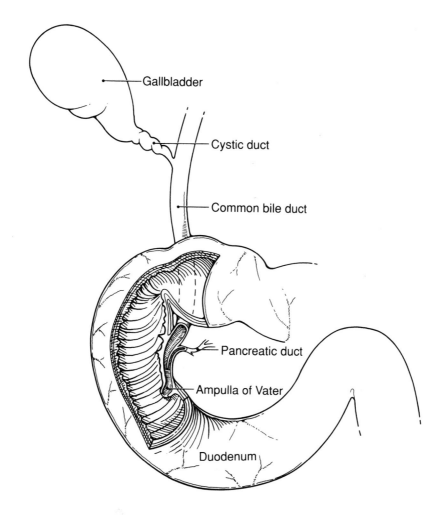

- Gallbladder
- Cystic duct
- Common bile duct
- Pancreatic duct
- Ampulla of Vater
- Duodenum

because the exocrine pancreas can be drained entirely by the so-called accessory pancreatic duct (of Santorini), which developmentally is the proximal part of the duct of the dorsal pancreatic bud, secretin injection may demonstrate the location of the termination of this duct but not that of the bile duct.

The orientation of and anatomic relationships between the intramural parts of the pancreatic duct and the common bile duct are important. The intramural parts of these ducts, whether fused or not, are typically about 1.5 cm long, but they can be as long as 2 cm. Prior to union, the bile duct is slightly superior to, and posterior to, the major pancreatic duct. Thus, the pancreatic duct is located at 3 o'clock with respect to the bile duct. The unfused, intramural parts of these ducts typically lie side by side, but they may partially twist around each other. Cautious advancement of the scissors is in order.

Completion of Sphincteroplasty (Fig. 60.2)

Technical Points

Continue the sphincteroplasty until the ampulla has been widely opened and the common duct will accept a large

FIGURE 60.1
VISUALIZATION OF THE AMPULLA

FIGURE 60.2
COMPLETION OF SPHINCTEROPLASTY

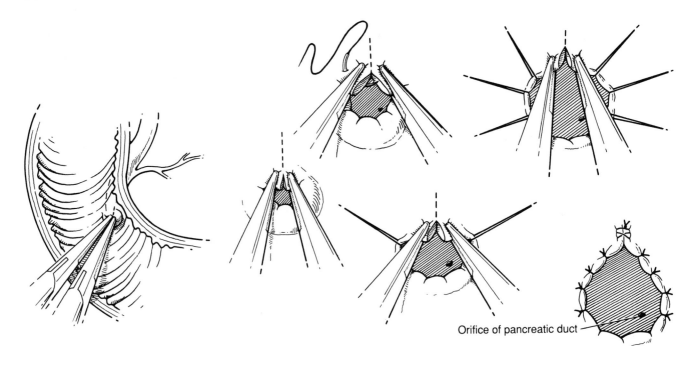

Orifice of pancreatic duct

Bakes dilator. Place interrupted sutures the entire length of the sphincteroplasty on both sides to suture the mucosa of the duodenum securely to the mucosa of the ampulla and to provide hemostasis. Place a horizontal suture at the apex of the sphincteroplasty. This suture not only provides hemostasis, but guards against a posterior perforation of the wall of the duodenum.

The length of the intraduodenal portion of the common duct varies from individual to individual. If the sphincteroplasty is long, it is possible to carry it out past the area where the common duct is intramural, resulting in posterior perforation of the duodenum. This may not be recognized initially, and can cause profound retroperitoneal sepsis several days after surgery. Carefully suturing the sphincteroplasty, especially at the apex, will guard against this complication. It may be helpful to think of the sphincteroplasty as a side-to-side choledochoduodenal anastomosis, suturing it with the same care.

Pass probes proximally and distally and confirm that the sphincteroplasty is widely patent and that the muscle of the ampulla has been divided adequately.

Visualize the pancreatic duct at approximately 3 o'clock inside the lumen of the ampulla. Identify it by its outpouring of clear pancreatic juice in response to the IV administration of secretin. A sphincteroplasty of the pancreatic duct can be performed, if indicated, over a lacrimal duct probe in a fashion similar to that described for the ampullary sphincteroplasty.

It is not necessary to leave a T tube in the common duct or to stent the sphincteroplasty. Close the choledochotomy primarily with a running suture of 4-0 Vicryl.

Close the incision in the duodenum in two layers. Generally, it is not possible to close this longitudinal incision in a transverse fashion. Lack of mobility in this portion of the duodenum and the length of incision necessary for adequate sphincteroplasty render this impractical. Therefore, simply close the incision in the same direction that it has been made, taking care not to narrow the lumen. Place omentum over the duodenal suture line and the choledochotomy. Place closed suction drains in the subhepatic space.

Anatomic Points

Regardless of the degree of union of the bile duct and major pancreatic duct, the intramural part of the bile duct does have a complex of sphincteric muscle that is embryologically and functionally distinct from the musculature of the duodenum. This sphincter complex varies in length from 6 to 30 mm, and can extend proximally into the pancreatic portion of the bile duct. It is this variability in length that makes it advisable to advance the sphincteroplasty by small increments of about 2 to 3 mm.

REFERENCES

1. Boyden EA. The anatomy of the choledochoduodenal junction in man. *Surg Gynecol Obstet* 1957;104:641.
2. Jones SA. Sphincteroplasty (not sphincterotomy) in the treatment of biliary tract disease. *Surg Clin North Am* 1973;53:1123.
3. Jones SA. The technique of transduodenal sphincteroplasty (not sphincterotomy). *Surg Rounds* 1979;2:14.
4. Moody FG, Vecchio R, Calabuig R, et al. Transduodenal sphincteroplasty with transampullary septectomy for stenosing papillitis. *Am J Surg* 1991;161:213–218. (Describes decompression of pancreatic duct by septectomy.)
5. Nussbaum MS, Warner BW, Sax HC, et al. Transduodenal sphincteroplasty and transampullary septotomy for primary sphincter of Oddi dysfunction. *Am J Surg* 1989;157:38–43.
6. Rattner DW, Fernandez-del Castillo C, Brugge WR, et al. Defining the criteria for local resection of ampullary neoplasms. *Arch Surg* 1996;131:366–371. (Describes technique of local excision.)
7. Reinhoff WF Jr, Pickerell KL. Pancreatitis: an anatomic study of the pancreatic and extrahepatic biliary systems. *Arch Surg* 1945;51:205.

CHAPTER 61

Portacaval and Distal Splenorenal Shunts

A variety of portasystemic shunt procedures have been devised, attesting to dissatisfaction with the side effects. Most patients with bleeding esophageal varices are managed by endoscopic control followed by TIPS; surgical shunts are employed only under special circumstances. Two procedures are discussed in this chapter: the end-to-side portacaval shunt and the distal splenorenal (Warren) shunt. Other shunting and non-shunting alternatives for control of variceal bleeding are described in the references cited at the end.

The end-to-side portacaval shunt immediately and reliably decreases portal pressure by completely diverting portal inflow into the systemic venous circulation. This shunt diminishes blood flow to the liver in cirrhotic patients with hepatopedal flow and may produce or worsen hepatic encephalopathy. Subsequent liver transplant is made much more difficult by this or any other central shunt. Technically, it is significantly easier and quicker than the distal splenorenal shunt.

These procedures depend upon an understanding of the anatomy of both the caval system and the hepatic portal system. In general, the caval system drains the body wall, extremities, head and neck, urogenital system, and liver; all components ultimately drain into the superior and inferior venae cavae. The hepatic portal system conveys blood from the capillary beds of the abdominal gastrointestinal tract, biliary apparatus, pancreas, and spleen to the sinusoids of the liver. After passing through the hepatic sinusoids, blood is conveyed to the inferior vena cava by the hepatic veins.

Although the caval and portal systems are functionally and morphologically considered to be separate entities, there are several actual or potential sites of anastomosis between the two that can provide collateral routes if the portal system is obstructed. These include the following:

1. The esophageal tributaries of the left gastric vein (portal) with the esophageal tributaries of the azygos or hemiazygos vein (caval)
2. The anal tributaries of the superior rectal (hemorrhoidal) vein (portal) with the anal tributaries of the middle and inferior rectal (hemorrhoidal) veins (caval)
3. The left umbilical and paraumbilical veins (portal) with the superficial epigastric veins (caval)
4. The veins of Retzius on bare areas of liver and the non-peritonealized surfaces of the colon, duodenum, and pancreas (portal) with the retroperitoneal branches of the intercostal, lumbar, and renal veins (caval)

These anastomotic sites are of great clinical importance, especially the esophageal anastomoses. Bleeding or ruptured varices at these sites can constitute a surgical emergency.

Portacaval Shunt

Incision and Mobilization of the Duodenum and Exposure of the Inferior Vena Cava (Fig. 61.1)

Technical Points

Position the patient supine. Place a folded towel under the lower thoracic spine or elevate the kidney rest slightly. Make a right subcostal incision and carry it across the midline, sloping it downward to follow the left costal margin. Divide the ligamentum teres hepatis with suture ligatures to secure

LIST OF STRUCTURES

Liver
Ligamentum teres hepatis
Falciform ligament
Hepatoduodenal ligament
Common bile duct
Common hepatic artery
Portal vein
    Splenic vein

Superior mesenteric vein
Gastroduodenal vein
Left gastric (coronary) vein
Right gastric (pyloric) vein
Prepyloric veins
Gastroepiploic arcade
    Left and right gastroepiploic veins
Ligament of Treitz

Pancreas
Duodenum
Colon
Left renal vein
    Left gonadal vein
    Left adrenal (suprarenal) vein

ORIENTATION

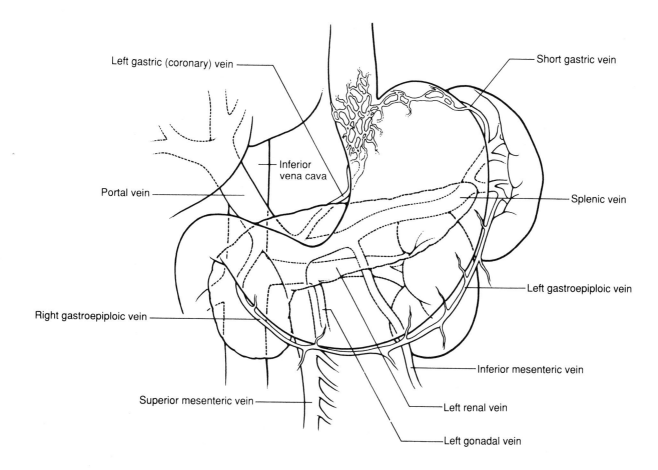

the umbilical vein. This is generally recanalized in patients with portal hypertension and may be quite large.

Measure portal pressure by cannulating an omental vein with a 20-gauge Angiocath and connecting this to a manometer calibrated for venous pressure measurements. Ligate the omental vein after you withdraw the cannula. Perform a needle biopsy of the liver (if this was not done preoperatively) and explore the abdomen.

Next, perform a wide Kocher maneuver to expose the inferior vena cava fully. Do this with caution, as dilated venous collaterals may have formed in the retroduodenal area. If the retroperitoneum is thickened and the inferior vena cava is not visible, first orient yourself by palpating the abdominal aorta. The inferior vena cava will lie immediately to the right of the aorta. Generally, it will be directly deep to the hepatoduodenal ligament, another useful landmark. Often, the invisible inferior vena cava is palpable as a large ballotable structure once the proper location has been identified. Clean the anterior surface of the vena cava by sharp dissection in the anterior adventitial plane to the level of the liver superiorly. Select a large clamp for partial occlusion, such as a Satinsky clamp, and verify that sufficient vena cava has been prepared for it to lie comfortably. Although it is not necessary to mobilize

the inferior vena cava fully and circumferentially, comfortable placement of the partial occlusion clamp is easier if an adequate segment of the vena cava has been cleared as far laterally as possible.

Anatomic Points

The ligamentum teres hepatis, located in the free edge of the falciform ligament, passes from the umbilicus to the umbilical portion of the left branch of the portal vein. This fibrotic remnant of the left umbilical vein retains a lumen that normally is completely occluded only close to the portal vein. In cases of portal hypertension, this occlusion can be opened, and the residual lumen can become greatly dilated. In addition to this, the ligamentum teres hepatis is accompanied by slender paraumbilical veins that provide a portacaval anastomosis; engorgement of these veins leads to the classic *caput medusae.* Thus, control of all these veins must be achieved prior to division of the ligamentum teres hepatis.

Omental veins are tributaries of the right or left gastroepiploic veins. Because of the proximal and distal communications between the omental veins, as well as the fact that the

FIGURE 61.1
INCISION AND MOBILIZATION OF THE DUODENUM AND EXPOSURE OF THE INFERIOR VENA CAVA

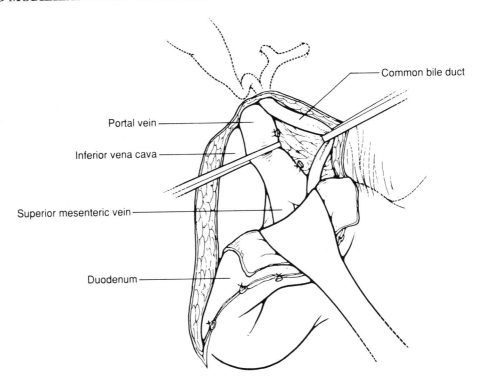

portal system is typically valveless, ligation on both sides of the cannula site is necessary for adequate hemostasis.

Visualization of the inferior vena cava in the upper abdomen is possible only if the duodenum and head of the pancreas are kocherized. The portal venous tributaries that will be mobilized with these organs are the retroduodenal vein, pyloric (right gastric) vein, supraduodenal vein, the pancreaticoduodenal veins, and the superior mesenteric vein. These will be engorged and fragile. In addition, several direct communications, via the veins of Retzius, between the portal and caval systems will most likely be enlarged and must be divided. These should be divided with care to prevent their avulsion from the inferior vena cava or its major tributaries.

Dissection of the Portal Vein (Fig. 61.2)

Technical Points

Rotate the duodenum medially to expose the posterior aspect of the hepatoduodenal ligament. Place a moist laparotomy sponge over the posterior duodenum and head of the pancreas and place a retractor there. Have your assistant apply gentle traction to maintain these structures up, in a fully kocherized position. Palpate the posterior surface of the hepatoduodenal ligament, which has been rotated upward toward you by retraction, and identify the portal vein. It is a large, soft, ballottable structure posterior to the common bile duct and hepatic artery. Incise the peritoneum overlying the posterolateral surface of the portal vein and enter the anterior adventitial plane of the vein.

All of the tributaries of the portal vein in this vicinity pass to the left (anteromedial). The right or "free" edge (that is, the edge of the vein corresponding to the free edge of the hepatoduodenal ligament) is without tributaries. Therefore, dissect proximally and distally along the vein in this region first. Use a peanut sponge to gently develop the plane partially around the portal vein. Use a vein retractor to elevate the common duct, hepatic artery, and soft tissues from the anterior surface of the portal vein. Carefully dissect in the adventitial plane of the portal vein until it can be gently elevated and surrounded by a vessel loop. Mobilize the vein cephalad to the hilum of the liver and caudad to the vicinity of the splenic vein. Divide several small tributaries that pass to the left.

Visualize the path that the portal vein will need to take to anastomose with the inferior vena cava. Divide and excise any thickened soft tissue lateral and posterior to the portal vein, if necessary, to create a groove in which the vein can lie without kinking.

Divide the portal vein between vascular clamps at the hilum of the liver, leaving sufficient length in the hilum to safely ligate or oversew the stump. A medium-sized, slightly angled vascular clamp provides good control over the portal vein and can be used by your assistant to hold the vein in the best possible position for anastomosis. Bulldog-type clamps are not useful in this situation because they allow too much mobility of the vein. Suture material will tend to catch in the spring of the clamp, as well.

Preoperative, venous-phase angiographic studies will generally have demonstrated patency of the portal vein.

FIGURE 61.2
DISSECTION OF THE PORTAL VEIN

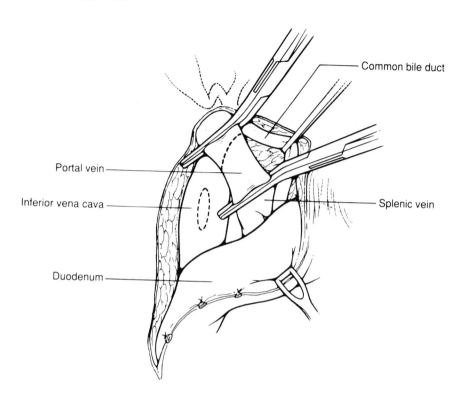

Sometimes, however, an unexpected thrombus is encountered. In such cases, an attempt at gentle extraction of the thrombus from the vein using forceps is often successful. Ligate the vein and then place a second transfixion suture ligature below the initial site of ligation for security.

Anatomic Points

The portal vein is formed dorsal to the neck of the pancreas by the union of the superior mesenteric and splenic veins. It then passes posterior to the first part of the duodenum and runs in the right border of the hepatoduodenal ligament to the porta hepatis, where it divides into left and right branches. From its origin to its terminal branches, this vein is 8 to 10 cm long and 8 to 14 mm in diameter. Initially, it is somewhat to the right of the beginning of the superior mesenteric artery and anterior to the inferior vena cava. As it ascends in the hepatoduodenal ligament, it lies posterior to both the common bile duct (closest to the free edge of the hepatoduodenal ligament) and the hepatic artery complex. The gastroduodenal artery usually arises from the common hepatic artery to the left of the portal vein, then crosses the anterior surface of the vein before it branches into the superior pancreaticoduodenal and right gastroepiploic arteries. Because of these relationships, the portal vein is most easily approached from its posterior surface. However, the surgeon should be aware that aberrant right hepatic arteries (eg, those arising from the superior mesenteric artery or independently from the celiac artery) almost invariably lie posterior to the portal vein.

Tributaries of the portal vein vary considerably. In addition to the splenic and superior mesenteric veins, frequently, the left gastric (coronary), right gastric (pyloric), prepyloric, paraumbilical, accessory pancreatic, and cystic veins drain directly into the portal vein. Of these, the only one of significant size is the left gastric vein, which enters from the left in approximately 25% of cases. In the remaining 75% of cases, it terminates in the splenic vein, usually very close to the confluence of the splenic and superior mesenteric veins. Other tributaries tend to enter the anterior surface of the vein. The right side, which is the side along the free edge of the hepatoduodenal ligament, usually has no tributaries.

Construction of Anastomosis (Fig. 61.3)

Technical and Anatomic Points

Trim the portal vein to a length that will reach comfortably to the inferior vena cava without kinking when the duodenum is allowed to fall back. Angle this cut obliquely (at approximately a 45-degree angle) to facilitate the anastomosis.

Place the partial occlusion clamp on the inferior vena cava. Position this clamp so that the handle is supported by soft tissues inferiorly. If properly placed, the clamp will lie comfortably and your assistant will not need to stabilize it. Make a longitudinal venotomy with a No. 11 blade on the left anterior aspect of the cava. Extend the venotomy with Pott's scissors.

Place stay sutures on the right side of the venotomy on the inferior vena cava (what will be the anterior wall of the

FIGURE 61.3
CONSTRUCTION OF ANASTOMOSIS

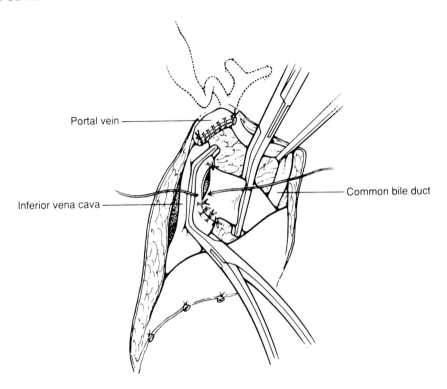

Portal vein

Inferior vena cava

Common bile duct

anastomosis) and the left side of the portal vein so that the venotomies can be held open atraumatically. Position the vascular clamp on the portal vein so that the cut edge of the portal vein is in close apposition to the venotomy of the inferior vena cava and have your assistant hold it there. Place two corner sutures and construct the back wall of the anastomosis with a running suture of 5-0 Prolene. Tie all knots on the outside. Use simple interrupted sutures for the front layer. This will avoid "pursestringing" and will allow the anastomosis to balloon outwardly.

Before tying the last suture, flush the inferior vena cava and portal vein by briefly opening the vascular clamps a little. Then tie the last suture. Open the partial occlusion clamp on the inferior vena cava first. Minor oozing from the suture line is to be expected and can be ignored. Bleeding from gaps in the suture line should be controlled by placing interrupted simple sutures. Next, open the portal vein clamp. Allow the duodenum and head of the pancreas to fall back into place. Observe the shunt for kinking.

Measure omental vein pressure at the beginning and end of the operation. It should be significantly lower (close to the central venous pressure) after placement of a successful shunt.

Check hemostasis. Generally, the operative field will dry up as soon as the shunt is opened and portal pressure is decreased. Just before closing the abdomen, palpate the portal vein and shunt. It should feel soft and should be easily collapsible with fingertip pressure. A thrombus within the

shunt will feel firm; sometimes, a thrombus will be palpated and then the vein will collapse as the clot is milked out. Thrombus formation indicates a technical problem, such as kinking, which must be corrected. Close the abdomen securely without drains.

Distal Splenorenal (Warren) Shunt

The distal splenorenal shunt was devised to maintain a high portal perfusion pressure while selectively decompressing esophageal varices. In this procedure, the splenic vein is disconnected from the portal vein and anastomosed in an end-to-side fashion to the left renal vein. Collateral pathways along the greater curvature of the stomach are interrupted, the coronary vein is ligated, and potential collaterals along the body and tail of the pancreas are interrupted. Hence, the esophageal varices are completely disconnected from the high-pressure portal system and are decompressed into the low-pressure systemic venous pathways via the left renal vein. Complete and meticulous interruption of collateral vessels is important. Small collateral connections between the portal system and the low-pressure caval system will dilate in time, causing loss of the selectivity of the shunt. Recurrent variceal bleeding and hepatic encephalopathy may also result.

Preoperative assessment of the patient for placement of a distal splenorenal shunt should include visceral angiography,

FIGURE 61.4
INCISION AND EXPOSURE OF THE PANCREAS

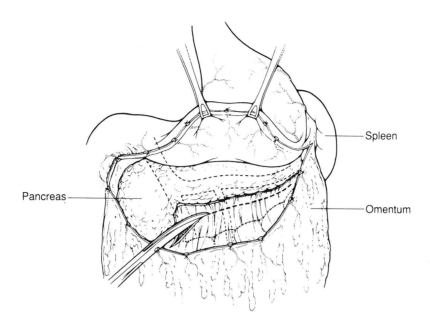

Pancreas

Spleen

Omentum

with venous-phase views to assess the patency of the splenic and portal veins, as well as left renal venography. A patent splenic vein measuring at least 1 cm in diameter (documented by angiography) and a single, unobstructed left renal vein are necessary for a successful shunt. In addition, the splenic vein must not be too high above the renal vein.

Incision and Exposure of the Pancreas (Fig. 61.4)

Technical Points

Position the patient supine. Place a folded sheet under the lower thoracic spine (or "break" the operating table) to produce slight hyperextension if the patient has a very deep abdominal cavity. Make a left subcostal incision. Extend the incision across the midline and downward so that it parallels the right costal margin for several centimeters.

Measure omental vein pressure as described in Fig. 61.1. Divide the gastrocolic omentum by sequentially clamping and ligating branches of the gastroepiploic arcade on the greater curvature of the stomach. Carry this dissection distally to the pylorus and proximally to the short gastric vessels. Secure the right gastroepiploic artery and vein with a suture ligature. This dissection not only provides a window through which the splenic vein can be exposed, but also interrupts the collateral vessels.

Place two or three figure-of-eight stay sutures through the posterior gastric wall and use these to elevate and retract the stomach cephalad. Identify the pancreas by its appearance and by palpation. Retract the duodenum downward by applying gentle traction with a laparotomy pad. Commence dissection in the (generally) avascular plane between the

inferior border of the pancreas and the upper border of the duodenum. This can usually be done by introducing the tips of a right-angle clamp, spreading them, and then displaying the tissue for your assistant to divide with electrocautery.

Anatomic Points

The gastroepiploic arcade, formed by the anastomosis of right and left gastroepiploic veins, lies in the gastrocolic ligament. The right gastroepiploic vein terminates by draining into the superior mesenteric or portal vein, whereas the left gastroepiploic vein drains into the splenic vein or one of its splenic tributaries. Several gastric and omental tributaries drain into this arcade.

Mobilization of the Pancreas and Identification of the Splenic Vein (Fig. 61.5)

Technical Points

Incise the peritoneum overlying the groove between the pancreas and the duodenum with electrocautery. Follow this out to the tail of the pancreas. Incise the ligament of Treitz and mobilize the fourth portion of the duodenum downward if necessary. If the spleen is greatly enlarged, beware of angulation and downward displacement of the tail of the pancreas and splenic vein. The inferior mesenteric vein will enter the field and empty either into the splenic vein or, occasionally, the superior mesenteric vein. Identify, ligate, and divide this vein.

Next, gently elevate the pancreas and its adherent splenic vein from the retroperitoneum. Generally, this can be done by careful blunt dissection in an avascular plane. Identify

FIGURE 61.5
MOBILIZATION OF THE PANCREAS AND IDENTIFICATION OF THE SPLENIC VEIN

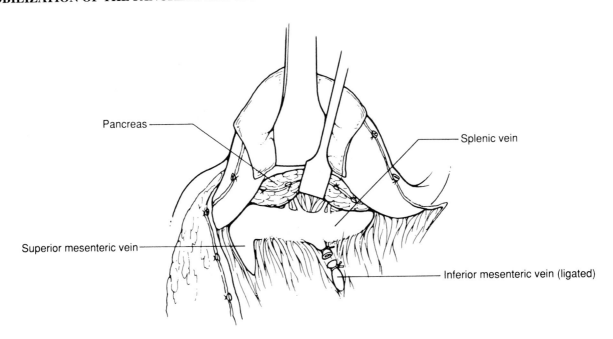

the splenic vein by palpation and carefully incise the overlying areolar tissue to enter the adventitial plane of the vessel.

Anatomic Points

The ligament of Treitz, or suspensory muscle of the duodenum, is typically composed of striated muscle from the right crus of the diaphragm near the esophageal hiatus, connective tissue in continuity with that around the celiac artery, and smooth muscle derived from the circular muscle layer of the gut at or near the duodenojejunal flexure. Despite its muscular components, it apparently has little contractile function, but rather serves to suspend the duodenojejunal flexure. However, because of its muscular components, division of this ligament should be done between clamps or with electrocautery.

Mobilization of the third (horizontal) and fourth (ascending) parts of the duodenum requires some knowledge of these portions of the duodenum. The third part, which is about 8 cm long, begins on the right side of the fourth lumbar vertebra and, with a slight cranial inclination, passes to the left to join the fourth part of the duodenum just anterior to the aorta. From right to left, it lies anterior to the right crus of the diaphragm, then to the inferior vena cava, and finally, to the aorta. Its anterior surface is covered by peritoneum except where it is crossed by the root of the mesentery and the superior mesenteric vessels. The fourth part of the duodenum, which is approximately 2.5 cm long, lies anterior and to the left of the aorta. It terminates opposite the second lumbar vertebra, where it turns abruptly anterior to become

continuous with the duodenum at the duodenojejunal flexure. This part of the duodenum is anterior to the left sympathetic trunk, left psoas major muscle, and left renal and gonadal vessels. To the right is the beginning of the root of the mesentery, whereas to the left are the left kidney and ureter.

These parts of the duodenum receive their blood supply primarily from the anterior and posterior pancreaticoduodenal arcades and (distally) the first jejunal artery. As these arteries approach the duodenum along its concavity, mobilization of both the duodenum and head of the pancreas can easily be accomplished by division of the peritoneum along the concave side of the duodenum, followed by blunt dissection in the avascular fusion plane posterior to the duodenum and pancreas. This maneuver, however, demands some familiarity with the posterior relationships of the duodenum and pancreas.

Mobilization of the Splenic Vein (Fig. 61.6)

Technical Points

Completely expose the posterior surface of the splenic vein by careful sharp dissection in the adventitial plane. Before you expose the vein by opening the anterior adventitial plane, it will appear whitish because of the overlying connecting tissue. When you are in the correct plane, the vein will appear blue and it will bulge into the field. The vein is extremely thin-walled and fragile, so it must be handled with care.

Multiple, short, fine tributaries connect the splenic vein to the posterior surface of the pancreas. These are relatively

FIGURE 61.6
MOBILIZATION OF THE SPLENIC VEIN

Left gastric (coronary) vein (ligated)

Pancreas

Splenic vein

Portal vein

Superior mesenteric vein

Inferior mesenteric vein (ligated)

sparse in the immediate vicinity of the juncture of the splenic vein and portal vein. Carefully develop the plane behind the splenic vein by gentle dissection with a right-angle clamp. Pass a Silastic loop around the vein. The coronary vein can sometimes be identified entering the superior aspect of the splenic vein at the splenic vein/portal vein juncture. Doubly ligate and divide it. If you cannot identify the coronary vein in this location, or do not feel you can safely approach it from this angle, it can be identified and ligated in the lesser omentum after completing the shunt. Ligation of this vein is critical for adequate portosystemic disconnection.

Next, divide the splenic vein at its termination on the portal vein. This will facilitate subsequent dissection and may "dry up" the field by disconnecting the left upper quadrant from the high-pressure portal system. However, pressure in the splenic vein stump will be high, and early division of the splenic vein precludes conversion to a proximal splenorenal (Linton-type) shunt as a bail-out maneuver if the splenic vein is injured near the hilum. Secure the splenic vein between two straight vascular clamps. Oversew the stump of the splenic vein at the portal vein with a running vascular suture. Alternatively, a relatively small splenic vein may be secured by simple ligature. If you decide to ligate the vein rather than to oversew it, place a second transfixion suture ligation distal to the first ligature for extra security.

Carefully identify, ligate, and divide the multiple, small, short, venous tributaries. Use small hemostatic clips to secure the pancreatic side of each tributary. Do not use these on the splenic vein, though, as they are apt to catch on laparotomy pads or sutures, resulting in tearing of the vein. If a tributary is accidentally avulsed, control bleeding from the splenic vein by direct pressure. Suture-ligate the pancreatic side using a figure-of-eight stitch if the vessel has retracted. Then place a delicate figure-of-eight 5-0 monofilament

vascular suture across the small hole in the splenic vein. Do not attempt to place clamps on a bleeding site on the vein, as the clamp is likely to either tear the vein, enlarging the hole, or to cause too much of the vein wall to be included, resulting in narrowing when the vein is stitched. Control bleeding from large avulsion injuries with a partial occlusion clamp.

Continue mobilizing the splenic vein until all tributaries to the pancreas have been divided.

Anatomic Points

The splenic vein begins by the confluence of the segmental splenic radicles. In the gastrosplenic ligament, four or five short gastric veins typically drain into one or more of these radicles, often by passing into the upper part of the spleen itself. In addition, the left gastroepiploic vein also drains into the distal splenic vein proper, or into one of its splenic tributaries. From its origin in the hilum of the spleen, the splenic vein courses medially posterior to the pancreas, from which it receives multiple, short, fragile tributaries. About 40% of the time, the inferior mesenteric vein will also drain into the splenic vein near its union with the superior mesenteric vein. The splenic vein is inferior to the artery and is straight, rather than tortuous. The splenic vein or retropancreatic part of the superior mesenteric vein receives the inferior mesenteric vein at approximately the vertebral level of L-2. Because the inferior mesenteric artery originates from the aorta at a significantly lower level (vertebral level of L-3), it should not be in the operative field. Furthermore, because of gut rotation and fixation, posterior tributaries of the splenic vein, and communications between it and the renal vein, are minor or lacking, thus allowing relatively bloodless mobilization of the pancreas and splenic vein.

FIGURE 61.7
PREPARATION OF THE LEFT RENAL VEIN

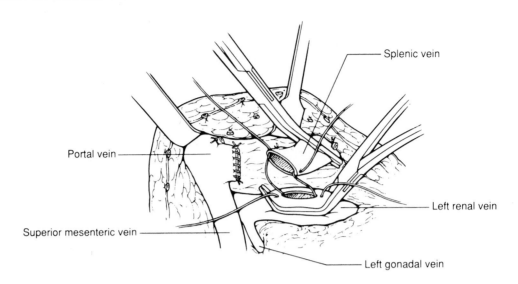

Preparation of the Left Renal Vein (Fig. 61.7)

Technical Points

Palpate the left kidney and the aorta to orient yourself in the retroperitoneum. The left renal vein will lie in the retroperitoneum between the kidney and aorta, at about the midkidney level. Continue dissection in the groove above the duodenum, mobilizing the duodenum downward if necessary. The renal vein will be encountered as a large, ballottable structure that often can be felt before it is seen. Develop the anterior adventitial plane of the renal vein. Operative ultrasonography is a useful adjunct if the vein is difficult to find in the thickened, boggy, cirrhotic retroperitoneum.

Identify and ligate the left adrenal vein. The anastomosis will generally be made in the region of the stump of the left adrenal vein, on the anterosuperior aspect of the renal vein. Dividing this vein will facilitate construction of the anastomosis by improving mobility of the vein and providing an area suitable for venotomy.

Preserve any gonadal veins that you might encounter on the inferior aspect of the left renal vein. Select a large, partial occlusion clamp, such as a Satinsky clamp, and verify that a sufficient length of renal vein has been prepared to use the clamp properly.

Anatomic Points

The left renal vein, ranging in length from 6 to 10 cm, passes from the hilum of the left kidney to the inferior vena cava. It crosses the aorta just inferior to the origin of the superior mesenteric artery. In its course, it tends to be anterior to the left renal artery and to associated retroperitoneal structures, but posterior to structures associated with the gastrointestinal tract. Thus, in a significant part of its course, it is posterior to the lower border of the pancreas and duodenum, and is in very close proximity to the splenic vein. Tributaries and communications of the left renal vein, in contrast to the right renal vein, are complicated. The left renal vein always receives the left gonadal vein relatively close to the renal hilum, and receives the left suprarenal (adrenal) vein, which usually combines with the left inferior phrenic vein, close to the midline. In addition, the left renal vein usually communicates with a variable number of lumbar veins or with the abdominal portion of the azygos system, and can have minor communications with the splenic vein.

Construction of Anastomosis (Fig. 61.8)

Technical and Anatomic Points

Plan the anastomosis so that the splenic vein approaches the left renal vein at a gentle angle, close to 45 degrees. Generally, it is advisable to trim the splenic vein. Do not hesitate to trim off 1 to 2 cm to improve the way the splenic vein lies. Remember that when the pancreas and stomach are allowed to return to their normal positions, the distance to the renal vein will decrease. Divide the splenic vein obliquely. Check the retroperitoneum between the renal vein and the splenic hilum. Divide as much of this tissue as necessary to create a groove in which the splenic vein can lie comfortably without kinking.

Place a partial occlusion clamp on the left renal vein and make a venotomy using a No. 11 blade. Extend the venotomy with Pott's scissors. Excise the stump of the divided adrenal vein if it is in the way.

Have your assistant stabilize the splenic vein so that the anastomosis can be sutured without tension. Place stay sutures in the anterior wall of the splenic vein and the left renal vein and use these to retract the veins, holding them open atraumatically.

FIGURE 61.8
CONSTRUCTION OF ANASTOMOSIS

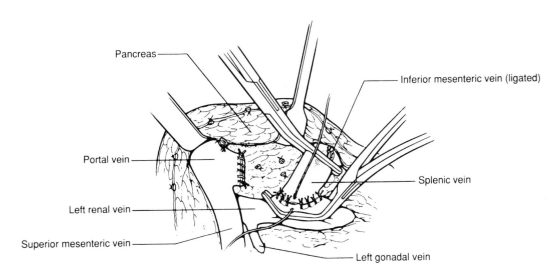

Sew the back wall of the anastomosis with a running suture of 5-0 Prolene. Start on the outside of one end of the suture line and place a simple suture through both veins. Run this suture across to the other side and pass it to the outside. Place another suture through both veins and tie it.

Suture the anterior row with multiple interrupted simple sutures to avoid pursestringing. Flush the anatomosis by flushing both the partial occlusion clamp on the renal vein and the splenic vein prior to tying the final suture. Then tie the last suture and cautiously open the renal vein clamp. Minor oozing from the suture line is to be expected and will stop. Major bleeding requires careful placement of additional simple interrupted sutures. If the anastomosis looks good, open the clamp on the splenic vein. If no major bleeding is noted from the anastomosis, place a topical hemostatic agent around it and check to make sure that it is not kinked when the pancreas and stomach are released and allowed to fall back into place. Ligate the coronary vein if this was not done earlier.

Palpate the shunt again before closing the abdomen. A patent shunt will feel soft and ballottable, compressing easily with fingertip pressure, and it will balloon out rapidly when the pressure is released. A clotted shunt will feel slightly firm and will not compress easily, or it may refill sluggishly. Correct any kinks or suspected technical problems at this time. Thrombosis of the shunt in the postoperative period results in an acute rise in venous pressure in the varices and causes massive variceal hemorrhage. Such thrombosis is generally attributable to a correctable technical error. Omental vein pressure is generally not significantly lowered by placement of the shunt. Hence, measurement of omental vein pressure is generally not performed at the conclusion of the operation and cannot be used to verify patency of the shunt.

Close the abdomen carefully without drains, remembering that ascites may accumulate in the postoperative period.

REFERENCES

1. Cameron JL, Harrington DP, Maddrey WC. The mesocaval shunt. *Surg Gynecol Obstet* 1980;150:401.
2. Cameron JL, Zuidema GD, Smith GW, et al. Mesocaval shunts for the control of bleeding esophageal varices. *Surgery* 1979;85:257. (Provides good description of interposition shunt.)
3. Drapanas T. Mesocaval shunt for portal hypertension. *Ann Surg* 1972;176:435.
4. Helton WS, Maves R, Wicks K, et al. Transjugular intrahepatic portasystemic shunt vs surgical shunt in good-risk cirrhotic patients: a case-control comparison. *Arch Surg* 2001;136:17–20.
5. Henderson JM, Nagle A, Curtas S, et al. Surgical shunts and TIPS for variceal decompression in the 1990s. *Surgery* 2000;128:540–547. (Discusses role of TIPS and surgical shunts.)
6. Knechtle SJ, D'Alessandro AM, Armbrust MJ, et al. Surgical portosystemic shunts for treatment of portal hypertensive bleeding: outcome and effect on liver function. *Surgery* 1999;126:708–713.
7. McDermott WV. The techniques of portal-systemic shunt surgery. *Surgery* 1965;57:778. (Provides good description of portacaval shunts.)
8. Millikan WJ Jr, Henderson JM, Galloway JR, et al. Surgical rescue for failures of cirrhotic sclerotherapy. *Am J Surg* 1990;160:117–121. (Discusses options including liver transplantation.)
9. Mucha P, van Heerden JA. EEA stapling for control of acute variceal hemorrhage: technique and indications. *Am J Surg* 1984;148:399. (Describes esophageal transection technique.)
10. Orloff MJ, Orloff MS, Orloff SL, et al. Experimental, clinical, and metabolic results of side-to-side portacaval shunt for intractable cirrhotic ascites. *J Am Coll Surg* 1997;184:557–570.

11. Orloff MJ, Daily PO, Orloff SL, et al. A 27-year experience with surgical treatment of Budd-Chiari syndrome. *Ann Surg* 2000;232:340–352. (Describes technical modifications for this situation.)

12. Orozco H, Mercado MA. The evolution of portal hypertension surgery: lessons from 1000 operations and 50 years' experience. *Arch Surg* 2000;135:1389–1394.

13. Sugiura M, Futagawa S. Further evaluation of the Sugiura procedure in the treatment of esophageal varices. *Arch Surg* 1977;112:1317. (Describes extensive devascularization coupled with esophageal transection.)

14. Warren WD, Millikan WJ. Selective transsplenic decompression procedure: changes in technique after 300 cases. *Contemp Surg* 1981;18:11. (Presents excellent distillation of long-term experience with the shunt that bears the first author's name.)

15. Warren WD, Millikan WJ, Henderson JM, et al. Ten years of portal hypertensive surgery at Emory: result and new perspectives. *Ann Surg* 1982;195:530. (Discusses Warren shunt.)

16. Wexler MJ. Treatment of bleeding esophageal varices by transabdominal esophageal transection with the EEA stapling instrument. *Surgery* 1980;88:406. (Describes esophageal transection technique.)

CHAPTER 62

Major Hepatic Resection

Major liver resections are occasionally performed for trauma but more commonly are performed for resection of primary or metastatic tumors within the liver. Resections are planned according to the segmental anatomy of the liver, outlined in the first section of this chapter. This segmental anatomy is based on the internal vascular and ductal branching pattern. External landmarks are deceptive; for example, the obvious external dividing point—the falciform ligament—does not separate the true left lobe from the right lobe. Rather, the dividing line between the two major lobes runs to the right of the falciform ligament, through the gallbladder fossa. The falciform ligament demarcates the left lateral segment of the liver.

In this chapter, the specific technical steps involved in performing right hepatic lobectomy and left lateral segmentectomy are detailed. Other anatomic resections, such as trisegmentectomy, are discussed in detail in the references at the end.

Segmental Anatomy of the Liver (Fig. 62.1)

Technical Points

Liver resection is planned to excise a pathologic lesion while maintaining an adequate margin if the resection is being performed for malignant disease with the aim of preserving the remaining liver. Resections that are done along segmental lines minimize bleeding and the risk for injury to adjacent structures. With the exception of major wedge resections, most resections are performed according to segmental anatomy.

Preoperative arteriography and computed tomography (CT) scans with portography are useful in planning the operative approach. Most resections will involve a right hepatic lobectomy or resection of segments II and III of the left lobe (formerly termed left lateral segmentectomy). Right hepatic lobectomies are discussed first in this chapter.

Anatomic Points

The segmental anatomy of the liver is based on ramifications of the portal triad structures. With few exceptions, the ramifications of these three structures (portal vein, hepatic artery, and biliary apparatus) accompany each other through the liver parenchyma. These triads interdigitate with the branches of the hepatic vein in much the way that the fingers of one hand, from above, might interdigitate with the fingers of the other hand from below.

On the basis of the first major division of portal triad structures, the liver can be divided into a right and left lobe of nearly equal size. The plane of division (line of Cantlie) runs from the inferior vena cava to the middle of the gallbladder fossa, parallel to the fissure of the round ligament.

Each of the two major lobes of the liver can be subdivided into segments. The left lobe is composed of medial and lateral segments, with the plane of division indicated by the falciform ligament and fissure of the round ligament. The right lobe is subdivided into anterior and posterior segments. Typically, no external features indicate the plane dividing the right lobe segments, although sometimes an intersegmental fissure is present.

LIST OF STRUCTURES

Liver	Caudate lobe	Left hepatic vein
Left lobe	Quadrate lobe	Middle hepatic vein
Left lateral segment	Gallbladder	Portal vein
Left medial segment	Cystic duct	Right branch
Right lobe	Falciform ligament	Left branch
Anterior segment	Ligamentum teres hepatis	Proper hepatic artery
Superior subsegment	Triangular ligaments	Right hepatic artery
Inferior subsegment	Coronary ligaments	Left hepatic artery
Posterior segment	Line of Cantlie	
Superior subsegment	Inferior vena cava	
Inferior subsegment	Right hepatic vein	

ORIENTATION

Left lobectomy

Right lobectomy

Left lateral segmentectomy

Trisegmentectomy

Finally, each segment can be divided into superior and inferior subsegments. Because there are no external features that can be used to demarcate these superior and inferior subsegments, the surgical importance of subsegments is considered to be minimal.

Segments IV and I, the quadrate and caudate lobes, are apparent on visual inspection of the liver. However, these externally apparent lobes do not correspond to functional anatomic subunits. The quadrate lobe is a part of the medial segment of the left lobe. The caudate lobe receives its portal supply from both the right and left lobar branches. The interlobar plane passes through the middle of the caudate lobe. Thus, this so-called lobe is not functionally distinct; rather, its right half is part of the right lobe, whereas its left half is part of the left lobe.

The caudate lobe has particular nuisance value during the performance of a side-to-side portacaval shunt (see Chapter 61). Enlargement of this region secondary to cirrhosis may make it difficult to bring the portal vein down to the inferior vena cava during shunt construction. Sometimes, partial wedge excision of this lobe is necessary to allow the shunt to be constructed.

The venous drainage of the liver is through the hepatic veins. It does not follow these divisions. Three major branches of the hepatic veins define the corresponding major scissurae. Thus, the right hepatic vein defines the right scissura between segments 6 and 7 to the right and 5 and 8 to the left of the right hepatic vein. The middle hepatic vein defines the main scissura between segments 5 and 8 to the right and segments 1 and 4 to the left. This main scissura corresponds to the line of Cantlie dividing the true left and right lobes of the liver. Finally, the left hepatic vein defines the left scissura between segments 1 and 4 to the right and segments 2 and 3 to the left.

Right Hepatic Lobectomy

Incision and Mobilization of the Liver (Fig. 62.2)

Technical Points

Right hepatic lobectomy can be performed through a midline or right upper quadrant incision. In most patients, a right upper quadrant incision that can be extended across the midline

FIGURE 62.1
SEGMENTAL ANATOMY OF THE LIVER

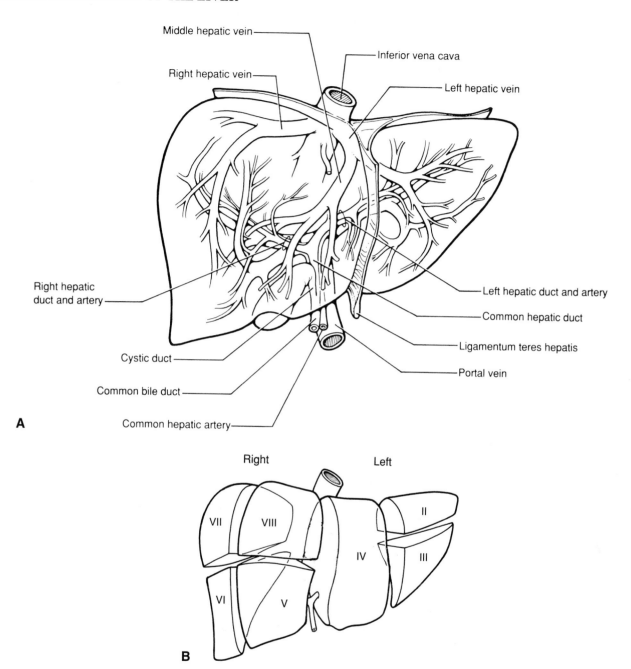

as a chevron provides superior exposure. Thoracoabdominal extension of the incision is rarely needed.

Fully expose the liver by mobilizing the hepatic flexure of the colon and lysing any adhesions from the gallbladder to the omentum and adjacent structures. Divide the ligamentum teres hepatis and incise the falciform ligament for a limited extent.

Reflect the liver medially and downward to expose the peritoneal reflections on the posterior aspect of the liver. Incise the attachments of the liver to the lateral abdominal wall and diaphragm sharply. If the tumor is adherent to a small area of the diaphragm, resect a portion of the diaphragm in continuity if it is otherwise resectable.

Anatomic Points

An upper midline extension, with or without removal of the xiphoid process, is frequently added to the chevron incision just described. The superior epigastric arteries usually lie immediately adjacent to the xiphoid process at this level.

FIGURE 62.2
INCISION AND MOBILIZATION OF THE LIVER

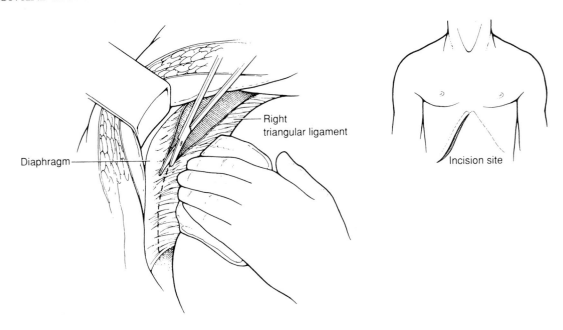

Diaphragm

Right triangular ligament

Incision site

Collateral flow from intercostal vessels and the inferior epigastric vessels allows safe control by suture ligation. These vessels are large enough to cause persistent bleeding.

Mobilization of the hepatic flexure is accomplished by incision of the peritoneum immediately lateral to the flexure, followed by dissection in the relatively avascular developmental fusion plane deep to the colon. Any bleeding that occurs will be minor because no large vessels will be encountered. Likewise, adhesions between the gallbladder and omentum, or other adjacent structures, should be relatively avascular. By contrast, division of the ligamentum teres hepatis should be done between clamps because this fibrous remnant of the left umbilical vein is always accompanied by paraumbilical veins and frequently retains a patent lumen.

The liver is attached to the diaphragm relatively posteriorly by a series of peritoneal reflections termed *ligaments*. As the peritoneal leaves of the falciform ligament reach the liver, they diverge to left and right to form the coronary ligaments that surround the bare area of the liver. This region of the liver is described as bare because it is not covered by peritoneum. On the right, the coronary ligament consists of anterior (superior) and posterior (inferior) layers that are widely separated from each other. On the left, the anterior and posterior layers are quite close, separated from each other only by a modest amount of connective tissue. Within this connective tissue run some variable vessels, nerves, and frequently, biliary radicles. The left triangular ligament forms the upper boundary of the superior recess of the omental bursa, whereas the superior layer of the right coronary ligament prevents the manual exploration of the diaphragmatic surface of the liver. Division of the coronary ligament and of the right or left triangular ligaments, or both, is necessary to mobilize the liver and expose the hepatic part of the inferior vena cava.

The coronary and right triangular ligaments are simply peritoneal reflections and can be sharply divided with no special precautions. The long, narrow, left triangular ligament always contains vessels or bile canaliculi, or both, and thus should be divided between clamps. As the incision of these peritoneal reflections progresses medially, the hepatic veins will begin to appear.

Dissection in the Hilum of the Liver (Fig. 62.3)

Technical Points

Incise the peritoneum in the region of Calot's triangle and identify the cystic duct and ligate it. Remove the gallbladder from its bed to define the anatomy of the gallbladder fossa, which will be used as a line of resection.

Trace the common hepatic duct up into the liver by carefully following its anterior surface and identify the confluence of the right and left hepatic ducts. Ligate and divide the right hepatic duct. The next structure to identify is the right hepatic artery. This will lie posterior to the hepatic duct, but its location is otherwise extremely variable. Review the arteriogram, particularly if there are any anomalies. Divide the right hepatic artery. Next, dissect in the areolar plane posterior to the hepatic artery and hepatic duct and identify the right branch of the portal vein. If it is difficult to surround the right portal vein, it is often safest to identify the main portal vein and the left portal vein first. Surround these vessels with Silastic loops. Gentle traction will help to expose the right portal vein, which is then divided and secured with a suture ligature.

Rotate the liver medially and inferiorly. Identify, ligate, and divide the multiple small branches of hepatic veins between the liver and the inferior vena cava. A major hepatic vein will

FIGURE 62.3
DISSECTION IN THE HILUM OF THE LIVER

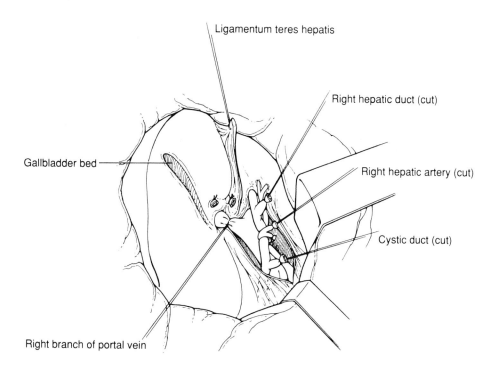

Ligamentum teres hepatis

Right hepatic duct (cut)

Gallbladder bed

Right hepatic artery (cut)

Cystic duct (cut)

Right branch of portal vein

be located in the superior aspect of the operative field. Secure this by suture ligature.

Rotate the liver cephalad to identify the small hepatic veins entering the vena cava near the inferior border of the liver. Often, tumor involvement renders the liver so rigid that it is extremely difficult to rotate and compress it in order to expose these hepatic veins.

Anatomic Points

The relative relationships of the major structures within the hepatoduodenal ligament are maintained up into the hilum of the liver, forming a pattern that is followed throughout the liver. The portal vein is posterior in the hepatoduodenal ligament and at the porta hepatis. The common hepatic duct is anterior and to the right, whereas the hepatic artery is anterior and to the left.

Calot's triangle is that triangle which is formed by the liver, common hepatic duct, and cystic duct. It usually contains the cystic artery and right hepatic artery and, when present, the accessory right hepatic arteries and accessory hepatic ducts. Remember that, although the arteries usually are posterior to the biliary ducts, a common anomaly involves the hepatic artery crossing anterior to the common hepatic duct.

The common hepatic duct is formed by the confluence of the right and left ducts at the porta hepatis. This union may be intrahepatic or extrahepatic; hence, parenchymal dissection may be necessary to allow ligation of the right duct. In about 28% of the cases, one of the two right segmental ducts crosses the interlobar plane to drain into the left hepatic duct.

Of the structures entering the porta hepatis, the arterial supply is probably the most variable. Typically, the common hepatic artery divides into left and right branches at the porta hepatis, before entering liver parenchyma. Thereafter, the right branch soon divides into anterior and posterior segmental branches. Seemingly, almost any conceivable variation from this pattern can—and does—occur. For example, the right hepatic artery frequently arises from the superior mesenteric artery (in 17% of cases), a middle hepatic artery (in reality, the artery supplying the left medial segment) may be visible extrahepatically and may arise from the right hepatic artery, and various accessory arteries can also be present. A hepatic arteriogram is almost obligatory.

The portal vein also usually divides into left and right branches extrahepatically. The right portal vein, like the right hepatic artery, travels only a short distance within the substance of the liver before it divides into its segmental branches. Although there is less variation in the portal venous system than in either the arterial supply or the biliary apparatus, the intrahepatic course of the right portal vein tends to be more variable than that of the left, and caution should be exercised.

Parenchymal Resection (Fig. 62.4)

Technical Points

Devascularization of the right lobe of the liver will produce an obvious line of demarcation between the right and left lobes. The devascularized right lobe will be visibly darker than the left. Incise the capsule of the liver along this dark line. By

FIGURE 62.4
PARENCHYMAL RESECTION

FIGURE 62.5
TECHNIQUE OF RESECTION

finger fracture technique, progress through the parenchyma of the liver, securing the bile ducts and vessels as they are encountered using hemoclips or suture ligatures.

Several finger fracture techniques are available, depending on individual preference. The simplest is a true finger fracture, in which the left thumb and index finger are rubbed together to crush intervening normal liver tissue. Vessels and bile ducts will be palpable and should be clipped. Alternatively, the central part of a pool suction tip can be used as a blunt dissector. Finally, a specially designed ultrasonic aspiration device is preferred by some surgeons. The overall goal is controlled crush of hepatic parenchyma to expose tubular structures that require direct control.

As the dissection progresses, the first assistant helps to hold the developing crevice open by rotating the right lobe strongly to the right as the left lobe is rotated to the left.

In the deep substance of the liver, large veins will be encountered that must be secured by careful ligature in continuity. Hepatic veins that were not ligated before parenchymal resection will need to be controlled at this point. Remove the lobe of the liver and check hemostasis in the hepatic remnant. Continued oozing from the raw surface of the remaining left lobe of the liver should be managed by suture ligature and hemostatic clips. When all obvious bleeding has been controlled, use Gelfoam or Surgicel to control any remaining oozing.

Place omentum over the raw edge of the liver and place closed-suction drains close to the operative field.

Anatomic Points

The liver drains through three major (right, left, and middle) veins and a variable number (12 to 15) of minor veins. The three major veins of the liver are intersegmental or interlobar.

The right hepatic vein lies between the anterior and posterior segments of the right lobe, the middle hepatic vein lies in the true interlobar fissure, and the left hepatic vein is located in the superior aspect of the umbilical fissure. Thus, the right hepatic vein must be ligated. Depending on the relationship of the resection plane to the middle hepatic vein, either tributaries or the middle vein itself will have to be ligated. Remember that, in most cases (84%), the middle vein drains into the terminal part of the left hepatic vein, rather than into the inferior vena cava directly, because ligation of the common trunk could be disastrous.

Resection of Segments II and III
(Left Lateral Segmentectomy)

Technique of Resection (Fig. 62.5)

Technical Points

This procedure is sometimes performed for trauma; the relative ease with which part or all of the left lateral segment can be resected leads many to favor resection for definitive control of complex injuries to this area. Less commonly, tumor limited to the extreme lateral edge of the liver is managed with this type of resection.

A midline or subcostal incision is appropriate. Divide the ligamentum teres hepatis and incise the falciform ligament to gain adequate access to the left lateral segment. Divide the free edge of the left triangular ligament between clips and incise the left triangular ligament medially to mobilize this portion of the liver fully.

Using electrocautery, draw a line of projected resection on Glisson's capsule. This line should pass just to the left of the falciform ligament and umbilical fissure. Use a finger fracture technique to divide the parenchyma, securing small vascular and ductal structures with clips. Ligate all major vascular and ductal structures in continuity.

Anatomic Points

Be careful to keep the dissection to the left of the umbilical fissure, rather than within the fissure. The umbilical part of the portal vein lies in the fissure and has branches on both the medial and lateral sides. Likewise, the arterial supply of the medial segment can be derived primarily from so-called retrograde branches arising from the left lateral segmental arteries. Thus, resection and subsequent control of portal vein branches and arterial branches on the right side of the umbilical fissure can result in devascularization of the left medial segment.

REFERENCES

1. Arnoletti JP, Brodsky J. Reduction of transfusion requirements during major hepatic resection for metastatic disease. *Surgery* 1999;125:166–171.
2. Bismuth H, Chiche L. Surgical anatomy and anatomical surgery of the liver. In: Blumgart, *Surgery of the Liver and Biliary Tract.* London: Churchill Livingston, 1994:1557–1578.
3. Blumgart LH. Liver resection: liver and biliary tumours. In: Blumgart, *Surgery of the Liver and Biliary Tract.* London: Churchill Livingston, 1994:1557–1578. (Provides comprehensive review of techniques.)
4. Chang YF, Huang TL, Chen CL, et al. Variations of the middle and inferior right hepatic vein: application in hepatectomy. *J Clin Ultrasound* 1997;25:175–182.
5. Delattre J-F, Avisse C, Flament J-B. Anatomic basis of hepatic surgery. *Surg Clin North Am* 2000;80:345–362. (Presents excellent summary of surgical anatomy and embryology.)
6. Kennedy PA, Madding GF. Surgical anatomy of the liver. *Surg Clin North Am* 1977;57:233. (Reviews segmental anatomy.)
7. Lin TY. Results in 107 hepatic lobectomies with a preliminary report on the use of a clamp to reduce blood loss. *Ann Surg* 1973;177:413. (Clamp may be of use in some situations.)
8. Michels NA. New anatomy of the liver and its variant blood supply and collateral circulation. *Am J Surg* 1966;122:337. (Reviews anomalies.)
9. Miller DR. Median sternotomy extension of abdominal incision for hepatic lobectomy. *Ann Surg* 1972;175:193. (Presents best way to get additional exposure.)
10. Petrelli NJ, Conte CC. Avoiding complications of hepatic resection. *Infect Surg* 1990;9:25. (Presents general discussion of complications and methods to avoid them.)
11. Scheele J, Stangl R. Segment orientated anatomical liver resections. In: Blumgart, *Surgery of the Liver and Biliary Tract.* London: Churchill Livingston, 1994:1557–1578.
12. Strong RW, Lynch SV, Wall DR, et al. Anatomic resection for severe liver trauma. *Surgery* 1998;123:251–257.
13. Starzl TE, Iwatsuki S, Shaw BW, et al. Left hepatic trisegmentectomy. *Surg Gynecol Obstet* 1982;155:21. (Describes uncommon resection.)
14. Starzl TE, Koep LJ, Weil R, et al. Right trisegmentectomy for hepatic neoplasms. *Surg Gynecol Obstet* 1980;150:208. (Provides good description of extensive resection.)
15. Sugarbaker PH, Nelson RC, Murray DR, et al. A segmental approach to computerized tomographic portography for hepatic resection. *Surg Gynecol Obstet* 1990;171:189. (Provides clear description of anatomy delineated by computed tomography scanning as related to segmental hepatic anatomy and the planning of resections.)
16. Suzuki T, Nakayasu A, Kawabe K, et al. Surgical significance of anatomic variations of the hepatic artery. *Am J Surg* 1971;122:505.

CHAPTER 63

Pancreatic Resections

In this chapter, distal pancreatectomy (resection of the tail of the pancreas) will be described first. Because of the close anatomic proximity of the tail of pancreas to the splenic vessels, splenectomy is generally performed when the tail of the pancreas is resected. When this operation is performed for benign tumors or for trauma, it may be possible to preserve the blood supply of the spleen. Both methods of performing the procedure are described in this section. Laparoscopic distal pancreatectomy is described in Chapter 64.

Resection of the head of the pancreas is done in combination with duodenal resection. This procedure is called pancreatoduodenectomy, or the Whipple procedure. It is described in the second part of this chapter. Total pancreatectomy, pylorus-preserving Whipple, and other specialized pancreatic resections are described in the references at the end.

Distal Pancreatectomy without Splenectomy

Exposure of the Body and Tail of the Pancreas (Fig. 63.1)

Technical Points

Make a window in the gastrocolic omentum by serially clamping and dividing the gastroepiploic vessels on the greater curvature of the stomach. Divide these from the region of the distal antrum to the short gastric vessels. Retract the portion of the stomach that is cephalad to the greater omentum inferiorly. Place retractors or stay sutures to maintain the stomach in an elevated position. Divide the avascular folds between the stomach and pancreas (gastropancreatic folds, or Allen's veil) to expose the body and tail of the pancreas fully. The splenic vessels may be palpable in the region of the distal pancreas. The splenic artery runs along the superior surface of the pancreas and is often visible, palpable, or both. The splenic vein lies posterior to the pancreas and cannot be seen until the pancreas is mobilized. Incise the peritoneum along the inferior border of the pancreas with electrocautery.

Elevate the pancreas out of the retroperitoneum by blunt dissection in an avascular (normally) plane. The splenic artery and vein will be elevated along with the body and tail of the pancreas. Identify the point at which the pancreas is to be divided. Generally, this point will be somewhat to the left of the superior mesenteric vein. Develop a plane between the pancreas and the splenic artery and splenic vein by careful blunt dissection. Use Silastic vessel loops on the two vessels to facilitate traction once the plane has been developed. Divide the pancreas using a TA-55 stapler with 3.5-mm staples. Place Allis clamps on the distal pancreas and lift up.

Multiple, short, fine vessels connecting the body and tail of the pancreas to the splenic artery and splenic vein must then be isolated and serially clipped or ligated. If these small vessels are inadvertently avulsed, use fine Prolene sutures to obtain hemostasis in the splenic artery and splenic vein.

LIST OF STRUCTURES

Pancreas
  Head
  Body
  Tail
  Uncinate process
  Pancreatic duct
Spleen
  Splenic artery
  Splenic vein
  Hilum of spleen
Colon
  Transverse mesocolon
  Transverse colon
  Middle colic artery and veins

Stomach
  Greater curvature
  Pylorus
  Antrum
Duodenum
  First, second, third, and fourth
    portions
Ligament of Treitz
Gallbladder
  Cystic artery
  Cystic duct
Common bile duct
Porta hepatis

Right hepatic artery
Portal vein
Superior mesenteric artery and vein
Inferior vena cava
Left and right gastroepiploic artery and
    vein
Gastropancreatic arteries
Inferior (transverse) pancreatic artery
Great pancreatic artery
Gastrocolic omentum (ligament)
Gastropancreatic folds
Gastrosplenic ligament
Splenocolic ligament

ORIENTATION

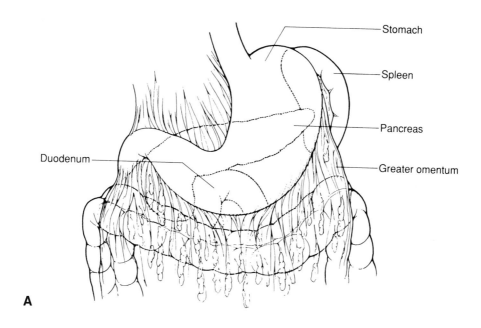

Stomach

Spleen

Pancreas

Greater omentum

Duodenum

A

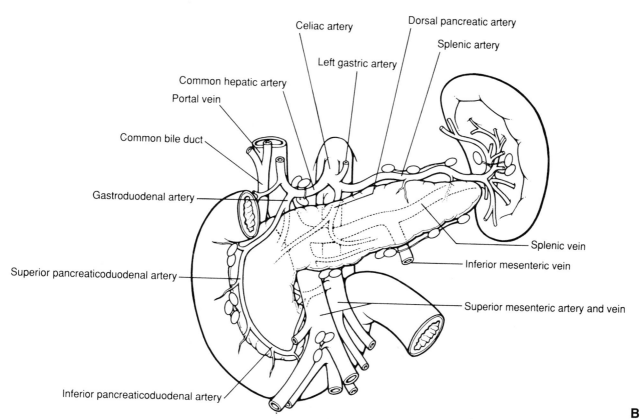

Celiac artery

Dorsal pancreatic artery

Splenic artery

Left gastric artery

Common hepatic artery

Portal vein

Common bile duct

Gastroduodenal artery

Superior pancreaticoduodenal artery

Splenic vein

Inferior mesenteric vein

Superior mesenteric artery and vein

Inferior pancreaticoduodenal artery

B

Continue the dissection out to the tail of the pancreas, pre-serving the splenic artery and splenic vein. Check the area for hemostasis and place omentum over the pancreatic stump. Closed-suction drains may be placed in the bed of the resec-tion if desired.

Anatomic Points

The greater omentum is attached to the greater curvature of the stomach and first part of the duodenum. On the left, it is continuous with the gastrosplenic ligament. The entire length

FIGURE 63.1
EXPOSURE OF THE BODY AND TAIL OF THE PANCREAS

Splenic artery

Splenic vein

A

B

C

D

of its posterior surface is adherent to the entire length of the transverse colon. That portion of the greater omentum connecting the stomach and transverse colon is the gastrocolic omentum (ligament). The gastroepiploic vessels, contained within the greater omentum, typically are close to the stomach, but may be 2 cm or more distant from the stomach.

On the left, the gastrosplenic and splenocolic ligaments are continuous with the greater omentum. Multiple, short, gastric arteries (commonly, four to six) arise from the splenic artery or its branches and run through the gastrosplenic ligament to the greater curvature of the stomach at the fundus. The left gastroepiploic artery has a similar origin and similar course, except that it parallels the greater curvature, running from left to right, ultimately anastomosing with the right gastroepiploic artery. There are no vessels of consequence in the splenocolic

ligament, although small communications may exist between the splenic vessels and branches of the middle or right colic vessels.

The lienorenal ligament attaches the spleen to the retroperitoneum. In this ligament are the major splenic vessels and the tail of the pancreas, which usually is either in contact with the splenic hilum or is no more than 1 cm distant from the hilum.

The gastropancreatic folds are formed by the left gastric artery as it passes from the celiac trunk to the upper part of the lesser curvature. Avascular, filmy connections can occur between the visceral peritoneum of the stomach and the parietal peritoneum covering the pancreas. These are common at the right extremity of the stomach, where the antrum is in close proximity to the head of the pancreas, and on the left,

FIGURE 63.2
RESECTION OF DISTAL PANCREAS

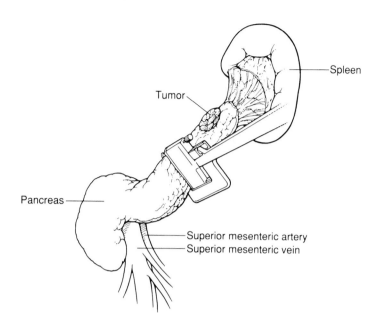

where the posterior surface of the stomach is very close to the tail of the pancreas. These avascular folds tether the stomach to the posterior wall of the lesser sac, as the duodenum starts to become retroperitoneal, and to the gastrosplenic ligament and its contained vasculature.

The splenic artery runs along the superior border of the pancreas from its celiac trunk origin to the hilum of the spleen. The celiac trunk lies superior and to the left of the neck of the pancreas. As it progresses toward the spleen, it has a characteristically tortuous course (in the adult) owing to tethering by pancreatic branches, and it frequently dips downward posterior to the pancreas. By contrast, the splenic vein should not be visible until the pancreatic tail and splenic hilum are explored because this vein is posterior to the pancreas. As these vessels approach the splenic hilum, both artery and vein have a variable number of splenic branches or tributaries (usually two or three) that serve the different splenic segments; this branching most commonly occurs about 4 cm from the splenic hilum, but the distance may range from 1 to 12 cm. Typically, the splenic vein tributaries are inferior and somewhat posterior to the corresponding arterial branches.

Posterior to the pancreas, an avascular plane exists as a result of the fusion of the mesogastrium with the posterior parietal peritoneum and the fact that those more proximal structures contained within the mesogastrium become retroperitoneal. As could be expected, the avascular fusion plane is also posterior to the splenic vessels.

The relationship of the major vessels posterior to the pancreas is also important. The portal vein, formed by the union of the superior mesenteric and splenic veins, lies to the right of the aorta and superior mesenteric artery. The splenic vein,

which lies more or less in the transverse plane, joins the superior mesenteric vein by passing between the superior mesenteric artery and pancreas; thus, in this region, the splenic vein is the most anterior major vascular structure.

As the splenic artery and vein travel along the length of the pancreas, several short, delicate radicles either supply or drain the pancreas. There are more pancreatic veins (15 to 31) than there are pancreatic arteries (4 to 11), and both appear to be distributed fairly evenly along the length of the vessels.

Distal Pancreatectomy with Splenectomy

Resection of Distal Pancreas (Fig. 63.2)

Technical Points

First, mobilize the spleen and tail of the pancreas into the operative field using the technique just described. Begin by dividing the short gastric vessels in the gastrosplenic ligament. Leave the spleen attached to the tail of the pancreas by the hilar vessels and mobilize the tail of the pancreas and splenic vessels with the spleen up into the incision. When the point of division has been determined, individually ligate and divide the splenic artery and splenic vein. Place 2-0 silk sutures in a figure-of-eight pattern at the superior and inferior border of the pancreas to secure the gastropancreatic arteries. Leave these long for traction. Divide the pancreas using a TA-55 stapler with 3.5-mm staples. Secure any bleeding points with fine suture ligatures. If the pancreatic duct is identified in the staple line, it may be secured with an additional 3-0 silk suture ligature. This is not required if a good staple line has been achieved. Place omentum over the stump of the pancreas and closed-suction drains in the region of the pancreatic bed if desired.

Anatomic Points

There are typically four to six short gastric arteries, plus the left gastroepiploic artery, in the gastrosplenic ligament. The number and origin of the short gastric arteries is quite variable, although their destination—the greater curvature of the stomach—is not.

Division of the body of the pancreas requires control of the intrapancreatic vasculature; in order to maintain a clear field, some control must be gained before sectioning. One major vessel is the inferior or transverse pancreatic artery; the origin of this artery is quite variable, but its inferodorsal course along the pancreas, either extraparenchymal or intraparenchymal, is fairly constant. The other main artery is a branch of the great pancreatic artery, a branch of the splenic artery that typically enters at the junction of the middle and distal thirds of this vessel; it then divides into one or more branches coursing to the tail and one or more branches coursing toward the head. The latter branches parallel the inferior pancreatic artery but lie more superiorly than the inferior pancreatic artery does. These arteries, or their ramifications, are the ones that must be hemostatically controlled with the figure-of-eight sutures.

The pancreatic duct, in the area to be resected, is approximately midway between the superior and inferior borders of the pancreas. It is slightly more posterior than anterior but is nevertheless anterior to the major pancreatic vasculature. Normally, the diameter of the duct in the body of the pancreas varies between 2 and 4 mm.

Pancreaticoduodenectomy

Initial Mobilization of Pancreas and Assessment of Tumor Resectability (Fig. 63.3)

Technical Points

Make a chevron-shaped left subcostal incision that extends across the midline. This will provide good access to the upper abdomen in most patients. Assess tumor resectability carefully before division of any major structures. Because of the intimate relationships between the head of the pancreas and superior mesenteric artery and portal vein, it is important to ascertain whether the tumor can be removed safely before beginning resection.

First, inspect the abdomen for signs of metastatic disease. If metastases are found in the liver or the omentum, confirm these by frozen-section analysis. In such cases, a biliary bypass procedure will provide excellent palliation without the morbidity and mortality associated with a major resection.

If no metastatic disease is identified, mobilize the hepatic flexure of the right colon downward to expose the duodenum and head of the pancreas fully. Perform a wide Kocher maneuver, incising the peritoneum lateral to the duodenum. Reflect the duodenum and head of the pancreas medially so that the inferior vena cava is fully exposed. Palpate the head of the pancreas between your fingers. Note the size and consistency of the head of the pancreas and the size of the tumor mass.

Open the gastrocolic omentum by dividing it along the greater curvature of the stomach. Serially clamp and tie branches of the gastroepiploic vessels. Inspect the body and tail of the pancreas. If the body and tail of the pancreas appear

FIGURE 63.3
INITIAL MOBILIZATION OF PANCREAS AND ASSESSMENT OF TUMOR RESECTABILITY

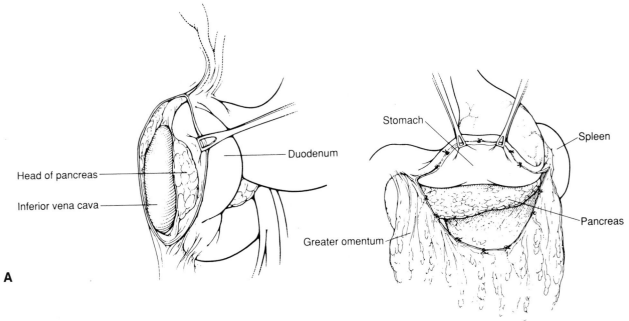

Head of pancreas

Inferior vena cava

Duodenum

A

Stomach

Spleen

Greater omentum

Pancreas

B

to be normal and the tumor feels small and is limited in size and location to the region of the head of the pancreas, it is next necessary to assess whether the pancreas can be mobilized off the portal vein. This is the most hazardous and treacherous part of the initial mobilization and must be done with care.

Identify the superior mesenteric vein passing deep to the body of the pancreas at the inferior border. By sharp and blunt dissection, enter the adventitial plane of the vein and follow it upward under the pancreas. No collateral vein should enter the anterior surface of the superior mesenteric vein from the substance of the pancreas. This plane is normally avascular. Identify the portal vein cephalad to the pancreas behind the common bile duct and develop the plane behind the portal vein. It should be possible for the body of the pancreas to be completely surrounded at the region of the portal vein and superior mesenteric vein. If tumor is found to be invading the portal vein or superior mesenteric vein, then either resection with a segment of portal vein or a biliary bypass procedure will need to be performed. If the portal vein is inadvertently injured during the course of this mobilization, causing massive, uncontrollable bleeding, obtain access to the portal vein by rapidly transecting the pancreas over the vein. Then pass a Penrose drain around the body of the pancreas in the region of the portal vein.

Anatomic Points

The anatomy pertinent to the preferred chevron incision has already been discussed. Mobilization of the hepatic flexure of the colon can be done with some impunity because the superolateral mesenteric attachments are devoid of significant vasculature. Likewise, performance of the Kocher maneuver should not result in significant bleeding. In both cases (colon mobilization and the Kocher maneuver), incision and division of the peritoneum is made on the antimesenteric side of the gut, and the goal is to find the avascular fusion plane that will allow blunt dissection and mobilization of gut derivatives toward the midline. As you reflect the duodenum and head of the pancreas, remember that the head of the pancreas and the third portion of the duodenum lie on the inferior vena cava, and use appropriate caution during their mobilization.

The superior mesenteric vein typically lies to the right of the superior mesenteric artery. It runs anterior to the third portion of the duodenum and the uncinate process of the pancreas. It then passes dorsal to the neck of the pancreas, where it unites with the splenic vein to form the portal vein, which then continues posterior to the duodenum to gain access to the gastroduodenal ligament. The plane between the anterior surface of the superior mesenteric vein or portal vein and the posterior surface of the neck of the pancreas is usually avascular. Small veins, which are smaller than the splenic or inferior mesenteric vein but still large enough to cause hemostatic problems, often enter the lateral side of the superior mesenteric–portal vein axis. Thus, caution is warranted. In addition, remember that variations in this region are legion; hence, almost any anatomic arrangement can and should be expected.

FIGURE 63.4
DIVISION OF THE STOMACH AND COMMON BILE DUCT

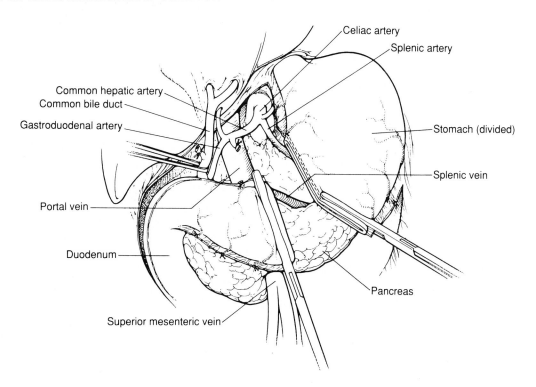

Division of the Stomach and Common Bile Duct (Fig. 63.4)

Technical Points

Choose a point of division in the greater curvature of the stomach and divide the stomach, constructing a Hofmeister shelf in the usual fashion (see Fig. 48.2 in Chapter 48). Divide the vessels in the lesser curvature, progressing down toward the pylorus. Identify and surround the common bile duct in the porta hepatis. Perform a cholecystectomy and ligate the cystic duct. Divide the common bile duct well above the substance of the pancreas. Place two stay sutures on the wall of the common duct for identification and subsequent anastomosis.

Anatomic Points

Division of the gastroepiploic arcade has already been accomplished, and because of the collateral circulation at this point, vascular control must be obtained on both sides of division. The same is true of division of the right gastric and left gastric vascular arcades, which lie in the lesser omentum. The arterial and venous arcades parallel the lesser curvature of the stomach and usually lie close to this border of the stomach. Bear in mind that, frequently (20% to 35% of cases), this arterial arcade can consist of two parallel arteries because both right and left gastric arteries can divide. In addition, the left gastric artery can supply the left lateral segment of the liver; this variant may provide the major or sole blood supply to this segment. Other than the gastric arcade and portal triad structures in the hepatoduodenal ligament, the lesser omentum contains the vagally-derived nerves of Latarjet (in close proximity to the arterial arcade) and the hepatic branch of the anterior vagal trunk. The nerves of Latarjet, which supply the stomach and pyloric region, also must be divided. The hepatic branch of the anterior vagal trunk, however, originates in the vicinity of the esophageal hiatus and traverses the lesser omentum very close to its hepatic attachment. It should not be at risk if the dissection is restricted to the lower, or gastric, part of the hepatogastric ligament.

Customary precautions prevail in performing cholecystectomy and common bile duct division. Remember that the cystic artery usually lies in the triangle of Calot, regardless of its origin (which is quite variable), and that the location of the union of cystic duct and common hepatic duct is also quite variable. For these reasons, the structures in this area should be skeletonized to allow adequate visualization before ligation or division.

Division of the Jejunum (Fig. 63.5)

Technical Points

Divide the jejunum at a convenient point just below the ligament of Treitz. Mobilize the ligament of Treitz and as much of the duodenum as feasible from the left side of the abdomen. Pass the divided jejunum through, under the transverse mesocolon and mesenteric small bowel, so that it comes out on the same side as the rest of the duodenum. At this point, the stomach and duodenum will be swung to the right.

Anatomic Points

Mention has already been made of the fact that the ligament of Treitz also contains muscle, derived either from the crus of the diaphragm or from the jejunal wall. As a consequence, its mobilization can cause unwanted bleeding unless measures are taken (using clamps or electrocautery) to prevent this.

When a window is made in the transverse colon, the middle colic artery should be identified. This is usually one of the first branches of the superior mesenteric artery, and it reaches the transverse colon by traveling through the transverse mesocolon.

Division of the Pancreas (Fig. 63.6)

Technical Points

Place figure-of-eight stay sutures in the upper and inferior border of the pancreas in the region of the superior and inferior pancreatic arcades. Divide the pancreas sharply. Secure bleeding points with electrocautery. Identify the pancreatic duct. Place Allis clamps on the portion of the pancreas to be resected and begin to peel it from right to left off the portal vein. Multiple small tributaries in the region of the pancreatic head and uncinate process will need to be secured with fine ligatures. At this point, this is the only remaining connection of the specimen to the abdomen. Proceed with caution to avoid injuring the portal vein or superior mesenteric vein. The right hepatic artery occasionally arises from the superior mesenteric artery. In this case, it will be encountered in the surgical field. Therefore, identify the origin and termination of any anomalous vessel before division. If you encounter an aberrant right hepatic artery, preserve it. Once the specimen has been removed, carefully check the bed for hemostasis.

Anatomic Points

The location of intrapancreatic arcades has already been discussed in this chapter, as has the location of the pancreatic duct. The multiple small portal tributaries in the pancreatic head and uncinate process drain into the lateral aspect of the superior mesenteric vein–portal vein axis. In addition, the right gastric vein may be encountered, again entering the lateral aspect of the portal vein. Frequently, one can identify the inferior mesenteric vein, either entering the superior mesenteric vein or at the angle between the superior mesenteric vein and splenic vein.

The head and uncinate process of the pancreas fill the concavity formed by the C loop of the pancreas. The head of the pancreas lies cranial and somewhat anterior to the root of the superior mesenteric artery and the termination of the superior mesenteric vein, whereas the uncinate process is inferior and more or less posterior to the superior mesenteric vessels. The blood supply to the head of the pancreas and duodenum is provided by the anastomosing superior pancreaticoduodenal artery (a terminal branch of the gastroduodenal artery, which arises either posterior to the duodenum or slightly more inferior) and inferior pancreaticoduodenal artery (typically, the first branch of the superior mesenteric artery).

FIGURE 63.5
DIVISION OF THE JEJUNUM

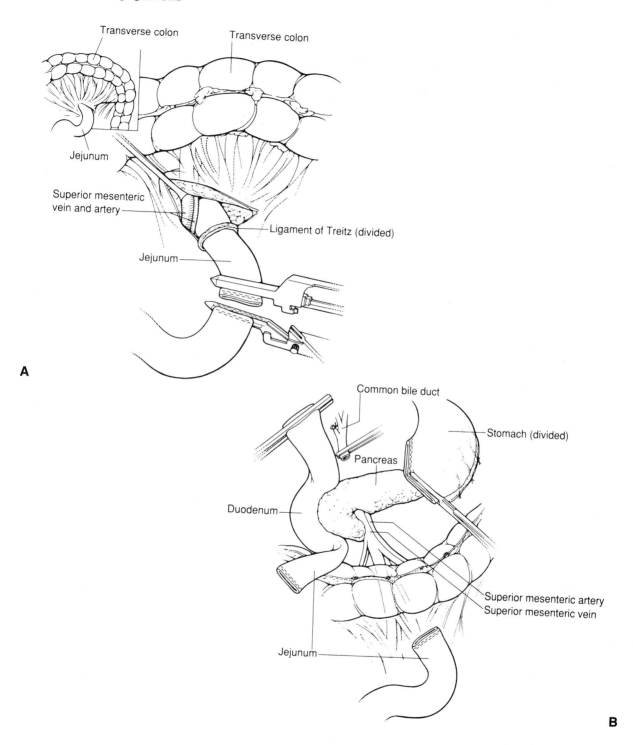

A

B

Reconstruction (Fig. 63.7)

Technical and Anatomic Points

Reconstruction is accomplished by a series of three anastomoses: pancreaticojejunostomy, choledochojejunostomy, and gastrojejunostomy. Generally, the tail of the pancreas is anastomosed onto the end of the piece of jejunum. The second anastomosis in line is an end-to-side anastomosis of the common bile duct to the jejunum. The third anastomosis consists of the gastrojejunostomy.

The pancreaticojejunostomy is constructed by invaginating jejunum over the tail of the pancreas. Alternatively, a mucosa-to-mucosa anastomosis may be constructed. If the pancreatic duct is fine, place a small, fine, Silastic cannula

FIGURE 63.6
DIVISION OF THE PANCREAS

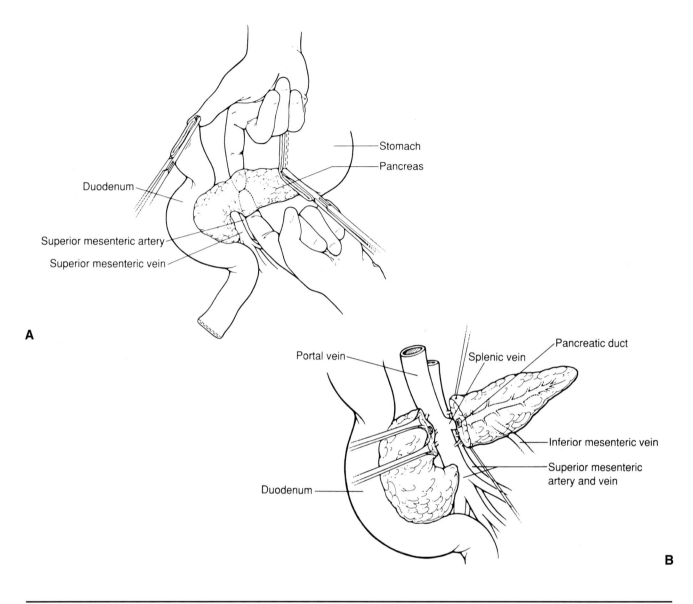

Stomach

Pancreas

Duodenum

Superior mesenteric artery

Superior mesenteric vein

A

Portal vein

Splenic vein

Pancreatic duct

Inferior mesenteric vein

Superior mesenteric artery and vein

Duodenum

B

FIGURE 63.7
RECONSTRUCTION

within it to stent the anastomosis open. Make an end-to-side choledochojejunostomy about 10 cm distal to the pancreaticojejunostomy. This anastomosis may also be stented if desired. Construct the gastrojejunostomy downstream in standard two-layer fashion. Place omentum around the suture line. Position closed-suction drains in the vicinity of the pancreatic and biliary anastomoses. Close the abdomen in the usual fashion.

REFERENCES

1. Beger HG, Krautzberger W, Bittner R, et al. Duodenum-preserving resection of the head of the pancreas in patients with severe pancreatitis. *Surgery* 1985;97:467.
2. Braasch JW, Rossi RL, Watkins E. Pyloric and gastric preserving pancreatic resection: experience in 287 patients. *Ann Surg* 1986;204:411.
3. Cameron JL, Crist DW, Sitzman JV, et al. Factors influencing survival after pancreaticoduodenectomy for pancreatic cancer. *Am J Surg* 1991;161:120.
4. Carey LC. Pancreaticoduodenectomy. *Am J Surg* 1992;164:153. (Provides good description of pylorus-preserving Whipple procedure.)
5. Cubilla AL, Fortner J, Fitzgerald PJ. Lymph node involvement in carcinoma of the pancreas area. *Cancer* 1978;41:880.
6. Dawson DL, Scott-Conner CEH. Distal pancreatectomy with splenic preservation: the anatomic basis for a meticulous operation. *J Trauma* 1986;26:1142.
7. Earnhardt RC, McQuone SJ, Minasi JS. Intraoperative fine needle aspiration of pancreatic and extrahepatic biliary masses. *Surg Gynecol Obstet* 1993;177:147.
8. Falconer CWA, Griffiths E. The anatomy of the blood vessels in the region of the pancreas. *Br J Surg* 1950;37:334.
9. Flanigan DP, Kraft RO. Continuing experience with palliative chemical splanchnicectomy. *Arch Surg* 1978;113:509. (Describes a useful palliative procedure for when resection is impossible.)
10. Fortner JG. Regional pancreatectomy for carcinoma of the pancreas, ampulla, and other related sites: tumor staging and results. *Ann Surg* 1984;199:418.
11. Jimenez RE, Warshaw AI, Rattner DW, et al. Impact of laparoscopic staging in the treatment of pancreatic cancer. *Arch Surg* 2000;135:414.
12. Katz LB, Aufses AH, Rayfield E, et al. Preoperative localization and intraoperative monitoring in the management of patients with pancreatic insulinoma. *Surg Gynecol Obstet* 1986;163:509. (Describes how to find small, often nonpalpable lesions.)
13. Lin PW, Lin YJ. Prospective randomized comparison between pylorus-preserving and standard pancreaticoduodenectomy. *Br J Surg* 1999;86:603.
14. Moossa AR, Altorki N. Pancreatic biopsy. *Surg Clin North Am* 1983;63:1205. (Describes how to biopsy the pancreas with minimal morbidity.)
15. Nagorney DM, Edis AJ. A use for the stapler in pancreatic surgery. *Am J Surg* 1981;142:384.
16. Pachter HL, Pennington R, Chassin J, et al. Simplified distal pancreatectomy with the auto suture stapler: preliminary clinical observations. *Surgery* 1979;85:166.
17. Sarr MG, Cameron JL. Surgical management of unresectable carcinoma of the pancreas. *Surgery* 1982;91:123.
18. Sitges-Serra A, Badosa F. The anterior approach to control the splenic vessels in distal pancreatectomy. *Surg Gynecol Obstet* 1985;161:183. (Describes direct approach to the splenic vessels through the transected pancreas.)
19. Skandalakis JE, Gray SW, Rowe JS, et al. Anatomical complications of pancreatic surgery: parts I and II. *Contemp Surg* 1979;15:17, 21. (Presents good general review.)
20. Skandalakis JE, Gray SW, Rowe JS, et al. Surgical anatomy of the pancreas. *Contemp Surg* 1979;15:1.
21. Telford GL, Mason GR. Pancreaticogastrostomy: clinical experience with a direct pancreatic duct-to-gastric mucosa anastomosis. *Am J Surg* 1984;147:832. (Describes alternative technique that may reduce leakage from the pancreatic anastomosis.)
22. Thompson E, Nagorney DM. Stapled cholecystojejunostomy and gastrojejunostomy for the palliation of unresectable pancreatic carcinoma. *Am J Surg* 1986;151:509.
23. Thompson NW, Eckhauser FE, Talpos G, et al. Pancreaticoduodenectomy and celiac occlusive disease. *Ann Surg* 1981;193:399. (Discusses complications secondary to arterial occlusive disease in the celiac system.)
24. Van Heerden JA. Pancreatic resection for carcinoma of the pancreas: Whipple versus total pancreatectomy—an institutional perspective. *World J Surg* 1984;8:880.
25. Yeo CJ, Cameron JL, Sohn TA, et al. Pancreaticoduodenectomy with or without extended retroperitoneal lymphadenectomy for periampullary adenocarcinoma: comparison of morbidity and mortality and short-term outcome. *Ann Surg* 1999;229:613.

CHAPTER 64

Laparoscopic Distal Pancreatectomy

Laparoscopic access to the lesser sac is gained by the same maneuver as that employed during open surgery. The gastrocolic omentum is opened widely and the stomach reflected cephalad, with the colon displaced caudad. Most laparoscopic pancreatic procedures are performed with the patient positioned with legs spread, as for Nissen fundoplication. This allows optimum alignment of the visual axis.

This chapter shows laparoscopic distal pancreatectomy with and without splenectomy. Hand-assisted techniques are referenced at the end of the chapter, as are less common pancreatic resections, such as enucleation of islet cell tumors and resection of head of pancreas.

Orientation and Exposure (Fig. 64.1)

Technical Points

Typically five ports are used for this procedure, placed as indicated in Fig. 64.1A. Introduce the laparoscope through a slightly supraumbilical port to facilitate visualization of the left upper quadrant. After thoroughly exploring the abdomen, create an opening in the lesser sac by detaching the gastrocolic omentum from the greater curvature of the stomach using ultrasonic shears. Continue the division proximal and distal along the greater curvature until a sufficiently large window has been developed to allow the stomach to be reflected cephalad, exposing the pancreas and splenic artery (Fig. 64.1B). Divide any filmy adhesions between posterior gastric wall and retroperitoneum with the ultrasonic scalpel. Identify the region of interest. The splenic vein lies behind the pancreas and will not generally be seen (Fig. 64.1C). Laparoscopic ultrasound may assist in identifying abnormalities that are not visually evident. Determine the site of proposed transection of the pancreas.

Anatomic Points

The detailed anatomy of the lesser sac is discussed and illustrated in the orientation figures introducing Chapter 63 and in the anatomic points accompanying Fig. 63.1. From the laparoscopic perspective, entry into the lesser sac is best gained by going through the anterior leaf of the greater omentum (Fig. 64.1D) to expose the pancreas and splenic vessels.

Mobilization of Pancreas (Fig. 64.2)

Technical and Anatomic Points

Fully expose the body and tail of the pancreas by elevating the stomach and incising any gastropancreatic folds (Fig. 64.2A). Incise the retroperitoneum along the inferior and superior borders of the pancreas (Fig. 64.2B; see also Fig. 55.3B). Gently elevate the inferior margin of the spleen. The splenic vein should be visible deep to the pancreas, with the splenic artery visible along the superior margin.

Distal Pancreatectomy with Splenectomy (Fig. 64.3)

Technical and Anatomic Points

Divide the splenic flexure of the colon and short gastric vessels as shown in Fig. 55.1A,B in Chapter 55. Tilt the operating table to the right (left side up) to allow gravity to assist in retraction.

Identify the splenic artery at a convenient point where it loops above the pancreas. Secure it with double clips and divide it (Fig. 64.3A). An endoscopic vascular stapler or a pretied ligature is an acceptable alternative. Elevate the pancreas and splenic vein as a unit and divide these structures with the endoscopic linear stapler. (Fig. 64.3B). Elevate the distal pancreas and splenic vessels from the retroperitoneum.

LIST OF STRUCTURES

Pancreas
  Head
  Body
  Tail
  Pancreatic duct
Spleen
  Splenic artery

Splenic vein
Hilum of spleen
Transverse colon
Stomach
Portal vein
Superior mesenteric artery and vein
Left and right gastroepiploic artery
  and vein

Gastropancreatic arteries
Inferior (transverse) pancreatic artery
Great pancreatic artery
Gastrocolic omentum (ligament)
Gastropancreatic folds
Gastrosplenic ligament
Splenocolic ligament

FIGURE 64.1

ORIENTATION AND EXPOSURE (**B** from Wind GG. The spleen. In: *Applied laparoscopic anatomy: abdomen and pelvis.* Baltimore: Williams & Wilkins, 1997:187–216, with permission; **C** from Scott-Conner CEH, Cuschieri A, Carter FJ. Spleen and pancreas. In: *Minimal access surgical anatomy.* Philadelphia: Lippincott Williams & Wilkins, 2000:139–163, with permission; **D** from Wind GG. Stomach and duodenum. In: *Applied laparoscopic anatomy: abdomen and pelvis.* Baltimore: Williams & Wilkins, 1997:79–100, with permission.)

FIGURE 64.1   (Continued)

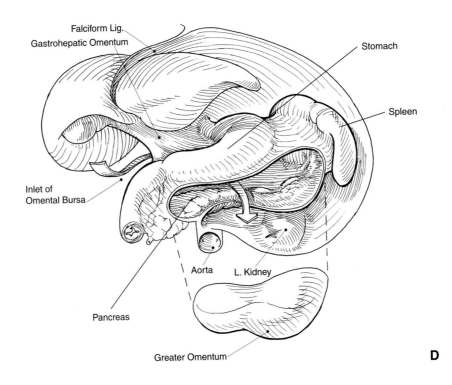

D

FIGURE 64.2
MOBILIZATION OF PANCREAS (**A** and **B** from Scott-Conner CEH, Cuschieri A, Carter FJ. Spleen and pancreas. In: *Minimal access surgical anatomy*. Philadelphia: Lippincott Williams & Wilkins, 2000:139–163, with permission.)

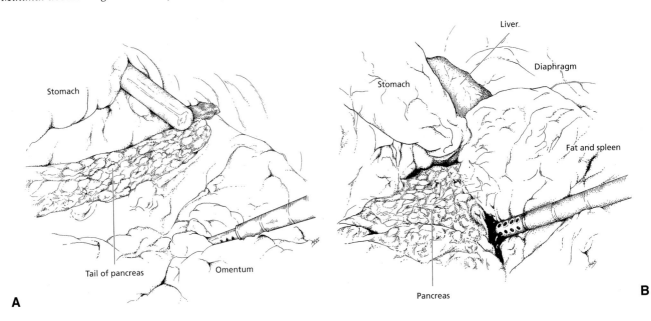

A   **B**

FIGURE 64.3
DISTAL PANCREATECTOMY WITH SPLENECTOMY (A from Scott-Conner CEH, Cuschieri A, Carter FJ. Spleen and pancreas. In: *Minimal access surgical anatomy.* Philadelphia: Lippincott Williams & Wilkins, 2000:139–163, with permission; **B** from Salky BA, Edye M. Laparoscopic pancreatectomy. *Surg Clin North Am* 1996;76:539–545, with permission.)

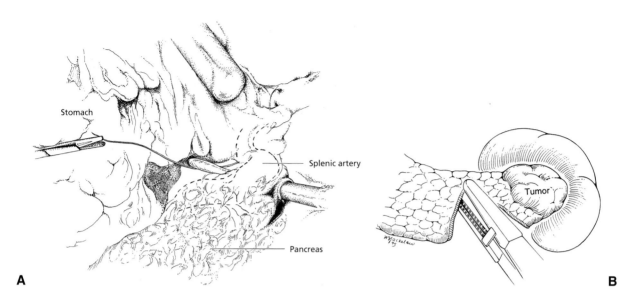

A   B

FIGURE 64.4
DISTAL PANCREATECTOMY WITHOUT SPLENECTOMY (From Scott-Conner CEH, Cuschieri A, Carter FJ. Spleen and pancreas. In: *Minimal access surgical anatomy.* Philadelphia: Lippincott Williams & Wilkins, 2000:139–163, with permission.)

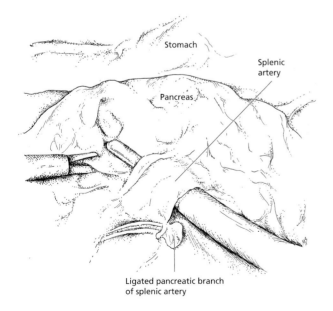

Divide the remaining peritoneal attachments of the spleen as described in Chapter 55.

Place the specimen in a retrieval bag. Make a short incision for intact removal. Attain hemostasis and close the incision and trocar sites.

Distal Pancreatectomy without Splenectomy (Fig. 64.4)

Technical and Anatomic Points

Develop a plane between pancreas and splenic vessels (Fig. 64.4). Divide the pancreas with the endoscopic cutting linear stapler as previously described. Use the ultrasonic scalpel to divide multiple small branches that tether the pancreas to the splenic vein and splenic artery. Preserve the main trunk of splenic artery and splenic vein.

REFERENCES

1. Gagner M, Pomp A. Laparoscopic pylorus-preserving pancreatoduodenectomy. *Surg Endosc* 1994;8:408–410.
2. Gagner M, Gentileschi P. Hand-assisted laparoscopic pancreatic resection. *Semin Laparosc Surg* 2001;8:114–125.
3. Lo CY, Lo CM, Fan ST. Role of laparoscopic ultrasonography in intraoperative localization of pancreatic insulinoma. *Surg Endosc* 2000;14:1131–1135. (Describes use of laparoscopic ultrasound before enucleation.)
4. Patterson EJ, Gagner M, Salky B, et al. Laparoscopic pancreatic resection: single-institution experience of 19 patients. *J Am Coll Surg* 2001; 193:281–287. (Includes experience with laparoscopic enucleation.)
5. Salky BA, Edye M. Laparoscopic pancreatectomy. *Surg Clin North Am* 1996;76:539–545.

CHAPTER 65

Internal Drainage of Pancreatic Pseudocysts

Pancreatic pseudocysts form when collections of fluid become loculated in the region of the pancreas and fail to reabsorb. Most pancreatic pseudocysts are found in a retrogastric location in the lesser sac. Proximity to the back wall of the stomach makes internal drainage by cyst gastrostomy the procedure of choice. Occasionally, a pseudocyst in the head of the pancreas may require drainage by anastomosis to the duodenum (cyst duodenostomy); in other cases, a very dependent pseudocyst that is not close to the back wall of the stomach may require drainage by Roux-en-Y cyst jejunostomy. These procedures are discussed at the end of this chapter.

Cyst Gastrostomy

Delineation of Anatomy and Preparation for Anastomosis (Fig. 65.1)

Technical Points

Use an incision that provides good exposure to the epigastric region. Generally, an upper midline or a chevron-type incision, depending on the build of the patient, is elected. Palpate the abdomen after the patient is asleep and plan an incision that is located directly over the palpable mass, if possible.

The typical retrogastric cyst is approached through the anterior wall of the stomach. Place stay sutures of 2-0 silk in the anterior wall of the stomach in a convenient and mobile location, well away from the pylorus. Incise the gastric wall longitudinally with electrocautery. A generous longitudinal gastrotomy, at least 5 to 6 cm in length, is needed. Secure all bleeding points. Place an 18-gauge needle into the pseudocyst through the posterior wall of the stomach. Aspirate and confirm that there is no blood in the cyst. If blood is obtained on aspiration, the possibility of a cyst eroding into the splenic artery should be strongly considered. (In this case, consider closing the abdomen and obtaining angiographic embolization. Alternatively, the cyst must be widely opened through the gastrocolic omentum and direct suture control of the splenic artery achieved. Splenectomy may be needed. Closed-suction drains must then be placed in the cyst to provide external drainage. Culture the cyst fluid.

Aspirate about 100 mL of cyst fluid and then inject 50 to 100 mL of water-soluble contrast material and obtain a radiograph. This will demonstrate the anatomy of the cyst and whether or not there are septations that must be treated. Depending on the adequacy of preoperative studies, this step may be omitted. Place stay sutures in the posterior gastric wall and prepare to make an incision into the back wall of the stomach.

Anatomic Points

The anatomic relationships of the pancreas, the location of the pancreatic pseudocyst, and the anatomic fusion of adjacent organs in response to inflammation allow internal drainage of pancreatic pseudocysts.

The head of the pancreas lies in the duodenal curve. Superiorly, it is overlapped anteriorly by the first part of the duodenum; elsewhere, its margin is indented by the duodenum. Its anterior anatomic relationships include the first part of the duodenum, the gastroduodenal artery (which makes a groove in the pancreas that delineates head from neck), the

LIST OF STRUCTURES

Pancreas	Colon	First and second portions
Head	Transverse mesocolon	Common bile duct
Body	Middle colic artery and vein	Left and right gastroepiploic artery and
Tail	Stomach	vein
Uncinate process	Greater curvature	Gastrocolic omentum
Spleen	Pylorus	Gastropancreatic folds
Splenic artery	Antrum	Gastroduodenal artery
Splenic vein	Duodenum	Inferior vena cava

ORIENTATION

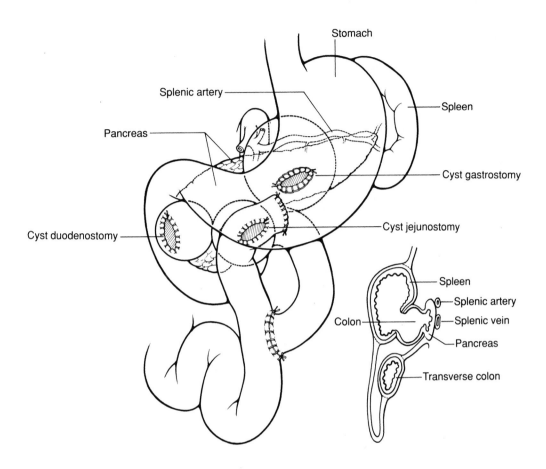

Stomach

Splenic artery

Spleen

Pancreas

Cyst gastrostomy

Cyst jejunostomy

Cyst duodenostomy

Spleen

Splenic artery

Splenic vein

Colon

Pancreas

Transverse colon

FIGURE 65.1
DELINEATION OF ANATOMY AND PREPARATION FOR ANASTOMOSIS

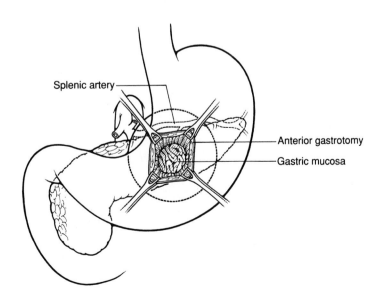

Splenic artery

Anterior gastrotomy

Gastric mucosa

transverse mesocolon, and jejunum. Posteriorly, the head of the pancreas lies on the right diaphragmatic crus, the inferior vena cava and terminal segments of the renal veins, and the aorta. The inferior part of the head is continuous with the uncinate process, which lies in the space between the superior mesenteric vessels and the aorta. The bile duct is either posterior to the head of the pancreas or embedded within the substance of this gland.

The neck of the pancreas begins on the right at the groove from the gastroduodenal artery and merges insensibly with the body. Anteriorly, it is related to the pylorus and omental bursa. Posteriorly, it is related to the superior mesenteric and splenic veins, which join to form the portal vein.

Anteriorly, the body of the pancreas is separated from the stomach by the omental bursa (lesser sac), and its peritoneal covering is continuous with the anterior leaf of the transverse mesocolon. Posteriorly, the body is in contact with the aorta, the beginning of the superior mesenteric artery, the left diaphragmatic crus, the left suprarenal gland, the left kidney and renal vessels, and the splenic vein. The inferior aspect of the body is in contact with the duodenojejunal flexure, coils of jejunum, and the left colic flexure. Where it is not in direct contact with these organs, the peritoneum covering it is directly continuous with the transverse mesocolon.

The tail of the pancreas is the narrow left termination of the pancreas. It extends to the splenic surface at the hilum. The tail lies in the lienorenal ligament and is in contact with the splenic flexure of the colon. Posteriorly, it is in contact with the left kidney.

In summary, remember that the pancreas is a retroperitoneal organ whose head is inferior to the root of the transverse mesocolon, but whose body and tail are predominantly superior to the transverse mesocolon. Thus, the body and tail are posterior to the peritoneum of the lesser sac and to the stomach. Because of these anatomic relationships, inflammatory processes involving the body and tail of the pancreas can easily result in adhesions between the pancreas and the posterior wall of the stomach.

The major blood supply to the stomach is provided by the gastric artery arcade along the lesser curvature, the gastroepiploic arcade along the greater curvature, and the short gastric arteries to the fundus. Thus, the anterior gastrotomy should be located about halfway between the greater and lesser curvatures to avoid dividing large vessels that could cause troublesome bleeding.

Construction of A Cyst Gastrostomy (Fig. 65.2)

Technical and Anatomic Points

Incise the back wall of the stomach and puncture through into the cysts with electrocautery or by poking through with a clamp. Decompress the cyst with suction. The retroperitoneal area should become completely flat so that no residual masses are palpable. If a residual mass is palpable, the possibility of a second pseudocyst should be considered. If a second pseudocyst is found, it, too, must be drained. Enlarge the opening in the back wall of the stomach until it is several centimeters across. Take a full-thickness piece of the back wall of the stomach and the anterior wall of the cyst for biopsy. Check the edges of the incision for hemostasis. Use electrocautery and suture ligatures to achieve hemostasis in the edge.

**FIGURE 65.2
CONSTRUCTION OF A CYST GASTROSTOMY**

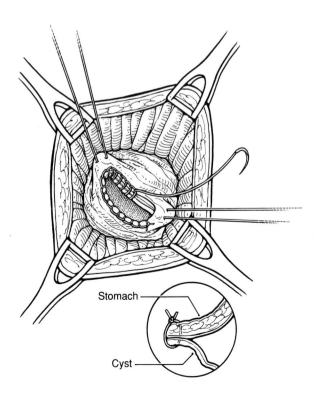

Stomach
Cyst

**FIGURE 65.3
CONSTRUCTION OF CYST DUODENOSTOMY**

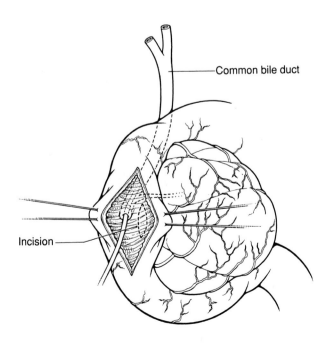

Common bile duct
Incision

Place a running lock-stitch of 2-0 Vicryl around the entire anastomosis to ensure adequate hemostasis. Note that this anastomosis is actually simply a fenestration. The inflammatory process in the lesser sac creates a fusion between the anterior wall of the pseudocyst and the back wall of the stomach. The suture is placed purely for hemostasis. At the conclusion of the procedure, hemostasis must be absolute. The retroperitoneum should be collapsed, and no residual masses should be palpable. A nasogastric tube should lie comfortably within the stomach.

Close the gastrotomy in two layers by suture, or by application of a linear stapling device. Place omentum over the gastrotomy.

Cyst Duodenostomy

Construction of Cyst Duodenostomy (Fig. 65.3)

Technical Points

Cyst duodenostomy is performed when a pseudocyst in the head of the pancreas is not in proximity to the back wall of the stomach. It is a procedure of second choice because it is more hazardous than cyst gastrostomy because of the potential for damage to the intraduodenal common duct.

Perform a Kocher maneuver, if possible, to elevate the duodenum and head of pancreas into the surgical field. Open the common bile duct and place a probe within it if there

FIGURE 65.4
ROUX-EN-Y DRAINAGE OF A PSEUDOCYST

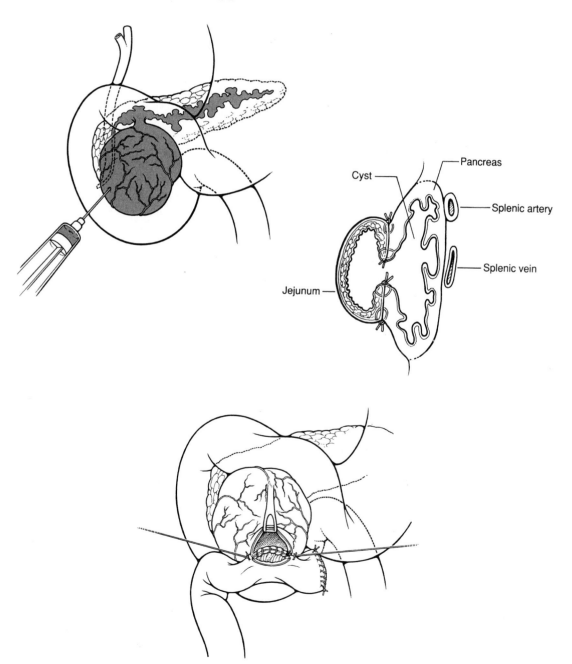

is any uncertainty about the relationship of the common bile duct to the cyst. Incise the anterior wall of the duodenum over the cyst. Place stay sutures on the back wall of the duodenum. Make certain that you know where the common bile duct lies within the surgical field.

Make an opening into the pseudocyst through the back wall of the duodenum. Perform an anastomosis in a similar fashion to that outlined for cyst gastrostomy. Perform a cholangiogram at the conclusion of the procedure to verify that no injury to the common duct has occurred.

Close the duodenostomy in two layers. Cover the duodenal suture line with omentum.

Anatomic Points

The infrapyloric segment of the bile duct is close to the duodenal edge of the pancreas. Here, it is either retropancreatic or, more commonly, is bridged posteriorly by pancreatic tissue. When the duodenum and pancreas are mobilized by the Kocher maneuver, this duct can be seen to be more closely associated with the parietal surface of the pancreas than with the peritoneal surface.

Roux-en-Y Drainage of a Pseudocyst

Roux-en-Y Drainage of a Pseudocyst (Fig. 65.4)

Technical Points

Expose the pseudocyst, which is generally located in the inferior portion of the lesser sac. Elevate the transverse colon and examine an avascular portion of the transverse mesocolon. If the pseudocyst can be identified in this region, this is the most convenient area for anastomosis. Confirm the location of the pseudocyst by palpation and by aspiration with an 18-gauge needle.

Construct a Roux-en-Y loop of jejunum. Place stay sutures into the pseudocyst in a dependent region. Make an opening into the pseudocyst and aspirate the cyst fluid. Obtain a full-thickness biopsy specimen of the wall of the pseudocyst. Construct a two-layer anastomosis between the pseudocyst and the blind end of the Roux loop. Use interrupted 3-0 silk for the outer layer and interrupted 3-0 Vicryl for the inner layer. In contrast to the cyst gastrostomy and cyst duodenostomy procedures previously described, this anastomosis is surgically created because previous fusion of the cyst to the Roux loop has not occurred. Therefore, the anastomosis must be constructed with the same meticulous care with which any intestinal anastomosis is performed. Do not stent the anastomosis.

Place omentum around the anastomosis. Closed-suction drains may be placed in the vicinity of the anastomosis, if desired, but are not necessary.

Anatomic Points

Because the pseudocyst is most often located in the inferior portion of the omental bursa, the most logical route to the cyst is through the posterior leaf of the transverse mesocolon. Exposure of the posterior leaf of transverse mesocolon is accomplished by elevating the transverse colon. If possible, place the Roux limb to the left of the middle colic artery, where the transverse mesocolon is essentially avascular.

REFERENCES

1. Beckingham IJ, Krige JEJ, Bornman PC, et al. Endoscopic management of pancreatic pseudocysts. *Br J Surg* 1997;84:1638–1645. (Presents alternative to surgical drainage.)
2. Bradley EL. Cystoduodenostomy: new perspectives. *Ann Surg* 1984;200:698.
3. Bradley EL, Austin H. Multiple pancreatic pseudocysts: the principle of internal cystocystostomy in surgical management. *Surgery* 1982;92:111.
4. Bradley EL, Clements JL. Transenteric rupture of pancreatic pseudocysts: management of pseudocyst enteric fistulas. *Am Surg* 1976;42:827. (Discusses uncommon complication of untreated pseudocysts.)
5. Johnson LB, Rattner DW, Warshaw AL. The effect of size of giant pancreatic pseudocysts on the outcome of internal drainage procedures. *Surg Gynecol Obstet* 1991;173:171.
6. Kuroda A, Konishi T, Kimura W, et al. Cystopancreaticostomy and longitudinal pancreaticojejunostomy as a simpler technique of combined drainage operation for chronic pancreatitis with pancreatic pseudocyst causing persistent cholecystasis. *Surg Gynecol Obstet* 1993;177:183.
7. Lohr-Happe A, Peiper M, Lankisch PG. Natural course of operated pseudocysts in chronic pancreatitis. *Gut* 1994;35:1479.
8. Taghizadeh F, Bower RJ, Kiesewetter WB. Stapled cystogastrostomy: a method of treatment for pediatric pancreatic pseudocyst. *Ann Surg* 1979;190:166.
9. Vitale GC, Lawhon JC, Larson GM, et al. Endoscopic drainage of the pancreatic pseudocyst. *Surgery* 1999;126:616–623. (Presents alternative method of drainage.)
10. Warshaw AL, Rattner DW. Facts and fallacies of common bile duct obstruction by pancreatic pseudocysts. *Ann Surg* 1980;192:33.

THE SMALL AND LARGE INTESTINE

In this section, common operations performed on the small and large intestine are described. First, small bowel resection and anastomosis are detailed in Chapter 66, in which the technique of double-layered, handsewn anastomosis is introduced. Strictureplasty for Crohn's disease is also described. Chapter 67 describes the equivalent laparoscopic procedure using a stapled technique. The general topography of the small intestine and the differences between the jejunum and ileum have already been illustrated in previous chapters. The appendix, a diverticulum of the gastrointestinal tract of uncertain significance, is described in Chapters 68 and 69, in which the common operations of traditional and laparoscopic appendectomy are presented. Because the operation for appendicitis sometimes discloses an unexpected Meckel's diverticulum, the procedures for resection of this diverticulum are included in these chapters.

As in other sections, endoscopy is used to introduce the topography and general layout of the colon (Chapter 70). This introduction to the colon is further expanded in the discussions of colostomy and colostomy closure (Chapter 71), often the first operations on the large intestine performed during surgical training. In this chapter, the blood supply and mesenteries of the colon are described. Finally, chapters on laparoscopic colostomy, open and laparoscopic colon resections, and right and left colon resections (Chapters 72 to 74) complete this part. Low anterior resection for carcinoma of the rectum is described in conjunction with abdominoperineal resection (Chapters 75 and 76) in the next part, *The Pelvis*.

CHAPTER 66

Small Bowel Resection and Anastomosis

Small bowel resection is performed when a segment of small intestine must be removed. The nature of the pathology dictates the extent of resection. Carcinoma of the small intestine is rare. Resection for carcinoma should encompass margins of at least 10 cm and a fan-shaped piece of mesentery containing regional nodes. Resection for benign disease is more common. In the latter case, margins should be conservative, and as much bowel as possible should be preserved. This is particularly true when reoperations may be necessary (e.g., in patients with Crohn's disease). Strictureplasty, a popular alternative to resection in patients with Crohn's disease, is briefly presented at the end of this chapter.

When a significant length of small intestine must be removed, measure the length of the remaining bowel. Take a wet umbilical tape and measure the length along the antimesenteric border, with the bowel under slight stretch. Record the measured length in the operative note.

Small Bowel Resection (Fig. 66.1)

Technical Points

Always "run" the entire small intestine before any resection. Grasp a section of small bowel and pass it from one hand to the other, "walking" your fingers proximally. You should be progressing in the general direction of the left upper quadrant. Identify the ligament of Treitz. Progressing distally from the ligament of Treitz, elevate a section of small bowel about 10 cm in length. Flip each section over so that both sides are examined. Then pass the section to your first assistant. Continue in this fashion to the ileocecal valve. If, by chance, the loop of bowel that you grasp in the beginning leads you to the ileocecal valve instead of the ligament of Treitz, it is perfectly acceptable to run the bowel from distal to proximal, finishing at the ligament of Treitz. Minimize the amount of time that the bowel is out of the abdomen. Interference with venous drainage, swelling, and hypothermia can result from

LIST OF STRUCTURES

Jejunum
Ileum
Cecum
Ileocecal valve
Ligament of Treitz

prolonged evisceration. Return all bowel, with the exception of the segment to be resected, to the abdomen.

Grasp the bowel between the thumb and forefinger of your nondominant hand and use your thumb to feel the mesenteric border of the bowel at one of the planned resection margins. Take a fine-pointed mosquito hemostat and pass it under one of the small vessels that supply the bowel. Double-clamp and ligate the vessel with fine silk. Do not try to break through on your first pass unless the mesentery is very flimsy. Divide the mesentery close to the bowel with precision to minimize the bulk of tissue included in ligatures next to the bowel. The mesenteric surface of the bowel will then be clean and ready for anastomosis.

Clamp the bowel with Allen clamps or similar straight clamps designed to hold bowel securely. Kocher clamps will work if nothing else is available. Divide the bowel between the clamps with a scalpel.

Repeat this process at the other end of the segment to be resected.

Lift the bowel up to display the mesentery and identify the line along which you plan to resect it. With the mesentery slightly stretched, place the opened blade of a pair of Metzenbaum scissors into the incision in the mesentery and lift up, elevating a flap of peritoneum with the tip of the blade. Push-cut the peritoneum by pushing with the crotch of the barely opened scissors, outlining a V-shaped segment of mesentery to be resected. This cut should not injure the underlying mesenteric vessels. Flip the bowel over and do the same thing on the other side of the mesentery. Use the thumb and forefinger of your nondominant hand to elevate the thin, fatty mesentery. A finger fracture technique is sometimes useful. Double-clamp and divide all mesenteric vessels, and remove the resected segment.

Secure the mesenteric vessels with suture ligatures of 3-0 silk.

Anatomic Points

Running the bowel allows the surgeon to inspect the entire length of small bowel for disease or incidental developmental anomalies. The most common anomaly is Meckel's diverticulum, which has been reported to be present (although is usually asymptomatic) as frequently as 4.5% of the time.

The ligament of Treitz, or the suspensory muscle of the duodenum, marks the beginning of the intraperitoneal jejunum. This ligament is present about 75% of the time. A

FIGURE 66.1
SMALL BOWEL RESECTION

A   B

band of smooth muscle running from the connective tissue around the celiac artery and right diaphragmatic crus blends with smooth muscle at the duodenojejunal flexure. It has little significance as a muscle but functions as a ligament to maintain the duodenojejunal flexure. However, because it is muscular and thus vascular, division of this ligament, if necessary, must be done between clamps and with appropriate hemostatic control.

As you run the bowel, note the blood supply and venous drainage of the small bowel. Numerous jejunal and ileal branches arise from the left side of the superior mesenteric artery. A few centimeters from the intestinal border, these arteries branch, and contiguous branches of the superior mesenteric artery anastomose to form arcades. There tends to be one order of arcades for the proximal jejunum, several orders in the middle third of the small bowel, and then a decrease in the number of orders so that the distal ileum may again be supplied by a single arcade. These anastomotic arches form the primary collateral blood supply for any given segment of small bowel. Multiple vasa recti of variable lengths arise from those arches closest to the bowel wall and directly supply the bowel. Each vasa recta typically (about 90% of the time) passes to one side of the bowel wall, rather than splitting to supply both sides; the side supplied alternates as one progresses along the bowel. The vasa recti are end arteries. An intramural plexus allows intestinal viability to be maintained for a small distance after division of these terminal vessels.

Intestinal veins follow a pattern similar to that of the arterial supply. Although there are no supporting statistics available, one gets the distinct impression that veins tend to lie on the upper side of the mesentery, whereas arteries tend to course on the lower side.

Although jejunum blends imperceptibly with ileum in the midportion of the small bowel, the following differences may help one to distinguish between jejunum and ileum:

1. Jejunum has a thicker wall and larger lumen than ileum; thus, the diameter of the small bowel decreases as one progresses distally.
2. In the jejunum, fat is restricted to the mesentery, but as one progresses distally, fat creeps up onto the wall of the ileum.
3. Jejunal arterial arcades tend to be less complex and vasa recti tend to be longer in the proximal jejunum; arcade complexity increases and vasa recti become shorter as one progresses distally. Arcade complexity reaches its maximum in the middle third of the small bowel, then becomes simpler more distally. However, the vasa recti do not lengthen.

Anastomosis (Fig. 66.2)

Technical Points

Inspect both ends of the bowel and verify that the color is normal, indicating a good blood supply. Occasionally, division of the mesentery compromises the circulation to one or both of the ends. If the color becomes dusky or bluish adjacent to the clamps, suspect vascular compromise and resect additional bowel.

Check the mesenteric border. The bowel should be cleaned of mesenteric fat for a distance of 2 to 3 mm from the clamp. Extension of this is unnecessary and may result in ischemia.

Align the mesenteric borders and confirm that the bowel is not twisted by tracing the V of the mesentery. Some surgeons

FIGURE 66.2
ANASTOMOSIS

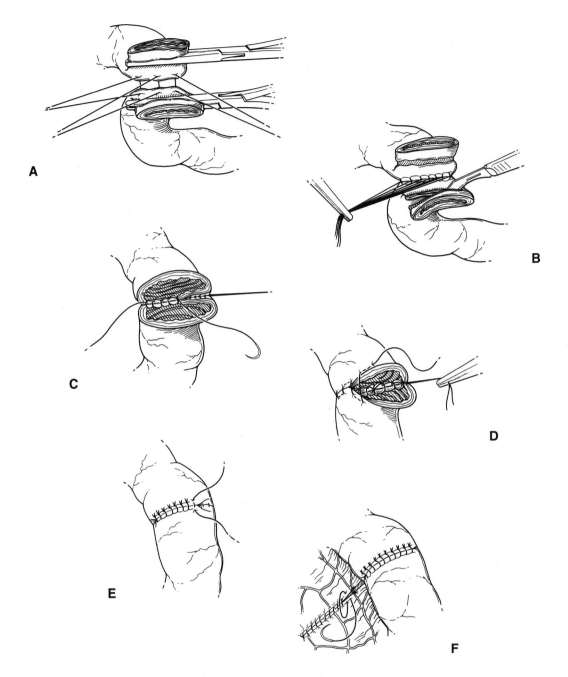

prefer to close the mesenteric defect first. This ensures that there are no twists and that vascular compromise does not occur in the process of mesenteric closure. Use wet laparotomy pads to isolate the two ends to be anastomosed.

Construct the anastomosis by placing a posterior row of interrupted Lembert sutures of 3-0 silk. Remove the clamps and excise the crushed ends of the bowel. It is advantageous to leave a small (0.5-mm) remnant of crush because it keeps all of the layers of the bowel wall together so that the mucosa does not "pout out."

Place the inner suture as a running lock-stitch of 3-0 Vicryl, beginning at the middle of the back wall and progressing

in each direction. Use two sutures and tie them together in the midline. Continue the suture line anteriorly as a running Connell suture to invert the outer row. Tie the two sutures together at the midpoint of the anterior row. Complete the anastomosis with an outer seromuscular layer of interrupted Lembert sutures of 3-0 silk.

Close the mesenteric defect by suturing the two sides of the V together. Either an interrupted or a continuous suture may be used. Take bites that extend through the peritoneum but that are not deep enough to "catch" the underlying vessels. Leave no defect through which a loop of small intestine could herniate. Wrap the anastomosis with omentum, if available.

Anatomic Points

The outer layer of the bowel wall is the serosa, which is visceral peritoneum. Just deep to this layer, one can see the vasculature to the bowel and, where appropriate, the fat encroaching on the ileal wall. The next layer is longitudinal smooth muscle, then circular smooth muscle; between them is Auerbach's myenteric nerve plexus. These two layers comprise the *tunica muscularis,* or *muscularis externa.* The next layer encountered is the *submucosa,* which is predominantly areolar connective tissue; it contains a plexus of blood vessels and Meissner's submucosal nerve plexus. The innermost layer—the *mucosa*—can be divided into an outer muscularis mucosa, middle lamina propria, and inner epithelium.

Of the four layers, it is the submucosa that provides the strength in bowel repairs. Moreover, although a time-honored theory holds that proper healing of bowel wounds depends on apposition of serosal layers, this is, in fact, not the case. Rather, accurate and watertight apposition of one surface to another, whether serosa or mucosa, coupled with sufficient time allowed for healing, is all that is necessary.

Strictureplasty for Crohn's Disease (Fig. 66.3)

Technical and Anatomic Points

Strictureplasty is an alternative to resection for management of a strictured segment. It is particularly useful for multiple strictured areas. It allows maximum preservation of bowel length with restoration of a widely patent lumen. Use the Heineke-Mikulicz approach for short segments, the Finney approach for longer areas.

Heineke-Mikulicz Strictureplasty

Open the strictured portion of bowel in a longitudinal fashion (Fig. 66.3A). Place two stay sutures of 3-0 silk at opposite sides to hold the bowel open—these may be used as corner stitches if placed as Lembert sutures. Close the incision in a transverse fashion with a running suture of 3-0 Vicryl placed as a Connell suture, followed by a layer of interrupted 3-0 silk Lembert sutures.

Finney-Type Strictureplasty

For longer strictured areas, again open the entire strictured area in a longitudinal fashion (Fig. 66.3B). Then loop the bowel at its midportion to approximate the proximal and distal edges of one side of the incision. Sew these together with interrupted 3-0 silk Lembert sutures. Begin an inner layer of running 3-0 Vicryl at the point where the bowel folds back on itself. Run this suture line as a locking stitch to the apex, then use it to approximate the two open ends of bowel as a Connell suture. Complete this functional side-to-side anastomosis with an outer layer of 3-0 Lembert sutures.

FIGURE 66.3
STRICTUREPLASTY FOR CROHN'S DISEASE (A and **B** from Scott-Conner CEH. Current surgical management of inflammatory bowel disease. *South Med J* 1994;87:1232–1241, with permission.

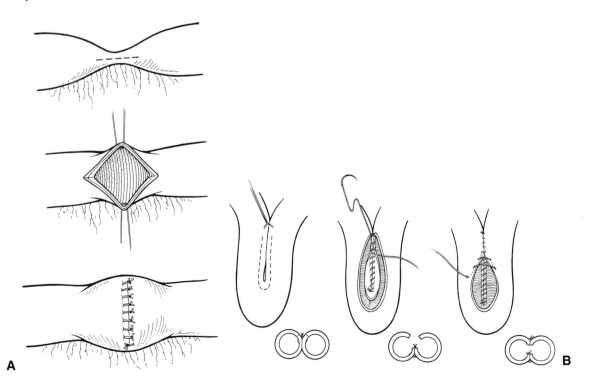

A   B

REFERENCES

1. Asensio JA, Berne JD, Chahwan S, et al. Traumatic injury to the superior mesenteric artery. *Am J Surg* 1999;178:235–239. (Discusses special considerations for management of rare injury.)

2. Barnes JP. The techniques for end-to-end intestinal anastomosis. *Surg Gynecol Obstet* 1974;138:433.

3. Bulkley GB, Zuidema GD, Hamilton ST, et al. Intraoperative determination of small intestinal viability following ischemic injury. *Ann Surg* 1981;193:628.

4. Getzen LC. Intestinal suturing. I. The development of intestinal sutures. *Curr Probl Surg* 1969;6:1.

5. Getzen LC. Intestinal suturing. II. Inverting and everting intestinal sutures. *Curr Probl Surg* 1969;6:1.

6. Mulholland M. Atlas of small intestinal surgery. In: Bell RH Jr, Rikkers L, Mulholland M, eds. *Digestive tract surgery: a text and atlas.* Philadelphia: JB Lippincott, 1996:1304–1305. (Discusses strictureplasty for Crohn's disease.)

7. Poth EJ, Gold D. Technics of gastrointestinal suture. *Curr Probl Surg* 1965;2:1.

8. Scott-Conner CEH. Current surgical management of inflammatory bowel disease. *South Med J* 1994;87:1232–1241.

9. Townsend MC, Pelias ME. A technique for rapid closure of traumatic small intestine perforations without resection. *Am J Surg* 1992;164:171. (Describes ingenious method of staple closure of perforations too large for primary closure.)

CHAPTER 67

Laparoscopic Small Bowel Resection and Anastomosis

Depending on the habitus of the patient, the nature of the pathology, and the mobility of the small bowel, there are several approaches that can be used. The technique that is shown here uses laparoscopic mobilization and mesenteric division, followed by extracorporeal completion of resection and anastomosis. It is also possible to construct a fully intracorporeal anastomosis. The advantages are minor, however, because an incision must be made to retrieve the specimen. In some circumstances, the entire mesenteric division and anastomosis may be done after exteriorizing the specimen—the laparoscope then is used simply to localize and elevate the relevant loop.

Orientation and Initial Mobilization (Fig. 67.1)

Technical Points

Place the first trocar at the umbilicus and explore the abdomen. If the lesion is in the proximal small intestine, set up the laparoscopic field and trocar sites to allow comfortable access to the left upper quadrant (Fig. 67.1A). For middle or distal small intestine, a right lower quadrant field is more appropriate (Fig. 67.1B). Explore the abdomen and trace the small bowel from the ligament of Treitz to the terminal ileum. Confirm the location of the segment to be resected. Identify the proximal and distal resection margins.

Pass two traction sutures—each through the anterior abdominal wall, through the mesentery at the two respective resection margins, and back through the anterior abdominal wall in such a fashion as to suspend the loop of bowel (Fig. 67.1C).

Anatomic Points

The base of the small bowel mesentery runs along a diagonal line from the left upper quadrant to the right lower quadrant

---

FIGURE 67.1

ORIENTATION AND INITIAL MOBILIZATION (D from Scott-Conner CEH, Cuschieri A, Carter FJ. Small intestine and appendix. In: *Minimal access surgical anatomy*. Philadelphia: Lippincott Williams & Wilkins, 2000:165–184, with permission.)

FIGURE 67.1 (Continued)

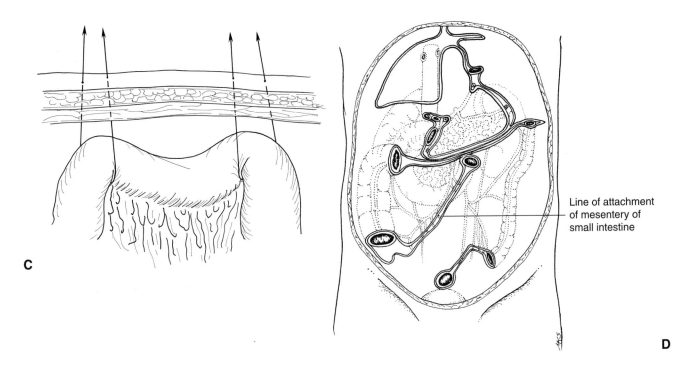

Line of attachment
of mesentery of
small intestine

C

D

(Fig. 67.1D). The length of the mesentery in the middle small intestine (see Fig. 44.5) makes it relatively easy to suspend a loop in a convenient working space.

Division of Mesentery and Extracorporeal Anastomosis (Fig. 67.2)

Technical and Anatomic Points

Mark or "score" the mesentery along the proposed line of division. This will generally consist of a fan-shaped portion of mesentery connecting the two points of proposed transection, as described in Chapter 66. Laparoscopic scissors with electrocautery work well for this. Then, sequentially divide the mesentery and associated vessels with the ultrasonic scalpel or a linear cutting endoscopic stapler (vascular cartridge) (Fig. 67.2A). Extend one of the trocar incisions or create a short midline incision and exteriorize the loop of bowel (Fig. 67.2B). Divide the bowel and create a

FIGURE 67.2
DIVISION OF MESENTERY AND EXTRACORPOREAL ANASTOMOSIS

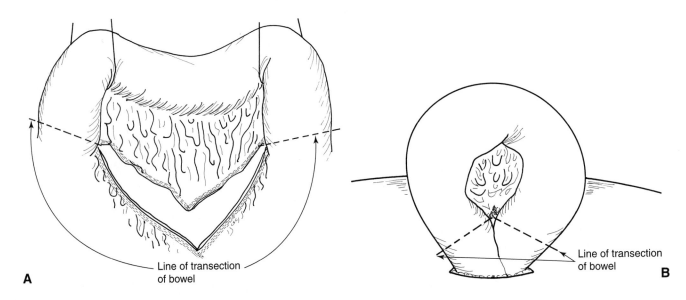

Line of transection
of bowel

A

Line of transection
of bowel

B

side-to-side stapled anastomosis (see Fig. 74.3, where this is illustrated for extracorporeal anastomosis after laparoscopic right colon resection). Close the mesenteric defect with sutures and return the loop of bowel to the abdomen. Close the abdominal incision and trocar sites in the usual fashion.

REFERENCES

1. Lange V, Meyer G, Schardey HM, et al. Different techniques of laparoscopic end-to-end small-bowel anastomoses. *Surg Endosc* 1995;10:1012–1015.
2. Schirmer BD. Small bowel resection, enterolysis, and enteroenterostomy. In: Scott-Conner CEH, ed. *The SAGES manual: fundamentals of laparoscopy and GI endoscopy.* New York: Springer-Verlag, 1999:254–266.
3. Schonleben K. Small-bowel resection. In: Kremer K, Platzer W, Schreiber HW, et al, eds. *Minimally invasive abdominal surgery.* New York: Thieme, 2001:316–320. (Illustrates intracorporeal anastomotic techniques.)
4. Scott-Conner CEH, Cuschieri A, Carter FJ. Small intestine and appendix. In: *Minimal access surgical anatomy.* Philadelphia, Lippincott Williams & Wilkins, 2000:165–184.

CHAPTER 68

Appendectomy and Resection of Meckel's Diverticulum

The anatomy of the lateral abdominal wall, including the rectus sheath and the right lower quadrant, is described in this chapter. The laparoscopic approach to the appendix and Meckel's diverticulum is given in Chapter 69.

Skin Incision (Fig. 68.1)

Technical Points

The skin incision is planned according to two fixed anatomic landmarks: the anterosuperior iliac spine and the umbilicus. Draw a line from the umbilicus to the anterosuperior iliac spine. McBurney's point lies one third of the distance from the anterosuperior iliac spine. The classic McBurney incision is made perpendicular to this line. The incision may be modified to follow the local lines of skin tension, as indicated, but it should pass through McBurney's point. A Rockey-Davis incision is made over McBurney's point but is directed in a nearly transverse direction. This incision yields a good cosmetic result because it parallels Langer's lines. It also more nearly approximates the direction of the major cutaneous nerves of the region, and it is easy to extend this incision should unexpected pathology be encountered at laparotomy.

If a mass is palpable in the right lower quadrant after induction of anesthesia, make the incision over the mass.

Anatomic Points

The anterosuperior iliac spine presents as a prominence in slender individuals but may take the form of a depression in obese patients. It is a constant, palpable landmark. The lateral border of the rectus abdominis muscle may be visible as the semilunar line. This begins inferiorly at the pubic tubercle and curves laterally as it ascends. At the level of the umbilicus, the semilunar line is about 7 cm from the midline and lies about halfway between the midline and the side of the body.

Generally in this region, one will be able to identify a distinct division of the superficial fascia into two layers: the more superficial layer of fatty areolar tissue, which is Camper's fascia, and the deeper, membranous layer, which is Scarpa's fascia.

Muscle-Splitting Incision (Fig. 68.2)

Technical Points

The external oblique muscle and its aponeurosis form the first layer of the abdominal wall (which is encountered as the incision is deepened). Open each layer of the abdominal wall by splitting, rather than cutting, the muscular and aponeurotic fibers. The resulting muscle-splitting incision is called a gridiron incision. Because each layer is opened parallel to the muscle fibers and hence in the direction of maximum tension when the fibers contract, the resulting incision is very strong, and hernias are rare.

Medially, the external oblique aponeurosis contributes to the anterior rectus sheath. Usually, the rectus sheath forms the medial boundary of the fascial incision. If necessary, the rectus sheath may be incised. The rectus muscle can then be retracted medially to achieve additional exposure.

Anatomic Points

The fibers of the external oblique muscle run obliquely from above downward, and from lateral to medial (i.e., in the same direction as you would put your hands into your

LIST OF STRUCTURES

Anterosuperior iliac spine
Umbilicus
McBurney's point
Camper's fascia
Scarpa's fascia
External oblique muscle and
  aponeurosis
Rectus abdominis muscle

Rectus sheath
Semilunar line
Arcuate line (of Douglas)
Transversus abdominis muscle
Transversalis fascia
Iliohypogastric nerve
Subcostal nerves
Cecum

Appendix
Mesoappendix
Appendicular artery
Ileocolic artery
Fold of Treves
Meckel's diverticulum

FIGURE 68.1
SKIN INCISION

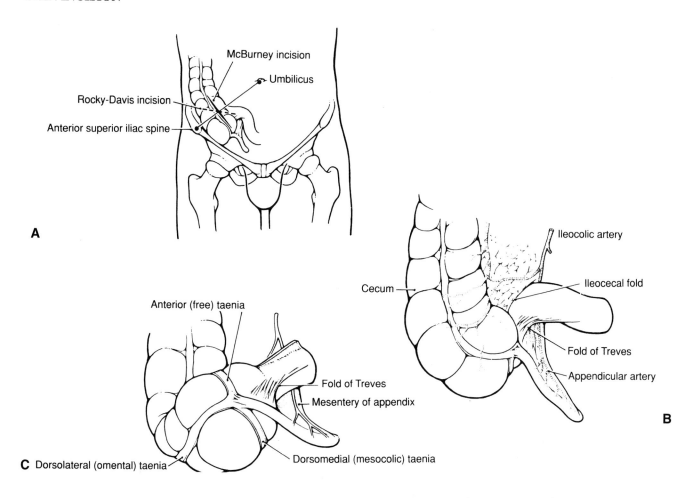

A

B

C

FIGURE 68.2
MUSCLE-SPLITTING INCISION

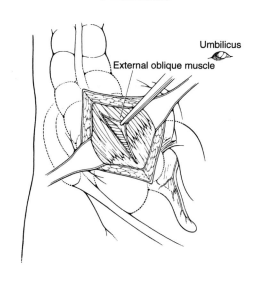

pockets). Fibers of the external oblique muscle terminate in its aponeurosis following a curved line from the semilunar line to approximately the anterosuperior iliac spine.

The major cutaneous nerves of the region are branches of the iliohypogastric and subcostal nerves.

Deepening the Incision (Fig. 68.3)

Technical Points

Split the fibers of the internal oblique and transversus abdominis muscles in turn by a combination of sharp and blunt dissection. Incise the fascia with a scalpel, cutting carefully, parallel to the fibers. Extend the cut by inserting partially closed Metzenbaum scissors and pushing, or by splitting bluntly with two fingers or a pair of hemostats. Medially, the sheath of the rectus abdominis muscle limits the extent of the split.

Anatomic Points

Note that the fibers of the internal oblique muscle are almost transverse at the level of this incision and that muscle extends

FIGURE 68.3
DEEPENING THE INCISION

much more medially than the muscular portion of the external oblique muscle. The aponeurosis of the internal oblique muscle contributes to the anterior rectus sheath along the entire length of this muscle and, by splitting, to the posterior rectus sheath above the arcuate line of Douglas.

Observe that fibers of the transversus abdominis muscle, in the operative field, almost parallel those of the internal oblique muscle. Muscle fibers proper terminate slightly more laterally than do those of the internal oblique muscle. The aponeurosis of the transversus abdominis muscle contributes fibers to the anterior rectus sheath below the line of Douglas as well as to the posterior rectus sheath above.

The plane between the internal oblique and transversus abdominis muscles should be approached with caution because the main branches of the nerves that innervate the lower rectus abdominis muscle (T-11, subcostal) and the skin of the lower abdominal wall (T-11, subcostal, iliohypogastric) lie within this plane.

Entry into the Peritoneum (Fig. 68.4)

Technical Points

Incise the peritoneum in any convenient direction. Generally, cutting in a vertical or oblique direction provides good exposure and avoids the possibility of inadvertent entry into the rectus sheath medially, injury to the inferior epigastric vessels medially, or injury to the cecum laterally. Obtain a culture of any turbid or purulent fluid that is encountered, and place retractors to obtain exposure.

Locate the cecum, which may be identified by its size, as well as the presence of taeniae, the terminal ileum, and the lateral peritoneal attachment (Fig. 68.4A). Cecum will commonly present into the wound, but occasionally, greater omentum, small intestine, or even sigmoid colon may be the first structure encountered. If small intestine presents into the incision and the cecum cannot be located easily, follow the small intestine distally to the terminal ileum, which leads to the cecum. Grasp the cecum firmly and pull it gently toward the patient's left shoulder with a rocking motion. If the cecum cannot be mobilized sufficiently by this maneuver, it may be necessary to incise the lateral peritoneal reflection and elevate the cecum from the retroperitoneum by blunt dissection (Fig. 68.4B).

Anatomic Points

Although typically transversalis fascia and peritoneum are fused at this point and thus can be cut as a unit, it is important to remember that these are two separate layers between which lie variable amounts of loose areolar connective tissue and fat. Note, too, that the peritoneum, which attaches the lateral side of the cecum and colon to the abdominal wall, is an embryonic fusion plane between parietal and visceral peritoneum. It is, therefore, an essentially bloodless plane and can be carefully cut with a minimum of bleeding.

The position of the appendix relative to the cecum and terminal ileum is extremely variable. The retrocecal and retroileal positions are most common (65%), but a pelvic position may also be found (31%).

FIGURE 68.4
ENTRY INTO THE PERITONEUM

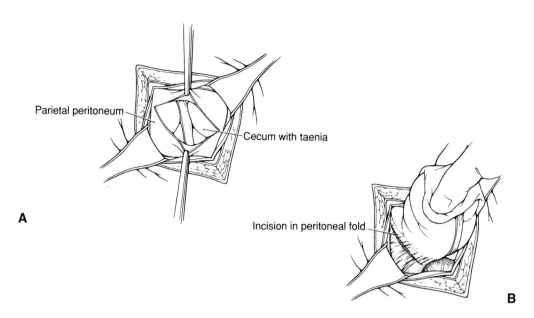

Developmentally, the appendix represents the original apex of the cecum. As a result of asymmetric growth of the cecum, the origin of the appendix is usually on the posteromedial side of the cecum. The appendix is usually intraperitoneal, even when it is retrocecal. Although a retroperitoneal location for the appendix has been reported, this is generally the result of inflammation.

Regardless of location, the appendix can reliably be located by following the taeniae downward along the cecum to their junction with each other. The base of the appendix is always located at this point.

Mobilizing the Appendix (Fig. 68.5)

Technical Points

Grasp the appendix with a Babcock clamp, taking great care not to cut through tissues that are inflamed and edematous. Do not pull on the appendix; if it is close to perforation, it

FIGURE 68.5
MOBILIZING THE APPENDIX

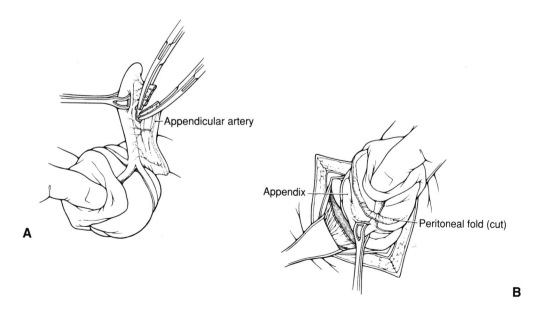

may come free in your hand, and the base will retract into the depths of the incision. Clamp and ligate the mesentery of the appendix, starting at the part that is visible and progressing more proximally. As the mesentery is divided, the appendix will become more mobile, and the tip will come up into the wound. Sometimes, the appendix is sufficiently mobile that the appendicular artery can be secured with a single clamp, without preliminary division of the mesoappendix. Always ligate the appendicular artery separately from the appendiceal stump. If the artery is included in the stump ligature or

inverted with the stump, troublesome postoperative bleeding may occur.

Anatomic Points

The mesoappendix transports the appendicular artery. This is a branch of the ileocolic artery, which arises from the superior mesenteric artery. The mesoappendix passes posterior to the terminal ileum and is of variable length. Commonly, it is so short that the appendix is significantly tethered behind

FIGURE 68.6
APPENDECTOMY

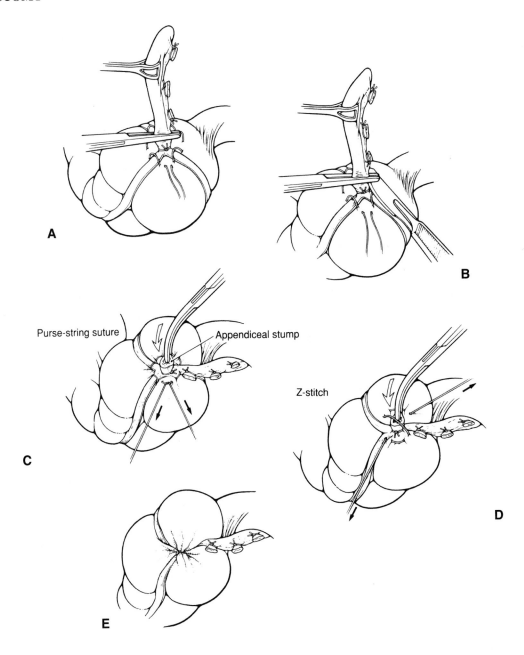

A

B

Purse-string suture   Appendiceal stump

C

Z-stitch

D

E

the cecum and ileum and may be folded upon itself. The appendicular artery frequently runs close to the base of the appendix and then passes away from the appendix to run in the free edge of the mesoappendix, sending out several small branches.

The mesoappendix forms the posterior wall of the inferior ileocecal fossa. A fold of fatty tissue (the inferior ileocecal fold, or bloodless fold of Treves) commonly runs from the antimesenteric border of the terminal ileum to the cecum. This can be cut safely.

Appendectomy (Fig. 68.6)

Technical Points

The most common cause of acute appendicitis is obstruction of the appendiceal lumen by a fecalith. In such cases, the appendix distal to the fecalith becomes inflamed and edematous; however, the portion proximal to the fecalith remains relatively normal. Thus, dissection of the appendix past the inflamed portion toward the cecum often yields a segment of appendix that may be ligated safely (Fig. 68.6A). Carefully dissect the appendix down to its origin from the cecum. Crush the appendix carefully with a clamp, then clamp it just distal to the crushed portion. Ligate the appendix through the previously crushed portion, clamp above the ligature, and cut through the base of the appendix (Fig. 68.6B).

If desired, invert the appendiceal stump by use of a purse-string suture or Z stitch (Fig. 68.6C,D). The inverting suture should be placed wide enough to allow the cecum to cover the stump completely when the suture is tied; however, it should not impinge on the ileocecal valve or appendicular artery. Because there is maximal mobility laterally, the suture may be placed wider laterally, allowing the cecum to roll medially over the stump of the appendix.

Anatomic Points

The ileocecal valve represents a protrusion of the mucosa, submucosa, and circular muscle layers of the terminal ileum into the cecal lumen. This valve may function both actively and passively. The base of the appendix is usually less than 2 cm from this valve.

Exploration in the Case of a Grossly Normal Appendix (Fig. 68.7)

Technical Points

If the appendix appears to be normal, direct your initial search toward adjacent organs. First, inspect the terminal ileum for signs of inflammatory bowel disease or enlarged mesenteric lymph nodes. Search for a Meckel's diverticulum by "running" the small bowel carefully for a distance of at least 5 feet from the ileocecal valve. Carefully palpate the right colon, sigmoid colon, and bladder, as well as the uterus and ovaries in female patients.

FIGURE 68.7
EXPLORATION IN THE CASE OF A GROSSLY NORMAL APPENDIX

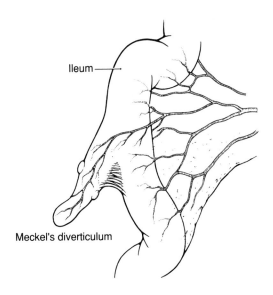

Ileum

Meckel's diverticulum

If you find an inflamed Meckel's diverticulum, excise the inflamed region by resecting a short segment of ileum and performing an end-to-end anastomosis (see Chapter 48).

Occasionally, a lesion in the upper abdomen, such as a perforated duodenal ulcer, will cause lower abdominal pain secondary to leakage of fluid down the right gutter. If pathology of the upper abdomen is suspected or confirmed, close the appendectomy incision and make a second (usually vertical midline) incision in the upper abdomen to gain adequate exposure.

Close the appendectomy incision in layers. Place drains only if a well-defined abscess cavity is encountered.

Anatomic Points

Meckel's diverticulum, the most common anomaly of the gastrointestinal tract, represents a persistent remnant of the vitelline duct (embryonic yolk stalk). Typically, this diverticulum is located on the antimesenteric border of the ileum, within 50 cm of the ileocecal valve. Occasionally, such diverticula have been found as far as 170 cm from the ileocecal valve. Thus, at least 200 cm of small bowel should be examined in order to avoid missing a Meckel's diverticulum. These diverticula also vary in length from 1 to 20 cm, although most (75%) are 1 to 5 cm long. Fibrous bands sometimes run from the diverticulum to the umbilicus, mesentery, omentum, or serosa of the gut. Rarely (2%), the lumen of the duct is retained from skin to bowel, resulting in a vitelline fistula. The mucosa of a Meckel's diverticulum is most commonly ileal; however, gastric, pancreatic, duodenal, colonic, and bile duct mucosa have been reported.

REFERENCES

1. Adams JT. Z-stitch suture for inversion of the appendiceal stump. *Surg Gynecol Obstet* 1968;127:1321.
2. Askew AR. The Fowler-Weir approach to appendicectomy. *Br J Surg* 1975;62:303.
3. Cullen JJ, Kelly KA, Hodge DO, et al. Surgical management of Meckel's diverticulum: an epidemiologic, population-based study. *Ann Surg* 1994;220:564–568. (Advocates removal of asymptomatic Meckel's diverticula found at laparotomy.)
4. Delany HM, Carnevale NJ. A "bikini" incision for appendectomy. *Am J Surg* 1976;132:126. (Presents alternative incision.)
5. Hale DA, Molloy M, Pearl RH, et al. Appendectomy: a contemporary appraisal. *Ann Surg* 1997;225:252–261.
6. Jelenko C, Davis LP. A transverse lower abdominal appendectomy incision with minimal muscle derangement. *Surg Gynecol Obstet* 1973; 136:451. (Presents alternative incision.)
7. Lewis FR, Holcroft JW, Bowy J, et al. Appendicitis: a critical review of diagnosis and treatment in 1,000 cases. *Arch Surg* 1975;110: 677.
8. Sandsmark M. Serious delayed rectal haemorrhage following uncomplicated appendicectomy. *Acta Chir Scand* 1977;143:385. (Discusses rare complication related to inversion of stump.)
9. Williamson WA, Bush RD. Williams LF. Retrocecal appendicitis. *Am J Surg* 1981;141:507.
10. Yalchouchy EK, Marano AF, Etienne JC, et al. Meckel's diverticulum. *J Am Coll Surg* 2001;192:658–662. (Reviews embryology and management.)

CHAPTER 69

Laparoscopic Appendectomy and Resection of Meckel's Diverticulum

This chapter describes both laparoscopic appendectomy (including mobilization of the right colon for retrocecal appendix) and resection of Meckel's diverticulum. Two methods of laparoscopic appendectomy—with and without the use of the endoscopic stapler—are presented.

Setup and Initial View (Fig. 69.1)

Technical Points

Position the patient supine with both arms tucked in. Set the room up with the primary monitor at the patient's right knee, and a secondary monitor, if desired, at the patient's left knee. Palpate the abdomen. A mass in the right lower quadrant generally implies complicated appendicitis; this can be managed laparoscopically if one is experienced.

Access the abdomen through a supraumbilical port. Inspect all four quadrants, looking for confirmation of the etiology. Aspirate and irrigate any purulent material, obtaining cultures if desired. If the appearance is consistent with appendicitis, place the operating table in Trendelenburg position with the right side elevated. The cecum should be visible in the right lower quadrant. Confirm cecum by taeniae and whiter color than adjacent loops of small intestine.

Place a working 10-mm port in the right upper quadrant at about the midclavicular line and pass an endoscopic Babcock clamp into the field. Gently retract the cecum toward the upper abdomen. The base of the appendix should roll into view. Note that the tip of the appendix is tethered by the mesoappendix, which passes behind the terminal ileum. Additional ports will be placed in the left lower quadrant or lower midline (12-mm), depending on the size of the patient, and optionally in the right lower quadrant for additional retraction in difficult cases (Fig. 69.1A).

LIST OF STRUCTURES

Cecum
Appendix
  Mesoappendix
  Appendicular artery
Terminal ileum
Meckel's diverticulum

Insert the 12-mm port next. If the patient is small, with a narrow abdomen, put this in the left lower quadrant, taking care to choose a site lateral to the rectus muscle to avoid the inferior epigastric vessels. If the patient is large, a lower midline site as shown will work well. As always, think in terms of working distance rather than fixed anatomic landmarks. Use an atraumatic grasper to manipulate cecum and appendix so that the appendix can be grasped by the Babcock clamp and elevated (Fig. 69.1B).

Anatomic Points

The outer muscular layer of the appendix is formed by longitudinal fibers, which are the continuation of the three taeniae of the colon. Thus, the appendix may be located by seeking the convergence of the taeniae. Location of the appendix varies, but it is always tethered to some extent by the mesoappendix, which passes behind the terminal ileum (Fig. 69.1C). In many individuals, the appendix is partially or completely retrocecal.

The laparoscopic approach (base before tip) is different from that commonly used during open appendectomy. The laparoscopic surgeon has the advantage of working from within the abdomen and approaches the appendix from a vantage point cephalad and to the right. Thus, as the cecum is pulled up, the base is the first part of the appendix to come into view. In all but the true retrocecal appendices (Fig. 69.4), the rest of the appendix generally then comes into view.

Appendectomy Using Endoscopic Stapling Device (Fig. 69.2)

Technical and Anatomic Points

Use a Maryland dissector to develop a window in the mesentery of the appendix at the base. Visualize the cecum funneling up toward the base to confirm that no residual appendiceal tissue will remain. The window needs to be about 1.5-cm wide. Enlarge it with an endoscopic right-angled forceps. Pass an endoscopic cutting linear stapler through the left lower quadrant port and staple across the base of the appendix (Fig. 69.2A). Remove the stapler. The appendix will now be hanging by the mesoappendix (Fig. 69.2B). Reload the stapler with a vascular cartridge and use it to divide the mesoappendix. A minimally inflamed appendix can be grasped at one

FIGURE 69.1
SETUP AND INITIAL VIEW (**B** from Scott-Conner CEH, Cuschieri A, Carter FJ. Small intestine and appendix. In: *Minimal access surgical anatomy.* Philadelphia: Lippincott Williams & Wilkins, 2000:165–184, with permission; **C** from Wind GG. The colon. In: *Applied laparoscopic anatomy: abdomen and pelvis.* Baltimore: Williams & Wilkins, 1997:217–246, with permission.)

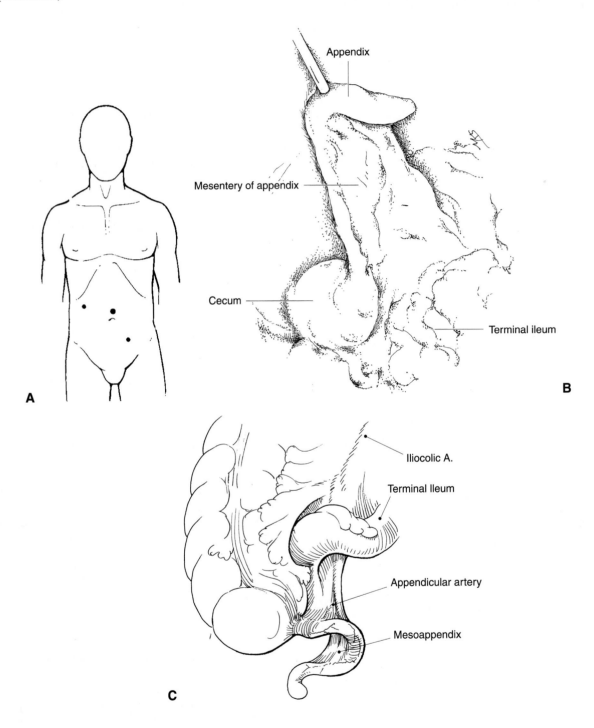

FIGURE 69.2
APPENDECTOMY USING ENDOSCOPIC STAPLING DEVICE (**A** from Apelgren KN. Laparoscopic appendectomy. In: Scott-Conner CEH, ed. *The SAGES manual: fundamentals of laparoscopy and GI endoscopy.* New York: Springer-Verlag, 1999:275–280, with permission; **B** from Scott-Conner CEH, Cuschieri A, Carter FJ. Small intestine and appendix. In: *Minimal access surgical anatomy.* Philadelphia: Lippincott Williams & Wilkins, 2000:165–184, with permission; **C** and **D** from Baker RJ, Fischer JE, eds. *Mastery of surgery.* 4th ed. Philadelphia: Lippincott Williams & Wilkins, 2001, with permission.)

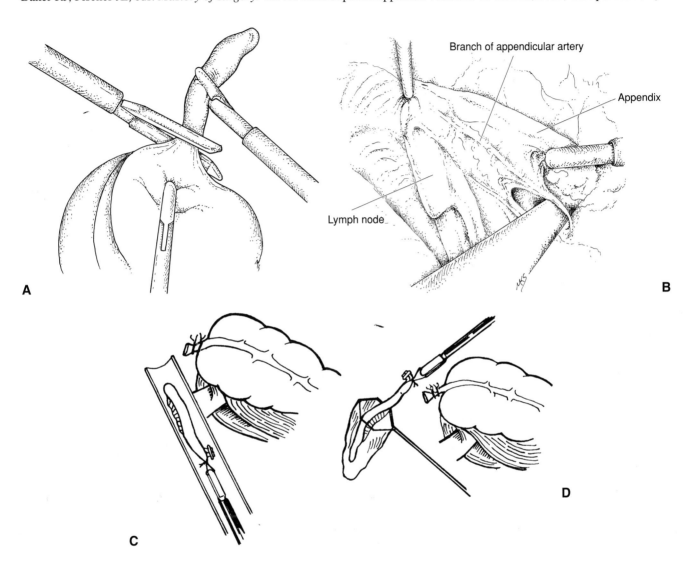

end (lengthwise) and withdrawn into the 12-mm trocar. Trocar and appendix can then be removed *en bloc* (Fig. 69.2C).

A purulent or perforated appendix is best placed in an endoscopic retrieval bag. To do this, pass the endoscopic retrieval bag through the 12-mm port and open it. Position the bag so that the opening faces the laparoscope. Maneuver the appendix into the bag and withdraw the grasper, shaking the grasper gently to encourage the appendix to drop off the grasper into the bag (Fig. 69.2D). Exercise caution during this maneuver because the appendix commonly adheres to the grasper and is pulled back out of the bag with the grasper. Once dropped into the pelvis among loops of bowel, the appendix may be difficult to impossible to find and recover. This is best prevented by caution during this phase of the

procedure. Visually confirm that the appendix is inside of the bag before closing and withdrawing the bag through the abdominal wall.

Irrigate the operative field. If desired, place a closed-suction drain in the pelvis or in an abscess cavity.

Appendectomy Using Endoloop (Fig. 69.3)

Technical and Anatomic Points

This method works best for a minimally inflamed appendix and a mesentery that is not too fatty. Elevate the appendix and inspect the mesentery. It will be necessary to divide the mesentery first. Either clips or an ultrasonic scalpel can be used to secure the mesentery. To use clips, first develop a

FIGURE 69.3

APPENDECTOMY USING ENDOLOOP (A and **B** from Scott-Conner CEH, et al. Laparoscopic appendectomy: initial experience in a teaching program. *Ann Surg* 1992;215:660–668, with permission.)

A   **B**

series of windows in the mesentery by dissecting with a Maryland dissector between the branches of the appendicular artery (Fig. 69.3A). Sequentially clip and divide these branches until the appendix is hanging by the base.

Pass an endoloop through the left lower quadrant port. Extend the loop into the field, taking care not to allow the endoloop to contact the bowel. The ligature is made of chromic catgut and will be limp (and difficult to manipulate) if it becomes wet. Shorten the loop slightly to facilitate manipu-

lation. Pass a grasper through the endoloop and grasp the appendix, pulling it through the loop (Fig. 69.3B). Manipulate the loop down to the base and slowly tighten the loop. Continue to adjust the position of the loop on the base of the appendix as the loop becomes smaller. Be aware that it will not be possible to open the loop and readjust it. Use the knot-pusher to position the loop at the exact base and cinch the loop down. Generally, two loops are placed on the base and a third is placed above (Fig. 69.3C). Cut between and remove

FIGURE 69.4

MANAGEMENT OF RETROCECAL APPENDIX (From Scott-Conner CEH, Cuschieri A, Carter FJ. Small intestine and appendix. In: *Minimal access surgical anatomy.* Philadelphia: Lippincott Williams & Wilkins, 2000:165–184, with permission.)

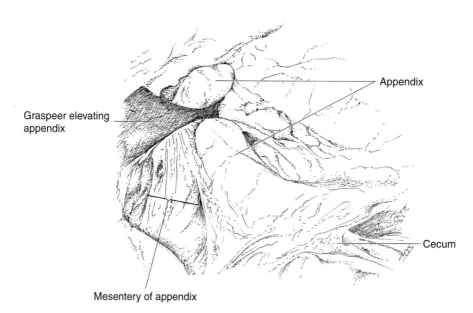

Appendix

Graspeer elevating appendix

Cecum

Mesentery of appendix

the appendix as previously described. Many surgeons place a clip over the knot of the endoloop for added security.

Management of Retrocecal Appendix (Fig. 69.4)

Technical Points

When the appendix is retrocecal, it is necessary to mobilize the cecum to gain exposure. Using scissors and electrocautery (or ultrasonic scalpel), incise the peritoneum lateral to the cecum and roll the cecum medially. The appendix will generally be adherent to the back wall of the cecum. Identify it by feel and grasp it with an endoscopic Babcock forceps as shown. Proceed with appendectomy as previously described.

Removal of Meckel's Diverticulum (Fig. 69.5)

Technical Points

Rarely, a normal appendix and an inflamed Meckel's diverticulum are found to coexist. Inspect the region of the Meckel's diverticulum and decide whether simple diverticulectomy or wedge excision of the segment of ileum containing the Meckel's diverticulum is required.

To perform simple diverticulectomy, first identify and control the blood vessel supplying the Meckel's diverticulum. This will generally be found in a fatty stripe that runs on the cephalad surface of the ileum (Fig. 69.5A). This stripe should be visible if the loop of ileum is held in the lower abdomen

FIGURE 69.5
REMOVAL OF MECKEL'S DIVERTICULUM (A from Scott-Conner CEH, Cuschieri A, Carter FJ. Small intestine and appendix. In: *Minimal access surgical anatomy.* Philadelphia: Lippincott Williams & Wilkins, 2000:165–184, with permission.)

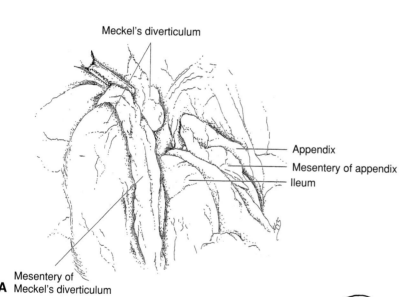

Meckel's diverticulum
Appendix
Mesentery of appendix
Ileum
A Mesentery of Meckel's diverticulum

B

(with the laparoscope looking down from above). Then pass an endoscopic stapler through the left lower quadrant port and staple across the base of the Meckel's diverticulum (Fig. 69.5B).

Proceed with appendectomy as previously described, if desired.

Anatomic Points

As discussed in detail in Chapter 68, a Meckel's diverticulum represents a remnant of the vitelline duct. The fatty stripe containing the blood supply may be a useful landmark when the diverticulum is difficult to identify.

REFERENCES

1. Apelgren KN. Laparoscopic appendectomy. In: Scott-Conner CEH, ed. *The SAGES manual: fundamentals of laparoscopy and GI endoscopy.* New York: Springer-Verlag, 1999:275–280.
2. Scott-Conner CEH, Cuschieri A, Carter FJ. Small intestine and appendix. In: *Minimal access surgical anatomy.* Philadelphia: Lippincott Williams & Wilkins, 2000:165–184.

CHAPTER 70

Colonoscopy

Colonoscopy is performed with the patient lying in the left lateral decubitus (Sims) position. Flexible sigmoidoscopy will not be discussed separately because it duplicates the initial maneuvers of colonoscopy. Concentrate on passing the scope safely and atraumatically. Inspect the region as the scope is withdrawn. Use as little air insufflation as possible to ensure patient comfort and to facilitate passage of the scope. This procedure is used to introduce the topography of the colon.

Rectosigmoid (Fig. 70.1)

Technical Points

Perform a digital rectal examination first to lubricate the anal canal and to confirm that no low obstructing lesions are present. If stool is encountered, consider rescheduling the examination after completion of a more adequate bowel prep.

Place the index finger of your dominant hand on the tip of the scope and press the tip, angled at about 45 degrees, against the anus. Instruct the patient to bear down. This will relax the sphincters and facilitate passage of the scope. Press the scope into the anal canal. Note that the rim of the scope is elevated, which makes insertion of the tip *en face* difficult, if not impossible.

The rectum curves posteriorly to hug the hollow of the sacrum. Insufflate enough air to identify its lumen. The valves of Houston may be visible.

At the pelvic brim, the relatively straight rectum blends imperceptibly with the mobile sigmoid. The length and mobility of this segment vary considerably from individual to individual and may be altered by prior surgery. Try to traverse the sigmoid using as little length of the scope and as little air insufflation as possible.

Anatomic Points

Flexible endoscopy has significantly decreased the incidence of perforation of the rectum. However, because perforations still occur, one should be aware of the anatomy and relationships of the rectum and anal canal. As the terminal rectum penetrates the pelvic diaphragm, it makes an approximate right-angled bend. From the standpoint of the endoscopist inserting an instrument into the anus, this bend occurs about 4 cm proximal to the anal verge (here defined as the transition zone where the dry, hirsute, perianal skin changes to the moist, squamous epithelium lining the anal canal). This necessitates directing the tip of the instrument toward the concavity of the sacrum. Immediately anterior to this point of angulation are the median prostate gland and paramedian seminal vesicle in male patients, and the vagina in female patients. In male patients, more proximally, the anterior rectal wall is in contact with the urinary bladder. Still further from the anal verge (about 7.5 cm in males and 5.5 cm in females), the peritoneum is reflected from the anterior surface of the rectum to the posterior surface of the urinary bladder (in males) or the uterus (in females), forming the rectovesical or rectouterine pouch (cul-de-sac of Douglas), respectively. This is the most dependent recess of the peritoneal cavity; thus, it can fill with peritoneal fluid, pus, or loops of bowel.

The terminal large bowel is divided into a proximal rectum and terminal anal canal. From the anal verge, the anal canal extends to the pectinate line, a distance of about 1.5 cm. At this line, the stratified squamous epithelium changes to columnar cells characteristic of large bowel mucosa. Approximately at this line, a number of changes occur: the arterial supply changes from the more caudal inferior rectal arteries to the more proximal middle and superior rectal (hemorrhoidal) arteries, the venous return changes from tributaries of the caval system to tributaries of the portal system, the lymphatic drainage pattern changes from drainage to the inguinal nodes to drainage to the internal iliac or inferior mesenteric nodes, and the nerve supply changes from somatic innervation by the pudendal nerves to autonomic innervation (sympathetic and parasympathetic) from hypogastric plexuses.

The rectum extends from the pectinate line to the level of the third sacral vertebra, a distance of about 12 to 15 cm.

LIST OF STRUCTURES

Rectum
  Transverse rectal folds (valves of Houston)
Sigmoid colon
Descending (left) colon
Splenic flexure
Transverse colon
Hepatic flexure
Ascending (right) colon
Cecum
Ileocecal valve

ORIENTATION

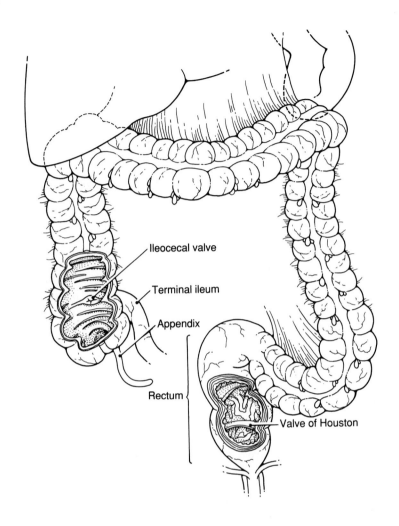

Ileocecal valve

Terminal ileum

Appendix

Rectum

Valve of Houston

FIGURE 70.1
RECTOSIGMOID

A

B

FIGURE 70.2
DESCENDING COLON

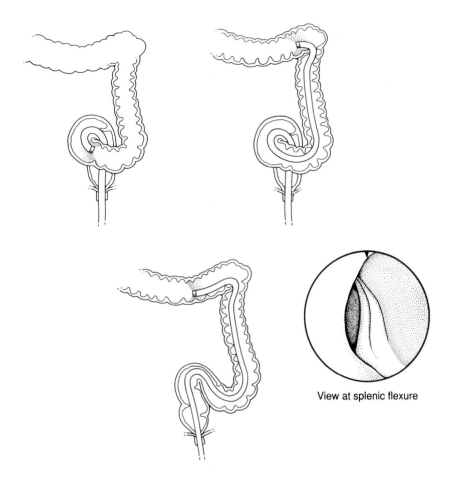

View at splenic flexure

The lowest part of the rectum, which is entirely below the peritoneal reflection, is significantly wider than the anal canal and is capable of great dilation; this is the rectal ampulla. It is the terminal ampulla that makes the approximate right-angled bend, termed the *perineal flexure.* The only features of note in the normal rectum are the transverse rectal folds (valves of Houston). Typically, there are three folds: the most distal one (4 to 7 cm from the anal verge) on the left, an intermediate one (8 to 10 cm from the anal verge) on the right, and the most proximal one (10 to 12 cm from the anal verge), again on the left. The number of transverse folds, however, can vary from one to five, and their placement may be reversed. Finally, it should be noted that the rectum lacks the characteristic haustra of the colon. This is a result of the dispersal of the musculature of the three taeniae coli to form a circumferential longitudinal muscle layer of uniform thickness.

Endoscopically, the sigmoid colon can be distinguished by well-marked semilunar folds. In addition, the mucosa in this region is velvety in appearance. Although the length and disposition of the sigmoid colon are variable, the fact that it is suspended on a mesentery enables it to be somewhat straightened by the passage of the endoscope. The first part

entered—the terminal sigmoid—typically lies to the right of the midline.

Descending Colon (Fig. 70.2)

Technical Points

Identify the left (descending) colon by its relative straightness compared with the tortuous sigmoid. Advancing the scope through this channel is relatively easy. If the scope does not advance easily, there is probably an excessively large loop in the sigmoid colon. Reduce this loop by simultaneously withdrawing the scope while having an assistant push gently on the left lower quadrant.

At the splenic flexure, a bluish shadow (the spleen) may be visible through the bowel wall. Often, the only clue is that the lumen of the bowel disappears. To traverse the splenic flexure, hook the tip of the scope around the flexure and then straighten the scope as it is advanced.

Anatomic Points

The retroperitoneal left colon is marked by circular folds that are located at more regular intervals than are the semicircular

FIGURE 70.3
TRANSVERSE COLON

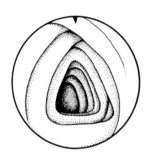

folds of the sigmoid colon. The mucosa here is smooth, somewhat shiny, and gray-pink in color.

Transverse Colon (Fig. 70.3)

Technical Points

The transverse colon usually has a characteristically triangular lumen. It is variable in both length and mobility. Imagine the bowel being "reefed up" and shortened over the scope as it is passed.

The hepatic flexure is generally not as angulated as the splenic flexure, but it may be more difficult to pass by. Often, so much scope has been inserted that a loop can form either in the sigmoid or in the transverse colon. Pull back on the scope and suction out some air to collapse the bowel partially. This may allow the tip to advance into the ascending (or right) colon. The bluish shadow of the liver may be visible through the bowel wall.

Anatomic Points

The approach to the splenic flexure, the proximal end of the left colon, is recognized endoscopically by the dome-like appearance of the lumen. This is the result of the sharp angulation of this flexure. The endoscope must be directed to the right and inferiorly for passage into the transverse colon.

FIGURE 70.4
RIGHT COLON AND CECUM

Ileocecal valve

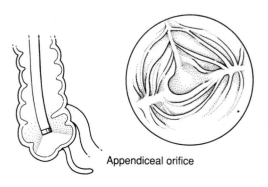

Appendiceal orifice

FIGURE 70.5
COMPLETION OF THE EXAMINATION

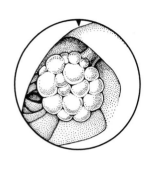

Although quite variable in length, the transverse colon is suspended by a mesentery (transverse mesocolon), which allows it to be manipulated endoscopically. The transverse colon is characterized by its triangular lumen, which is reflected in both haustra and mucosal folds.

The hepatic flexure is not as acute as the splenic flexure, and the mucosal folds here have been described as pagoda shaped. The lumen and folds at this flexure are triangular, and the extremities of the folds overlap somewhat, rather than being continuous like those of the rest of the transverse colon.

Right Colon and Cecum (Fig. 70.4)

Technical Points

Continue to advance the scope by a series of withdrawal and advance maneuvers until the ileocecal valve and convergence of the taeniae at the cecum are visible. You must be certain that you have visualized the cecum. Many endoscopists use fluoroscopy to confirm the location of the scope within the cecal air shadow, injecting Hypaque into the bowel through the scope if necessary. If fluoroscopy is not available, confirm that the cecum has been reached on the basis of (a) endoscopic appearance, (b) the appearance of a light in the right lower quadrant, and (c) a visible indentation of the bowel wall when the right lower quadrant is palpated.

Cannulation of the terminal ileum can be achieved in many patients by angling the tip of the scope and pulling back, engaging the tip within the ileocecal valve. Several centimeters of terminal ileum can often be examined in this way.

Anatomic Points

On endoscopic examination, the retroperitoneal right (ascending) colon will be seen to have semicircular mucosal folds. Generally, it is larger in diameter than the left colon.

The cecum is greater in diameter than the rest of the colon, and its wall seems to be thinner. Because of these anatomic characteristics and LaPlace's law, overinsufflation of the colon can cause the cecum to rupture more easily than other regions of the colon. The orifice of the appendix is not at the most dependent part of the cecum. Instead, it is usually on the posteromedial side of the cecum, as is the ileocecal valve. Of the two, the appendix is more caudal. It is always circular and is usually concealed by a mucosal fold.

The shape of the ileocecal valve is variable. It can present as a circular or oval protrusion into the lumen of the cecum, or it may be bilabial. In the latter case, the orientation of the lips is similar to that of the semilunar folds of the right colon. Typically, the valve is 2 to 3 cm in diameter and about 10 cm superior to the blind end of the cecum.

Completion of the Examination (Fig. 70.5)

Technical and Anatomic Points

As the colonoscope is withdrawn, carefully and systematically examine the bowel. Advance the scope to reexamine areas that are missed if the tip of the scope "jumps back" too fast for adequate inspection of the mucosa.

Note the position of any abnormalities by referring to fixed landmarks whenever possible. Distances vary from examination to examination; it is much more meaningful to state that a lesion is "just proximal to the splenic flexure" than to characterize it as being "at 100 cm."

REFERENCES

1. Catalano MF. Normal structures on endoscopic ultrasonography: visualization measurement data and interobserver variation. *Gastrointest Endosc Clin North Am* 1995;5:475–486.
2. Church JM. *Endoscopy of the colon, rectum, and anus.* New York: Igaku-Shoin, 1995.
3. Sugarbaker PH, Vineyard GC, Peterson LM. Anatomic localization and step by step advancement of the fiberoptic colonoscope. *Surg Gynecol Obstet* 1976;143:457.

CHAPTER 71

Loop Colostomy and Colostomy Closure

A loop colostomy is the easiest colostomy to make and to take down. It is used in situations in which temporary (often emergency) decompression or diversion of colonic contents is required. In this chapter, the construction and closure of a right transverse colostomy is illustrated. Loop ileostomy, an alternative technique of fecal diversion, is described in the references at the end. The equivalent laparoscopic procedure is shown in Chapter 72.

Isolation of Loop (Fig. 71.1)

Technical Points

Make a short (about 10 cm in length) transverse incision in the right upper quadrant. Do not make the incision too far laterally. The transverse colon becomes deeper and higher in the vicinity of the hepatic flexure (lateral) and more mobile in the midsection (medial).

Identify the colon by its overlying greater omentum. Mobilize a greatly distended and dilated colon with caution to avoid spillage of enteric contents. If the incision is not large enough to deliver the loop comfortably, enlarge the incision. Observe the character of the peritoneal fluid. If it is turbid or purulent, a colonic perforation may have occurred. In this case, proceed with a full laparotomy.

Divide the omentum to expose the colon by serially clamping and tying it. Develop a mesenteric window under the colon by passing a clamp or finger through an avascular portion of the mesocolon. Pass a Penrose drain under the colon and use it to elevate the colon.

Anatomic Points

The incision is typically made about halfway between the umbilicus and costal margin, 3 to 5 cm lateral to the linea

LIST OF STRUCTURES

Greater omentum
Transverse colon
   Hepatic flexure
Middle colic artery
Marginal artery (of Drummond)
Rectus abdominis muscle
   Anterior rectus sheath
Superior epigastric artery

alba. At this site, all or part of the incision will cross the rectus abdominis muscle. First, cut the anterior rectus sheath, exposing the rectus fibers. Then divide the rectus fibers with electrocautery. Bleeding difficulties may result if the superior epigastric artery is not identified and controlled. This artery (and its venae comitantes) is immediately posterior to the rectus abdominis muscle, about midway between its medial and lateral borders. It usually enters the muscle, anastomosing with the inferior epigastric artery, about halfway between the umbilicus and the xiphoid cartilage.

Once the peritoneum is opened, the colon must be identified with certainty. As the anterior layer of the greater omentum forms the gastrocolic ligament, omentum overlies the colon and thus must be divided to visualize the colon clearly. Use clamps and ties to divide the omentum. Look for the distinguishing haustra, epiploic appendages, and taeniae coli to identify colon positively.

Division of the transverse mesocolon, which is necessary to encircle the colon, cannot be done blindly. Look for an avascular region and avoid trauma to the middle colic artery or the marginal artery (of Drummond). The middle colic artery arises from the superior mesenteric artery to supply the transverse colon. It should not be at risk for injury if the mesocolon is divided close to the bowel. The marginal artery, an anastomotic channel ultimately connecting the colonic branches of the inferior and superior mesenteric arteries and from which the vasa recti originate to supply the colon directly, lies at a variable distance from the wall of the colon. Its distance from the colon has been reported to range from less than 1 cm to 8 cm.

Anchoring and Maturing the Colostomy (Fig. 71.2)

Technical Points

Tack the colostomy to the fascia with multiple interrupted sutures. Pass a colostomy bridge under the loop. Close the skin, if necessary, until the loop comes out through a hole of appropriate size. If the bowel is greatly distended, place a pursestring suture through the region to be opened. Open the bowel and pass a pool-tipped suction tube into the bowel to decompress it. Then, open the bowel more widely by incising along a taenia. Mature the colostomy by suturing full thickness of the bowel to the dermis of the skin with multiple interrupted fine absorbable sutures.

If desired, a linear stapling device may be used to close the distal bowel, thereby ensuring total diversion of colonic

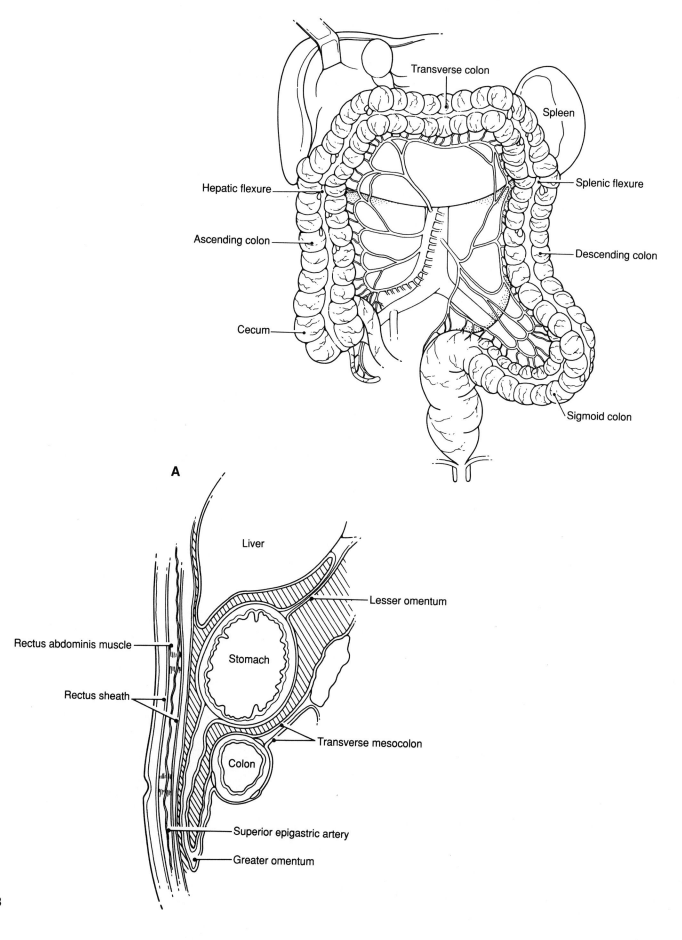

FIGURE 71.1
ISOLATION OF LOOP

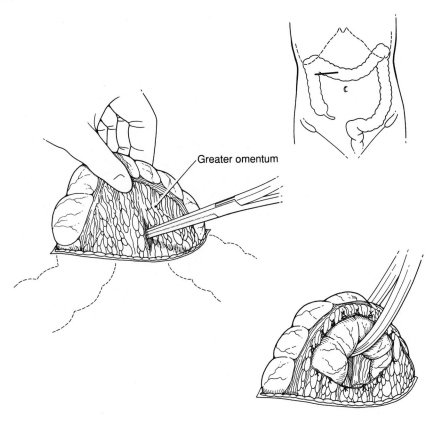

Greater omentum

FIGURE 71.2
ANCHORING AND MATURING THE COLOSTOMY

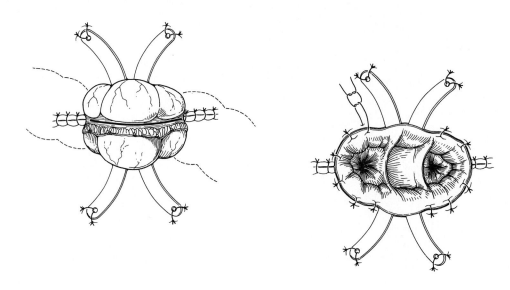

contents. However, keep in mind that this may recanalize in time, allowing bowel contents to flow distally again. It will also require resection of this segment for closure.

Anatomic Points

The parietal layers to which the colon is sutured, at this level, include the parietal peritoneum, fascia transversalis, rectus abdominis muscle, and both anterior and posterior rectus sheaths. If the lateral end of the incision is lateral to the rectus abdominis muscle, then the layers included are the parietal peritoneum, fascia transversalis, and transversus abdominis muscle and the aponeuroses of the internal oblique and external oblique muscles.

The taenia selected will generally be the so-called omental taenia, from which the greater omentum arises. The accumulation of longitudinal muscle fibers at the taeniae coli provides additional bowel wall thickness to be included in the coloparietal suture and includes layers at right angles to each other.

Closure of A Loop Colostomy (Fig. 71.3)

Technical Points

Incise the mucocutaneous border around the colostomy. Place

Allis clamps on the cut edge of the bowel and dissect in the plane between bowel and subcutaneous tissues. Identify and cut any sutures tacking the bowel to fascia. When the loop of bowel is completely free of the abdominal wall, pull sufficient bowel up to ensure that an anastomosis can be made without tension.

Under favorable conditions, the colostomy can be closed by simple suture of the open anterior wall (plastic closure) in a transverse fashion. Check the pliability and mobility of the cut ends of the bowel and carefully clean it. Place a running Connell suture of 3-0 Vicryl to invert the open bowel and then an outer layer of interrupted 3-0 silk Lembert sutures. Check the anastomosis for patency and cover with omentum if available.

Close the fascia in the usual manner. Loosely close the skin or pack it open. Tight closure of skin and subcutaneous tissue in a former ostomy site is generally ill advised.

Anatomic Points

Here, as is true almost everywhere else in the gastrointestinal tract, inverted closures can result in significant luminal narrowing. For this reason, inverted closures of longitudinal incisions are often done in a transverse fashion.

FIGURE 71.3
CLOSURE OF A LOOP COLOSTOMY

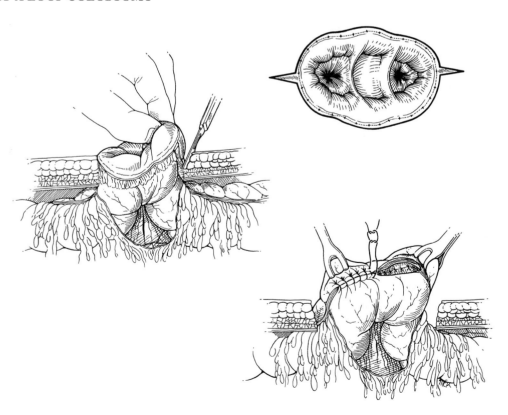

REFERENCES

1. Abcarian H, Pearl RK. Stomas. *Surg Clin North Am* 1988;68:1295.
2. Barker WF, Benfield JR, deKernion JB, et al. The creation and care of enterocutaneous stomas. *Curr Probl Surg* 1975;12:1. (Provides comprehensive review.)
3. Corman ML, Veidenheimer MC, Coller JA. Loop ileostomy as an alternative to end stoma. *Surg Gynecol Obstet* 1979;149:585. (Provides good description of technique.)
4. Doberneck RC. Revision and closure of the colostomy. *Surg Clin North Am* 1991;71:193. (Provides good review of complications and pitfalls.)
5. Dozois RR, ed. *Alternative to conventional ileostomy.* Chicago: Year Book Medical Publishers, 1985.
6. Eng K, Localio A. Simplified complementary transverse colostomy for low colorectal anastomosis. *Surg Gynecol Obstet* 1981;153:735. (Describes simple technique that is easily constructed and closed.)
7. Hines JR, Harris GD. Colostomy and colostomy closure. *Surg Clin North Am* 1977;57:1379.
8. Keighley MRB. Ileostomy; Colostomy. In: Keighley MRB, Williams NS. *Surgery of the anus, rectum and colon.* London: WB Saunders, 1993:139–244.
9. Kretschmer KP. *The intestinal stoma: indications, operative methods, care, rehabilitation.* Philadelphia: WB Saunders, 1978. (Provides good source of information about stomas and their care.)
10. Madira JA, Fiore AC. Reanastomosis of a Hartmann rectal pouch: a simplified procedure. *Am J Surg* 1983;145:279. (Describes use of a circular stapler to close a colostomy with Hartmann's pouch.)
11. Prasad ML, Pearl RK, Orsay CP, et al. End-loop ileocolostomy for massive trauma to the right side of the colon. *Arch Surg* 1984;119:975. (This technique, which can be adapted for divided colostomies, allows easy closure by a local plastic procedure.)
12. Turnbull RB, Weakley FL. *Atlas of intestinal stomas.* St. Louis: CV Mosby, 1967. (This is the classic reference.)
13. Wolff LH, Wolff WA, Wolff LH Jr. A re-evaluation of tube cecostomy. *Surg Gynecol Obstet* 1980;151:257.

CHAPTER 72

Laparoscopic Colostomy

Amanda M. Metcalf

A laparoscopic approach for a transverse loop colostomy can be helpful in the elective situation when construction of a diverting colostomy is the aim of the procedure and when the bowel is not extremely distended.

Laparoscopic Identification and Delivery of Bowel (Fig. 72.1)

Technical and Anatomic Points

Use an umbilical port site to insufflate the abdomen to 12 mm Hg and insert a 10-mm cannula. Inspect the peritoneal

---

FIGURE 72.1
LAPAROSCOPIC IDENTIFICATION AND DELIVERY OF BOWEL (From Bogen GL, Mancino AT, Scott-Conner CEH. Laparoscopy for staging and palliation of gastrointestinal malignancy. *Surg Clin North Am* 1996;76:557–569, with permission.)

LIST OF STRUCTURES

Colon
    Transverse colon

---

cavity with a straight viewing laparoscope. Ensure that the proposed stoma site is free of adhesions and that it lies over a mobile loop of colon.

The advantage of a laparoscopic approach to a transverse colon loop colostomy is that one can directly visualize the portion of the transverse colon to be used. If patients have had previous surgery, with adhesions between the omentum and lower abdominal wall that limit colon mobility, another section of the colon can be used. Alternatively, an additional port site in the lower abdomen can be placed and adhesions lysed, to allow improved colonic mobility.

Place an additional 10- to 12-mm trocar through the proposed stoma site. Pass an atraumatic bowel clamp through this port site and grasp and elevate the most appropriate portion of transverse colon. Withdraw the grasper into the trocar to raise the loop of colon toward the anterior abdominal wall. If the colon can reach the anterior abdominal wall with pneumoperitoneum, the length should be adequate to construct a colostomy.

Release the pneumoperitoneum and excise an elliptical portion of skin. Advance the trocar over the Babcock to allow dissection through the subcutaneous tissues. Enlarge the fascial incision over a right-angled clamp for a length of 3 to 4 cm, retract the rectus muscle, and incise the posterior fascia. Draw the bowel through the fascial defect. Mature the colostomy as described in Chapter 71.

REFERENCES

1. Beagley MJ, Poole G, Peat BG, et al. The use of temporary loop ileostomy in lumbosacral burns. *Burns* 2000;26:298–301.
2. Bogen GL, Mancino AT, Scott-Conner CEH. Laparoscopy for staging and palliation of gastrointestinal malignancy. *Surg Clin North Am* 1996;76:557–569.

CHAPTER 73

Right and Left Colon Resections

Resections of the colon are planned according to arterial supply and venous and lymphatic drainage. For lesions of the cecum or ascending colon up to and including the hepatic flexure, the standard resection is a right hemicolectomy. This includes resection of the terminal ileum, ascending colon, and right transverse colon. An end-to-end anastomosis is then performed between the ileum and transverse colon.

Left hemicolectomy is performed for lesions in the sigmoid or descending colon. The colon is resected from the middle of the transverse colon to the peritoneal reflection. This wide field of resection is needed when the inferior mesenteric vein and artery are ligated at their origin in order to resect lymph nodes along the inferior mesenteric artery. An end-to-end anastomosis is then performed between the middle of the transverse colon and the rectosigmoid.

Lesions involving the transverse colon can be managed by transverse colon resection, whereby the transverse colon, including both flexures, is removed and the ends are reanastomosed. In this chapter, right and left hemicolectomy is discussed, and transverse colon resection is mentioned briefly. In each case, the arterial and venous drainage of the segment determines the extent of resection.

More limited resections are occasionally performed for localized perforations or trauma. These are done in much the same manner but require a less extensive dissection. Chapter 74 describes laparoscopic colon resection. References at the end give additional information on specialized procedures.

Right Hemicolectomy

Incision and Exploration of the Abdomen (Fig. 73.1)

Technical Points

The hepatic flexure of the colon is quite close to the cecum, so that a right colon resection can conveniently be performed through a right transverse incision. Consider using this incision in patients who have not had previous subcostal or right lower quadrant incisions (that might compromise the vascularity of the transected rectus muscle). This incision is particularly good for obese patients. Alternatively, a midline or right paramedian incision may be chosen.

Outline a right transverse incision by palpating two landmarks: the costal margin at the anterior axillary line and the anterosuperior iliac spine. Divide the distance between these two points in half and mark it with a pen. Draw a straight transverse line from this point to a point just beyond the midline. Generally, this line will pass above the umbilicus, although occasionally, it will pass below. If it passes straight through the umbilicus, redraw it slightly above. Make the incision through skin and subcutaneous tissue and achieve hemostasis. Divide the muscular and fascial layers of the abdominal wall with electrocautery in a straight line with the skin incision. Enter the abdomen and explore it thoroughly.

A complete and thorough exploration of the abdomen is a necessary preamble to all abdominal surgery cases. In the case of colon cancer, special attention should be paid to possible sites of metastases: the liver, the lymph nodes draining

LIST OF STRUCTURES

Ascending (right) colon
  Cecum
  Ileocecal valve
  Hepatic flexure
Transverse colon
Descending (left) colon
  Splenic flexure
  Sigmoid colon
Rectum
White line of Toldt
Celiac artery

Superior mesenteric artery
  Middle colic artery
  Jejunal arteries
  Right colic artery
  Ileocolic artery
Inferior mesenteric artery
  Left colic artery
  Sigmoid arteries
  Superior rectal (hemorrhoidal) artery
Middle rectal (hemorrhoidal) arteries

Marginal artery (of Drummond)
Ileum
Duodenum
Spleen
Gastrocolic omentum
Ureter
Gonadal vessels
Iliac vessels
Genitofemoral nerve

ORIENTATION

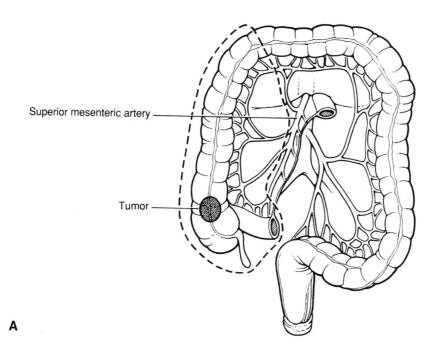

Superior mesenteric artery

Tumor

A

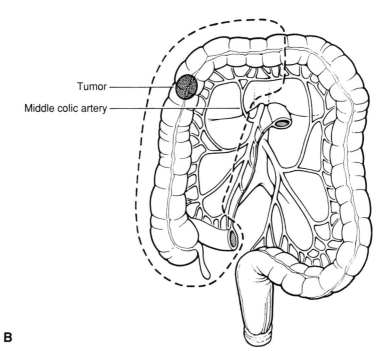

Tumor

Middle colic artery

B

C

D

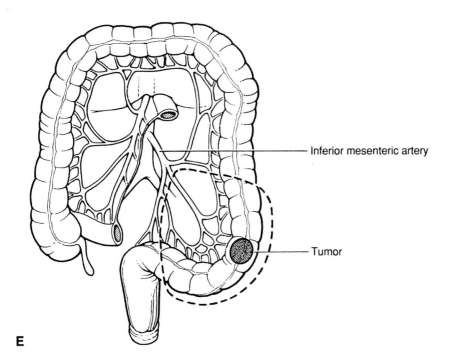

Inferior mesenteric artery

Tumor

E

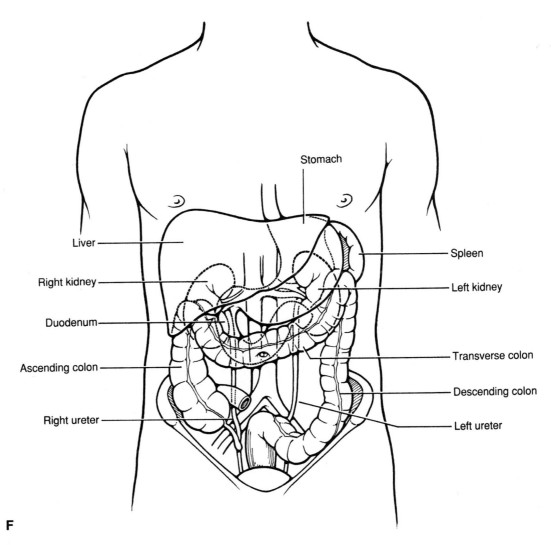

Stomach

Liver

Spleen

Right kidney

Left kidney

Duodenum

Ascending colon

Transverse colon

Descending colon

Right ureter

Left ureter

F

FIGURE 73.1
INCISION AND EXPLORATION OF THE ABDOMEN

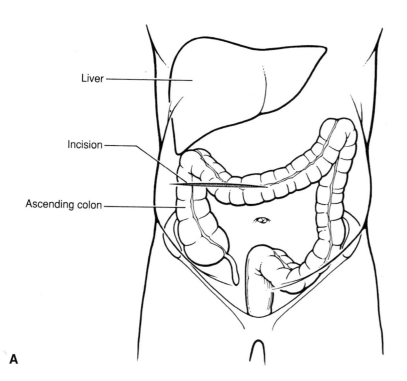

Liver

Incision

Ascending colon

A

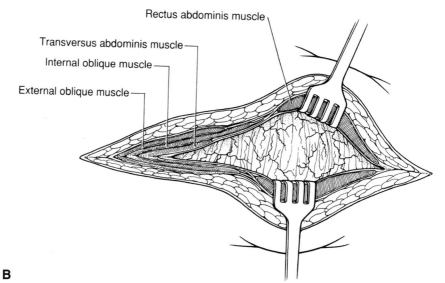

Rectus abdominis muscle

Transversus abdominis muscle

Internal oblique muscle

External oblique muscle

B

the segment of colon to be resected, the pelvis, the ovaries (in women), and the peritoneal surfaces. Tumor extending beyond the field of resection does not preclude colectomy, but any such metastatic disease should be documented carefully by biopsy. Palpate the entire colon. Second primary lesions are common and may be missed on preoperative screening studies.

Anatomic Points

Transverse incisions were briefly discussed in Chapter 36. The transverse incision recommended here should not divide

more than one segmental nerve and, thus, should not result in anesthesia, paresthesia, or paralysis of any part of the anterior abdominal wall, including the rectus abdominis muscle. This incision approximates the direction of the muscle fiber bundles laterally but is more or less transverse to the direction of rectus abdominis muscle fibers. Often, one of the tendinous inscriptions (usually the lowest) occurs at the level of the umbilicus. The incision should pass either above or below the umbilicus, thereby avoiding cutting through this tendinous inscription because segmental vessels are invariably encountered in the inscriptions and may cause bleeding. If the incision is extended across the midline above the umbilicus,

FIGURE 73.2
MOBILIZATION OF THE COLON

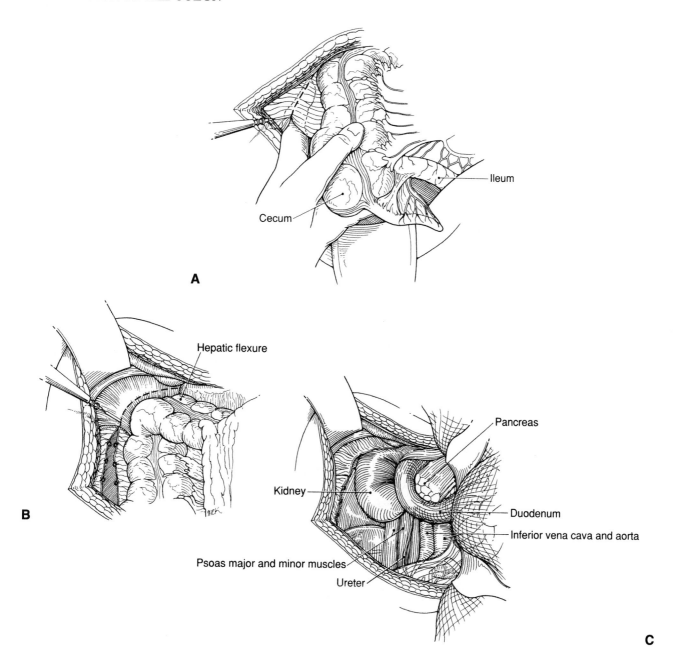

the falciform ligament and ligamentum teres hepatis must be divided. This should be done between clamps, and ligatures should be placed both proximally and distally owing to the paraumbilical veins that accompany the round ligament. These veins can be quite large if the portal system is obstructed and portal blood is shunted to the caval system.

Mobilization of the Colon (Fig. 73.2)

Technical Points

Place a self-retaining retractor, such as a Balfour, in the incision. Elevate the cecum and pull it medially. Incise the peri-

toneum lateral to the cecum and pass your nondominant hand behind the colon. Pass the index finger of your nondominant hand laterally to display the peritoneal reflection, thinning it out along the edge of the right colon. Incise it, using scissors or electrocautery, from the cecum to the hepatic flexure. In the region of the hepatic flexure, the peritoneal attachments will become increasingly thick and vascularized. Generally, these can be divided with electrocautery, although some of these vascular adhesions may require clamping and tying or clipping.

Sharply divide the filmy adhesions between the colon and retroperitoneum. Elevate the right colon up into the wound from the cecum to the hepatic flexure. As the colon is reflected medially and upward, the terminal ileum will come up as well. Identify the right ureter where it crosses the common iliac vessels just distal to their bifurcation. The colon will come up with minimal dissection in the avascular retroperitoneal plane. As you proceed up toward the hepatic flexure, search for and identify the duodenum, which is adherent to the transverse mesocolon and frequently will be tented up by traction on the colon. Mobilize the colon off the duodenum with care, sharply incising filmy adhesions and pushing the duodenum down and back into the retroperitoneum. Then place laparotomy pads in the bed of the colon and turn your attention to the region of the hepatic flexure.

At the hepatic flexure, one must begin taking the greater omentum with the specimen. The greater omentum connects the greater curvature of the stomach and the transverse colon.

Identify the area of the middle transverse colon that is planned for anastomosis. Preserve the middle colic artery to ensure a good blood supply to the anastomosis. Elevate the transverse colon and palpate the middle colic artery in the mesocolon. Select an area just to the right of the middle colic artery. Divide the omentum from this point up to the greater curvature of the stomach using clamps and ties. Take the greater omentum off the greater curvature of the stomach from this point distally toward the pylorus using clamps and ties. It should then be possible to elevate the entire colon, including the hepatic flexure and middle transverse colon (which will be tethered only by its mesentery).

Anatomic Points

Remember that, initially, all of the colon was intraperitoneal and that its blood supply developed during this intraperitoneal state. The ascending (right) and descending (left) colon are retroperitoneal because of fusion of apposing visceral and parietal serosal surfaces. The mesentery of the colon, with vessels derived from the superior and inferior mesenteric arteries, is retroperitoneal but lies anterior to other important retroperitoneal structures, such as the kidneys and ureters. By careful blunt dissection in the fusion plane, the retroperitoneal segments of the colon and their blood supply can be mobilized toward the midline with minimal blood loss.

Although significant variation in detail exists, there is a basic pattern of blood supply. The entire right colon, from the appendix to the junction of the middle and distal thirds of the transverse colon, is supplied by branches of the superior mesenteric artery. The superior mesenteric artery, arising just distal (1.5 cm) to the celiac trunk posterior to the pancreas, passes anterior to the third part of the duodenum to enter the root of the mesentery of the small bowel. Before it emerges from behind the pancreas, or just as it emerges, it gives rise to the middle colic artery, which usually passes into the transverse mesocolon at the inferior border of the pancreatic neck and then curves to the right. About 5 to 7 cm from the colon, the middle colic artery divides into right and left branches that parallel the transverse colon. These branches

anastomose with branches of other arteries, ultimately forming the marginal artery (of Drummond).

In the root of the small bowel mesentery, the superior mesenteric artery is accompanied on its right by the superior mesenteric vein. Typically, the jejunal and ileal branches arise from the left side of the superior mesenteric artery and run in the mesentery to the small bowel, which has been displaced to the right. The right colic and ileocolic arteries arise from the right side of the superior mesenteric artery and run along the posterior abdominal wall, initially posterior to the superior mesenteric vein, to the right colon. The right colic and ileocolic arteries usually divide into two main branches—an ascending and a descending branch—that approximately parallel the colon. These branches ultimately anastomose with other arteries to complete the right portion of the marginal artery of Drummond. (The descending branch of the ileocolic artery anastomoses with the termination of the superior mesenteric artery, whereas the ascending branch of the right colic artery anastomoses with the right branch of the middle colic artery.) It should be noted that it is the descending branch of the ileocolic artery that supplies the cecum, appendix, and terminal ileum. Right colon resections typically include the last few inches of the ileum in order to ensure an adequate blood supply to the area of anastomosis.

The marginal artery is located 1 to 8 cm from the bowel wall. Regardless of its formation, it gives rise to vasa recti that supply the colon. These arteries rarely anastomose because they run to the wall of the large bowel, alternately supplying the anterior or posterior side of the bowel, and enter the bowel wall in close proximity to taeniae coli. Although the vasa recti ultimately form a rich submucosal plexus, there is only limited longitudinal blood flow. Inadvertent destruction of the vasa recti that supply the anastomosis site can result in ischemia and anastomotic leak.

With few exceptions, the venous return essentially parallels the arterial supply. The major exception is the inferior mesenteric vein. Although the inferior mesenteric artery arises close to the bifurcation of the abdominal aorta, approximately at vertebral level T-4, the inferior mesenteric vein ascends to the left of the aorta and empties into the splenic vein or superior mesenteric vein posterior to the pancreas.

Lymphatics also parallel the arteries. Epicolic nodes, located on the wall of the colon, receive afferents from the colon. Efferents from these drain into paracolic nodes, which are typically found between the marginal artery and the bowel. Efferents from these parallel the branches of the superior mesenteric artery and inferior mesenteric artery and are periodically interrupted by intermediate nodes, named according to the artery with which they are associated. Lymph vessels from the intermediate nodes ultimately drain into nodes located at the origin of the superior mesenteric artery and inferior mesenteric artery. From these principal nodes, which again are named according to the artery with which they are associated, efferents ascend to the celiac nodes or to periaortic nodes on either side of the aorta. These ultimately drain into the cisterna chyli, typically lying just to the right of the aorta and slightly inferior to the celiac artery origin.

Resection of the terminal ileum, the cecum with its attached appendix, the ascending colon, and the proximal part of the transverse colon can be done with minimal bleeding if care is taken to enter the fusion plane immediately deep to the colon and its vasculature. Access to this plane is gained by way of a relatively avascular zone of peritoneum, called *the white line of Toldt,* which is visible when medial tension is placed on the ascending colon. As the fusion plane is entered and the colon is mobilized, care must be taken

to identify other retroperitoneal structures. The largest and most lateral structure in the upper right retroperitoneal space is the kidney, whereas in the lower right retroperitoneal space, the psoas major muscle, upon which the genitofemoral nerve rests, will be visualized. The ureter runs inferomedially from the renal hilum to the pelvic brim (crossing the iliac vasculature just distal to the division of the common iliac artery into the internal and external iliac arteries). The gonadal artery and vein cross the ureter as the latter structure passes over the psoas major muscle. With continued medial reflection, the duodenum and pancreas will be visualized.

FIGURE 73.3
RESECTION OF THE COLON AND CONSTRUCTION OF THE ANASTOMOSIS

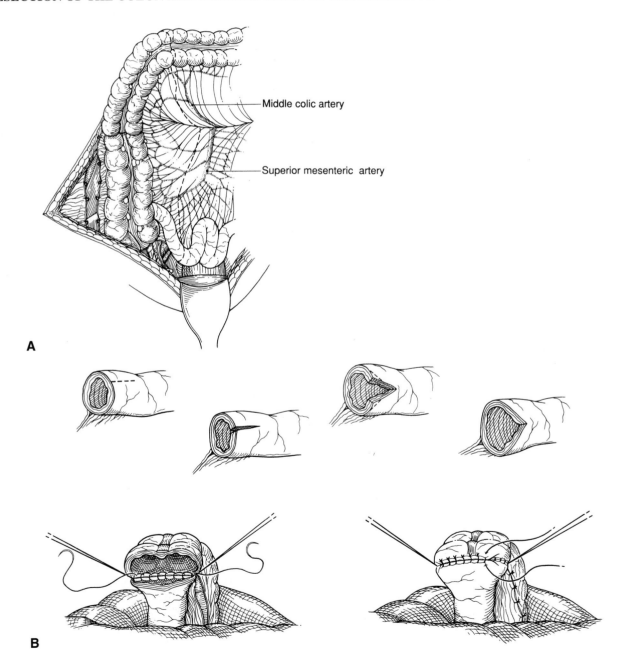

Resection of the Colon and Construction of the Anastomosis (Fig. 73.3)

Technical Points

Elevate the right colon and terminal ileum into the incision and look at the pattern of the mesenteric vascular arcades of the terminal ileum. Usually, about 5 to 10 cm of terminal ileum will be taken with the specimen. The length of terminal ileum is determined by its blood supply. Choose a point on the terminal ileum about 10 cm from the ileocecal valve where there appears to be good blood supply. Make a window through the ileal mesentery using hemostats. Divide the ileum with Allen clamps. Incise the peritoneum overlying the mesentery from this point to the middle transverse colon, taking the V of this peritoneal incision down to the base of the ileocolic artery. Clean the middle transverse colon and the area selected for anastomosis and divide it between Allen clamps. Then divide the mesentery of the colon serially with clamps and secure it with suture ligatures. Be sure to take the ileocolic artery and vein close to their origin to ensure that the lymph nodes associated with these vessels are taken as well.

After resection is completed, check the bed of the colon for hemostasis. Construct a two-layer, sutured, end-to-end anastomosis in the usual fashion. If there is a size discrepancy between the terminal ileum and the middle transverse colon, make a Cheatle slit along the antimesenteric border of the colon. This will effectively lengthen the area for anastomosis and eliminate the discrepancy. Close the hole in the mesentery by suturing the peritoneal surfaces of the mesentery together with a running suture of 3-0 Vicryl. Wrap omentum around the anastomosis.

Anatomic Points

The ileocolic artery divides into an ascending branch, which anastomoses with the right colic artery, and a descending branch, which supplies the terminal ileum, appendix, cecum, and proximal ascending colon. The ileal branch ultimately anastomoses with the termination of the superior mesenteric artery. Thus, the surgeon must select the point of division, based on visualization and selection of appropriate vasa recti, and divide the artery only after proximal and distal control of the anastomosis is achieved.

FIGURE 73.4
INCISION AND MOBILIZATION OF THE COLON

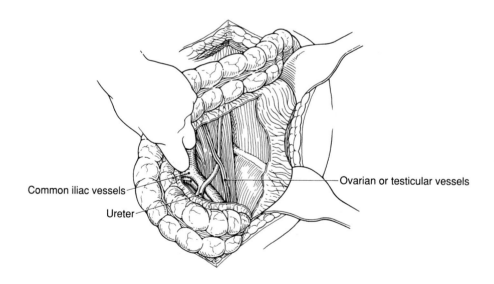

Common iliac vessels

Ureter

Ovarian or testicular vessels

Left Hemicolectomy

Incision and Mobilization of the Colon (Fig. 73.4)

Technical Points

Left hemicolectomy is best performed through a left paramedian or long midline incision. Alternatively, some surgeons prefer an oblique left lower quadrant incision. This incision is

not generally recommended, however, because it will present difficulties if a colostomy is subsequently required.

Make a long vertical incision to provide adequate exposure of both the splenic flexure and the pelvis. Palpate the colon and assess the tumor for mobility. Place a self-retaining retractor in the incision. Begin by mobilizing the sigmoid colon.

Lift the sigmoid colon medially and in an upward direction. Incise adhesions between the left colon and lateral peritoneum. (This is generally not the true white line of Toldt, which lies beneath these adhesions.) Once the colon is mobilized, the white line of Toldt, which corresponds to the peritoneal reflection, will become visible. Incise this peritoneal reflection and elevate the sigmoid colon and its mesentery up into the wound.

Identify the left ureter where it crosses the bifurcation of the iliac artery. If you anticipate a difficult pelvic dissection because of tumor involvement or an inflammatory process, surround the ureter and place a Silastic loop around it to facilitate reference to it later in the dissection. Avoid extensive mobilization of the ureter that might strip it of its blood supply, causing ischemia and stricture formation. Mobilize the colon from the distal sigmoid up to the region of the splenic flexure. Generally, mobilization will become more difficult as the splenic flexure is approached. Do not pull down on the splenic flexure—this only increases the probability of injuring the spleen. Instead, when this dissection becomes difficult, place a pack in the retrocolic space and begin dissection of the splenic flexure from the transverse colon (Fig. 73.5).

Anatomic Points

Adhesions can develop between the terminal descending colon or proximal sigmoid colon and the parietal peritoneum; frequently, these involve the epiploic appendages. Because these are lateral to the white line of Toldt, they can obscure this landmark for access to the avascular peritoneal fusion plane. Cautious dissection, coupled with medial traction of the sigmoid and descending colon, should allow identification of the proper fusion plane.

The root of the sigmoid mesocolon is variably located but typically is disposed as an inverted V, with its apex near the division of the left common iliac artery. Its left limb parallels the medial side of the psoas major muscle, whereas the right limb, which is in the true pelvis, passes inferomedially, ending in the midline at the midsacral region. This mesentery contains the sigmoid colon, sigmoid vessels, and superior rectal (hemorrhoidal) vessels. In addition, the apex of this mesentery marks the point where the left ureter enters the true pelvis. Identification and control of all vessels will facilitate mobilization, and identification here (and more proximally) of the ureter will prevent iatrogenic trauma to this structure.

Skeletonization of the ureter can deprive it of its blood supply. The blood supply of the ureter, on both sides, is provided by branches from the renal artery, aorta, gonadal artery, common and internal iliac arteries, and inferior vesical arteries. Because most of its blood supply enters its medial aspect, if either side must be mobilized, it is safest to mobilize its lateral portion.

During mobilization of the descending and left colon, the following retroperitoneal structures, all of which are posterior to the colon and its blood supply, should be identified: left kidney, left gonadal vein draining into the left renal vein, left gonadal artery, left ureter, left genitofemoral nerve on the left psoas major muscle, and the iliac vessels.

FIGURE 73.5
MOBILIZATION OF THE SPLENIC FLEXURE

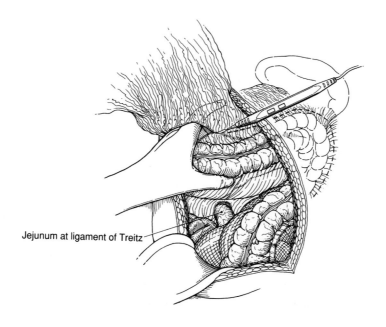

Jejunum at ligament of Treitz

Mobilization of the Splenic Flexure (Fig. 73.5)

Technical Points

Mobilization of the splenic flexure is often the most challenging part of left hemicolectomy. Generally, the left colon dives deeply retroperitoneal and passes quite high in the vicinity of the spleen. Approach this mobilization from below (proceeding upward along the retroperitoneal reflection) and from above (proceeding from right to left along the transverse colon).

Begin by continuing to incise the white line of Toldt and elevate the colon up out of the retroperitoneum. When you have gone as high as you can comfortably go from below, incising the peritoneal reflection from the vicinity of the descending colon, pack this area off and turn your attention to the transverse colon. Lift up on the greater omentum and separate it from the middle transverse colon by sharp dissection in the avascular fusion plane. As this plane is developed, you can pass the fingers of your nondominant hand behind the omentum and use it to display the plane. Leave the small fat tabs that protrude 5 to 10 mm from the colon on the colon. These contain small looping vessels that will bleed if divided. The proper plane is avascular and can be incised with Metzenbaum scissors, although many surgeons prefer to use electrocautery. In any event, be especially careful if this segment of the colon contains diverticula because diverticula may protrude into the fat tabs and be injured if the cut is too deep. Proceed up toward the region of the splenic flexure, pushing up on the omentum and down on the colon as you go. By pushing up on the omentum rather than pulling down, you minimize the risk for injuring the spleen by traction. You will soon reach a point at which it is possible to pass your nondominant hand completely around behind the splenic flexure of the colon. You can then divide the few remaining attachments with hemoclips. The attachments in the immediate vicinity of the splenic flexure frequently contain small vessels that will bleed if taken sharply. Mobilize the colon by sharp and blunt dissection into the midportion of the wound.

Anatomic Points

The anatomic relationships, as well as the peritoneal attachments, of the splenic flexure must be appreciated. The splenic flexure is quite sharp and is attached to the diaphragm by the phrenicocolic ligament. This peritoneal fold, which is continuous with the greater omentum, is inferolateral to the lower pole of the spleen and forms a "splenic shelf." Thus, the splenic flexure is typically immediately inferior and anterior to the hilum of the spleen and tail of the pancreas. This flexure is usually so sharp that the descending limb is overlaid by the terminal transverse limb. Reflection (see the previous discussion of technique) of the posterior side of the greater omentum from the anterior side of the transverse mesocolon, accomplished by dissecting in an avascular fusion plane, prevents the surgeon from placing undue traction on the spleen.

Identification of the Right Ureter and Division of the Colon Distally (Fig. 73.6)

Technical Points

Pack the sigmoid colon to the left and examine the peritoneum overlying the right common iliac artery. Often, the ureter is visible in the retroperitoneum. Incise the retroperitoneum and identify the ureter where it crosses just distal to the bifurcation of the common iliac artery. If you expect difficulty dissecting in the pelvis, surround the ureter with a Silastic loop. Identify the point of the distal colon that has been chosen for resection. Generally, this will be an area just above the peritoneal reflection. Mobilization of the rectosigmoid below the level of the peritoneal reflection is discussed in greater detail in Chapter 53. Clean the colon circumferentially and divide it between clamps. Incise the peritoneum from the point of division of the colon up along the point of origin of the inferior mesenteric artery to a portion of the middle transverse colon just to the left of the middle colic artery. Clean the portion of the middle transverse colon selected for anastomosis and divide the mesentery with clamps, securing the vessels with suture ligatures of 2-0 silk. Remove the specimen.

Anatomic Points

The terminal transverse colon and left colon, to the level of the lower rectum, are supplied by the inferior mesenteric artery, which usually arises from the front of the aorta, about 3 to 4 cm distal to the origin of the superior mesenteric artery and the same distance proximal to the bifurcation of the aorta. This artery (which is directed inferiorly and to the left) and its branches are largely retroperitoneal. Within a few centimeters of its origin, it gives rise to its first major branch, the left colic artery. More distally, arteries lie lateral to their corresponding veins. The left colic artery divides into ascending and descending branches that parallel the colon. The ascending branch ultimately forms part of the marginal artery (of Drummond) before anastomosing with the left branch of the middle colic artery, whereas the descending branch anastomoses with the first sigmoid artery. Either the inferior mesenteric artery or the left colic artery passes anterior to the main trunk of the inferior mesenteric vein.

A variable number of sigmoid arteries (range of one to five, but usually two or three) next arise from the inferior mesenteric artery, enter the sigmoid colon, and, like the arteries previously discussed, divide into ascending and descending branches. These branches anastomose with each other and with arteries derived from other branches (e.g., the descending branch of the left colic artery, the superior rectal artery), thus continuing the marginal artery (of Drummond).

The superior rectal (hemorrhoidal) artery is the termination of the inferior mesenteric artery. This artery crosses the left common iliac vessels in the base of the sigmoid mesocolon and enters the pelvis, where it lies posterior to the rectum. In this location, it soon divides into right and left branches that anastomose with branches of the paired middle rectal (hemorrhoidal) arteries. In addition, this artery usually forms

FIGURE 73.6
IDENTIFICATION OF THE RIGHT URETER AND DIVISION OF THE COLON DISTALLY

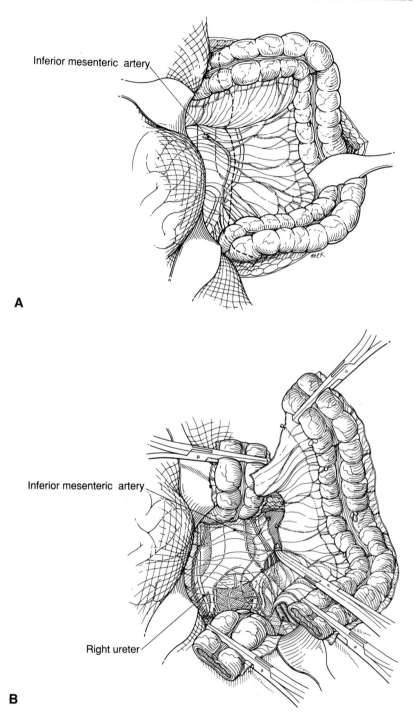

Inferior mesenteric artery

A

Inferior mesenteric artery

Right ureter

B

FIGURE 73.7
CONSTRUCTION OF THE ANASTOMOSIS

an anastomosis with the last sigmoid artery, thereby negating the importance of Sudeck's critical point and essentially completing a marginal artery of Drummond from the beginning of the cecum to the rectum.

Construction of the Anastomosis (Fig. 73.7)

Technical and Anatomic Points

Generally, the transverse colon will swing easily down to anastomose without tension to the sigmoid. Occasionally,

however, further mobilization is necessary. Mobility is ultimately limited by the middle colic artery and vein. If the middle transverse colon will not reach to the distal sigmoid, it may be necessary to resect back to the terminal ileum; however, this is only very rarely warranted. Construct an end-to-end anastomosis between the middle transverse colon and the sigmoid in the usual fashion. Generally, the mesenteric defect is broad and cannot be closed. If the colon has been mobilized out of the pelvis, leaving a raw surface in the hollow of the sacrum, place closed-suction drains in the pelvis.

REFERENCES

1. Baker JS. Low end to side rectosigmoidal anastomosis. *Arch Surg* 1950; 61:143.
2. Beahrs JR, Beahrs OH, Beahrs MM, et al. Urinary tract complications with rectal surgery. *Ann Surg* 1978;187:542.
3. Goligher JC, Lee PWR, Macfie J, et al. Experience with the Russian model 249 suture gun for anastomosis of the rectum. *Surg Gynecol Obstet* 1979;148:517. (This paper is historically interesting.)
4. Hays LV, Davis DR. A technic for restoring intestinal continuity after left hemicolectomy for cancer of the distal colon and rectum. *Am J Surg* 1976;131:390.
5. Jordan WP, Scaljon W. Anatomic complications of abdominal surgery with special reference to the ureter. *Am Surg* 1979;45:565.
6. Lee JF, Maurer VM, Block GE. Anatomic relations of pelvic autonomic nerves to pelvic operations. *Arch Surg* 1973;107:324.
7. Localio SA, Baron B. Abdomino-transsacral resection and anastomosis for mid-rectal cancer. *Ann Surg* 1973;178:540.
8. Lyttle JA, Parks AG. Intersphincteric excision of the rectum. *Br J Surg* 1977;64:413.
9. Weist JW, Kestenberg A, Becker JM. A technique for safe transanal passage of the circular end-to-end stapler for low anterior anastomosis of the colon. *Am J Surg* 1986;151:512.
10. Williams NS. Surgical principles. In: Keighley MRB, Williams NS, et al. *Surgery of the anus, rectum and colon.* London: WB Saunders, 1993:102–127.

CHAPTER 74

Laparoscopic Colon Resection

Amanda M. Metcalf

Since the specimen must be extracted through an incision, a laparoscopic approach to colon resection is most useful when the specimen is not unduly bulky. Large tumors or inflammatory phlegmons that require a large excision for extraction will negate the value of a laparoscopic approach. Another important preoperative consideration is to ensure that the precise anatomic location of the lesion is established. This is especially important for smaller lesions because a laparoscopic approach minimizes palpatory clues to location.

Right Colon Resection—Trocar Placement and Exploration of the Abdomen (Fig. 74.1)

Technical Points

Place the patient on the operating table with arms tucked to the sides, in a modified lithotomy position. The hips should be only minimally flexed with the thighs at the level of the abdominal wall. This allows the surgeon and assistants to have unrestricted access to the patient from both sides and between the legs. Securely fasten the patient to the table because laparoscopic exposure often relies on exaggerated table positioning. Place monitors on either side of the head of the table. The surgeon will stand on the side opposite to the side of resection, and the assistant will stand on the other side.

For a right colon resection, three basic port sites are used: umbilical, left upper quadrant, and left lower quadrant (Fig. 74.1A). Additional sites that may be useful intraoperatively are located in the right upper quadrant, right lower quadrant, and occasionally in the high left upper quadrant just inferior to the costal margin. After a pneumoperitoneum has been established and 10- to 12-mm cannulas are placed in the three basic sites, laparoscopic exploration should be performed.

Anatomic Points

Injury to the superior or inferior epigastric vessels from trocar placement can be avoided by placing these sites lateral to the rectus muscle. Injury to these vessels can result in brisk bleeding that can be difficult to control without suture ligature. A Kroner device can be used to place a hemostatic suture that encompasses a bleeding vessel. Because this technique effectively closes the port site, an additional port site will need to be placed.

Initial exploration will reveal the ascending and descending colon. The hepatic flexure and transverse colon may be obscured by overlying omentum (Fig. 74.1B). Attachments to the abdominal wall are more prominently seen than during open surgery, possibly because the colon "hangs" from the abdominal wall (Fig. 74.1C).

Right Colon Resection—Mobilizing the Colon (Fig. 74.2)

Technical Points

Place a straight (0-degree) laparoscope through the umbilical port site. Optimal passive exposure is obtained by placing the patient in a steep Trendelenburg position with the table rotated to the left. Retract the cecum medially using

LIST OF STRUCTURES

Colon
  Right colon
    Cecum
    Ascending colon
    Hepatic flexure
  Transverse colon
  Left colon
    Splenic flexure
    Descending colon
    Sigmoid colon

Line of Toldt
Hepatocolic ligament
Gastrocolic ligament
Phrenicocolic ligament
Splenocolic ligament
Omentum
Lesser sac
Superior epigastric artery and vein
Inferior epigastric artery and vein
Ileocolic artery and vein

Middle colic artery and vein
Inferior mesenteric artery and vein
  Left colic artery and vein
  Sigmoidal vessels
Sacral promontory
Ureters
Gonadal vessels
Gerota's fascia

FIGURE 74.1
RIGHT COLON RESECTION—TROCAR PLACEMENT AND EXPLORATION OF THE ABDOMEN (B and C
from Scott-Conner CEH, Cuschieri A, Carter FJ. Colon and rectum. In: *Minimal access surgical anatomy.* Philadelphia:
Lippincott Williams & Wilkins, 2000:185–210, with permission.)

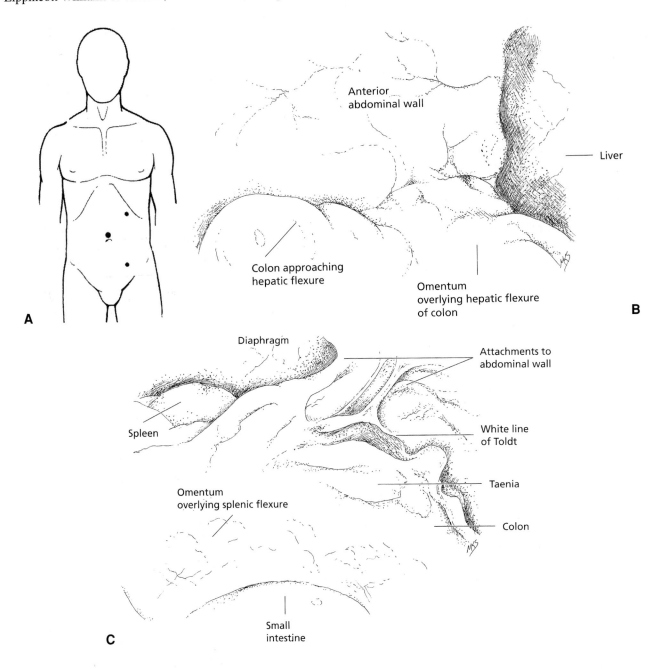

atraumatic bowel clamps. Elevate and incise the peritoneum along the line of Toldt with electrocautery scissors or ultrasonic shears (Fig. 74.2A). As the dissection continues, more distal portions of the right colon will need to be retracted to maintain good traction and countertraction. Divide all adhesions, however flimsy, to allow complete mobilization.

Continue this dissection to the region of the hepatocolic ligament. This region is more vascular and is divided hemostatically most easily with the ultrasonic scissors. With full mobilization, visualize the ureter, Gerota's fascia, and the duodenum.

Place the patient in reverse Trendelenburg position with the table in neutral rotation. Grasp the transverse colon and retract it inferiorly to place the gastrocolic ligament on traction. The omentum forming the gastrocolic ligament can be divided most easily from the region of the middle colic vessels to the hepatocolic ligament using the ultrasonic scissors.

If intracorporeal ligation of the vessels is planned, grasp the hepatic flexure and retract it superiorly toward the anterior abdominal wall. This places the right mesocolon on traction, and the right colic vessels can be observed tenting the mesentery. Divide the mesentery lateral to the vessels with

FIGURE 74.2
RIGHT COLON RESECTION—MOBILIZING THE COLON (**A** and **B** from Metcalf A. Laparoscopic colon resection. In: Scott-Conner CEH, ed. *The SAGES manual: fundamentals of laparoscopy and GI endoscopy.* New York: Springer-Verlag, 1999, with permission.)

the ultrasonic scissors. Introduce an endoscopic vascular linear cutting stapling device from the left lower quadrant port. Pass the vascular pedicle into the jaws of the stapler, taking care to visualize the tips of the stapling device behind the vascular pedicle to avoid inadvertent incorporation of adjacent structures into the staple line (Fig. 74.2B).

After division of the pedicle, move the laparoscope to a different port site, and grasp the cecum through the umbilical port site. Create a vertical 3- to 5-cm skin incision, incorporating this site, and incise the fascia. Deinsufflate the abdomen and retrieve the specimen through the incision. Clamp, divide, and ligate the ileocolic and right branch of the middle colic vessels as well as any smaller vessels near the proposed site of transection.

Anatomic Points

Division of all adhesions in the right gutter to the right colon is imperative to mobilize the colon fully. The retroperitoneal structures can then be pushed posteriorly out of harm's way. The lesser sac is often obliterated in the region of the hepatic flexure of the colon. Division of the omentum in the gastrocolic ligament toward the midportion of the transverse colon usually allows easy entry into the lesser sac and prevents inadvertent damage to the underlying transverse mesocolon.

Right Colon Resection—Extracorporeal Anastomosis (Fig. 74.3)

Technical Points

Clear several centimeters of both ileum and colon of fat circumferentially at the proposed transection sites. For a stapled

anastomosis, use a linear cutting stapling device to transect the ileum and the colon and allow removal of the surgical specimen (Fig. 74.3A). Next, align the antimesenteric borders of the ileum and colon, and close the mesenteric defect (Fig. 74.3B). Excise a corner of the antimesenteric side of the staple line to allow placement of the linear cutting stapling device (Fig. 74.3C). Place one limb of the linear stapling device in the colon, the other in the small bowel (Fig. 74.3D). While closing the stapler, take care to ensure that the staple line will be on the antimesenteric side of both bowel limbs and that the entire length of the staple line is used to construct an adequately sized aperture (Fig. 74.3E). Fire the stapler. Inspect the staple lines for hemostasis (Fig. 74.3F). Close the enterotomy left after firing the linear cutting stapler by approximating the edge of the ileum to the colon with Allis clamps. Place these so that the previous staple lines are staggered, thus avoiding an unnecessary number of intersecting staple lines (Fig. 74.3G). Place a linear stapling device below the Allis clamps and fire it (Fig. 74.3H). Remove excess tissue distal to the staple line before removing the stapler (Fig. 74.3I). Reduce the bowel back into the abdomen and close the incisions.

Laparoscopic Left Hemicolectomy—Mobilization of the Left Colon and Splenic Flexure (Fig. 74.4)

Technical Points

Position the patient as described for laparoscopic right colon resection. Trocar placement for a left colon resection includes an umbilical port site and three other port sites: right upper and lower quadrants and a left upper quadrant site

FIGURE 74.3
RIGHT COLON RESECTION—EXTRACORPOREAL ANASTOMOSIS (A–I from Gordon PH, Nivatvongs S. *Principles and practice of surgery for the colon, rectum, and anus.* 2nd ed. St Louis: Quality Medical Publishing, 1999:632–634, with permission.)

FIGURE 74.4
LAPAROSCOPIC LEFT HEMICOLECTOMY—MOBILIZATION OF THE LEFT COLON AND SPLENIC
FLEXURE (**B** and **C** from Scott-Conner CEH, Cuschieri A, Carter FJ. Colon and rectum. In: *Minimal access surgical anatomy.* Philadelphia: Lippincott Williams & Wilkins, 2000:185–210, with permission; **D** and **E** from Wind GG. The colon. In: *Applied laparoscopic anatomy: abdomen and pelvis.* Baltimore: Williams & Wilkins, 1997:217–246, with permission.)

FIGURE 74.4 (Continued)

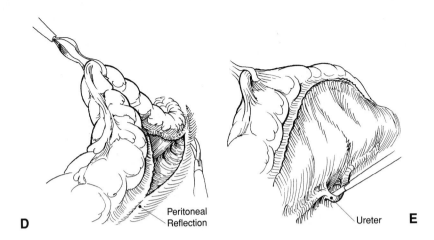

D — Peritoneal Reflection

E — Ureter

(Fig. 74.4A). Occasionally, additional port sites in the left lower quadrant and high right upper quadrant sites are needed. Place the patient in steep Trendelenburg position with the table rotated to the right. The surgeon stands on the right side of the patient or between the patient's legs, and the assistant stands on the left side.

Grasp the sigmoid colon with an atraumatic bowel clamp, and retract it toward the midline. Incise any adhesions and the peritoneum along the line of Toldt (Fig. 74.4B). Sequentially grasp and regrasp the colon to provide sufficient traction to allow dividing all adhesions to the splenic flexure. With full mobilization, one should be able to visualize the sacral promontory, the ureter, the gonadal vessels, and Gerota's fascia (Fig. 74.4C–E).

Next, place the patient in reverse Trendelenburg position and grasp the transverse colon. Retract it inferiorly to allow division of the omentum in the gastrocolic ligament from the middle transverse colon to the region of the spleen. It is often helpful for the surgeon to stand between the patient's legs during this portion of the procedure. It may also be helpful to use a 30-degree scope rather than a 0-degree scope. Visible adhesions between the omentum and the spleen are often most easily managed by early division to prevent traction injuries (see Fig. 55.1). Dissection of the last portion can be quite difficult. It may be helpful to alternate between retracting the left transverse colon and dividing the gastrocolic ligament, and retracting the descending colon and dividing the phrenicocolic ligament to complete the dissection. The ultrasonic shears are invaluable in performing this portion of the procedure.

Anatomic Points

The important anatomic points for a safe laparoscopic dissection of the splenic flexure are those as described for the open approach. Of paramount importance in either situation is to ensure that one has achieved entry into the key anatomic planes with division of all adhesions, even those that appear inconsequential, before dividing the remaining attachments in the region of the splenic flexure.

Resection of the Colon (Fig. 74.5)

Technical Points

After complete mobilization of the left colon, the vascular pedicle must be ligated intracorporeally. Grasp the sigmoid colon and retract it toward the anterior abdominal wall (Fig. 74.5A). If necessary, the sigmoid mesocolon can be grasped to obtain adequate traction. With adequate traction, the location of the inferior mesenteric artery and its main branches, the left colic and the sigmoidal, can be identified as cordlike structures tenting the mesentery. Transillumination by a second laparoscope is occasionally useful.

Create a window through the mesentery on either side of these vessels. Use the vascular endoscopic linear cutting stapler, passed through a right lower quadrant port site, to divide these vessels. As always, take care to visualize the tip of the stapling instrument in order to avoid incorporation of adjacent structures into the staple line.

Choose the distal site for resection, and divide the remaining mesocolon using the ultrasonic scissors. After completely dividing the mesocolon, divide the bowel with the endoscopic linear cutting stapler (Fig. 74.5C), again visualizing the tips of the instrument to avoid incorporating adjacent structures.

Circular Stapled Anastomosis (Fig. 74.6)

Technical Points

Grasp the proximal staple line through the left upper quadrant port site and retract it up to the anterior abdominal wall in this region. Advance the cannula over the clamp and lengthen the skin incision to 3 to 4 cm in size. Deepen this incision through all layers of the abdominal wall. Retrieve the end of the colon and complete an extracorporeal resection.

Place a pursestring suture in the proximal end of the bowel and insert the anvil of the circular stapling device

FIGURE 74.5
RESECTION OF THE COLON (**A** and **B** from Wind GG. The colon. In: *Applied laparoscopic anatomy: abdomen and pelvis.* Baltimore: Williams & Wilkins, 1997:217–246, with permission; **C** from Weiss EG, Wexner SD. Laparoscopic segmental colectomies. In: Scott-Conner CEH, ed. *The SAGES manual: fundamentals of laparoscopy and GI endoscopy.* New York: Springer-Verlag, 1999, with permission.)

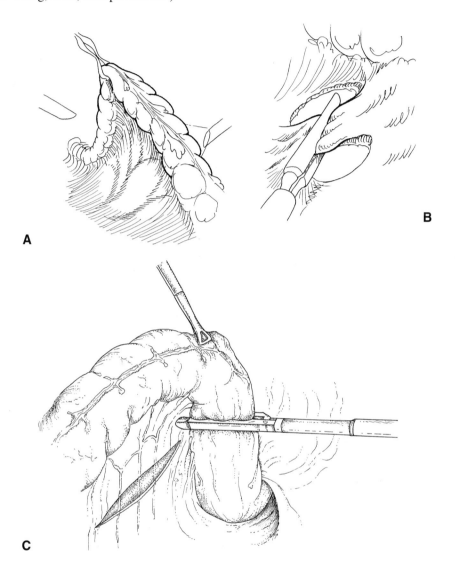

(Fig. 74.6A,B). Tie the pursestring and replace the bowel into the abdominal cavity. Close the fascial incision around the original cannula and reestablish pneumoperitoneum. Grasp the anvil with an anvil-grasping clamp and bring it down to the proposed anastomotic site. Take care to ensure that the bowel is not rotated as it is brought down to the anastomotic site. If the length is inadequate, obtain greater mobility by dividing additional omentum in the left upper quadrant.

Pass the circular stapler transanally and advance it to the distal staple line. Extrude the trocar of the circular stapler through the staple line of the distal rectum under direct vision (Fig. 74.6C). Attach the anvil and approximate it to the cartridge under direct vision. Fire and remove the circular stapler. Inspect the donuts for completeness. Test the anastomosis by filling the pelvis with saline and occluding the bowel proximal to the anastomosis with a noncrushing bowel clamp. Next insufflate the rectum with air and observe for any bubbles, indicating a leak. Check hemostasis, irrigate the operative field, and close all port sites.

Anatomic Points

Abnormal rotation or torsion of the proximal bowel is surprisingly easy during manipulation of the anvil. If not corrected, it can lead to colonic obstruction proximal to the anastomosis. Mesenteric defects that are created during laparoscopic left-sided colon resection are usually not repaired.

FIGURE 74.6
CIRCULAR STAPLED ANASTOMOSIS (A–C from Weiss EG, Wexner SD. Laparoscopic segmental colectomies. In: Scott-Conner CEH, ed. *The SAGES manual: fundamentals of laparoscopy and GI endoscopy.* New York: Springer-Verlag, 1999, with permission.)

A   B   C

REFERENCES

1. Darzi A. Hand-assisted laparoscopic colorectal surgery. *Semin Laparosc Surg* 2001;8:153–160. (Describes technical aspects of using hand to assist in dissection, retraction, and hemostasis.)
2. Gordon PH, Nivatvongs S. *Principles and practice of surgery for the colon, rectum, and anus.* 2nd ed. St. Louis: Quality Medical Publishing, 1999:632–634.
3. Lauter DM, Froines EJ. Initial experience with 150 cases of laparoscopic assisted colectomy. *Am J Surg* 2001;181:398–403.
4. Milsom JW, Bohm B, Hammerhofer KA, et al. A prospective, randomized trial comparing laparoscopic versus conventional techniques in colorectal cancer surgery: a preliminary report. *J Am Coll Surg* 1998; 187:46–57.
5. Pandya S, Murray JJ, Coller JA, et al. Laparoscopic colectomy: indications for conversion to laparotomy. *Arch Surg* 1999;134:471–475. (Presents good review of large experience.)
6. Scott-Conner CEH, Cuschieri A, Carter FJ. Colon and rectum. In: *Minimal access surgical anatomy.* Philadelphia: Lippincott Williams & Wilkins, 2000:185–210. (Provides color photographs and line drawings of laparoscopic anatomy.)
7. Tomita H, Marcello PW, Milsom JW. Laparoscopic surgery of the colon and rectum. *World J Surg* 1999;23:397–405.
8. Wexner SD, Moscovitz ID. Laparoscopic colectomy in diverticular and Crohn's disease. *Surg Clin North Am* 2000;80:1299–1319.
9. Young-Fadok TM, Nelson H. Laparoscopic right colectomy: five-step procedure. *Diseases Colon Rectum* 2000;43:267–271.

THE PELVIS

This part includes open and laparoscopic abdominoperineal resection and the related low anterior resection (Chapters 75 and 76), continuing the discussion of colon anatomy that was begun in the previous part. More complex sphincter-sparing procedures, such as ileoanal anastomosis, are detailed in the references at the end of these chapters.

The remaining two chapters—total abdominal hysterectomy and oophorectomy (along with related procedures) (Chapter 77) and laparoscopic surgery of the female pelvis (Chapter 78)—present the anatomy of the female reproductive tract. The references listed at the end of these chapters provide descriptions of pelvic lymphadenectomy (both open and laparoscopic) and other, less common, pelvic operations.

CHAPTER 75

Abdominoperineal Resection, Low Anterior Resection

Abdominoperineal resection is performed for treatment of cancer of the lower rectum. Sometimes after extensive mobilization, a tumor is found to be resectable with preservation of the anal sphincters, and an end-to-end anastomosis can be done by low anterior resection. In this chapter, abdominoperineal resection will be considered along with the closely related low anterior resection. This dissection will be described as it is done for a male patient. The modifications necessary for a female patient are described at the end of this section. The corresponding laparoscopic procedures are described in Chapter 76.

Position of the Patient and the Incision (Fig. 75.1)

Technical Points

Position the patient supine on the operating table. Use either specially constructed leg supports or homemade outrigger "skis" to support the legs in moderate abduction with mild flexion at the hips and knees. The buttocks should extend slightly over the end of the operating table. Comfortable access to the perineal region should be available for the operating surgeon. Avoid the use of standard lithotomy stirrups

because these produce excessive flexion at the hip and knee and have been associated with vascular complications when used for lengthy procedures. Close the anus securely with a pursestring suture. Prepare and drape the anterior abdomen and perineal region. Place a towel over the perineum to provide temporary coverage until access is required. The initial phase of the dissection is done through the abdomen, with the second assistant standing between the legs of the patient. The instrument nurse should stand on a stool. Do not proceed with the perineal dissection unless you are certain that sphincter preservation will not be possible.

A lower midline incision provides good exposure to the lower abdomen and pelvis. Make the incision from just above the umbilicus to the level of the pubis. Explore the abdomen. Mobilize the left colon as described in Chapter 73. Carry the peritoneal incisions anteriorly, about 1 cm up on the bladder, meeting in the midline between the bladder and the rectum.

Identify both ureters and surround them with Silastic loops. After the peritoneal incision has been completed and both ureters have been identified, divide the sigmoid colon at the point selected. Pass a hand behind the inferior mesenteric artery in the avascular plane just anterior to the vertebral

LIST OF STRUCTURES

Sigmoid colon
Rectum
   Lateral rectal ligaments
Anal canal
Ureters
Bladder
Sacrum
Coccyx
Pelvic diaphragm
Levator ani (levator sling)
   Iliococcygeus muscle
   Pubococcygeus muscle
Coccygeus muscle
Ischiorectal fossa
Pubic symphysis
Ischial tuberosities
Perineum

Anterior (urogenital) triangle
Posterior (anal) triangle
Anococcygeal raphe
Perineal body
Pudendal nerve
Pudendal (Alcock's) canal
Aorta
Inferior mesenteric artery
   Superior rectal (hemorrhoidal)
   artery
Middle rectal (hemorrhoidal) arteries
Internal pudendal artery
   Inferior rectal (hemorrhoidal)
   arteries
Middle sacral artery
Common iliac arteries
   Internal iliac arteries

Presacral venous plexus
Superior hypogastric plexus
In the male:
   Prostate
   Seminal vesicles
   Membranous urethra
   Bulb of penis
   Rectovesical fascia (of
      Denonvilliers)
   Rectovesical pouch
   Transverse perineal muscles
In the female:
   Uterus
   Ovaries
   Vagina
   Rectouterine pouch (of Douglas)

ORIENTATION

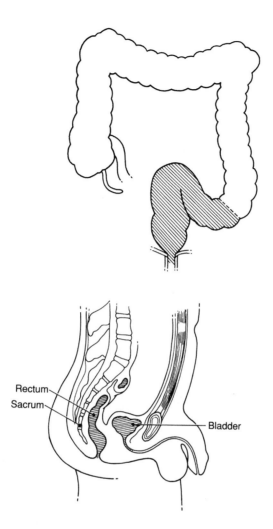

bodies. Locate both ureters and confirm that they have not been included with the mesentery of the colon. Serially divide the mesentery of the colon with clamps. Using laparotomy pads, pack the proximal left colon up in the left upper quadrant.

The distal sigmoid is now completely free and can be circumferentially elevated from the pelvis, allowing access to the rectum. First, complete the posterior dissection. Elevate the sigmoid colon and pass your hand behind it into the hollow of the sacrum. The aorta and common iliac vessels should be seen through a very light veil of areolar tissue. A few bands passing directly posterior between the colon and the presacral space can be divided using electrocautery or scissors. A middle sacral artery usually is present and should be secured with hemoclips. The colon should elevate easily, and a glistening layer of retroperitoneal areolar tissue should be left intact over the presacral venous plexus. You should be able to dissect this plane easily by hand. If difficulty is encountered, it is possible that you are in the wrong plane; stop and

reassess the situation. Torrential bleeding from the presacral venous plexus may follow inadvertent entry into this plexus. Conversely, remaining in the correct plane of dissection not only minimizes bleeding but also helps preserve autonomic nerves in the region. Dissection in the hollow of the sacrum should proceed readily until the tip of the coccyx is palpable and the rectosigmoid is elevated up on the hand. Check the hollow of the sacrum for hemostasis.

Next, turn your attention to the anterior dissection. Place three long hemostats, such as Crile hemostats, on the peritoneal reflection overlying the bladder. By sharp and blunt dissection, free the rectum from the posterior wall of the bladder until the seminal vesicles (in the male) are encountered. Carry this dissection down below the seminal vesicles, remaining in a plane posterior to Denonvilliers' fascia to minimize the chances of nerve injury. As noted in Fig. 75.5, the posterior wall of the vagina is commonly excised with the specimen in a female. In this case, the anterior dissection need only proceed to a convenient point below the uterine cervix.

FIGURE 75.1
POSITION OF THE PATIENT AND THE INCISION

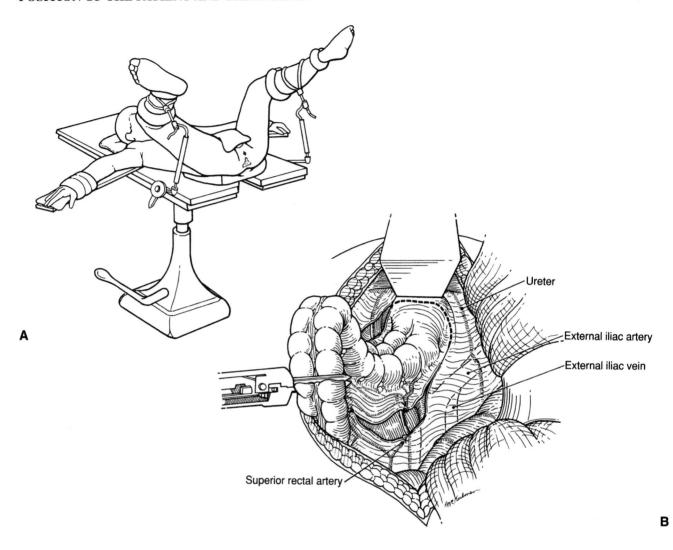

A

Ureter

External iliac artery

External iliac vein

Superior rectal artery

B

Anatomic Points

Identification of the ureters is easily accomplished if one re-
members where the ureters lie as they enter the pelvis. Both
left and right ureters are retroperitoneal and cross the peritoneal surface of the iliac vasculature in the vicinity of the
origin of the internal iliac artery. The left ureter enters the
pelvis at the apex of the sigmoid mesocolon, being crossed
here by the descending limb of the mesocolon and its contained vasculature, the superior rectal (hemorrhoidal) vessels.
Thus, its course in the pelvis is lateral to the pelvic limb of
the sigmoid mesocolon and anterior (medial) to the internal
iliac artery. The right ureter is similarly related to the internal
iliac artery. Further, in the female, the ureter lies posterior
to the ovarian vessels, which pass into the pelvis through
the suspensory ligaments. In the female pelvis proper, the
ovaries typically lie just anterior to the ureters. At this stage
in the operation, it is also worthwhile to note that the blood

supply of the pelvic portion of the ureters, derived from the
internal iliac arteries or its branches, enters the ureter from
its lateral side; hence, dissection to isolate the ureters should
be done medially and the ureters gently mobilized laterally.
Be careful not to skeletonize the ureters because the vascular
anastomoses are tenuous at best. The ureters are at particular risk for injury during the following three phases of the
operation:

1. Ligation of the inferior mesenteric artery
2. Incision of the pelvic peritoneum lateral to the rectum
3. Division of the lateral stalks of the rectum deep in the
   pelvis (particularly if this phase is done from below during
   abdominoperineal resection)

Early identification, safe mobilization out of the operative
field, and gentle marking with Silastic loops (to facilitate
repeated verification of integrity) help minimize the risk for
injury.

In its initial stage of development, the inferior mesenteric artery was originally located in the mesentery of the colon. However, with the fixation of the descending colon and the fusion of the left side of the mesentery with parietal peritoneum, the inferior mesenteric artery came to be primarily retroperitoneal. It can, however, be mobilized easily by blunt dissection in the fusion plane just posterior to the artery. The superior rectal (hemorrhoidal) artery, the pelvic continuation of the inferior mesenteric artery, passes into the pelvis in the base of the sigmoid mesocolon. It branches into right and left vessels approximately at the level of the rectosigmoid junction (third sacral vertebra), and these branches continue distally on the posterolateral sides of the rectum. Typically, the right branch is larger than the left. As the sigmoid and rectum are mobilized, the superior rectal (hemorrhoidal) artery and its branches will mobilize with it.

Mobilization of the rectum from the presacral space is not without risk. If the wrong plane is entered, one can easily avulse veins of the presacral venous plexus or avulse the middle sacral artery. In 15% of individuals, the presacral venous plexus anastomoses with the vertebral plexus, usually at the level of S-3 to S-5. These individuals are prone to torrential bleeding if the presacral venous plexus is torn. The middle sacral artery originates from the posterior side of the aorta, just proximal to its bifurcation into the common iliac arteries. Although small, it is large enough to cause significant bleeding if not controlled. The key to avoiding this artery and the presacral venous plexus is to dissect in a plane anterior to the superior hypogastric plexus, which itself is immediately anterior to the terminal aorta, the roots of the common iliac arteries, and the middle sacral artery.

The technical objective of the anterior dissection of the rectum is to dissect in the avascular plane provided by the rectovesical fascia (of Denonvilliers). This septum, located in the male between the prostate (and seminal vesicles) and rectum, is attached above to the peritoneum of the rectovesical pouch, laterally to the pelvic diaphragm, and inferiorly to the perineal body. In the embryo, the peritoneal cavity extends inferiorly to the perineal body. As the prostate and rectum increase in size, the peritoneum covering the posterior prostate and anterior rectum is apposed. Subsequent fusion of the apposed serosal surfaces results in the definitive rectovesical fascia. The fusion plane is relatively avascular.

FIGURE 75.2
DIVISION OF THE LATERAL RECTAL LIGAMENTS

A   B

Division of the Lateral Rectal Ligaments (Fig. 75.2)

Technical Points

The remaining attachments to be taken from above are the mesentery of the rectum and the lateral rectal ligaments. These include the middle rectal (hemorrhoidal) vessels. Secure the left lateral ligament first. Place your nondominant hand on the sigmoid colon, passing two fingers anterior and two fingers posterior to the rectosigmoid. Pull the colon to the right to define a pedicle of thickened tissue between your fingers. Take this tissue serially with hemoclips or with sutures and ligatures. Proceed down to the pelvic diaphragm.

Next, pull the colon to the left and divide the right lateral ligament in the same fashion. The colon should now be totally free to the level of the pelvic diaphragm. At this point, it is possible to palpate the tumor to determine whether an anterior resection with anastomosis might be possible.

Anatomic Points

The ill-defined lateral rectal ligaments are often described as consisting of the connective tissue around the middle rectal (hemorrhoidal) artery and nerves. However, these ligaments are posterolateral, but the middle rectal artery approaches the rectum from a more anterolateral direction. In actuality, the ligaments consist primarily of the nerves to the rectum, accompanied by connective tissue and, in 25% of the cases, an accessory rectal artery.

The true middle rectal (hemorrhoidal) artery is quite variable in origin. It has been reported to be a branch of the internal pudendal (41%), inferior gluteal (23%), obturator, umbilical, and internal iliac arteries, among others in the vicinity. It is rarely absent. Typically, it reaches the rectum very close to the pelvic diaphragm, not in the lateral ligaments. The middle rectal (hemorrhoidal) artery has been described as being associated with the rectovesical fascia (of Denonvilliers) in the male, and just deep to the peritoneum of the rectouterine pouch in the female. Although the middle rectal (hemorrhoidal) artery primarily supplies the muscles of the rectum, it also anastomoses freely with the superior rectal (hemorrhoidal) artery, and it may anastomose with the inferior rectal (hemorrhoidal) artery. Most surgeons and anatomists would agree that there is an arterial "watershed" at about the pectinate line of the rectum.

FIGURE 75.3
LOW ANTERIOR RESECTION

Low Anterior Resection (Fig. 75.3)

Technical and Anatomic Points

If, after complete mobilization of the rectum to the level of the pelvic diaphragm (levator sling), the tumor appears to be in a higher position than initially appreciated, a low anterior resection using the EEA stapling device may be performed. Place a right-angled rectal clamp across the distal rectum just above the level of transection. Place two stay sutures of 2-0 silk below the level of transection, one on each side. These will allow you to maintain control of the rectal remnant, avoiding its retraction into the perineum. Transect the rectum and remove the specimen. Have suction ready as you do this to avoid soilage. Check the pelvis for hemostasis. Place a pursestring suture of 2-0 Prolene on the distal rectum.

Place this suture as a whipstitch, running it over and over to incorporate all layers of the bowel wall. Start from the upper surface on the outside so that it will be easy to tie the pursestring over the EEA.

Alternatively, divide the distal rectum with a linear stapling device. This allows secure closure. The EEA can then be "spiked" through the closed rectal segment.

Pack off the pelvis. Place a pursestring suture on the proximal sigmoid. Check to make sure that you have sufficient mobility for the sigmoid to reach easily to the selected area of the distal rectum. If you are not certain that mobility is adequate, mobilize the splenic flexure to bring down the colon. From below, an assistant should then cut the pursestring suture that has been placed on the anus. The lubricated EEA stapling device can then be introduced through the anus. Tie both pursestring sutures securely around the instrument and close the instrument, checking to make sure that the bowel is circumferentially inverted and completely incorporated at both ends. Fire the EEA and then open it. Place a traction suture of 2-0 silk in a Lembert fashion and close the anterior wall of the anastomosis. Use this traction suture to elevate the anastomosis and remove it atraumatically from the EEA after opening the instrument. Check the anastomosis by injecting povidone-iodine solution (Betadine) into the distal rectal segment. Carefully reinforce any areas of leakage with interrupted 3-0 silk Lembert sutures. Surround the anastomosis with omentum and place closed-suction drains in the pelvis.

FIGURE 75.4
PERINEAL PHASE OF ABDOMINOPERINEAL RESECTION

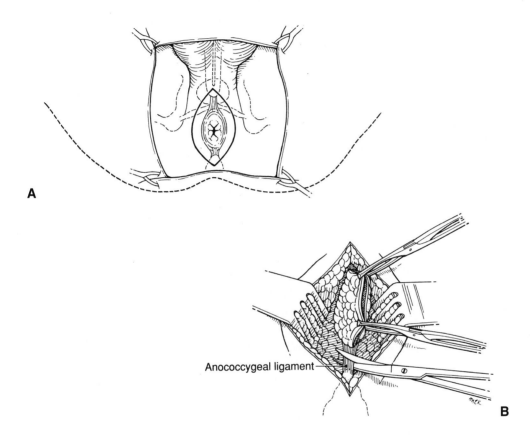

Anococcygeal ligament

Perineal Phase of Abdominoperineal Resection (Fig. 75.4)

Technical Points

If, even after mobilization, the tumor is too low for anterior resection, proceed with the perineal phase of the abdominopelvic resection. Remove the towel from the perineum and diagram an elliptical skin incision. In the male, palpate the transverse perineal muscle, which will form the anterior limit of the dissection. Incise the skin and subcutaneous tissues. Place Allis clamps on the skin edges of the specimen to approximate them. Begin the dissection laterally and posteriorly, deepening it through subcutaneous tissue until the tip of the coccyx is reached. With strong scissors, cut the fascia anterior to the coccyx. Have an assistant pass a hand through the abdominal incision and down posterior to the rectum to help you identify the correct plane. Cut with scissors until you have entered the peritoneal cavity just anterior to the coccyx.

Place a finger of your nondominant hand into the peritoneal cavity and hook the puborectalis portion of the pubococcygeus muscle. Divide this muscle anteriorly using electrocautery, progressing upward to about 2 o'clock and 10 o'clock on each side.

The anterior phase of the dissection must be done with extreme care because this is the area where injury to the urethra and prostate is possible. Divide the fat anterior to the rectum carefully using Metzenbaum scissors, and look for and identify the transverse slips of the transverse perineal muscles. If dissection remains posterior to this muscle, injury to the urethra is unlikely. Carefully deepen the dissection, using Metzenbaum scissors, until the prostate is identified. At this point, it is helpful to pass the specimen out through

FIGURE 75.4   (Continued)

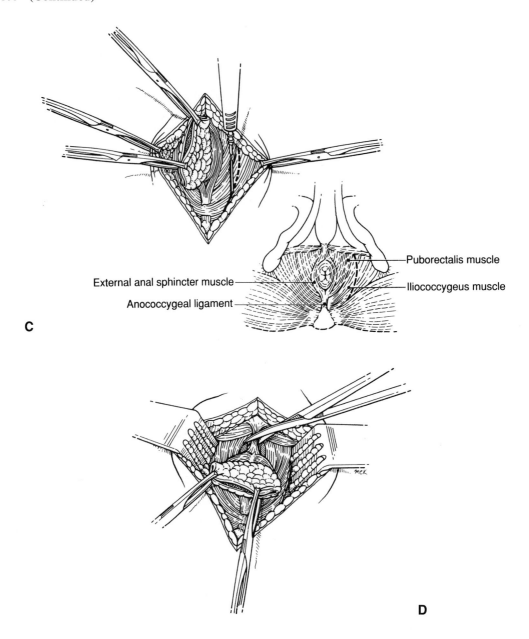

Puborectalis muscle

External anal sphincter muscle

Iliococcygeus muscle

Anococcygeal ligament

C

D

the perineum. This is possible unless the tumor is extremely bulky. Have an assistant hand you the distal resected end of the sigmoid through the posterior opening. Roll the colon down until it is hanging out the bottom like a tail. It should be suspended only by the remaining attachments to the prostate. These can be divided by sharp and blunt dissection. Slips of the puborectalis muscle must be divided laterally. Be careful not to extend the dissection too far anteriorly because strong traction on the specimen will bring the prostate down farther than expected, and injury to the prostate will still be possible. After the specimen is removed, check hemostasis from above and below. Irrigate through with copious amounts of warm saline.

As an assistant closes the perineal wound, close the abdominal wound and fashion an end-sigmoid colostomy in the left lower quadrant of the abdomen in the usual fashion. The perineal wound is closed in layers with running 2-0 Vicryl. Generally, it is not possible to reapproximate the puborectalis muscle. With adequate tumor resection, these muscles are often taken so widely that they cannot be brought back together. Soft tissues can, however, be approximated in several layers. Place closed-suction drains in the pelvis, bringing them out either lateral to the perineal incision or through the anterior abdominal wall.

Anatomic Points

The diamond-shaped perineum is bounded by imaginary lines connecting the anterior pubic symphysis, the lateral ischial tuberosities, and the posterior coccyx. The superior limit of the perineum is the pelvic diaphragm, composed of the paired levator ani (remember that the iliococcygeus, pubococcygeus, and puborectalis muscles are component parts of the levator ani) and coccygeus muscles and their associated fascia. The perineum can be divided into an anterior urogenital triangle and a posterior anal triangle by a horizontal line connecting the two ischial tuberosities. This line passes through the central tendon of the perineum (perineal body) and approximates the posterior edge of both the superficial and deep transverse perineal muscles, the latter being enclosed in the fascia of the superficial urogenital diaphragm. Because the anterior apex of the skin incision (described in the technical discussion) overlies the central tendon, the required dissection is limited to the anal triangle.

The central structure of the anal triangle is the anus. Anteriorly, the anal canal is anchored to the adjacent perineal body, and posteriorly it is anchored to the anococcygeal raphe (ligament), which attaches it to the tip of the coccyx. The lateral ischiorectal fossae are filled with fat and connective tissue. Rectal branches of the pudendal neurovascular structures pass through these spaces. Medially and superiorly, each ischiorectal fossa is limited by the pelvic diaphragm. This diaphragm is not flat, but funnel shaped. Its rim is attached to the midportion of the bony pelvis and the fascia covering the overlying obturator internus muscle, and its spout is the anus. Muscular fibers of the levator ani converge on fibers of the external anal sphincter, which some researchers consider to be an expression of the puborectalis part of the levator ani. The lateral boundary of the ischiorectal fossa is the obturator internus muscle and fascia.

Dissection in the anal triangle for removal of the rectum and anus proceeds from safe to dangerous, or from posterior to anterior. Detachment of the anococcygeal ligament from

the coccyx, followed by division of the pelvic diaphragm muscles close to their insertion on this ligament and on the anal canal, preserves most of the pelvic diaphragm and the nerve supply to the retained muscle fibers because the nerves pass from posterolateral to anteromedial on the pelvic surface of these muscles. The pudendal nerve, located in a split (pudendal, or Alcock's, canal) in the obturator fascia of the lateral wall of the ischiorectal fossa, supplies the external anal sphincter and all structures in the urogenital triangle. This nerve is also preserved if division of the pelvic diaphragm fibers is done close to the anorectal specimen.

Technically, dissection anterior to the anus is most difficult because of the proximity of the urethra and prostate gland and because of the anatomic characteristics of the perineal body. This anatomically ill-defined, pyramidal structure is a fibromuscular mass lying between the anal canal and the prostate gland (in the male) or vagina (in the female). It represents the fusion of all fascial layers in the perineum and pelvic floor (e.g., Colles' fascia, both layers of urogenital diaphragm fascia, and Denonvilliers' fascia). In addition, muscle fibers of essentially all of the muscles in that area (such as the pubococcygeal fibers of the levator ani, the deep and superficial transverse perineal muscles, the anterior fibers of the external anal sphincter, and the bulbospongiosus fibers) have some or all of their insertion on the perineal body. Because the superficial transverse perineal muscles mark the posterior edge of the urogenital diaphragm, through which the membranous urethra must pass, this muscle is the landmark that limits the anterior extent of the dissection. Posterior traction on the anorectal specimen will allow the surgeon to dissect in the plane of Denonvilliers' fascia, thereby avoiding injury to the prostate, membranous urethra, and bulb of the penis.

FIGURE 75.5
MODIFICATION OF ABDOMINOPELVIC RESECTION FOR FEMALE PATIENTS

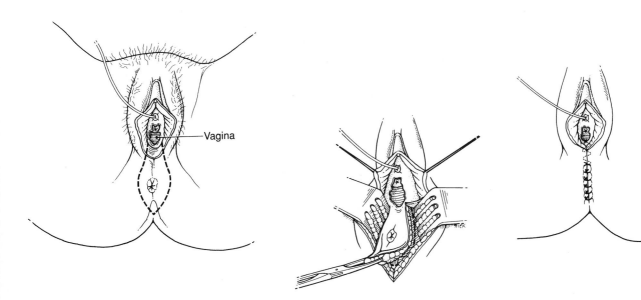

Modification of Abdominopelvic Resection for Female Patients (Fig. 75.5)

Technical Points

Abdominopelvic resection in the female patient is performed in essentially the same way as in the male patient. The only exception is that the posterior wall of the vagina is commonly resected with the specimen. This allows a better margin of the tumor to be obtained. Dissection in the rectovaginal septum is difficult and bloody, and a considerable amount of the posterior vaginal wall can be removed without compromising the vaginal lumen. As dissection progresses in the perineal region, a tongue of posterior vaginal wall is excised as part of the initial skin incision. The extent of this tongue depends on the location of the tumor, but commonly it will go back 5 to 10 cm. After resection of the specimen, the vaginal epithelium is closed with a subcuticular suture of 3-0 Vicryl, and the soft tissues are approximated in the normal fashion.

Anatomic Points

The primary anatomic difference that is pertinent to the abdominal phase of this operation in the female patient is the interposition of the vagina and uterus between the rectum and bladder. In the female patient, a rectouterine pouch (of Douglas), not a rectovesical pouch, is the lowest extent of the peritoneal cavity. In addition, a homologue to the rectovesical fascia (of Denonvilliers) is less easily demonstrated in female patients, although a cleavage plane between the rectum and posterior vaginal wall can be developed. Finally, complications can occur if one does not keep in mind that the uterine artery, a branch of the internal iliac artery (or one of its branches), passes forward, medially, and downward along the lateral wall in close proximity to the uterus. In the base of the broad ligament, lateral to the cervix, it turns medially, crossing the ureter close to the uterus. In this part of its course, it is bound to the lateral cervical ligament, contributing to this ligament's apex.

In the perineal phase of this operation, removal of part of the vaginal wall with the anorectal specimen necessitates removal of the perineal body, the more medial part of the superficial transverse perineal muscle, and a posteromedial part of the urogenital diaphragm. As in the male patient, major neurovascular structures are avoided by division of the perineal structures close to the midline.

REFERENCES

1. Cherry DA, Rothenberger DA. Pelvic floor physiology. *Surg Clin North Am* 1988;68:1217.
2. Dehni N, Schlegel RD, Cunningham C, et al. Influence of a defunctioning stoma on leakage rates after low colorectal anastomosis and colonic J pouch-anal anastomosis. *Br J Surg* 1998;85:1114–1117. (Confirms protective value of defunctionalizing stoma for extremely low anastomoses.)
3. Enker WE, Merchant N, Cohen AM, et al. Safety and efficacy of low anterior resection for rectal cancer: 681 consecutive cases from a specialty service. *Ann Surg* 1999;230:544–554.
4. Fazio VW, O'Riordain MG, Lavery IC, et al. Long-term functional outcome and quality of life after stapled restorative proctocolectomy. *Ann Surg* 1999;230:575–584.
5. Ger R. Surgical anatomy of the pelvis. *Surg Clin North Am* 1988;68:1201. (Provides good description of anatomy and physiology along with surgical considerations.)
6. Localio SA, Eng K, Coppa GF. Anorectal, presacral and sacral tumors: anatomy, physiology, pathogenesis and management. Philadelphia: WB Saunders, 1987. (Provides excellent discussion of transsacral approach.)
7. McCourtney JS, Finlay IG. Totally stapled restorative proctocolectomy. *Br J Surg* 1997;84:808–812.
8. Michelassi F, Hurst R. Restorative proctocolectomy with J-pouch ilioanal anastomosis. *Arch Surg* 2000;135:347–353.
9. Parks AG, Nicholls RJ, Belliveau P. Proctocolectomy with ileal reservoir and anal anastomosis. *Br J Surg* 1980;67:533.
10. Rothenberger DA, Vermeulen FD, Christenson CE, et al. Restorative proctocolectomy with ileal reservoir and ileoanal anastomosis. *Am J Surg* 1983;145:82. (Describes ileoanal anastomosis.)
11. Schoetz DJ. Complications of surgical excision of the rectum. *Surg Clin North Am* 1991;71:1271. (Presents good description of problems and management as well as strategies to avoid.)
12. Thompson-Fawcett MW, Warren BF, Mortensen NJ. A new look at the anal transitional zone with reference to restorative proctocolectomy and the columnar cuff. *Br J Surg* 1998;85:1517–1521.
13. Vignali A, Fazio VW, Lavery IC, et al. Factors associated with the occurrence of leaks in stapled rectal anastomoses: a review of 1,014 patients. *J Am Coll Surg* 1997;185:105–113.
14. Wong WD, Rothenberger DA, Goldberg SM. Ileoanal pouch procedures. *Curr Probl Surg* 1985;22:1.
15. Zaheer S, Pemberton JH, Farouk R, et al. Surgical treatment of adenocarcinoma of the rectum. *Ann Surg* 1998;227:800–811. (Advocates wide excision of mesorectum for tumor control.)

CHAPTER 76

Laparoscopic Low Anterior and Abdominoperineal Resection

Adam J. Dinnewitzer and Steven D. Wexner

Indications for laparoscopic colorectal surgery do not differ from those for open procedures. The only difference should be the method of access. As in open procedures, laparoscopic abdominoperineal resection is appropriate only for carcinomas that invade the anal sphincter or that are so close to the sphincter that a clamp or a stapler cannot be placed 2 cm or more to the distal edge of the tumor. Laparoscopic low anterior resection is appropriate for cancers in the mid (5 to 10 cm from the dentate line) or low rectum (less than 5 cm from the dentate line); in these cases, a total mesorectal excision with a coloanal anastomosis should be performed.

Preoperative evaluation, mechanical and antibiotic bowel preparation, and thromboembolic prophylaxis are also identical to those measures employed for open procedures. Preoperatively, an enterostomal therapist selects and marks the preferred site for a temporary or permanent stoma.

Unlike laparoscopy for benign disease, the benefits of laparoscopy for cancer have not yet been proved. Therefore, laparoscopic surgery for curative resection of rectal cancers should be done only in the context of a peer-reviewed externally monitored prospective randomized trial.

In this chapter, we describe both laparoscopic low anterior resection and laparoscopic abdominoperineal resection; use of a coloanal anastomosis as the intraabdominal component of the procedure is identical in both. Regardless of the procedure and technique, performance of a total mesorectal excision is of paramount importance in the cure of tumors in the lower two thirds of the rectum.

Laparoscopic Low Anterior Resection

Preoperative Setup and Trocar Placement (Fig. 76.1)

Technical Points

Place the patient in a modified lithotomy position with the hips and knees gently flexed at a maximum 15-degree angle. Greater elevation of the thighs may not allow the surgeon to move the instruments freely. The buttocks should extend slightly over the end of the operating table. This position gives proper access to the anus for endoscopy and insertion of a circular stapling device and also allows access to the

perineal region in case of abdominoperineal resection. Place the right arm of the patient alongside the trunk (rather than out on an armboard) to allow room for the surgeon and second assistant, who stand on the right side of the patient. Place an orogastric tube and a urinary catheter to minimize the risk for gastric or bladder injury, respectively, during trocar insertion. Prepare and drape the abdomen and perineal region for an open procedure for the eventuality that the laparoscopic procedure cannot be safely completed. The surgeon stands on the right side of the patient, the first assistant surgeon on the left, and the second assistant, who controls the camera, to the left of the surgeon.

A CO_2 pneumoperitoneum of 12 to 15 mm Hg is established in the usual fashion, through a small vertical infraumbilical incision. A 0- or 30-degree laparoscope is then introduced, and the abdomen is thoroughly explored to assess other pathology and to determine any metastatic dissemination. To inspect the liver, the patient is brought into a steep reverse Trendelenburg position; if the technology is available, a laparoscopic ultrasound of the liver should be performed.

If the proposed operation is deemed feasible, the other ports will be positioned. The operation is facilitated by the camera and the instruments being interchangeable to all ports. For this reason, only 10- to 12-mm trocars are used; three operating port sites are usually sufficient. Place the additional trocars under direct endoscopic visualization in the right lower quadrant and at the level of the umbilicus, both along the right midclavicular line. Another port is inserted in either the left midclavicular line, also at the level of the umbilicus, or in the right upper quadrant in the midclavicular line. The port positioning takes into account the patient's anatomy, the location of the incision for specimen retrieval, and the site of any planned stoma.

The following additional instruments are required:

- Four 10- to 12-mm trocars with reducer caps
- Ultrasonic scalpel
- One 10-mm bowel clamp
- Two 10-mm Babcock graspers
- Both 30- and 45-mm endoscopic linear cutting staplers
- A 29-mm or 33-mm endoscopic curved intraluminal stapler

FIGURE 76.1
PREOPERATIVE SETUP AND TROCAR PLACEMENT

Second
assistant

First assistant

Surgeon

Monitor, irrigation
suction system

Electrosurgical unit

Monitor, light
source, VCR,
Camera System,
CO_2 insufflator

- A 75-mm linear cutting stapler
- A 5-inch plastic wound protector

Mobilizing the Sigmoid and Descending Colon (Fig. 76.2)

Technical Points

Place the patient in a steep Trendelenburg position with the table tilted to the right side so that the small bowel gravitates toward the right upper quadrant of the abdomen and no retraction to the small bowel is required. Gently grasp the sigmoid colon with a Babcock clamp through the right paraumbilical port and move the bowel to the patient's right side. This maneuver places traction on the posterior peritoneum overlying the iliac vessels. Incise the peritoneum with the ultrasonic scalpel placed through the right lower quadrant port. Sequentially slide the ultrasonic scalpel under the peritoneum, and advance it down the pelvic sidewall toward the anterior peritoneal reflection, using it to push the mesorectum and mesosigmoid medially away from retroperitoneal structures. Identify the ureter as it crosses the iliac vessels and trace it proximally as far as possible. Continue this separation of the sigmoid colon from the lateral wall

cephalad along the descending colon until the splenic flexure is reached.

Anatomic Points

The abdominal and pelvic part of the ureter lies in extraperitoneal areolar tissue. The abdominal part, which descends on the medial part of the psoas major muscle, enters the lesser pelvis anterior to either the end of the common or the beginning of the external iliac vessels. The left ureter lies beneath the root of the sigmoid mesocolon. The right ureter lies behind the lower part of the mesentery and the terminal ileum. In the pelvis, the ureter is anterior to the internal iliac artery and covered by the parietal endopelvic fascia. Laterally, it lies on the fascia of the musculus obturator internus. In males, the ureters pass between the internal iliac vessels and the ascending vas deferens. Then they turn anteriorly, pass along the levator ani, and penetrate the base of the bladder in front of the seminal vesicles. In females, the pelvic part at first has the same relations as in males, but anteriorly to the ureters lay the ovaries. At the pelvic floor, the ureter turns anteriorly on the levator ani, turns forward slightly above the lateral vaginal fornix, and then inclines medially to reach the bladder.

FIGURE 76.2
MOBILIZING THE SIGMOID AND DESCENDING COLON

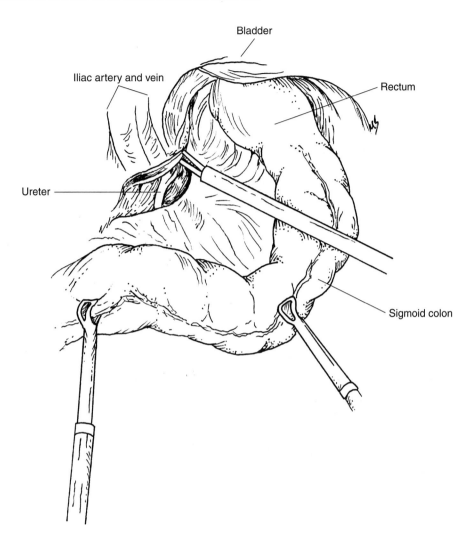

Mobilizing the Splenic Flexure (Fig. 76.3)

Technical Points

Place the patient in a steep reverse Trendelenburg position. This allows the transverse colon and viscera to fall away from the spleen and stomach. While the assistant retracts the splenic flexure toward the umbilicus with the Babcock clamp, separate the mesentery of the descending colon from Gerota's fascia until the splenic flexure is reached.

Next, approach the splenic flexure along the transverse colon. Displace the greater omentum toward the stomach and retract the transverse colon caudad to expose the avascular plane between the omentum and the transverse colon. Incise this avascular plane with the ultrasonic scalpel to enter the lesser sac and continue the dissection until the splenocolic ligament is completely divided. The sigmoid colon, the descending colon, and the transverse colon have now been fully mobilized to the midline.

Anatomic Points

Several structures must be divided to mobilize the splenic flexure. The splenic flexure is attached to the diaphragm and to the spleen. The phrenicocolic ligament is beneath the lower pole of the spleen. The ligament between the lower pole of the spleen and the splenic flexure is called the *splenocolic ligament*. For full mobilization, the greater omentum must be separated from the transverse colon in the vicinity of the splenic flexure. For this, the plane between the greater omentum and the colon must be divided to enter the lesser sac.

Division of the Inferior Mesenteric Vessels (Fig. 76.4)

Technical Points

To dissect the inferior mesenteric vessels, place the patient in the Trendelenburg position. The inferior mesenteric artery

FIGURE 76.3
MOBILIZING THE SPLENIC FLEXURE

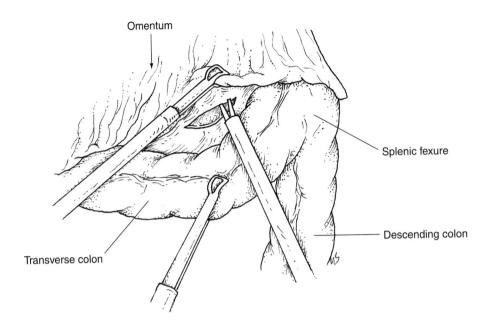

Omentum

Splenic fexure

Descending colon

Transverse colon

will be divided at its origin from the aorta. This allows complete mobilization of the left colon for a tension-free coloanal anastomosis. Additional dissection must be performed on the right side of the mesocolon. The assistant surgeon grasps the proximal sigmoid colon and reflects the colon toward the left side, causing tension on the peritoneum along the right side. Divide the peritoneum using the ultrasonic scalpel. Continue this division vertically toward the pelvis and proximally toward the root of the mesentery. Create a window between the inferior mesenteric artery and the aortic bifurcation. Follow

FIGURE 76.4
DIVISION OF THE INFERIOR MESENTERIC VESSELS

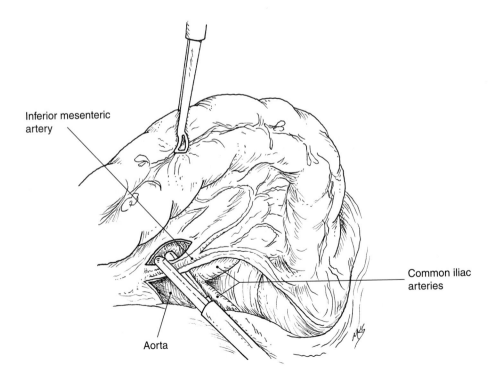

Inferior mesenteric
artery

Common iliac
arteries

Aorta

this dissection plane cephalad to the origin of the inferior mesenteric artery.

Identify and traverse the avascular window cephalad to the origin of the inferior mesenteric artery. The ideal point of transection is about 1 cm distal to the aorta to avoid injury to the sympathetic nerves. These nerves can usually be visualized through the developed window. Insert a vascular stapling device and position it at the level of the planned transection. Visualize the ureter and ensure that no extraneous tissue is enclosed within the jaws of the stapler. Fire the stapler to secure and divide the artery. The vein is usually divided at the tail of the pancreas. Additional mobility can be gained from dividing the mesocolon from the inferior mesenteric artery stump to the root of the middle colic vessels.

Anatomic Points

The inferior mesenteric artery originates from the ventral aorta at the level of L-3. The artery courses to the left and provides vessels to the left part of the transverse, descending, and sigmoid colon. The left colic artery, which is the first branch of the inferior mesentery artery, joins the middle colic artery, which arises from the superior mesenteric artery. These collateral vessels between the superior and the inferior mesenteric arteries supply the splenic flexure. The superior rectal artery is the terminal branch of the inferior mesenteric artery and supplies the rectum.

Similarly, the venous drainage of the rectum is to the inferior mesenteric vein. The lymphatic drainage of the rectum is to nodes in the mesorectum, and then to nodes along the superior rectal and ultimately, the inferior mesenteric artery.

FIGURE 76.5
PERITONEAL INCISION AND INITIAL MOBILIZATION OF THE RECTUM

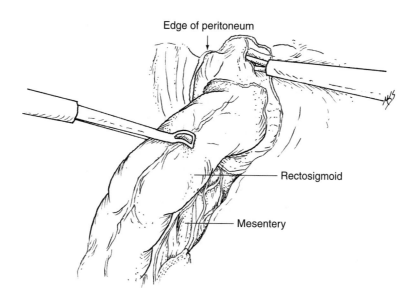

Edge of peritoneum

Rectosigmoid

Mesentery

Peritoneal Incision and Initial Mobilization of the Rectum (Fig. 76.5)

Technical Points

Attention is now turned to the rectum and pelvic dissection. In female patients, the uterus and adnexa need to be elevated to facilitate the subsequent steps. For this purpose, introduce a suture with a straight needle through the abdominal wall one fingerbreadth above the pubis. Then pass the needle through the broad ligament on the right side, turn it 180 degrees, and pass it through the broad ligament on the left side. Again pass the needle through the abdominal wall to the anterior abdominal surface. Draw the uterus and adnexa up to the abdominal wall and secure them in place by pulling the suture taut and clipping the ends with two Mosquito clamps. Alternatively, a

Babcock clamp can be used to elevate the uterus through the abdomen or a uterine sound to perform transvaginal elevation.

Gently grasp the rectum as distal as possible by alternatively carefully grasping, retracting, and then repositioning the clamps. Ultimately, the rectum is retracted cephalad and anteriorly. Using the ultrasonic scalpel, extend the peritoneal incisions on the left and right sides caudally and then join these incisions transversely at the peritoneal reflection. Identify the right ureter as it crosses the iliac vessels. Divide the lateral attachments with the ultrasonic scalpel in the avascular plane along the internal iliac vessels.

Anatomic Points

The mesorectum, derived from the dorsal mesentery, is the

visceral mesentery surrounding the rectum. For total mesorectal excision, the dissection is performed along the presacral fascia, a thickened part of the parietal endopelvic fascia, without violation of the smooth outer surface of the mesorectum, which is covered by a thin layer of visceral fascia. The presacral fascia covers the concavity of the sacrum and coccyx, hypogastric nerves, median sacral artery, and presacral veins. The middle sacral artery originates from the posterior side of the aorta, just proximal to its bifurcation into the common iliac arteries, and it supplies the posterior wall of the anorectal junction and of the anal canal. The presacral veins are avalvular and communicate with the internal vertebral venous system. Bleeding from these veins is difficult to control: the veins partly retract into the sacral foramina and remain open because their adventitia is fused to the sacral periosteum at the opening of the foramina. Sacral thumbtacks are generally the best way to control such hemorrhage.

The anterior aspect of the midrectum is covered by Denonvilliers' fascia and is situated behind the seminal vesicles in males and behind the vaginal wall in females. Denonvilliers' fascia arises from the fusion of the two walls of the embryologic peritoneal cul-de-sac and reaches from the deepest point of the rectovesical or rectovaginal pouch to the pelvic floor.

FIGURE 76.6
COMPLETION OF RECTAL MOBILIZATION

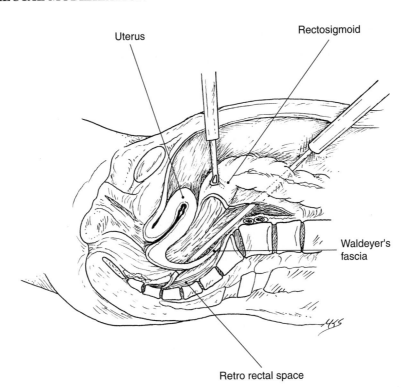

Completion of Rectal Mobilization (Fig. 76.6)

Technical and Anatomic Points

The assistant surgeon carefully grasps the rectosigmoid above the sacral promontory and provides anterior and left lateral traction. Undertake dissection with the ultrasonic scalpel close to the posterior aspect of the superior rectal artery as it crosses the pelvic brim and nears the rectal wall, thereby avoiding damage to the left hypogastric nerves. This dissection at the promontory of the sacrum behind the superior rectal artery exposes the fascia propria of the rectum in front and the presacral fascia with the superior hypogastric plexus behind. Perform the dissection along the presacral fascia using the ultrasonic scalpel while the rectum is retracted cephalad and anteriorly. An intact presacral fascia and an encapsulated mesorectum ensure that there will be no sacral venous hemorrhage. Divide the rectosacral fascia (Waldeyer's fascia), which fuses the parietal and visceral fascia, and continue the dissection until the levator muscles have been identified.

Follow this plane laterally. No significant nerves or vessels should cross this space.

Finally, mobilize the anterior rectum. The bladder is retracted anteriorly, and the plane between the prostate (or vagina) and the rectum is entered. The dissection is performed between Denonvilliers' fascia and the prostate and seminal vesicles in a caudad direction. The seminal vesicles can clearly be seen attached to the bladder. In female patients, the anterior mesorectum is less substantial, and Denonvilliers' fascia is less obvious. The dissection is undertaken between Denonvilliers' fascia and the posterior vaginal wall. Proper dissection is along the areolar plane between the anterior rectal and posterior vaginal walls. The rectum and

FIGURE 76.7
RECTAL EXCISION AND ANASTOMOSIS

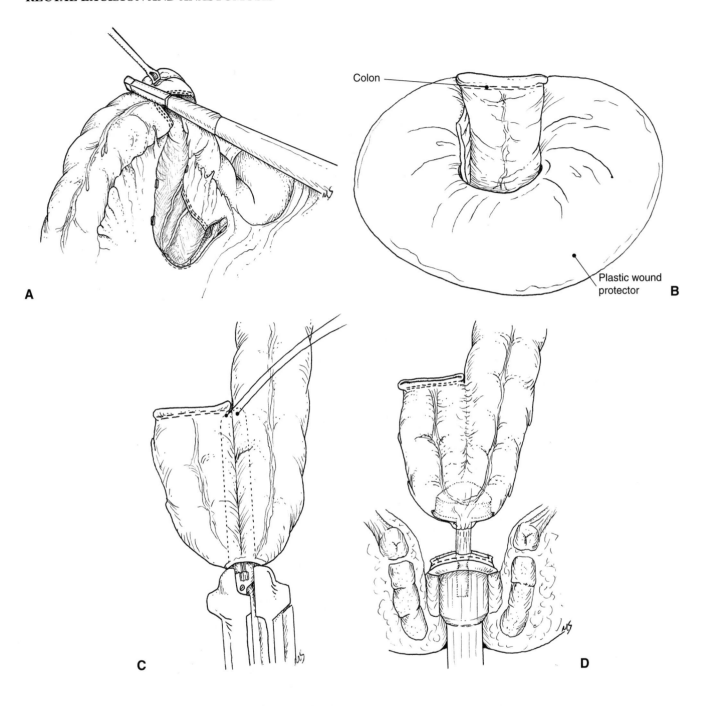

A

B

Colon

Plastic wound protector

C

D

mesorectum have now been fully mobilized all around, and the rectum is ready for transection.

Rectal Excision and Anastomosis (Fig. 76.7)

Technical and Anatomic Points

The most important part of laparoscopic rectal extirpation is to ensure that cure of the patient is not being jeopardized. Both long-term survival and local recurrence must be considered. Accordingly, all the steps outlined thus far are paramount to this goal and include high ligation of the inferior mesenteric artery and vein to ensure a tension-free anastomosis, total mesorectal excision, and wide lateral dissection without any clamping, suturing, or ligation of residual lateral pelvic sidewall tissue. Lateral tissue that remains may harbor mesorectal deposits of tumor. However, in addition to all of these steps, it is now incumbent on the surgeon to ensure that a minimum of a 2-cm tumor-free distal margin can be obtained in the fresh unfixed, unpinned state.

Place a noncrushing clamp across the rectum at least 2 cm distal to the lower extent of the tumor. Then pass a Babcock clamp through either the left paramedian (if placed) port or the right upper quadrant. Close the noncrushing clamp and irrigate the rectum. Insert a 30- or 45-mm laparoscopic linear cutting stapling device through the right iliac fossa port, and place it in a perpendicular position (Fig. 76.7A). Retraction in a cephalad direction with the noncrushing clamp below the tumor concurrent with cephalad pushing of the perineum by the perineal assistant can facilitate this maneuver. However, two stapler firings are often necessary.

Remove the left or right lower quadrant port and lengthen the incision to 5 cm, or the diameter of the tumor. Protect the incision by a plastic sleeve (wound protector) to avoid tumor cell implantation, and exteriorize the specimen (Fig. 76.7B). Excise the rectum and sigmoid colon to the sigmoid-descending junction and create a colonic J pouch using a 75-mm linear cutting stapler (Fig. 77.7C). Place a pursestring suture to secure the anvil of the circular stapler into the lumen (Fig. 76.7D). Return the colon into the abdominal cavity and close the incision.

If a 2-cm margin cannot be safely ensured, either an alternate procedure, as described later, or conversion to laparotomy should be undertaken. It would also not be considered appropriate to convert the procedure to an abdominoperineal resection because of an inadequate laparoscopic margin.

If the stapler or staplers can be safely applied to obtain an acceptable tumor-free distal margin, make a 4-cm long Pfannenstiel incision to introduce the jaws of the Proximate Access 55 stapler (Ethicon Endosurgery Inc., Cincinnati, OH). Reestablish pneumoperitoneum by closing the fascia with sutures. Place a pursestring suture around the flexible portion of the shaft of the stapler. Under direct vision, place the stapler jaws around the rectum at the level of the plane of the levator ani muscle. This procedure can be facilitated by pushing the perineum from the outside. Once the correct position is obtained, fire the stapler. Introduce the Endoscopic

Linear Cutter (Ethicon Endosurgery Inc., Cincinnati, OH) 60-mm stapler from the lateral trocar and use it to staple and divide the rectum proximally to the previously applied staple line. The portion of rectum between the two suture lines is divided and removed. After removing the sutures and the pursestring suture holding the stapler shaft, open the jaws of the Proximate Access 55 and remove the stapler. Protect the wound with a plastic sleeve and then exteriorize the rectum and sigmoid colon through the Pfannenstiel incision. Excise the rectum and part of the sigmoid colon and create a colonic J pouch using the 75-mm linear cutter. Place a pursestring suture to secure the anvil of the circular stapler into the lumen. Return the colon into the abdominal cavity and close the incision.

Reinsufflate the abdomen and introduce the circular stapler transanally so that the trocar pierces the stapled stump near the center of the stapler line. Grasp the anvil with the anvil-grasping clamp and connect the anvil with the trocar. Close the stapler under direct vision and fire it. Gently remove stapler and assess the donuts for completeness.

Place the patient in a reverse Trendelenburg position. Fill the pelvis with saline and test the anastomosis by insufflating air into the anus with the descending colon occluded by a clamp. If there is no leak, aspirate the irrigation fluid. Alternatively, instead of insufflating air through a bulb syringe, perform rigid or flexible endoscopy to assess the mucosa of the pouch and visualize the staple line to ensure hemostasis.

Creation of A Loop Ileostomy (Fig. 76.8)

Technical and Anatomic Points

Introduce a Babcock clamp into the right lower quadrant port. Select the most distal portion of the ileum that reaches the anterior abdominal wall without tension for creation of a loop ileostomy. Gently grasp the bowel with the Babcock clamp and draw bowel and trocar out as a unit. To facilitate passage of the loop of ileum, incise the fascia in a vertical direction. Once the ileum is exteriorized, partially reestablish pneumoperitoneum and verify hemostasis. Insert a drain through one of the other ports and direct it in the pelvis. Remove all ports under direct laparoscopic vision, release pneumoperitoneum, and mature the stoma.

Laparoscopic Abdominoperineal Resection

Modification for Abdominoperineal Resection (Fig. 76.9)

Technical and Anatomic Points

The abdominal phase of abdominoperineal resection is identical to that of a low anterior resection. After mobilizing the left and sigmoid colon and rectum, circumferentially clear the fat from the bowel at the level of the sigmoid descending junction. Divide the bowel with the linear stapling device.

Once the laparoscopic dissection is completed, begin the perineal phase of the operation in the standard manner.

FIGURE 76.8
CREATION OF A LOOP ILEOSTOMY

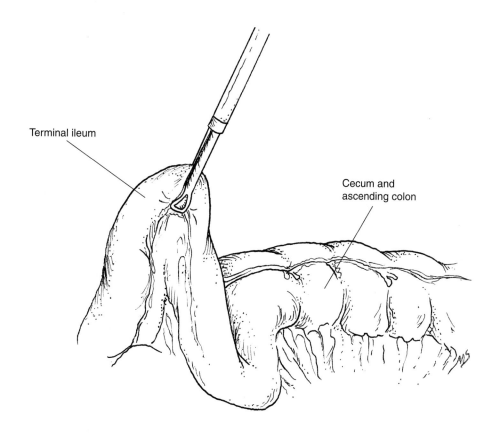

Terminal ileum

Cecum and
ascending colon

FIGURE 76.9
MODIFICATION FOR ABDOMINOPERINEAL RESECTION

Remove the specimen through the perineal wound. Close the perineal wound, leaving one suture untied. Introduce a closed Babcock clamp through this small opening into the abdominal cavity. Approximate the skin by crossing the suture ends, and reestablish pneumoperitoneum. Under laparoscopic view, guide the closed instrument into the right trocar sleeve. When the tip of the Babcock clamp is outside the abdominal wall, gently remove the trocar. Use the Babcock to grasp the distal end of the drain and withdraw it into the abdominal cavity. Clamp the proximal part of the drain to prevent gas leakage. Position the drain under direct vision. Assess the abdomen and pelvis for hemostasis and completely close the perineal wound. Desufflate the abdomen and deliver the colon out through the left port site after incising the fascia. Fashion an end-colostomy.

It is important to emphasize that laparoscopic proctectomy may be one the most difficult laparoscopic colorectal procedures. As such, the reported conversion rates in the literature certainly exceed the rates reported for other types of laparoscopic colorectal operations for other indications. At all steps, the surgeon should have a low threshold to convert to laparotomy and the patient should have been preoperatively apprised of the possibility of a laparotomy. Conversion to a laparotomy should be deemed prudent rather than regarded as a failure. Basically, there are two types of conversion: reactive and preemptive. Preemptive conversions occur when dense adhesions, obesity, bleeding, or unclear anatomy precludes the continuation of the operation in a timely, safe, and efficient manner. In this instance, the surgeon may try alternative maneuvers to improve the progress of the operation; if unsuccessful, however, conversion to a laparotomy may be in the patient's best interest. Conversely, the reactive conversion occurs when a problem such as massive hemorrhage, bowel perforation, ureteric transection, or tumor cell spillage has occurred. Patients who undergo preemptive conversion have outcomes that are quite favorable; however, not surprisingly, patients who have undergone reactive conversion do not fare as well.

Whether the procedure is performed as an anterior resection or abdominoperineal resection, and whether by laparotomy or laparoscopy, the patient's outcome and safety rather than the ability to complete a certain procedure by a certain technique must prevail. If the surgeon routinely adheres to this precept, the outcome should always be optimal.

REFERENCES

1. Ballantyne GH, Leahy PF, Modlin IM. *Laparoscopic surgery.* Philadelphia: WB Saunders, 1994.
2. Beck DE, Wexner SD. *Fundamentals of anorectal surgery.* 2nd ed. London: WB Saunders, 1998.
3. Brune IB. *Laparo-endoscopic surgery.* 2nd ed. Berlin: Blackwell, 1996.
4. Milsom JW, Boehm B. *Laparoscopic colorectal surgery.* New York: Springer, 1996.
5. Phillips EH, Rosenthal RJ. *Operative strategies in laparoscopic surgery.* Heidelberg: Springer, 1995.
6. Wexner SD. *Laparoscopic colorectal surgery.* New York: Wiley-Liss, 1999.
7. Wind GG. *Applied laparoscopic anatomy: abdomen and pelvis.* Baltimore: Williams & Wilkins, 1997.

CHAPTER 77

Total Abdominal Hysterectomy and Oophorectomy

Hysterectomy may be performed transabdominally or vaginally. One or both ovaries may be removed with the uterus. In this chapter, total abdominal hysterectomy with bilateral salpingo-oophorectomy is described. Modification of the technique to preserve one or both ovaries is also discussed. Chapter 78 provides an introduction to laparoscopic surgery of the female pelvis.

Incision and Initial Exposure (Fig. 77.1)

Technical Points

Position the patient in a dorsal lithotomy position. Empty the bladder by straight catheterization or by placing an indwelling Foley catheter. Once general anesthesia has been administered, perform a pelvic examination to confirm the anatomy. A Trendelenburg position of about 15 degrees will facilitate pelvic exposure.

Total abdominal hysterectomy may be performed through a lower midline incision. However, the more cosmetically appealing Pfannenstiel incision is described here.

Make a transverse incision in the natural skin crease where the skin incision will be hidden by regrowth of pubic hair. Make the incision about 10 to 15 cm long, depending on the habitus of the patient. Carry this incision through skin and subcutaneous tissue to the underlying rectus sheath. Incise the anterior rectus sheath in line with the skin incision. Develop flaps between the anterior rectus sheath and the underlying rectus muscle until the muscle is exposed well in the midline to about the level of the umbilicus. Retract the rectus

muscles laterally to expose the midline fascia and underlying peritoneum. Incise the fascia and peritoneum vertically from the umbilicus to the pubis. Identify the bladder in the inferior aspect of the incision and gently retract it downward, out of harm's way. Exposure through this incision is quite limited. Use it only when you do not anticipate a need for access to the upper abdomen.

Anatomic Points

The infraumbilical vertical midline incision exposes a very narrow linea alba, from which fibers of the rectus abdominis muscle originate and upon which the more anterior pyramidalis muscle inserts; this makes a true midline incision technically difficult. If the exact midline is not divided, then this becomes a muscle-splitting incision through the pyramidalis and rectus abdominis muscles. Surgically, the posterior rectus sheath ends approximately halfway between the umbilicus and pubis, at the arcuate line. Inferior to this line, the posterior surface of the rectus abdominis muscle is in contact with the transversalis fascia.

The Pfannenstiel incision, a transverse incision in the infraspinous crease, follows Langer's lines and is low enough (about 5 cm superior to the pubic symphysis) to allow the scar to be hidden by pubic hair. Retraction of the rectus sheath superiorly and inferiorly may necessitate sharp dissection because one or more infraumbilical tendinous inscriptions (where the sheath becomes adherent to the rectus muscle) may be present. When the linea alba is split vertically, caution should be used to avoid the deeper urinary bladder and

LIST OF STRUCTURES

Uterus
  Cervix
Vagina
Fallopian (uterine) tubes
Ovaries
Round ligament
Broad ligament
Suspensory (infundibulopelvic)
  ligament
Ovarian ligament

Lateral cervical (cardinal) ligament
Uterosacral ligament
Bladder
Ureter
Urachus
Vesicouterine pouch (anterior
  cul-de-sac)
Rectouterine pouch (posterior
  cul-de-sac, pouch of Douglas)
Rectovaginal fascia

Internal iliac artery
Uterine artery
  Tubal branch
  Ovarian branch
Ovarian artery
Rectus abdominis muscle
Anterior rectus sheath
Linea alba
Pyramidalis muscle
Transversalis fascia

FIGURE 77.1
INCISION AND INITIAL EXPOSURE

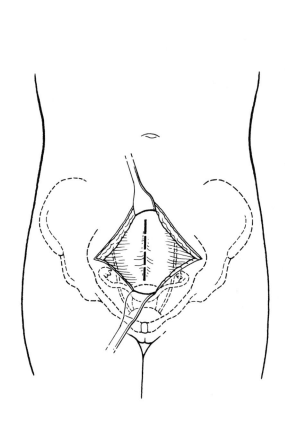

the urachus. The latter is usually entirely fibrotic but can retain a partially patent lumen in continuity with the lumen of the urinary bladder; this has been reported to occur in as many as 33% of the cases.

The uterus is positioned between the urinary bladder and rectum. Both the uterus and the uterine tubes are invested by the broad ligament, an expression of peritoneum. Normally, the uterus is anteverted so that the fundus lies superior to the urinary bladder. Between the uterus and bladder is a shallow recess, the vesicouterine pouch or anterior cul-de-sac, whereas posterior to the uterus, between it and the rectum, is the much deeper rectouterine pouch (of Douglas), or posterior cul-de-sac.

Immediately inferior to the junction of the uterine tube and uterus, and causing a fold on the anterior leaf of the broad ligament, is the round ligament of the uterus. The lower homologue of the gubernaculum testis, it runs lateral to the deep inguinal ring, where it enters the inguinal canal; it then exits the superficial inguinal ring and finally blends with the connective tissue of the labium majus.

The peritoneal layers of the broad ligament are closest along its uterine attachment. As one progresses inferolaterally, the anterior and posterior leaves diverge to become continuous with peritoneum of the vesicouterine pouch and rectouterine pouch, respectively. In the lower part of the broad ligament are the ureter and uterine artery, both of which must be clearly distinguished.

Division of the Round Ligaments and Development of Pelvic Dissection (Fig. 77.2)

Technical Points

Place Kelly clamps on the uterine fundus on each side and use these to provide upward traction. Divide the round ligaments between clamps and secure the ends with suture ligatures of heavy chromic. Incise the peritoneum along the anterior and posterior surfaces of the broad ligament. If the uterine tube and ovary are to be removed with the uterus, incise the broad ligament lateral to the tube and ovary, retracting these structures medially with the uterus. If an ovary is to be spared, the uterine tube and ovarian ligament must be divided. Pass a finger behind the tube and ovary, elevating these structures with the ovarian ligament, away from the broad ligament. Clamp and suture-ligate this pedicle of tissue. Allow the ovary and distal uterine tube to retract laterally, and continue the dissection.

FIGURE 77.2
DIVISION OF THE ROUND LIGAMENTS AND DEVELOPMENT OF PELVIC DISSECTION

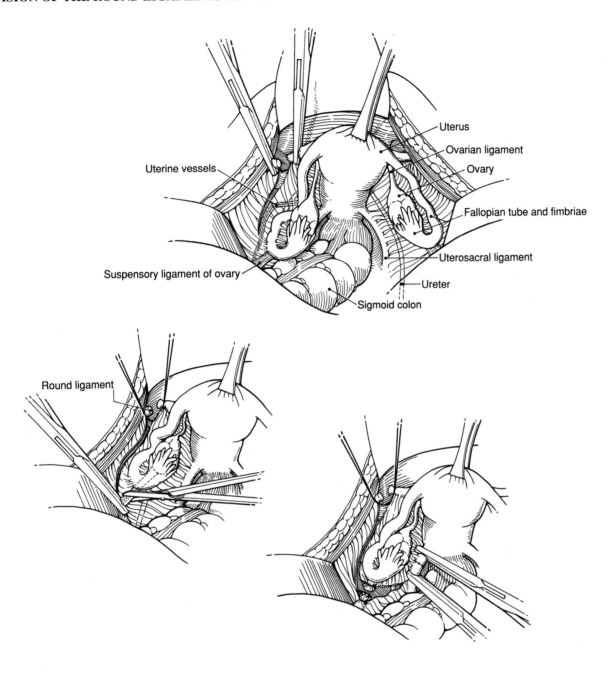

Identify the ureter on each side where it crosses the common iliac vessels at the bifurcation. As the dissection is carried down parallel to the cervix, the uterine vessels will be encountered at the isthmus of the uterus. Secure these with Heaney clamps and divide them. Skeletonize these vascular pedicles so that they can be securely divided and secured with suture-ligatures.

Place retractors to expose the bladder and the anterior cul-de-sac. Continue the anterior incision of the broad ligament across the peritoneum overlying the bladder. By sharp and blunt dissection, develop the flap of bladder and free this from the underlying uterus and cervix.

Anatomic Points

The uterine tubes, which occupy the superior free edge of the broad ligament curve, pass laterally from the body of the uterus, loop superiorly over the ovary, and then curve downward and posteriorly to allow the fimbriae to "embrace" the ovary. The suspensory ligaments run from the bend of the uterine tube to the lateral pelvic wall, transmitting the ovarian vessels. From the medial end of the ovary, and visible on the posterior surface of the broad ligament, the ovarian ligament runs from the ovary, between the two peritoneal layers of the broad ligament, to the lateral border of the uterus just inferior to the uterine tube. This fibrous cord is the upper homologue of the male gubernaculum testis. The angle made by the ovarian ligament and the uterine tube is quite acute.

Tubal and ovarian branches of the uterine artery are also located in the broad ligament close to both the uterine tube and the ovarian ligament. The ovarian branch has a functional anastomosis with the ovarian artery.

As the ureter crosses the iliac vessels, it is in close proximity to the more lateral suspensory ligament. Thus, incision of the peritoneum in this area should be done with some caution.

The origin of the uterine arteries is variable, although in all cases, it ultimately is derived from the internal iliac artery. From its origin, it courses inferomedially along the lateral pelvic wall in close proximity to the ureter. Lateral to the cervix of the uterus, this medially-directed artery crosses over the ureter to reach the lateral aspect of the uterus at the level of the uterine isthmus. Here, it divides into ascending and descending trunks that parallel the uterus and vagina and, through short branches, supply these organs. The ascending trunk has broad anastomoses with the ovarian artery. Typically, the point where the uterine artery crosses the ureter is about 1.5 to 2 cm lateral to the cervix, but this can be quite variable. Further, the oblique course of the ureter with respect to the uterine artery renders the two structures in contact or closely adjacent to each other for a distance of 1 to 2.5 cm. These two facts make a meticulous dissection of the uterine artery mandatory.

Completion of the Hysterectomy (Fig. 77.3)

Technical Points

Retract the uterus upward to expose the rectovaginal fascia. Incise the peritoneum overlying the uterosacral ligaments and free the vagina from the rectum, especially on the medial aspect of these ligaments. The rectovaginal fascia should dissect easily. Divide any remaining lateral attachments and secure them with suture ligatures. Palpate the cervix and divide the

FIGURE 77.3
COMPLETION OF THE HYSTERECTOMY

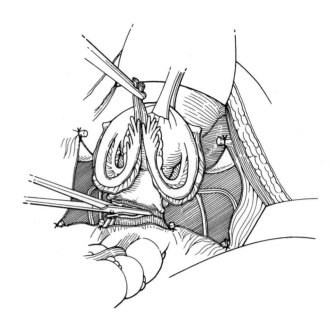

vagina just below the cervix. Place clamps on the two lateral corners of the vagina and suture-ligate them.

Anatomic Points

Between the anterior wall of the rectum and posterior wall of the vagina, the rectovaginal fascia extends from the peritoneum to the pelvic floor and laterally to the pelvic walls. This fascia, the homologue of the male rectovesical fascia, is attached, but separable, from the vagina; it is easily separable from the rectum. This fascia provides a plane of dissection between the rectum and the vagina.

The fibromuscular uterosacral ligaments—the more posterior and medial parts of the extraperitoneal pelvic supporting tissue—are broadly continuous with the lateral cervical

FIGURE 77.4
CLOSURE OF THE PERITONEUM

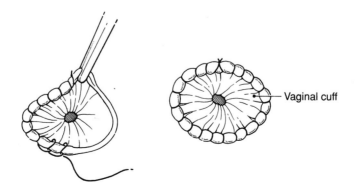

Vaginal cuff

or cardinal ligaments. The uterosacral ligaments attach to the cervix and upper vagina and, with a gentle lateral curve, course posteriorly to attach to the sacrum on either side of the rectum. They form the rectouterine folds (of Douglas), which are the lateral boundaries of the rectouterine pouch (of Douglas) or posterior cul-de-sac. The rectouterine folds contain smooth muscle, fibroelastic connective tissue, and neurovascular structures.

Closure of the Peritoneum (Fig. 77.4)

Technical and Anatomic Points

The vaginal cuff is commonly left open for drainage. Overrun the edge of the cuff with a running lock-stitch of absorbable suture to ensure hemostasis. Reperitonealize the pelvic floor with a running suture of 2-0 Vicryl. Close the abdominal incision in the usual fashion.

REFERENCES

1. Aslan P, Brooks A, Drummond M, et al. Incidence and management of gynaecological-related ureteric injuries. *Aust N Z J Obstet Gynaecol* 1999;39:178–181.
2. Bateman BG, Taylor PT Jr. Reproductive considerations during abdominal surgical procedures in young women. *Surg Clin North Am* 1991;71:1053. (Presents good review of conservative surgical options for ectopic pregnancy and ovarian cyst.)
3. Brubaker LT, Wilbanks GD. Urinary tract injuries in pelvic surgery. *Surg Clin North Am* 1991;71:963.
4. Daly JW, Higgins KA. Injury to the ureter during gynecologic surgical procedures. *Surg Gynecol Obstet* 1988;167:19.
5. Grainger DA, Soderstrom RM, Schiff SF, et al. Ureteral injuries at laparoscopy: insights into diagnosis, management, and prevention. *Obstet Gynecol* 1990;75:839.
6. Harkki-Siren P, Sjoberg J, Tiitinen A. Urinary tract injuries after hysterectomy. *Obstet Gynecol* 1998;92:113–118. (Risk for ureteral injury is higher with laparoscopic than with conventional hysterectomy.)
7. Masterson BJ. Selection of incisions for gynecologic procedures. *Surg Clin North Am* 1991;71:1041.
8. Radley S, Keighley MR, Radley SC, et al. Bowel dysfunction following hysterectomy. *Br J Obstet Gynaecol* 1999;106:1120–1125.
9. Summitt RL Jr. Laparoscopic-assisted vaginal hysterectomy: a review of usefulness and outcomes. *Clin Obstet Gynecol* 2000;43:584–593.

CHAPTER 78

Laparoscopic Surgery of the Female Pelvis

This chapter provides an introduction to the laparoscopic anatomy of the female pelvis and uses several simple procedures to illustrate that anatomy. Obviously, a single chapter cannot do full justice to an entire subspecialty, but basic information about these procedures and the relevant laparoscopic anatomy will be useful to the general surgeon. References at the end give further technical details of more advanced procedures.

The laparoscopic view of the pelvis (see the orientation figure) is similar to that obtained with the uterus elevated and retracted for transabdominal hysterectomy (see also Fig. 77.2). The round ligaments arch up and laterally to exit through the internal (deep) inguinal rings. The uterus lies between bladder (anterior) and rectosigmoid colon (posterior). The white color of the ovaries contrasts sharply with the pink color of the encircling fallopian tubes. Crossing the pelvic brim, the ureters, gonadal vessels, and round ligament (from posterior to anterior) are found. The right ureter is generally visible under the pelvic peritoneum as it crosses over the iliac vessels, and will vermiculate if touched. The left is generally hidden by overlying sigmoid colon and mesentery.

Orientation and Exposure of the Adnexal Structures (Fig. 78.1)

Technical Points

Position the patient supine with the legs in stirrups (Fig. 78.1A). Empty the urinary bladder by straight catheterization (for short procedures) or indwelling Foley catheter (for long procedures). Drape the perineum to provide access to the vagina. Manipulation of the cervix (upward pressure using a cervical retractor) will displace the pelvic viscera closer to the laparoscope or to one side or the other, facilitating visualization.

Identify the round ligaments, crossing over the pelvic brim to exit through the internal inguinal rings (Fig. 78.1B). The fallopian tubes are generally somewhat pinker than the round ligaments and lie beneath them. Note the ureters crossing medially over the iliac vessels and then passing obliquely under the ovarian vessels. When gently touched with a probe or closed grasper, the ureter will vermiculate under the peritoneum and can thus be positively identified.

To display the adnexal structures (ovary and fallopian tube) on one side and create a larger working space, use the cervical retractor to displace the uterus up out of the pelvis and over to the contralateral side. Alternatively, a probe passed gently under the uterus or adnexae can provide some exposure, generally of one adnexa at a time (Fig. 78.1C,D). Ovary and fallopian tubes lie between the round and infundibulopelvic ligaments.

Anatomic Points

The pelvic sidewall triangle (Fig. 78.1C) consists of the round ligament, the infundibulopelvic ligament, and the external iliac artery. The ureter enters the pelvis medial to this triangle. The right ureter is often visible under the peritoneum overlying the external iliac artery; the left ureter is frequently obscured by the overlying sigmoid colon or its mesentery.

LIST OF STRUCTURES

Uterus
  Cervix
Vagina
  Posterior fornix
Fallopian (uterine) tubes
Ovaries
Round ligament
Broad ligament

Suspensory (infundibulopelvic)
  ligament
Ovarian ligament
Lateral cervical (cardinal) ligament
Uterosacral ligament
Bladder
Ureter
Urachus

Vesicouterine pouch (anterior
  cul-de-sac)
Rectouterine pouch (posterior
  cul-de-sac, pouch of Douglas)
Internal iliac artery
Uterine artery
Ovarian (gonadal) artery

(From Wind GG. The pelvis. In: *Applied laparoscopic anatomy: abdomen and pelvis.* Baltimore: Williams & Wilkins, 1997:249–299, with permission.)

ORIENTATION

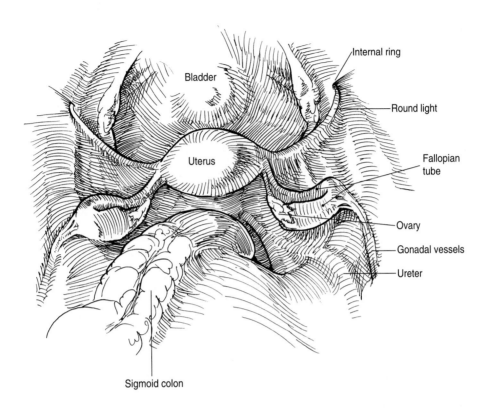

Laparoscopic Tubal Ligation (Fig. 78.2)

Technical Points

Identify the fallopian tubes. Elevate one with an atraumatic grasper. Numerous techniques for tubal ligation exist, none perfect. The simplest method uses a clip to occlude and gradually cut through the tubes. Place the clip on the tube and lock it closed. Repeat this on the other side.

Anatomic Points

As previously mentioned, it is imperative to differentiate round ligament from fallopian tubes. The round ligaments extend beyond the pelvic brim to the region of the internal inguinal ring. In contrast, the pinker fallopian tubes are initially less visible and terminate in the fimbriated regions, which are in close proximity to the ovaries.

Excision of Ovarian Cyst (Fig. 78.3)

Technical and Anatomic Points

Place secondary trocars lateral to the rectus sheaths as shown

(Fig. 78.3A). A small cyst may be excised with preservation of the ovary, particularly in a young woman. Define the plane between cyst and adjacent normal ovarian tissue and excise the cyst completely using ultrasonic shears or scissors with electrocautery (Fig. 78.3B). Take care not to puncture the cyst; dermoid cysts in particular contain material that may be highly irritating to the peritoneum. Place a small cyst in a retrieval bag and remove it through a trocar site. The defect in the ovary may be closed for hemostasis, as shown, or left open.

Salpingo-Oophorectomy (Fig. 78.4)

Technical Points

Salpingo-oophorectomy is performed by elevating the ovary to expose the infundibulopelvic ligament (Fig. 78.4A). Secure the contained gonadal (ovarian) vessels (Fig. 78.4B). Intervening peritoneal reflections between fallopian tube, ovary, and uterus must be divided and the fallopian tube secured at the uterine isthmus.

When a torsed gangrenous adnexa is encountered, a relatively slender pedicle can often be identified (or torsion would not have occurred). Thus, although in theory multiple structures must be divided, in practice, a torsed adnexa generally can be removed by simply dividing the twisted structures with an endoscopic cutting linear stapler (Fig. 78.4C) along the line shown.

Generally, the cyst will be too large to remove through a specimen retrieval pouch. Aspiration risks spillage of contents. Retrieval through a posterior culdotomy is a highly acceptable alternative. Place a moist sponge stick in the posterior fornix of the vagina and use it to elevate the posterior cul-de-sac into the operative field. Cut directly over the sponge stick with electrocautery or scissors.

Push the intact cyst down into the cul-de-sac and pop it through the culdotomy. Close the culdotomy through a vaginal (or laparoscopic) approach with 2-0 Vicryl sutures. Confirm hemostasis and close the trocar sites in the usual fashion.

Anatomic Points

The cul-de-sac (rectouterine recess) between the uterus and rectum is the deepest part of the female pelvis. Pelvic peritoneum is in close proximity to the posterior fornix of the vagina, allowing easy access from below.

Ectopic Pregnancy (Fig. 78.5)

Technical and Anatomic Points

Ectopic pregnancies commonly occur at the locations shown in Fig. 78.5A. Again, numerous options for management exist, but when an ectopic pregnancy is identified at laparoscopy, one option is salpingostomy with evacuation of the contents of the tube (Fig. 78.5B). The small incision is left unsutured.

FIGURE 78.1

ORIENTATION AND EXPOSURE OF THE ADNEXAL STRUCTURES (**A** from Apelgren KN, Cowan BD, Metcalf AM, et al. Laparoscopic appendectomy and the management of gynecologic pathologic conditions found at laparoscopy for presumed appendicitis. *Surg Clin North Am* 1996;76:469–482, with permission; **B** and **C** from Hedican SP. Pelvis. In: Scott-Conner CEH, Cuschieri A, Carter FJ, eds. *Minimal access surgical anatomy.* Philadelphia: Lippincott Williams & Wilkins, 2000:211–238; **D** from Peritoneal cavity. In: Scott-Conner CEH, Cuschieri A, Carter FJ. *Minimal access surgical anatomy.* Philadelphia: Lippincott Williams & Wilkins, 2000:23–43, with permission.)

FIGURE 78.1   (Continued)

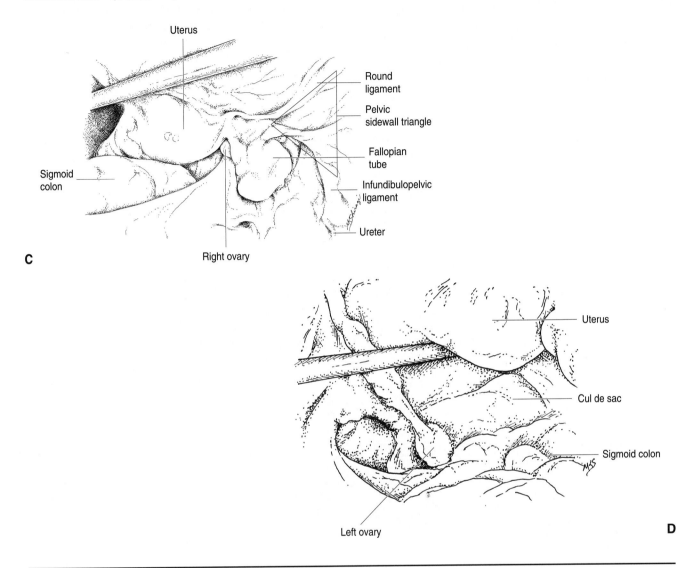

C

D

FIGURE 78.2
LAPAROSCOPIC TUBAL LIGATION (From Apelgren KN, Cowan BD, Metcalf AM, et al. Laparoscopic appendectomy and the management of gynecologic pathologic conditions found at laparoscopy for presumed appendicitis. *Surg Clin North Am* 1996;76:469–482, with permission.)

FIGURE 78.3
EXCISION OF OVARIAN CYST (**A** and **B** from Apelgren KN, Cowan BD, Metcalf AM, et al. Laparoscopic appendectomy and the management of gynecologic pathologic conditions found at laparoscopy for presumed appendicitis. *Surg Clin North Am* 1996;76:469–482, with permission.)

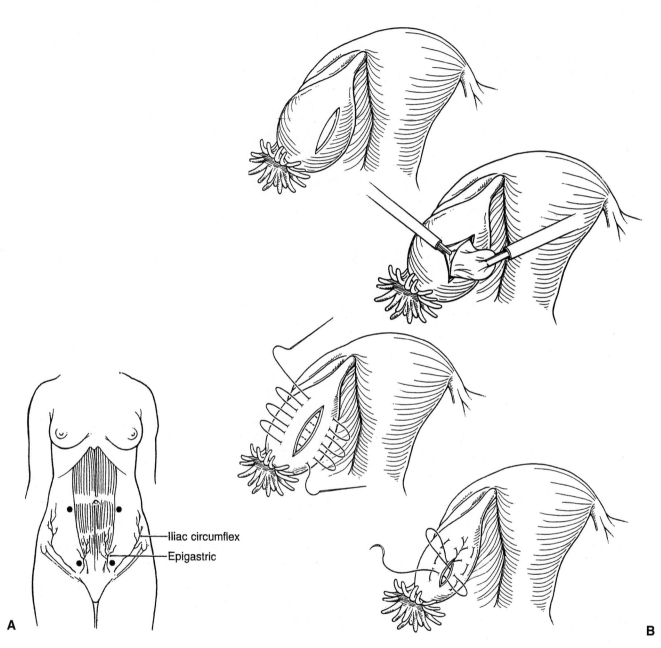

Iliac circumflex

Epigastric

A

B

FIGURE 78.4
SALPINGO-OOPHORECTOMY (**A** and **B** from Wind GG. The pelvis. In: *Applied laparoscopic anatomy: abdomen and pelvis.* Baltimore: Williams & Wilkins, 1997:249–299, with permission.)

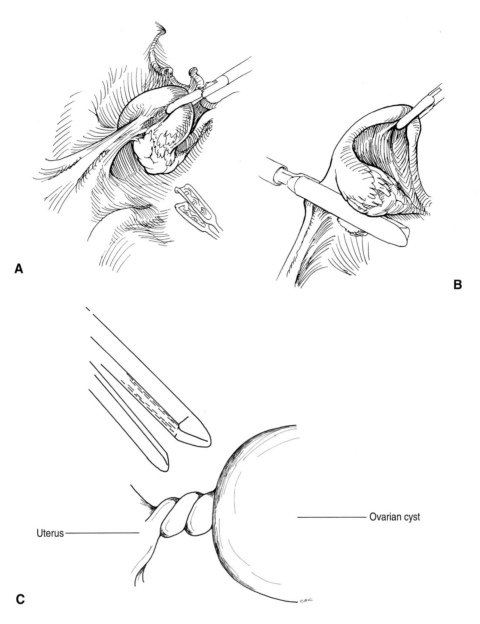

Uterus

Ovarian cyst

FIGURE 78.5
ECTOPIC PREGNANCY (**A** and **B** from Apelgren KN, Cowan BD, Metcalf AM, et al. Laparoscopic appendectomy and the management of gynecologic pathologic conditions found at laparoscopy for presumed appendicitis. *Surg Clin North Am* 1996;76:469–482, with permission.)

FIGURE 78.6
LAPAROSCOPIC HYSTERECTOMY: DISSECTION IN THE BROAD LIGAMENT AND INCISION IN THE ANTERIOR CUL-DE-SAC (**A** and **B** from Meeks GR. Advanced laparoscopic gynecologic surgery. *Surg Clin North Am* 2000;80:1443–1164, with permission; **C** and **D** from Wind GG. The pelvis. In: *Applied laparoscopic anatomy: abdomen and pelvis.* Baltimore: Williams & Wilkins, 1997:249–299, with permission.)

FIGURE 78.6   (Continued)

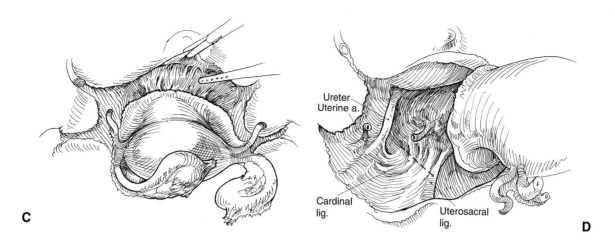

C   **D**

Ureter
Uterine a.
Cardinal lig.
Uterosacral lig.

FIGURE 78.7

COMPLETION OF HYSTERECTOMY AND CLOSURE OF VAGINA (**A** and **B** from Wind GG. The pelvis. In: *Applied laparoscopic anatomy: abdomen and pelvis.* Baltimore: Williams & Wilkins, 1997:249–299, with permission.)

Vagina (anterior wall)

A

Uterosacral lig.
Cardinal lig.
Vaginal mucosa

B

Laparoscopic Hysterectomy: Dissection in the Broad Ligament and Incision in the Anterior Cul-de-sac (Fig. 78.6)

Technical Points

Laparoscopic hysterectomy involves laparoscopic mobilization of the uterus with transvaginal extraction. Numerous variations exist, and only the general principles are given here. This is a difficult and advanced laparoscopic procedure with a steep learning curve. Laparoscopic hysterectomy with preservation of both tubes and ovaries is described first; salpingo-oophorectomy is easily added by first performing the mobilization described in Fig. 78.4.

Make an incision within the pelvic sidewall triangle between the fallopian tubes (medially) and the iliac vessels (laterally). It is imperative that the ureter be positively identified and mobilized away from the uterine vessels, where it passes toward the bladder. Sequentially divide the round ligament, fallopian tubes, and highly vascular broad ligament close to the uterus (Fig. 78.6A).

Extend the peritoneal incisions anteriorly and join these in the anterior cul-de-sac to allow access to the plane behind the bladder (Fig. 78.6B). Elevate the bladder flap by sharp and blunt dissection (Fig. 78.6C). Posteriorly, the uterosacral and cardinal ligaments must be divided (Fig. 78.6D).

Completion of Hysterectomy and Closure of Vagina (Fig. 78.7)

Technical and Anatomic Points

The hysterectomy may be completed transvaginally or from above as shown here. Make a circumferential incision in the wall of the vagina to divide the remaining attachment of the uterus (Fig. 78.7A). As described in Fig. 78.4, begin this incision in the posterior cul-de-sac. The vagina may be closed by laparoscopic suture (Fig. 78.7B) or sutured from below. Suture from below must be done with care to avoid inadvertent inclusion of bladder in the suture line.

Check hemostasis and close the trocar sites in the usual fashion.

REFERENCES

1. Apelgren KN, Cowan BD, Metcalf AM, et al. Laparoscopic appendectomy and the management of gynecologic pathologic conditions found at laparoscopy for presumed appendicitis. *Surg Clin North Am* 1996;76:469–482.
2. Grainger DA, Soderstom RM, Schiff SF, et al. Ureteral injuries at laparoscopy: insights into diagnosis, management, and prevention. *Obstet Gynecol* 1990;75:839–844.
3. Hsieh Y-Y, Lin W-C, Chang C-C, et al. Laparoscopic radical hysterectomy with low paraaortic, subaortic, and pelvic lymphadenectomy: results of short-term follow-up. *J Reprod Med* 1998;43:528–534.
4. Kadar N. Surgical anatomy and dissection techniques for laparoscopic surgery. *Curr Opin Obstet Gynecol* 1996;8:266–277. (Provides excellent detailed description of points for safe dissection.)
5. Maher PJ, Wood EC, Hill DJ, et al. Laparoscopically assisted hysterectomy. *Med J Aust* 1992;156:316–318.
6. Parker WH. Management of adnexal masses by operative laparoscopy: selection criteria. *J Reprod Med* 1992;37:603–606.
7. Possover M, Krause N, Plaul K, et al. Laparoscopic para-aortic and pelvic lymphadenectomy: experience with 150 patients and review of the literature. *Gynecol Oncol* 1998;71:19–28.
8. Reich H, McGlynn F, Sekel L, et al. Laparoscopic management of ovarian dermoid cysts. *J Reprod Med* 1992;37:640–644.
9. Spiritos NM, Schlaerth JB, Kimball RE, et al. Laparoscopic radical hysterectomy (type III) with aortic and pelvic lymphadenectomy. *Am J Obstet Gynecol* 1996;174:1763–1768.
10. Summit RL, Stovall TG, Libscomb GH, et al. Randomized comparison of laparoscopy-assisted vaginal hysterectomy with standard vaginal hysterectomy. *Obstet Gynecol* 1992;80:895–901.
11. Wind GG. The pelvis. In: *Applied laparoscopic anatomy: abdomen and pelvis.* Baltimore: Williams & Wilkins, 1997:249–299.

THE RETROPERITONEUM

The complex retroperitoneum technically includes anything that is not suspended upon a mesentery. To the surgeon, only the genitourinary tract, major vascular structures, and sympathetic chain are generally considered to be retroperitoneal because of the way in which these structures are approached. The pancreas, also a retroperitoneal organ, has been discussed in previous chapters (Chapters 63 to 65).

The general approach to structures in this region involves mobilizing portions of overlying gastrointestinal tract by returning them to their original midline (embryonic) location. The complex anatomy of the underlying structures is first described by presenting the genitourinary tract. Chapters 79 and 80 describe the anatomy of the adrenal (suprarenal) glands through a discussion of adrenalectomy, performed by (open) anterior and posterior approaches and laparoscopically. Chapter 79 also presents some anatomy of the back muscles in the section on the posterior approach to the adrenals. Renal anatomy is described through a discussion of radical nephrectomy (Chapter 81) and renal transplantation (Chapters 82 and 83).

Two related operations—abdominal aortic aneurysm repair and aortobifemoral grafting—are described in Chapter 84. Both standard and retroperitoneal approaches to the aorta are illustrated. Lumbar sympathectomy (Chapter 85) is rarely performed now, but is included to show the anatomy of the sympathetic chain and to illustrate the manner in which deep structures can be approached through a lateral extraperitoneal route.

CHAPTER 79

Adrenalectomy

Most adrenalectomies are performed transabdominally. In this chapter, the transabdominal approach to the adrenal glands will be described first because it is the one that is appropriate for tumors, such as pheochromocytomas, that may well be bilateral. A complete examination of the abdominal cavity, as well as removal of the adrenal (suprarenal) glands, is possible only through this approach.

The posterior approach to the adrenals is used only when

LIST OF STRUCTURES

Adrenal (suprarenal) glands
    Left and right suprarenal veins
    Inferior phrenic vein
    Inferior phrenic artery
    Superior suprarenal arteries
    Middle suprarenal artery
    Inferior suprarenal artery

Kidneys
    Left renal vein
        Left gonadal vein
Gerota's fascia
Inferior vena cava
Organ of Zuckerkandl
Trapezius muscle

Latissimus dorsi muscle
Erector spinae muscles
Internal oblique muscle
Transversus abdominis muscle
Quadratus lumborum muscle
Lumbodorsal fascia
Eleventh and twelfth ribs

ORIENTATION

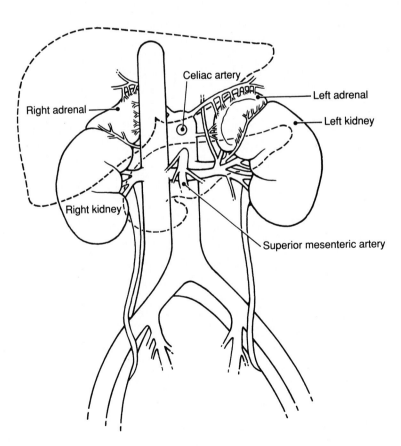

FIGURE 79.1
TRANSABDOMINAL ADRENALECTOMY INCISION

adrenalectomy is performed for endocrine ablation or for resection of a small, isolated aldosteronoma. It is described at the end of this chapter.

A lateral or flank approach provides excellent exposure, especially for the right adrenal gland. However, it is rarely used. References at the end of this chapter provide details of exposure using this method. Occasionally, large adrenal tumors require a thoracoabdominal incision for adequate exposure. Again, this is rare.

Laparoscopic adrenalectomy is described in Chapter 80.

Transabdominal Adrenalectomy Incision (Fig. 79.1)

Technical Points

Position the patient supine on the operating table with a roll under the lower costal margin, or break the operating table slightly to elevate the upper abdomen. Plan a bilateral subcostal or midline incision, depending on the physical habitus of the patient. For most patients, a subcostal approach is best. It may be necessary to make this incision quite long to obtain adequate exposure, especially in obese patients. Thoroughly explore the abdomen in the usual fashion.

Anatomic Points

The right adrenal lies slightly lower than the left and is conveniently approached through a right subcostal incision. Access to the left adrenal is more difficult because the gland occupies a more cephalad position. Although both adrenal glands are covered by overlying structures of the gastrointestinal tract, mobilization of these structures is easier on the right than on the left.

Left Adrenalectomy (Fig. 79.2)

Technical Points

Divide the gastrocolic omentum widely by taking the omentum off the greater curvature of the stomach. Serially clamp and tie the multiple branches of the gastroepiploic artery and vein that extend from the omentum to the greater curvature. Elevate the stomach cephalad with a retractor. Incise the peritoneum lying along the inferior border of the pancreas and gently elevate the pancreas by blunt dissection. Place a Harrington retractor on a moist laparotomy pad to elevate the pancreas. Reflect the transverse colon downward to improve exposure. Rarely, it may be necessary to mobilize the splenic flexure to achieve adequate exposure. Generally, the adrenal gland lies far enough medially that simple downward traction on the colon suffices.

Exposure obtained through the lesser sac is limited and is appropriate only for small tumors. If wider exposure is required, fully mobilize the spleen and tail of the pancreas up into the midline to expose the underlying retroperitoneal structures.

Palpate the kidney and use this as a guide to the left adrenal, which lies just cephalad and medial. Incise Gerota's fascia just medial to the superior aspect of the left kidney. The adrenal gland should be palpable and visible in this region. Identify the left renal vein and open the tissues overlying it to expose its anterior surface. The left gonadal vein is a useful landmark. The left adrenal vein generally lies just medial to it, on the superior aspect of the left renal vein. Begin to mobilize the adrenal gland by clipping small branches from the inferior phrenic artery and vein, which may enter the superior and medial borders of the adrenal. Secure these with hemoclips and divide them. It should then be possible to slip

FIGURE 79.2
LEFT ADRENALECTOMY

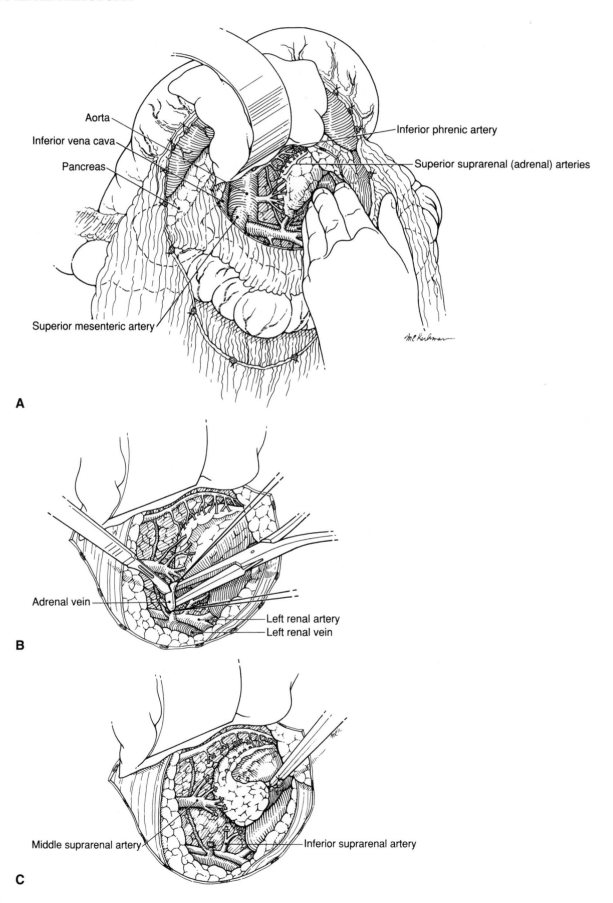

A

B

C

a finger behind the adrenal and elevate it. This posterior plane is generally avascular.

The adrenal vein passes inferiorly. Trace the superior aspect of the left renal vein to identify the relatively long adrenal vein passing off the superior surface just medial to the entrance of the gonadal vein. Ligate it in continuity and divide it. Leave the tie on the adrenal side long and use it to further elevate the adrenal into the field. Divide any remaining connections at the superior aspect of the gland (more or less blindly) with hemoclips. Because these contain only multiple, small arterial twigs, no major structures are at risk for injury.

Anatomic Points

The middle colic artery may be at risk for injury when the peritoneum along the caudal border of the pancreas is divided, or when the transverse colon is retracted inferiorly. This artery, an early branch of the superior mesenteric artery, usually arises posterior or just inferior to the neck of the pancreas and passes to the right. However, it can divide into left and right branches shortly after its origin, with the left branch then being in potential danger; alternatively, an accessory middle colic artery passing toward the splenic flexure can be present (occurring about 10% of the time). The inferior or transverse pancreatic artery runs along, or in, the caudal border of the pancreas, giving off posterior epiploic arteries that run in the anterior leaf of the transverse mesocolon, or sometimes giving off a fairly significant colic branch to the left colic flexure.

The left adrenal (suprarenal) gland is located within a subdivision of Gerota's fascia and is surrounded by perirenal fat and connective tissue. In contrast to the pyramidal right adrenal gland, the left gland is semilunar or leaf shaped, flattened, and broadly in contact (through its posterior surface) with the medial surface of the kidney, superior to the renal vasculature and to the left crus of the diaphragm. The anterior surface of this gland is related to the posterior wall of the omental bursa and, more inferiorly, to the body of the pancreas. Inferiorly, the gland may be in contact with the renal vasculature. Laterally, it can be in contact with the renal surface of the spleen. Medially, it is closely related to the left greater splanchnic nerve and celiac ganglion.

The arterial supply of the left adrenal gland is derived from three different sources. The superior suprarenal arteries, which are always multiple (ranging in number from 3 to 30), arise from the inferior phrenic artery as this artery passes close to the medial and superior borders of the gland. The middle suprarenal artery arises as a single vessel from the anterolateral aspect of the aorta, superior to the origin of the renal artery. The inferior suprarenal artery arises from the superior aspect of the renal artery. The middle and inferior suprarenal arteries may be multiple or may have branches, especially at the periphery of the suprarenal gland. In addition to these constant sources, the suprarenal gland can also receive blood from accessory renal arteries, the upper ureteric artery, and

the gonadal artery. Almost all of the arteries, regardless of their origin, enter the periphery of the gland. These multiple, small vessels are not individually ligated, but are secured in clips together with a mass of surrounding soft tissue.

The venous drainage of the left suprarenal gland is usually through a single, comparatively large vein that emerges from the central region of the anterior surface of the gland. From here, it passes inferiorly, joins the inferior phrenic vein, and empties into the superior aspect of the left renal vein. Typically, its termination is medial to the termination of the left gonadal vein.

Right Adrenalectomy (Fig. 79.3)

Technical Points

Reflect the hepatic flexure of the colon downward. Fully mobilize the duodenum with a wide Kocher maneuver and expose the inferior vena cava. Retract the liver cephalad with a Harrington retractor. The right adrenal gland should be palpable just above and medial to the kidney in the region between the superior pole of the kidney and the inferior vena cava. Make a peritoneal incision overlying the adrenal and expose it. Free the lateral border of the adrenal by serially clamping and tying or dividing with electrocautery. The medial border is dissected next. This dissection should be done directly on the vena cava.

Anatomic Points

The right adrenal gland is pyramidal in shape and is located, like its counterpart, in a subcompartment within Gerota's fascia. It is related to the anteromedial aspect of the upper pole of the kidney. Anteriorly, its upper part is in contact with the bare area of the liver, and frequently, with the inferior vena cava, whereas its lower part is covered by the parietal peritoneum lateral to the duodenum. Posteriorly, it is related to the right crus of the diaphragm.

The blood supply to the right adrenal gland is similar to that of the left, in that it receives a multitude of branches derived from the inferior phrenic artery, aorta, and renal artery. These branches enter the periphery of the gland. Dissection along the lateral side of the gland should be relatively avascular because the small arterial branches tend to enter superiorly, inferiorly, and medially.

Division of the Right Adrenal Vein (Fig. 79.4)

Technical Points

The right adrenal vein is short and fat and enters directly into the vena cava. It may be difficult to secure this vein, and it is important to avoid injuring the vena cava. Gently skeletonize the vein and divide it in continuity. If bleeding occurs in the course of this dissection, avoid the temptation to apply a clamp blindly. The vena cava is fragile and easily torn, and a small hole can rapidly enlarge into a disastrous rent. Control the bleeding with your finger until you can either suture the

FIGURE 79.3
RIGHT ADRENALECTOMY

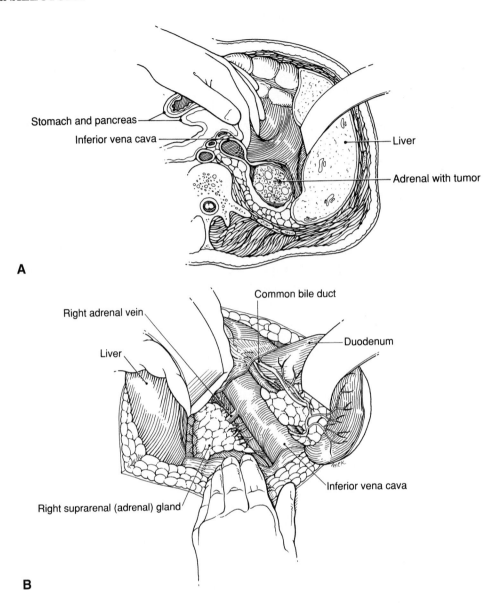

Stomach and pancreas

Inferior vena cava

Liver

Adrenal with tumor

A

Common bile duct

Right adrenal vein

Duodenum

Liver

Inferior vena cava

Right suprarenal (adrenal) gland

B

tear directly or apply a partial occlusion vascular clamp (such as a Satinsky clamp) to the inferior vena cava. Divide the remaining attachments to the adrenal with hemoclips.

Anatomic Points

Right adrenalectomy is comparatively difficult because part of the gland is frequently posterior to the inferior vena cava and because the single right suprarenal vein typically drains directly into the posterior aspect of the inferior vena cava. The right adrenal vein may enter the inferior vena cava at the angle between the renal vein and the inferior vena cava or may terminate directly into the inferior vena cava at the level of the adrenal. To expose the right adrenal vein, it is usually necessary to retract the inferior vena cava carefully to the left. The surgeon should be aware that this vein is usually

less than 1 cm in length and that its diameter, which measures about 3 mm, is unexpectedly large. In addition, it is said to be particularly fragile, as is this segment of the vena cava. To further complicate exposure of the right suprarenal vein, frequently, small hepatic tributaries drain directly into the vena cava, and these, too, can be avulsed. Because of the anatomic relationships of the structures in this area, especially the liver, hemorrhage in this region is difficult to control.

Exploration of the Retroperitoneum (Fig. 79.5)

Technical Points

Bilateral or extraadrenal pheochromocytomas are not rare. Therefore, both adrenal glands and the retroperitoneum

FIGURE 79.4
DIVISION OF THE RIGHT ADRENAL VEIN

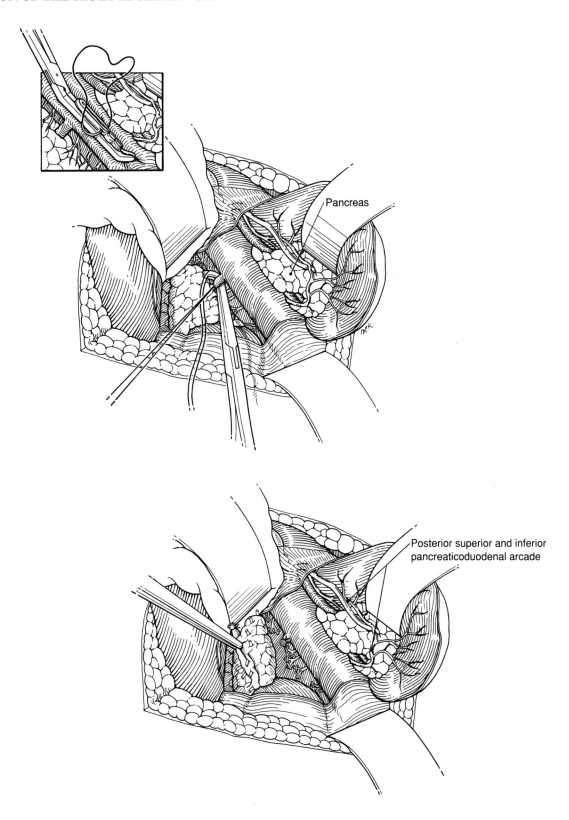

Pancreas

Posterior superior and inferior
pancreaticoduodenal arcade

FIGURE 79.5
EXPLORATION OF THE RETROPERITONEUM

Masses

Organ of Zuckerkandl

Masses

cells) migrate into the developing adrenal cortex, assuming a central position.

Accessory adrenocortical tissue of mesodermal origin can occur almost anywhere in the abdomen. The most frequent locations for cortical nodules are deep to the renal capsule, in the broad ligament of the female, and in the spermatic cord of the male.

Extramedullary chromaffin tissue (of neural crest origin) is normally found in proximity to all of the sympathetic chain ganglia and in discrete masses in the region of the abdominal sympathetic plexuses. The largest of these—the organ of Zuckerkandl—is located about the origin of the inferior mesenteric artery. These extramedullary chromaffin cells, especially those of the organ of Zuckerkandl, occur normally. They are, however, subject to the same disease processes (eg, pheochromocytoma) as the adrenal medulla; hence, exploration of the retroperitoneum must be considered when diseases of the adrenal medulla are diagnosed.

Posterior Adrenalectomy (Fig. 79.6)

Technical Points

Position the patient face down on the operating table with rolls beneath the hips and the chest to allow the abdomen to sag. This will avoid placing pressure on the vena cava and will increase the distance from the posterior abdominal wall to the intraabdominal viscera. Jackknife the operating table slightly to straighten the curvature of the spine. Plan an incision that extends straight from the tenth rib downward, parallel to the midline, and that then curves gently down toward the iliac crest. Carry this down through fascia and through the latissimus dorsi muscle.

Divide the attachments of the erector spinae muscle to the twelfth rib and resect this rib subperiosteally. Open the lumbodorsal fascia longitudinally along the lateral margin of the quadratus lumborum. Expose Gerota's fascia. Clamp and tie the subcostal artery and vein and retract the subcostal nerve out of the operative field. Bluntly elevate the diaphragm and pleura off of the underlying retroperitoneal tissues. Gently push the pleura out of the way, and divide the diaphragm with clamps and ties. Pull downward on the kidney to expose the adrenal gland. Divide lateral and superior attachments with hemoclips until only the adrenal vein (inferior on the right, medial on the left) remains. Ligate the adrenal vein in continuity with 2-0 silk and divide it. Achieve hemostasis and close the incision in layers.

Anatomic Points

The incision, as described, will first divide those fibers of the trapezius muscle that originate from the eleventh and twelfth thoracic vertebrae and that overlap the upper fibers of the latissimus dorsi muscle. The latter muscle originates from the lower six thoracic vertebrae and, through an aponeurosis, from all lumbar and sacral vertebrae and the posterior iliac crest. Muscular slips also arise from the lower three or four

should be palpated when an adrenalectomy is being performed. Incise the peritoneum overlying the aorta and the bifurcation of the common iliac arteries, and palpate the region of the paraaortic and parailiac lymph nodes for tumor masses. Also check the region of the bladder for tumor masses. Achieve hemostasis in the operative field and close the incision in the usual fashion, without drains.

Anatomic Points

A logical plan for exploration of the retroperitoneum must be based on an understanding of the development of the suprarenal glands. The adrenal cortex develops from mesoderm. Initially, the elongated primordium develops bilaterally on either side of the midline dorsal mesentery adjacent to the cranial end of the mesonephros. As the developing metanephric kidney "ascends," it contacts the lower pole of the suprarenal gland; later ascent causes the glands to assume their definitive shapes.

The primordia of the adrenal medullae develop at the same time. These are derived from neural crest cells associated with future ganglia from T-6 through T-12. As the peripheral neural tissue develops, the future medullary cells (or chromaffin

FIGURE 79.6
POSTERIOR ADRENALECTOMY

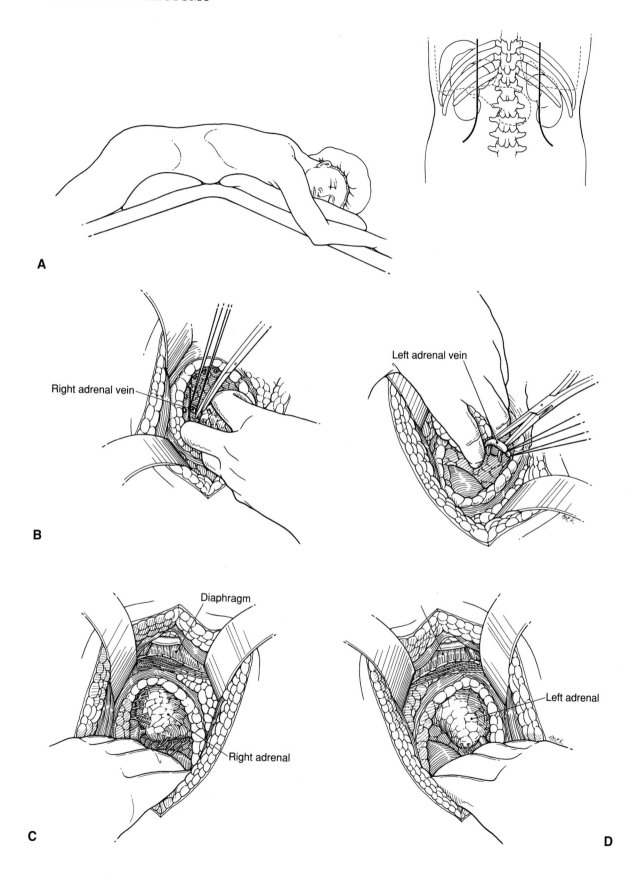

A

B

Right adrenal vein

Left adrenal vein

Diaphragm

Right adrenal

Left adrenal

C

D

ribs, interdigitating with slips of the external oblique muscle. Thus, as the incision is carried inferiorly, fibers of the latissimus dorsi muscle will be divided, as will sensory branches of the posterior primary divisions of spinal nerves superiorly and the anterior divisions inferiorly.

The lumbodorsal (thoracolumbar) fascia is the investing (deep) fascia of the back. It is composed of the fused aponeuroses of the latissimus dorsi, internal oblique, and transversus abdominis muscles. The aponeuroses of the two abdominal muscles fuse at the lateral edge of the erector spinae muscle mass, then split to encompass both anterior and posterior surfaces of the erector spinae, ultimately attaching to both spinous and transverse processes of the lumbar vertebrae. Fibers of the internal oblique muscle begin close to the site of fusion, whereas the transversus abdominis muscle fibers remain aponeurotic for some distance laterally. Thus, recognition of muscle fibers can afford the surgeon an indication of the depth of the incision because all else should be aponeurotic.

The quadratus lumborum muscle lies anterior to the anterior lamella of the lumbodorsal fascia. Branches of the spinal nerves that may be encountered in this dissection (subcostal, iliohypogastric, and ilioinguinal) pass laterally, anterior to the quadratus lumborum muscle. At variable distances laterally, they gain access to the plane between the transversus abdominis and internal oblique muscles to continue their course to the anterior midline. Because the kidney and suprarenal gland,

within Gerota's fascia, lie in tissue planes anterior (deep) to the quadratus lumborum muscle, caution must be exercised to avoid traumatic injury to the nerves and accompanying vascular structures.

Division of the latissimus dorsi muscle should expose the twelfth rib. Because some 12 muscles have at least a partial origin or insertion to the periosteum of this rib, it is most expedient to resect it subperiosteally.

In this region, the diaphragm originates from the twelfth rib and the lateral lumbocostal arch, a fibrous fascial thickening over the quadratus lumborum muscle that extends from the tip of the transverse process of vertebra L-2 to the tip of rib 12. Resection of the last rib allows access to the superior side of the diaphragm medially and to its inferior aspect laterally. The parietal pleura reflects from the dome of the diaphragm to the posterior and lateral aspect of the ribs, forming the costodiaphragmatic recess. The pleura of the costodiaphragmatic recess, attached to the ribs and diaphragm by endothoracic fascia, can be gently elevated, allowing division of the diaphragm. The adrenal gland will be exposed if the kidney is gently pulled inferiorly. This latter maneuver is necessary because the upper pole of the kidney, and thus the adrenal gland, lies superior to the T-12 vertebra and the last rib.

Because the adrenal gland lies cephalad to this incision, some prefer more direct exposure through the bed of the eleventh rib. In this case, more of the diaphragm must be divided and the pleura entered.

REFERENCES

1. Avisse C, Marcus C, Patey M, et al. Surgical anatomy and embryology of the adrenal glands. *Surg Clin North Am* 2000;80:403–416.
2. Carey LC, Ellison EH. Adrenalectomy: technique, errors, and pitfalls. *Surg Clin North Am* 1966;46:1283. (Emphasizes potential problems and how to avoid them.)
3. Chini ES, Thomas CG. An extended Kocher incision for bilateral adrenalectomy. *Am J Surg* 1985;149:292. (Describes extended bilateral subcostal approach.)
4. Geelhoed GW, Dunnick NR, Doppman JL. Management of intravenous extensions of endocrine tumors and prognosis after surgical treatment. *Am J Surg* 1980;139:844.
5. Godellas CV, Prinz RA. Surgical approach to adrenal neoplasms: laparoscopic versus open adrenalectomy. *Surg Clin North Am* 1998;7:807–817.
6. Johnstone FRC. The surgical anatomy of the adrenal glands with particular reference to the suprarenal vein. *Surg Clin North Am* 1964;44:1315. (Presents good review of vascular anatomy.)
7. Nash AG, Robbins GF. The operative approach to the left adrenal gland. *Surg Gynecol Obstet* 1973;137:670.
8. Pezzulich RA, Mannix H. Immediate complications of adrenal surgery. *Ann Surg* 1970;172:125.
9. Russell CF, Hamberger B, van Heerden JA, et al. Adrenalectomy: anterior or posterior approach? *Am J Surg* 1982;144:322. (Discusses pros and cons of two approaches.)
10. Thompson GB, Grant CS, van Heerden JA, et al. Laparoscopic versus open posterior adrenalectomy: a case-control study of 100 patients. *Surgery* 1997;122:1132–1136.

CHAPTER 80

Laparoscopic Adrenalectomy

James R. Howe

Adrenalectomy is performed for primary and metastatic tumors of the adrenal gland and for adrenal hyperplasia. The open transabdominal, flank, posterior, and thoracoabdominal approaches, described in Chapter 79, have largely been supplanted by laparoscopic adrenalectomy. The principal advantages of the laparoscopic approach are the same as those described for other minimal access procedures: smaller incisions, a magnified view of the operative field, less postoperative pain, shorter hospital stay, and a quicker return to work. The disadvantages are that it is more technically demanding in terms of equipment and the experience of the surgeon, that bilateral adrenalectomy cannot be performed without repositioning the patient, and that it is not recommended for the treatment of malignant neoplasms.

There are two principal laparoscopic approaches to the adrenal gland: transperitoneal and retroperitoneal. In the transperitoneal approach, the anatomic relationships are clearer because insufflation of the peritoneal cavity allows for visualization of the liver, spleen, colon, and stomach, which are helpful anatomic landmarks. The retroperitoneal approach leaves the intraperitoneal organs undisturbed, but creating a working space in the retroperitoneum can be difficult. This chapter describes the transperitoneal flank approach to adrenalectomy. References at the end detail alternatives, including the retroperitoneal and posterior approaches.

LIST OF STRUCTURES

Adrenal (suprarenal) glands
    Left and right adrenal veins
Kidney
    Left renal vein
Gerota's fascia
Inferior vena cava
Colon
    Splenic flexure
    Hepatic flexure
Liver

Patient Positioning and Incisions (Fig. 80.1)

Technical Points

Place a Foley catheter and an orogastric tube, and apply pneumatic compression stockings. Access to the adrenals by the transperitoneal approach requires four ports, and if these ports are placed too close to one another, instruments from one port are likely to interfere with those from another. For this reason, place ports 9 to 12 cm apart, depending on the size of the patient. This requires that the most lateral port be inserted through the flank. To make this possible, place the patient on a beanbag in the lateral decubitus position, with the area between the iliac crest and eleventh rib lying over the kidney rest. Raise the kidney rest to its highest position in order to open up this space, and then flex the table. Tilt the patient slightly backward to about 15 degrees, and then inflate the beanbag. Support the ipsilateral arm on a mobile upper arm rest and place a roll under the dependent axilla and a pillow between the legs. Lay towels over the nondependent hip and shoulder, and use adhesive tape over the towels to secure the patient to the table.

Mark a line two fingerbreadths caudad to the costal margin before insufflation. The lateral ports will be positioned in this line (Fig. 80.1A). The most medial port will be placed in the linea alba, 10 to 15 cm caudad to the xiphoid (port 1), with a supraumbilical incision being used in smaller patients. The next port (port 2) will be placed about 10 cm further laterally, in the midclavicular line. The third (port 3) will be placed 10 cm lateral to port 2, in the anterior axillary line.

Begin with an open insertion through the second port, then place ports 1 and 3 under direct vision after insufflation. The most lateral port (port 4) is placed through the flank between the iliac crest and the eleventh rib after the splenic flexure of the colon has been mobilized for left adrenalectomy or the hepatic flexure of the colon taken down for right adrenalectomy.

Anatomic Points

The adrenal glands are retroperitoneal organs; hence, transperitoneal access to these organs requires reflecting intraperitoneal structures medially. This includes mobilization of the splenic flexure of the colon, the spleen, and pancreas

FIGURE 80.1
PATIENT POSITIONING AND INCISIONS

A   B

on the left. On the right, the right lobe of the liver must be mobilized and retracted. The right adrenal gland is slightly more caudad than the left and is bordered by the kidney inferiorly, the diaphragm posteriorly, the liver superiorly, and the vena cava medially. The left adrenal rests on the superior pole of the left kidney, is adjacent to the aorta medially, and lies posterior to the tail of the pancreas and spleen; the diaphragm is located superiorly and posteriorly (Fig. 80.1B). Accessory adrenal tissue may be present near the gland or may even migrate in the vicinity of the testes or ovaries.

The adrenal glands have two components: the outer cortex, which gives rise to cortical adenomas and carcinomas, and the inner medulla, which gives rise to pheochromocytomas. The cortex develops from coelomic mesenchyme from the urogenital ridge during embryogenesis. The medulla develops from neural crest ectodermal cells, which migrate into the adrenal cortex during week 7 or 8 of development. These glands come to lie superomedially to each kidney—thus the older designation, "suprarenal glands." The right gland tends to be more triangular in shape, whereas the left is more crescenteric. The average adrenal gland is 3 to 5 cm in length and 5 to 10 mm in width, with a weight of 3 to 6 g. The yellow-orange color of the adrenal is quite distinct from the paler yellow of the perinephric fat.

Left Adrenalectomy (Fig. 80.2)

Technical Points

Insufflate to 15 mm Hg with CO_2 and pass a 30-degree laparoscope through port 1. Explore the abdomen. Pass a Babcock clamp through port 3 and grasp the splenic flexure of the colon. Divide the peritoneal attachments of the cephalad 15 to 20 cm of the descending colon with ultrasonic shears. At

this point, the fourth port can be placed under direct vision, angled to point toward the adrenal. Introduce the Babcock clamp through this port and retract the splenic flexure. Move the camera to the second port and the ultrasonic shears to the third port, and divide the peritoneal attachments of the spleen as high as possible.

Once this plane is entered, the kidney is visualized as it bulges anteriorly. Confirm this by palpation with a grasper or harmonic scalpel. Open Gerota's fascia vertically starting at the midpole and clear the anterior surface of the kidney by dividing the overlying perinephric fat (Fig. 80.2A). Next, pull the medial border of the fascia upward, and dissect Gerota's fascia from the underlying perinephric fat and rotate it medially (Fig. 80.2B).

Place a fan retractor through the first port, and use it to retract the spleen and peritoneal edge medially. Because the adrenal gland is superomedial to the upper pole of the kidney, divide the perinephric fat just above the superior pole, and then work toward the diaphragm, separating the lateral perinephric fat from the medial fat and adrenal gland. Next, continue the dissection medially and posteriorly in the general direction of the aorta.

During this dissection, larger tumors (>2 cm) will be readily visible as orange-yellow rounded masses, whereas smaller tumors will be difficult to distinguish from the pale yellow fat. The adrenal is more solid and flat than the surrounding fat, but palpation alone is not of much help in revealing the gland. Some surgeons use laparoscopic ultrasonography to help localize the position of the adrenal, but this is not available in most hospitals and adds expense to the procedure. Dissection along the superior aspect of the perinephric fat and superomedial edge of the kidney will eventually uncover an area of yellow-orange tissue that can be recognized as the adrenal gland. This dissection requires frequent

FIGURE 80.2
LEFT ADRENALECTOMY (C from Hedican SP. Kidneys and adrenal glands. In: Scott-Conner CEH, Cuschieri A, Carter FJ, eds. *Minimal access surgical anatomy.* Philadelphia: Lippincott Williams & Wilkins, 2000:267–292, with permission.)

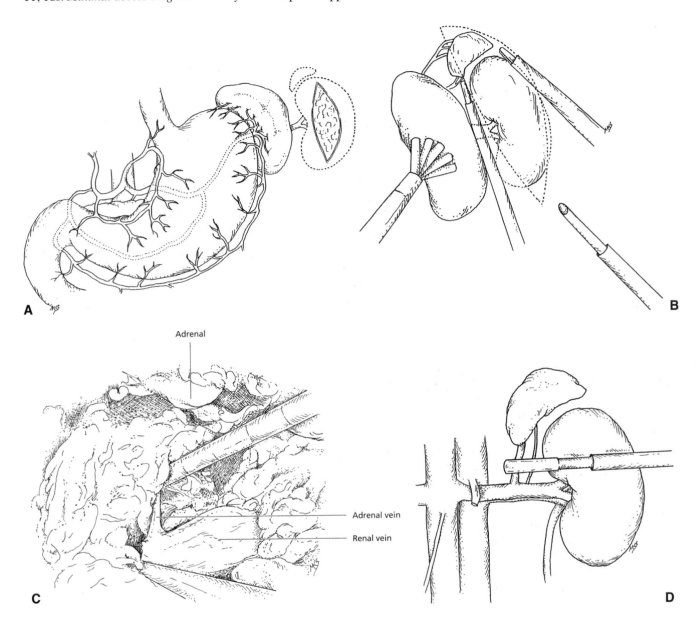

switching of the camera and instrument ports to optimize traction and visualization.

Next, work along the lateral and superior borders of the gland, leaving some adjacent fat, which can be used to grasp the gland. Retract the gland anteriorly, which facilitates clearing the superomedial attachments. The arterial branches are often not clearly visualized. Divide these with the ultrasonic shears.

Approach the adrenal vein last because misadventure in this region is the most likely cause for conversion to an open approach (Fig. 80.2C). Not only can the adrenal vein be torn, but also the superior pole vessels to the kidney can

be injured if the dissection is carried out 1 to 2 cm too far inferiorly or medially. Once a plane along the aorta is developed medially and also between the adrenal and kidney inferiorly, the remaining tissue at the inferior border of the adrenal can be divided using an endoscopic lineal stapler with a 2.5-mm load, or the vein can be directly clipped (Fig. 80.2D).

At this point, the adrenal is free. Pass an endoscopic retrieval bag through port 2 and retrieve and remove it. Inspect the operative bed for hemostasis, observe the color of the superior pole of the kidney, and examine the region for the presence of residual or accessory adrenal tissue. Irrigate the area, then remove the ports and close the fascia with 0-0 Vicryl sutures.

Anatomic Points

The arterial blood supply to each adrenal is derived from three sources: (a) branches from the aorta, (b) renal artery, and (c) inferior phrenic artery. These vessels are not generally seen during the dissection and are adequately controlled with the ultrasonic shears. The left adrenal vein drains into the left renal vein. Injury to the superior pole vessels of the kidney may occur when the left adrenal vein is ligated. This will manifest as a purple demarcation of the superior renal pole from the normal pink parenchyma. This most dangerous step in the procedure is rendered safer by dividing the vein last, having obtained as complete a dissection as possible. This requires that patients with pheochromocytoma be well blocked before the procedure, and most patients who have received 2 weeks of gradually increasing α blockade preoperatively will generally not have dramatic fluctuations in blood pressure. Care must be taken to avoid the pancreas by incising Gerota's fascia and reflecting it with the spleen. Care must also be taken not to injure the spleen while retracting it medially.

FIGURE 80.3
RIGHT ADRENALECTOMY (C from Hedican SP. Kidneys and adrenal glands. In: Scott-Conner CEH, Cuschieri A, Carter FJ, eds. *Minimal access surgical anatomy.* Philadelphia: Lippincott Williams & Wilkins, 2000:267–292, with permission.)

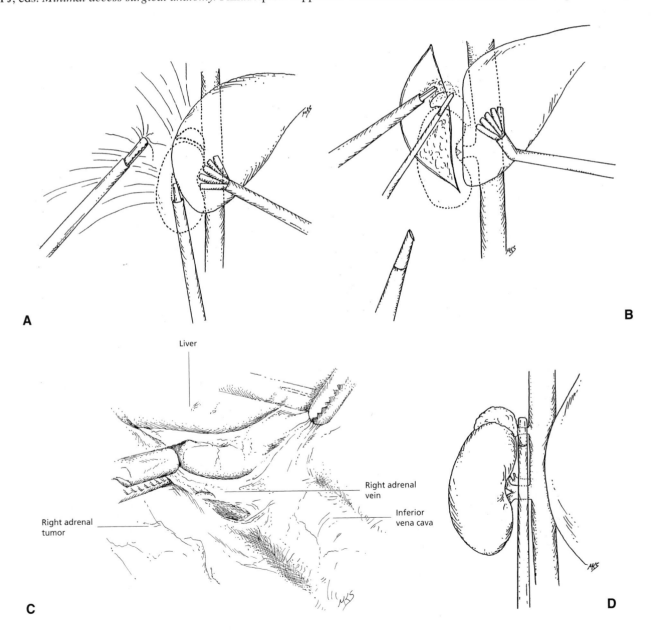

Right Adrenalectomy (Fig. 80.3)

Technical Points

The ports are placed in the same positions as described for left adrenalectomy, except on the right side. The hepatic flexure is visualized while pushing down on the abdominal wall from the fourth port site. If there is adequate space, introduce the port under direct vision. If not, mobilize the hepatic flexure. Place the 30-degree camera through port 2 and a fan retractor through port 1. Use the fan retractor to retract the liver medially (Fig. 80.3A).

Elevate the lateral peritoneum with a grasping clamp, and divide the peritoneal reflection of the right triangular ligament with the ultrasonic shears as high as possible. As the dissection proceeds, retract the liver medially and elevate it to improve exposure of the kidney and adrenal gland.

Open Gerota's fascia vertically overlying the midportion of the kidney to a point 4 to 6 cm above the superior pole of the kidney. Bisect the perinephric fat vertically beginning at the superior pole of the kidney. Dissect the fascia medially over this entire vertical length until the vena cava is visualized. This forms the medial extent of the dissection. Place the fan retractor on this fascial edge and the liver, elevating it and rotating it medially (Fig. 80.3B). Larger adrenal tumors may be visible at this time, which makes finding the edge of the adrenal gland easier.

Once the flattened edge of the yellow-orange adrenal gland is seen, dissect the superior and lateral surfaces first with the ultrasonic shears, freeing the gland from the surrounding fat. If the gland is not visualized, then continue to dissect through the perinephric fat in a superior and medial direction from the earlier point of bisection. The edge of the adrenal will eventually be encountered. If the lateral edge is still not found, dissect in the plane between the vena cava and above the superior pole of the kidney until it is encountered.

Once the superior and lateral portions of the adrenal are dissected, clear the groove between the kidney and adrenal, being careful not to dissect too far inferomedially, where the superior pole renal vessels are located. Once this is achieved, gently retract the gland laterally (Fig. 80.3C). Carefully divide the areolar tissue between the inferior aspect of the adrenal and vena cava using the ultrasonic shears. Also, clear the areolar tissue from the superomedial border of the adrenal, being careful to stay at the level of the top of the gland to avoid inadvertent injury to the adrenal vein.

The last remaining connection is the adrenal vein, which can be divided using an endoscopic cutting linear stapler with a 2.5-mm vascular cartridge placed adjacent and parallel to the vena cava through the openings made in this areolar tissue inferiorly and superiorly (Fig. 80.3D). The adrenal gland is placed in an endoscopic bag and removed through port 2. The area of dissection is inspected for hemostasis and irrigated, and closure is performed as described for left adrenalectomy.

Anatomic Points

To expose the superior aspects of the right adrenal and vena cava, the liver must be well mobilized. Once this is achieved, the fan retractor can be used to suspend the liver out of the way, above the adrenal. As on the left side, the three arteries are divided using the ultrasonic shears and are seldom visualized. The adrenal vein on the right is extremely short (about 1 cm), wide, and drains directly into the vena cava. Any misadventure with this vein will result in significant blood loss, which will be difficult or impossible to control laparoscopically. These events can be minimized if one uses an endoscopic lineal stapler and dissects out the inferior and superomedial aspects of the adrenal gland. Care should be taken not to encroach on the lateral wall of the vena cava using this technique.

REFERENCES

1. Bonjer HJ, Sorm V, Berends FJ, et al. Endoscopic retroperitoneal adrenalectomy: lessons learned from 111 consecutive cases. *Ann Surg* 2000;232:796–803.
2. Hedican SP. Kidneys and adrenal glands. In: Scott-Conner CEH, Cuschieri A, Carter FJ, eds. *Minimal access surgical anatomy.* Philadelphia: Lippincott Williams & Wilkins, 2000:267–292.
3. Siperstein AE, Berber E, Engle KL, et al. Laparoscopic posterior adrenalectomy. *Arch Surg* 2000;135:967–971.
4. Wind GG. *Applied laparoscopic anatomy: abdomen and pelvis.* Baltimore: Williams & Wilkins, 1997:301–367.

CHAPTER 81

Radical Nephrectomy

Sean P. Hedican and Richard D. Williams

Radical nephrectomy remains the primary treatment option for renal parenchymal malignancies. As classically described, radical nephrectomy involves the *en bloc* resection of the structures contained within Gerota's fascia, including the kidney, ipsilateral adrenal gland, perinephric fat, upper portion of the ureter, and regional lymphatics. This chapter focuses on the technical aspects and critical anatomic features of this operation. Important differences between right- and left-sided procedures and alternative surgical options are outlined.

Patient Positioning and Choice of Incision (Fig. 81.1)

Technical Points

Radical nephrectomy can be performed through a variety of incisions. The choice depends to a large extent on surgeon preference, patient body habitus, tumor size, and location of the lesion within the kidney. The need for additional procedures such as caval tumor thrombectomy, contralateral renal surgery, or simultaneous resection of limited metastatic disease in the liver or lungs may also determine which incision is the most efficacious. The technical aspects, rationale, and patient positioning of each of the primary surgical approaches are discussed later. For all incisions, we prefer a multiposi-tional self-retraining retractor such as the Omni-Tract, which allows simultaneous deep and superficial retraction.

Flank or Semiflank Incision. This approach is best suited for tumors of almost any size that are not primarily located in the upper pole and do not have associated tumor thrombus extending into the vena cava. It is especially useful in obese patients with a large abdominal pannus because the flank tends to have less subcutaneous fat than the abdomen. This incision provides direct extrapleural retroperitoneal exposure, avoiding contact with the intraperitoneal contents and, as a result, reduces the risk for postoperative ileus. Another benefit of this incision is direct posterior access to the main renal artery. Exposure can, however, be limited with larger tumors owing to the finite amount of space available for medial rotation of the kidney.

Position the patient in a semiflank position rotated 15 to 30 degrees posterior of vertical to allow extension of the incision medially across the rectus to give greater exposure when necessary. Center the patient with the kidneys over the break in the operative table and elevate the kidney rest. The legs and arms should be well padded using pillows both below the down extremity and in between. Alternatively, a sling can be used to support the upper arm. An axillary roll is

LIST OF STRUCTURES

Abdominal wall
  External oblique
  Internal oblique
  Transversus abdominis
  Rectus abdominis
Back
  Latissimus dorsi
  Serratus posterior inferior
Chest
  Ribs
  Intercostal muscles
  Intercostal vessels and nerve
  Diaphragm
  Pleura

Gerota's fascia
Perinephric fat
Kidneys
  Ureter
  Regional lymphatics
Adrenal gland
Vasculature
  Aorta
  Vena cava
  Renal artery
  Renal vein
  Ascending lumbar vein
  Gonadal vein
  Adrenal vein

Superior mesenteric artery
Inferior mesenteric artery
Liver
  Cardinal ligaments
  Triangular ligaments
  Hepatocolic ligaments
  Accessory hepatic veins
Spleen
  Lienocolic ligaments
Ascending and descending colon
  Line of Toldt
Duodenum
Pancreas

540

placed to prevent excess traction on the brachial plexus. As with all approaches, the patient is secured to the table with Velcro straps or wide cloth adhesive tape.

The incision can be made in several locations but usually begins off of the tip of the twelfth rib or the eleventh intercostal space for smaller tumors. Often, the higher incision is preferred because the renal hilum is deceptively cephalad in its location, despite indications on imaging studies. Division of the intercostal ligament provides excellent exposure even without resection of a rib. It is preferable to maximize exposure for larger tumors (>7 cm) by performing an incision directly over the eleventh or twelfth rib and resecting it. Rib resections are performed in a subperiosteal plane, which allows bone to regenerate from the periosteum. Take care to preserve the   neurovascular bundle that underlies the inferior edge of the rib. After dividing the anterior edge of the latissimus dorsi and underlying serratus posterior inferior muscle, incise the anterior periosteal layer using the cautery

FIGURE 81.1
PATIENT POSITIONING AND CHOICE OF INCISION

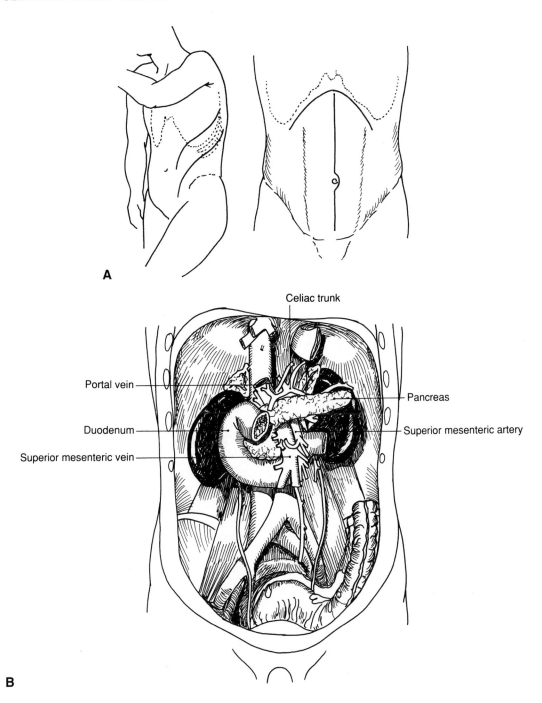

A

B

FIGURE 81.1 (Continued)

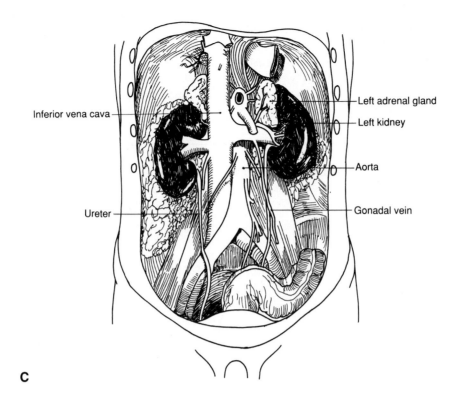

Inferior vena cava

Left adrenal gland

Left kidney

Aorta

Ureter

Gonadal vein

C

beginning at the edge of the sacrospinal muscle and extending along the entire rib. Raise anterior periosteal flaps with an Alexander periosteal elevator. Then elevate the rib from the posterior periosteal layer with Doyen rib elevators. Transect the rib laterally using a right-angled rib cutter and a bone rongeur to remove sharpened corners of the cut surface. Use electrocautery or apply bone wax to stop bleeding from the cut end of the rib. Release the diaphragm and pleural attachments and sweep these cephalad to avoid entering the pleural space.

Close any small inadvertent pleurotomies primarily with fine absorbable suture around a small red rubber catheter brought out through the fascial closure. After the skin is closed, submerge the open end of the red rubber catheter in a basin of water held below the level of the flank while the anesthesiologist performs several deep positive-pressure ventilations to evacuate entrapped air before tube removal.

Anterior Subcostal (Half-Chevron) Incision. This transperitoneal approach allows direct access to the vasculature without initial renal mobilization. It is particularly useful for larger tumors in almost any portion of the kidney. It may not be the optimum access, however, for extremely large upper pole tumors or in morbidly obese patients. The incision can, if necessary, be extended into a full-chevron incision to accommodate the largest renal tumors, to provide bilateral renal access, or to optimize exposure of the great vessels. This direct access to the peritoneum also facilitates exploration

for metastatic disease. As with any transperitoneal approach, there is a slightly higher risk for postoperative ileus and injury to adjacent organs such as the spleen and liver than is seen with retroperitoneal exposure. Depending on surgeon preference, the patient may be placed in a supine position with a rolled sheet beneath the upper lumbar spine or with a 45-degree angle of the chest and upper abdomen while the lower abdomen is kept as supine as possible. In this latter position, sandbags may be used behind the chest to support the position and the kidney rest and flexion of the table applied as described previously. Pillows are used to pad the lower extremities, and an airplane arm support is used to support the ipsilateral arm, which is brought across the body. The incision is begun just off the tip of the twelfth rib and extends two fingerbreadths below the costal margin with a gentle upward curve across the midline, usually ending at the contralateral rectus.

Thoracoabdominal Incision. This transthoracic transperitoneal exposure is ideal for large upper pole lesions or in cases in which an ipsilateral pulmonary wedge resection of limited metastatic disease is required. It is particularly helpful for large, right-sided, upper pole tumors of which visualization and exposure may otherwise be limited owing to the overlying liver. Right-sided renal cancers with associated supradiaphragmatic tumor thrombus requiring cardiac bypass techniques can also be approached in this fashion. The disadvantage of this incision is that it requires placement of a chest tube and is often associated with increased post-operative pain. In this approach, the patient is positioned as described previously for the flank incision.

Make the initial skin incision overlying the eighth to tenth ribs or within the associated interspaces. Begin at the posterior axillary line and carry the incision across the costal cartilage to the midline, extending it as far down toward the umbilicus as necessary. Perform a subperiosteal rib resection and divide the bridging costal cartilage. Incise the diaphragm using electrocautery along the periphery in the direction of the muscle fibers and several centimeters proximal to its attachment to the chest wall. Take care to avoid major branches of the phrenic nerve. After the incision is carried out through the abdominal wall musculature, both the thoracic and peritoneal cavities are widely exposed. Further exposure of the right kidney may be achieved by releasing the right coronary and triangular ligaments and elevating the liver into the diaphragmatic defect.

Place a small, cephalad-directed chest tube through a separate stab incision below a rib just behind the posterior axillary line. Direct it into the chest over that rib. If a concomitant pulmonary wedge resection is performed, a larger chest tube to facilitate evacuation of pleural fluid should be placed. Close the chest and abdomen separately. Interrupted figure-of-eight permanent closure sutures are preferable on the diaphragm to prevent distortion, and knots are placed on the peritoneal side of the closure (see also Fig. 28.6 in Chapter 28).

Midline Incision. The midline approach may be optimum when bilateral renal operations or simultaneous intraperitoneal surgery is planned. Place the patient supine and begin the incision just below the xiphoid. Extend it to the region of the umbilicus or below, if necessary. Cephalad extension of this incision into a median sternotomy can also be performed to provide cardiac bypass access for renal tumors with associated tumor thrombus extending into the supradiaphragmatic vena cava. Although this approach provides excellent exposure of the great vessels, cephalad and lateral regions of the kidney can be difficult to access depending on the patient's body habitus and the size of the tumor. Therefore, it is not one of our preferred approaches for routine radical nephrectomy.

Anatomic Points

The flank and upper abdominal musculature that is incised when making most of these incisions includes the fascia and muscular layers of the external oblique, internal oblique, transversus abdominis, and the rectus abdominis. These muscles vary greatly in thickness depending on the age and condition of the patient. Often, the transversus may appear as only thin straps of muscle fibers, which can be teased apart to reveal the underlying transversalis fascia that extends posterior to cover the anterior surface of the musculature of the retroperitoneum. This layer must be punctured laterally to enter the retroperitoneum and avoid the medially located peritoneum. Complete exposure of the retroperitoneal space is

gained by carefully sweeping the peritoneal envelope medially off the surface of Gerota's fascia. Incisions extended across the rectus abdominis should include the anterior and posterior fascial sheath as well as the muscle body to maximize exposure. It is important to remember that the pleural space often extends as far as the tenth rib laterally with inferior attachments to the diaphragm, which in turn attaches to the inner aspect of the twelfth rib. Careful incision and cephalad release of these structures must be performed to prevent inadvertent entry into the pleural cavity. The intercostal space contains three muscle layers and their associated membranes, including the external intercostal, internal intercostal, and innermost intercostal with attached transversus thoracis. The neurovascular bundle associated with each rib and supplying sensory innervation to the ipsilateral dermatomal segment lies in the inferior costal groove beneath each rib and should be preserved whenever possible.

Retroperitoneal Exposure, Isolation of the Hilar Vessels, Removal of the Standard Specimen, and Closure (Fig. 81.2)

Technical Points

Once access has been gained through the flank or abdominal wall, the next step is to expose the kidney and its vasculature. This requires thorough medial mobilization of the peritoneal envelope and its contents during direct retroperitoneal exposure or release of the line of Toldt and associated hepatocolic or lienocolic ligaments for a transperitoneal right- or left-sided nephrectomy, respectively. Release of the lateral colonic attachments allows the corresponding ascending or descending colon to be swept medially (Fig. 81.2A). Right-sided dissections also require a Kocher maneuver (medial mobilization of the second portion of the duodenum) to expose the underlying inferior vena cava (Fig. 81.2B). It is best to gain access to the main renal vessels early, especially for large highly vascularized tumors. In general, there is a single large renal artery that lies directly posterior to the main renal vein. Once all of the fibrofatty tissue is dissected from the surface of the vein using electrocautery, the vein may be elevated using a vein retractor or vessel loop to expose the underlying artery. This maneuver is facilitated during left-sided nephrectomy by initial ligation and division of the gonadal, adrenal, and ascending lumbar vessels, which drain into the inferior, superior, and posterior surfaces of the main renal vein, respectively. Early ligation and division of the renal artery followed by the main renal vein leaves only the blood flow through tumor and capsular vessels to address when mobilizing the remainder of the kidney. Initial ligation of the main renal vein before the artery is discouraged because it can result in significant arterial engorgement, resultant tumor or capsular rupture, and profound hemorrhage. When a left-sided dissection is being performed, caution must be exercised to avoid mistaking the superior mesenteric artery for the main renal artery. This can occur most commonly in association with large tumors that distort the anatomy. Complete dissection and identification of the lateral border of the

FIGURE 81.2
RETROPERITONEAL EXPOSURE, ISOLATION OF THE HILAR VESSELS, REMOVAL OF THE STANDARD SPECIMEN, AND CLOSURE (From Radical nephrectomy. In: *Stewart's operative urology.* 2nd ed. Baltimore: Williams & Wilkins, 1989, with permission.)

A   B

aorta both above and below the level of the renal vein helps to prevent this potential catastrophic error.

Routine removal of the adrenal gland is controversial. Because of the low risk for metastases, some surgeons prefer to exclude the adrenal gland from the removed specimen for T-1 lesions involving the middle or lower pole regions of the kidney if the adrenal is radiologically and palpably normal. This does, however, require violation of Gerota's fascia. For right-sided dissections, the adrenal gland is separated from the upper pole of the kidney with cautery after ligating the renal vein as it enters the inferior vena cava. The harmonic scalpel has recently been found to be ideal for this maneuver. If the left adrenal gland is being spared, the left adrenal vein can be preserved but is more commonly ligated to facilitate renal vein mobilization. The plane between the upper pole and the adrenal gland is separated using the electrocautery to provide adequate hemostasis of the small arterial branches supplying the adrenal. If the adrenal gland is to be included in the *en bloc* left-sided specimen, the renal vein is ligated and divided between the inferior vena cava medially and the adrenal vein branch laterally, and the medial edge of the adrenal gland is dissected using electrocautery. On the right side, the adrenal

vein is short and often substantial as it enters the right lateral edge of the inferior vena cava. After ligation of the right main renal vein, the fibrofatty and lymphatic tissue overlying the inferior vena cava are divided using electrocautery, and clips or small ties are placed on the more substantial lymphatic vessels. As the dissection is carried cephalad, the distinct border of the yellow-orange adrenal gland is identified, the short adrenal vein is carefully ligated and divided, and the adrenal is dissected with the kidney as described previously.

Once these primary vascular structures have been divided, the remainder of the kidney can be dissected rather rapidly in the plane surrounding Gerota's fascia. Substantial tumor vessels are clipped or ligated before division with electrocautery. The harmonic shears or scalpel can be used instead of clips or ties. Superiorly, on the right side, Gerota's fascial attachments at the diaphragm can be clipped, or cautery can be used to divide the tissue. Only occasionally are substantial periphrenic vessels encountered. This dissection frequently requires marked liver retraction for an optimum view. On the left side, superior dissection requires careful division of adhesions or vessels from the spleen to the colon and tissue surrounding Gerota's fascia and then blunt and sharp separation of the peritoneum surrounding the spleen from Gerota's fascia. Splenic damage from vigorous retraction on the peritoneal surface must be avoided. Likewise, dissection and retraction of the pancreas from the adrenal and superior pole of Gerota's fascia must be done cautiously to avoid injury of this unforgiving organ. Inferiorly, the ureter is identified as one of two tubular retroperitoneal structures running parallel to the aorta and is usually located lateral to the gonadal vein. It is readily distinguished by the peristaltic wave that can be induced by briefly compressing the structure with operative forceps. The ureteral stump is tied with nonabsorbable suture or clipped before division, usually as low as the operative incision will allow. This facilitates future identification of the upper extent of the pelvic stump should it require removal. The specimen is removed, and the retroperitoneum is irrigated. We typically do not place a drain unless there is a concern regarding pancreatic or hepatic trauma and a period of observation for pancreatic or biliary leakage is desired. Depending on surgeon preference, the fascial layers are reconstituted by an interrupted figure-of-eight suture or a running continuous suture of number 0 or 1 PDS, incorporating the innermost two layers and using a similar running or interrupted figure-of-eight suture to close the external oblique and anterior rectus fascia. The first layer or closure can incorporate the fascial layers of the transversus abdominis and internal oblique together, and the second layer closes the external oblique and anterior rectus fascia. The skin edges are reapproximated using wound clips.

Special Considerations: Regional Lymphadenectomy. Controversy exists surrounding the extent of regional lymphadenectomy that should be performed in association with a radical nephrectomy. Extensive dissection beyond the perihilar lymphatic tissue for low-stage tumors is probably unwarranted. The long-term survival for patients with lymph node metastasis is dismal, with 5-year survival rates of 5% to 20% arguing against significant advantage from removal of involved nodes. More thorough dissections may prove advantageous, however, even in cases of gross nodal disease, when the primary tumor is being removed before treatment with a biologic response modifier or other adjuvant treatment protocol. Regional lymphadenectomy can be performed as part of the *en bloc* specimen or separately after removal of the kidney. This later approach simplifies the dissection, especially for large tumors. The lymphatic tissue overlying, beneath, and lateral to the aorta is removed for left-sided dissections, and that surrounding all surfaces of the inferior vena cava is removed for right-sided tumors. A standard "split-and-roll" technique is employed by splitting the lymphatic tissue overlying the aorta or vena cava, ligating all major lymphatic channels, and rolling the tissue laterally and medially off the surface of the vessel. Ligating and dividing the posterior lumbar branches, allowing elevation of the great vessel, facilitates removal of retroaortic and retrocaval lymphatic tissue. The extent of the dissection is usually carried out from the crus of the diaphragm to the common iliac on the right and to just below the takeoff of the inferior mesenteric artery on the left. The packet includes all of the intervening fibrofatty tissue out lateral to the ipsilateral ureter.

Special Considerations: Tumor Thrombectomy (Fig. 81.3)

Technical Points

Tumor thrombus with extension into the inferior vena cava is seen in about 4% to 10% of cases of renal carcinoma. In the absence of metastatic disease, perinephric fat involvement, or direct vascular wall invasion, the presence of tumor thrombus does not appear to affect survival rates greatly, and complete extirpation has been reported to yield 10-year survival rates as high as 60%. Vena caval tumor thrombus is staged based on the cephalad extent of the thrombus, as follows:

Level I: infrahepatic extension less than 2 cm from the renal ostium

Level II: infrahepatic extension more than 2 cm from the ostium

Level III: infradiaphragmatic extension that achieves the level of the major hepatic veins

Level IV: supradiaphragmatic caval or atrial involvement

The surgical approach to renal tumors with associated thrombus depends primarily on the level of the thrombus, but also on surgeon preference and experience.

In cases of level I extension, the thrombus can usually be swept back into the renal vein by compressing the vena cava between the fingers and drawing the thrombus back inside the ostium. A Satinsky or similar vascular clamp is then placed with its convexity extending onto the caval surface after first securing and dividing the main renal artery. The main renal vein is then circumscribed on the caval side of the ostium using a scalpel, and the defect is oversewn using 4-0 or 5-0 cardiovascular suture.

Level II thrombus is addressed by first ligating and dividing all branches draining into the ipsilateral renal vein and involved caval segment. Rumel tourniquets are placed on the proximal and distal inferior vena cava as well as the contralateral main renal vein before circumscribing the ostium of the involved renal vein. Scissors are used to extend the cavotomy over the thrombus in an anterior longitudinal direction. The thrombus is then extracted from the involved caval segment. If areas of attachment to the endothelium are encountered that do not release easily with gentle elevation using an endarterectomy spatula, then the involved region may need to be excised. Reduction of caval lumen by more than 50% in the absence of significant collateral vessels usually requires caval reconstruction using patch grafting or, in rare cases, replacement. Small hepatic veins draining the caudate lobe can also be ligated and divided as shown, allowing further elevation of the liver to improve exposure of the more cephalad aspect of the thrombus. This maneuver facilitates full encirclement of the vena cava with a Rumel tourniquet.

Controversy exists regarding the management of level III thrombus, with some surgeons preferring cardiac or venous

FIGURE 81.3
SPECIAL CONSIDERATIONS: TUMOR THROMBECTOMY (From Marshall FF, Dietrick DD, Baumgartner WA, et al. Surgical management of renal cell carcinoma with intracaval neoplastic extension above the hepatic veins. *J Urol* 1988;139:1169, with permission.)

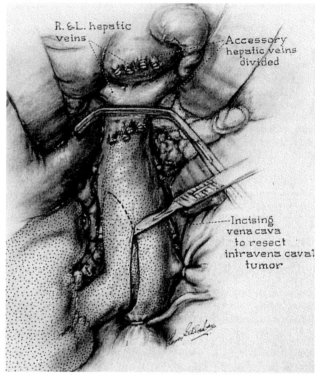

(caval–atrial) bypass techniques and others favoring clamping of the suprahepatic vena cava with occlusion of the porta hepatis and superior mesenteric artery.

Cardiopulmonary bypass with hypothermic arrest and exsanguination is the preferred approach to managing renal cell carcinomas with level IV thrombus. It is usually preferable to ligate the artery and perform as much of the dissection as possible before placing the patient on bypass. This reduces the amount of time on bypass and the postbypass bleeding that can occur if the entire dissection is performed in the exsanguinated state.

Anatomic Points

The right kidney typically lies 1 to 2 cm below the left in its cephalad extent in the retroperitoneum because of presence of the liver. The adrenal gland is found medial to the kidney on the left, with the right adrenal being more cephalad in location. The right renal artery, which arises slightly higher on the aorta, courses in a downward direction to reach the hilum of the corresponding kidney, as contrasted to the shorter, more horizontal course of the left renal artery. Small branches arise from the superior surface of both main renal arteries to supply the adrenal glands before dividing into five main segmental branches in the hilum. The vascular anatomy of the kidney

can differ from this classic description in as many as one third of patients, with separate upper or lower pole renal arteries being the most common finding.

There is extensive collateral venous drainage of the left renal vein through its gonadal, adrenal, and lumbar branches, with drainage also occurring into the inferior phrenic vessels. An understanding of this extensive venous network is important because all of these branches usually require ligation during radical nephrectomy. The size and significance of each of these vessels can change drastically depending on the vascularity of the tumor, its location, and the presence of associated thrombus. The right renal vein is significantly shorter and lacks the multiple accessory branches typically seen on the left. In general, there are several small veins draining from the caudate lobe of the liver (accessory hepatic veins) into the inferior vena cava. These can be ligated and divided to allow elevation of the liver for greater cephalad exposure to the vena cava below the main hepatic veins, which must remain intact.

Primary lymphatic drainage of the kidney can be altered by the presence of a large hypervascular tumor but typically follows the vasculature. In addition to several hilar nodes usually found adjacent to the renal vein, the first-echelon drainage of the left kidney is to the paraaortic, preaortic, and retroaortic lymphatics, and on the right it is to the perihilar, interaortocaval, paracaval, precaval, and retrocaval lymphatics. Some lymphatic channels can extend to the retrocrural nodes or into the thoracic duct. These represent the primary areas of involvement for renal parenchymal malignancies with associated lymphatic metastases and, as such, are the areas removed during regional lymphadenectomy.

Postoperative Care. Consideration should be given to pain control and gastrointestinal secretions postoperatively. We have found that epidural infusion analgesia is ideal for postoperative pain control. This decreases the need for substantial amounts of intravenous narcotics, which delay the return of bowel function. The only drawbacks of epidural pain control include the occasional effects on blood pressure, local pruritus, and the need to leave in a urethral catheter until the epidural is removed. If epidural analgesia is contraindicated, liberal use of bupivacaine intercostal nerve blocks during the closure is helpful. A nasogastric tube is rarely necessary when there has been minimal manipulation of the bowels and pancreas, particularly with epidural analgesia. Finally, it is important to be certain there is a radiographically normal contralateral adrenal gland when removal of the ipsilateral adrenal is planned. If there is not, sparing the adrenal should be considered, or postoperative steroid coverage must be provided.

REFERENCES

1. Marshall FF, Dietrick DD, Baumgartner WA, et al. Surgical management of renal cell carcinoma with intracaval neoplastic extension above the hepatic veins. *J Urol* 1988;139:1169.
2. Marshall FF. Radical nephrectomy: flank approaches. In: Marshall FF, Kavoussi LR, McAninch JW, et al, eds. *Textbook of operative urology.* Philadelphia: WB Saunders, 1996:248.
3. Sandlow JI, Williams RD. Anatomic and surgical considerations in radical nephrectomy. *Atlas Urol Clin North Am* 1998;6:25.

CHAPTER 82

Cadaveric Donor Nephrectomy and Renal Transplantation

You Min Wu

In this chapter, harvesting of kidneys and renal transplantation are described as a means of illustrating the anatomy of the retroperitoneum. The *en bloc* nephrectomy specimen consists of a segment of aorta, a segment of vena cava, the kidneys and their vessels, the ureters, and a generous amount of perinephric tissue, including the adrenal glands.

Cadaveric Donor Nephrectomy

Cadaveric Donor Nephrectomy: Incision and Exposure of the Chest and Abdomen (Fig. 82.1)

Technical and Anatomic Points

After appropriate pronouncement of brain death, the donor is placed on the operating table in the supine position and ventilated with 100% oxygen. Exposure for organ harvesting is provided by a longitudinal midline incision that extends from the suprasternal notch to the symphysis pubis. This incision provides sufficient exposure of and access to the heart, lungs, and abdominal viscera because a multiorgan harvest is always planned.

The sternum is split with an electric saw or a Lebsche knife; hemostasis of the cut surface is achieved with electrocautery and bone wax. A sternal retractor with spikes is placed in the lower third of the sternum and spread laterally. A special large Balfour retractor with teeth is used for the abdomen. The heart and liver teams usually start the dissection simultaneously. The kidneys can be dissected free and easily removed after flushing of the graft and the liver and pancreas are removed.

Preparation and Flushing of the Graft (Fig. 82.2)

Technical Points

Dissect the terminal aorta free. Divide the inferior mesenteric artery between ligatures and place two umbilical tapes around the terminal aorta (Fig. 82.2A). When the heart and liver teams start the preparatory dissection at the same time, this division can be performed initially. As a last step in the preparatory dissection, encircle the supraceliac aorta with an umbilical tape after separating the muscle fibers of the diaphragmatic crura longitudinally in a blunt fashion and incising the preaortic fascia. This step is omitted if the heart is not procured because the descending aorta can be cross-clamped in the left pleural cavity without preliminary dissection.

Heparin at a dose of 100 to 300 U/kg should be administered intravenously 3 minutes before cross-clamping. For a non–heart-beating donor, the dosage of heparin should be doubled. Tie the terminal aorta with an umbilical tape. The perfusate is temporarily stopped during the aortotomy to maintain exposure. Insert the aorta cannula into the terminal aorta (Fig. 82.2B). Position the tip of the aorta cannula below the renal artery to avoid blocking perfusion of renal artery. Fix the aorta cannula by another umbilical tape.

Apply a vascular clamp on the supraceliac aorta to continue cold perfusion of the kidneys through the terminal aorta cannula with 2 L of UW solution. At the same time, position a vent in the vena cava, usually above the diaphragm and just below the heart, to prevent venous engorgement and to drain flush solution from the operative field.

LIST OF STRUCTURES

Kidneys	Aorta	Diaphragm
Renal artery and vein	Celiac artery	Left and right crura
Ureter	Superior mesenteric artery	Inferior phrenic artery
Bladder	Inferior mesenteric artery (and vein)	Stomach
Gerota's fascia	Common iliac artery (and vein)	Duodenum
Gonadal artery and vein	Internal iliac artery (and vein)	Pancreas
Adrenal (suprarenal) gland	External iliac artery (and vein)	Spleen
Right adrenal (suprarenal) vein		Colon

FIGURE 82.1
CADAVERIC DONOR NEPHRECTOMY: INCISION AND EXPOSURE OF THE CHEST AND ABDOMEN

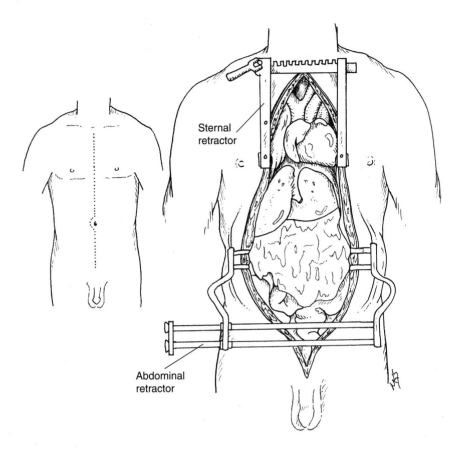

Sternal retractor

Abdominal retractor

FIGURE 82.2
PREPARATION AND FLUSHING OF THE GRAFT

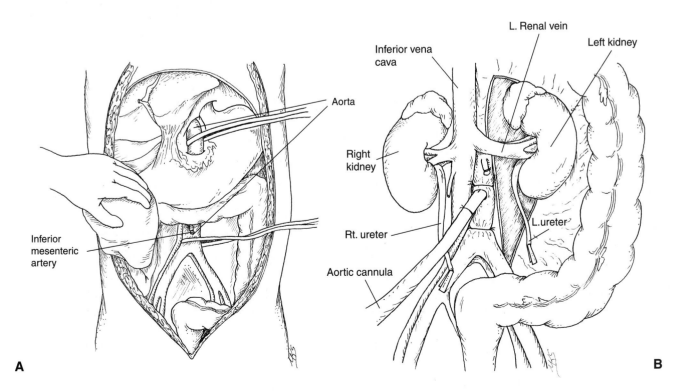

Aorta

Inferior mesenteric artery

Inferior vena cava

L. Renal vein

Left kidney

Right kidney

Rt. ureter

Aortic cannula

L. ureter

A

B

Anatomic Points

The paracolic gutters lie lateral to the colon and are limited medially by the retroperitoneal colon (ascending or descending) and its serosal covering, which became fused with parietal peritoneum during development. The white line of Toldt, visible in the angle between the parietal peritoneum and the lateral colon, marks the location of the fusion plane between original serosa or mesocolon and parietal peritoneum. Dissection in the fusion plane, from colon to midline, results in no damage to structures and minimal blood loss.

The gonadal vessels are the first major retroperitoneal structures encountered just superior to the pelvic brim. The right gonadal vein (a tributary of the inferior vena cava) and artery (an anterolateral branch of the aorta slightly inferior to the renal arteries) should be encountered as they cross the external iliac vessels somewhat lateral to the ureter. The ureter is just medial to these vessels.

More superiorly, Gerota's fascia (enclosing the right kidney, suprarenal gland, and perirenal fat) will be exposed as the hepatic flexure is mobilized. Further medial mobilization of the colon will expose the C loop of the duodenum, encompassing the head of the pancreas. These retroperitoneal structures are in direct contact with the anterior surface of Gerota's fascia. Further medial mobilization of the right colon, terminal ileum, duodenum, and head of the pancreas will expose the entire infrahepatic inferior vena cava lying to the right of the midline. Encirclement of the infrahepatic inferior vena cava should be done with some degree of caution because the short, fragile right adrenal vein typically drains into the posterolateral aspect of the inferior vena cava at a variable distance superior to the renal vein. When visualized, this should be doubly clamped and divided. Inferiorly, no special precautions are necessary before encircling the beginning of the inferior vena cava because the right ureter and gonadal vessels should have already been identified.

Encirclement of the distal aorta, just proximal to its bifurcation, is aided by lateral retraction of the inferior mesenteric artery because this parallels, to the left, the distal aorta. Skeletonization of the distal aorta, however, should be done with some care to avoid inadvertent laceration of the left fourth lumbar vein, which passes to the left posterior to the aorta.

As the abdominal aorta is skeletonized from inferior to superior, the first structure to be encountered should be the inferior mesenteric artery. More superiorly, again from the anterior surface of the aorta, small gonadal arteries can be identified. These may arise as a common trunk, separately and at the same or different levels, or they may arise from a renal or suprarenal artery. The next structure to be encountered should be the left renal vein, which typically crosses the anterior surface of the aorta just inferior to the origins of the superior mesenteric artery and left renal artery. However, retroaortic left renal veins or circumaortic left renal veins do occur, as commonly as 6% of the time. The superior mesenteric artery usually originates about 1 cm distal to the celiac artery; however, both of these major arteries can arise from a common trunk. Ligation of the last major visceral artery can be somewhat complicated if, as sometimes happens, one or more of its three branches (left gastric, splenic, or common hepatic) arise independently from the aorta.

Nephrectomy (Fig. 82.3)

Technical Points

Once the hepatectomy and pancreatectomy are complete, dissection is carried out in a bloodless field. The kidneys have already been flushed *in situ*. Mobilize the right colon and duodenum and sweep these up into the left upper abdomen. Divide the lesser splanchnic nerves and left mesocolon to expose the left kidney. Mobilize both kidneys medially with Gerota's fascia, using sharp dissection. Identify both ureters and transect these near the bladder. Tag and dissect the ureters up to the level of the lower pole. Divide the inferior vena cava and aorta just below the level of the aortic cannula. Complete the *en bloc* excision by incising the prevertebral fascia cephalad with a pair of heavy scissors, while the aorta and the inferior vena cava are retracted upward together with the kidneys and ureters (Fig. 82.3A). Five to 10 minutes are required for this *en bloc* dissection.

Once removed, immerse the kidneys in an ice basin and separate them. Divide the left renal vein first, including a cuff of the inferior vena cava. Of note, the entire inferior vena cava is left with the right kidney. Turn the kidneys posteriorly and incise the aorta between the paired lumbar arteries (Fig. 82.3B). After identifying the renal arteries from within, split the aorta anteriorly and separate the kidneys. Insert a fistula tip in each renal artery and flush a total of 250 to 300 mL of chilled UW solution through each kidney. Split Gerota's fascia along the convex surface of the kidney and partially dissect it off the kidney, particularly if there is a considerable amount of perinephric fat, to ensure good cooling. Package the kidneys separately and store them in UW solution. All remaining back-table preparation is left for the recipient surgeon.

If perfusion preservation is attempted, the proximal aorta is closed with sutures, and perfusion is through a cannula inserted through the distal aorta.

The kidneys are not separated if the donor is younger than 2 years of age—they are recovered and transplanted *en bloc*.

Anatomic Points

The paracolic gutters lie lateral to the colon and are limited medially by the retroperitoneal colon (ascending or descending) and its serosal covering, which became fused with parietal peritoneum during development. The white line of Toldt, visible in the angle between the parietal peritoneum and the lateral colon, marks the location of the fusion plane between original serosa or mesocolon and parietal peritoneum. Dissection in the fusion plane, from colon to midline, results in no damage to structures and minimal blood loss.

The gonadal vessels are the first major retroperitoneal structures that will be encountered just superior to the pelvic

FIGURE 82.3
NEPHRECTOMY

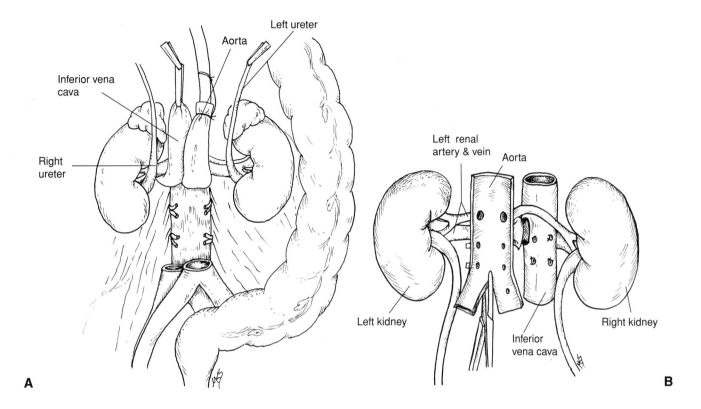

A

B

brim. The right gonadal vein (a tributary of the inferior vena cava) and artery (an anterolateral branch of the aorta slightly inferior to the renal arteries) should be encountered as they cross the external iliac vessels somewhat lateral to the ureter. The ureter is just medial to these vessels.

More superiorly, Gerota's fascia (enclosing the right kidney, suprarenal gland, and perirenal fat) will be exposed as the hepatic flexure is mobilized. Further medial mobilization of the colon will expose the C loop of the duodenum, encompassing the head of the pancreas. These retroperitoneal structures are in direct contact with the anterior surface of Gerota's fascia. Further medial mobilization of the right colon, terminal ileum, duodenum, and head of the pancreas will expose the entire infrahepatic inferior vena cava lying to the right of the midline. Encirclement of the infrahepatic inferior vena cava should be done with some degree of caution because the short, fragile right adrenal vein typically drains into the posterolateral aspect of the inferior vena cava at a variable distance superior to the renal vein. When visualized, this should be doubly clamped and divided. Inferiorly, no special precautions are necessary before encircling the beginning of the inferior vena cava because the right ureter and gonadal vessels should have already been identified.

Encirclement of the distal aorta, just proximal to its bifurcation, is aided by lateral retraction of the inferior mesenteric artery because this parallels, to the left, the distal aorta. Skele-

tonization of the distal aorta, however, should be done with some care to avoid inadvertent laceration of the left fourth lumbar vein, which passes to the left posterior to the aorta.

The blood supply to the right ureter is provided by branches from the renal arteries, aorta, gonadal arteries, iliac (common or internal) arteries, and vesical arteries. The longitudinal anastomosis between these vessels, on the surface of the ureter, is usually good. Typically, ureteric branches of arteries superior to the pelvic brim approach the ureter from its medial side. In the pelvis, because the ureters lie medial to the internal iliac arteries, the blood supply approaches from its lateral side. This is essentially true for as far as the ureters can be exposed in the pelvis.

Mobilization of the kidneys and ureters is facilitated by a conceptual understanding of Gerota's fascia. This perirenal fascia has been variously interpreted as being either continuous with the transversalis fascia or a "condensation" of retroperitoneal tissue. Regardless of its derivation, this facial layer encloses the kidney, suprarenal gland, and perirenal fat. The anterior layer of Gerota's fascia is rather poorly developed, whereas the posterior layer is significantly thicker. Anterior and posterior layers fuse around the lateral and superior aspects of the kidney and suprarenal gland. Medially and inferiorly, anterior and posterior layers do not fuse (or at least not firmly), so that the capsule is continuous with pericaval and periaortic tissue across the midline and is "open" inferiorly, essentially anterior and posterior to the ureter. Mobilization of the kidney is easiest if the plane posterior to the posterior layer of Gerota's fascia is developed, rather than trying to develop a plane between the true capsule of the kidney and Gerota's fascia.

Exposure of the left kidney and ureter follows most of the colon mobilization procedures done with performing a left hemicolectomy. On the antimesenteric side of the colon, incision along the white line of Toldt, a comparatively avascular line formed by embryonic fusion of the serosa and parietal peritoneum, enables entrance to the relatively avascular plane that results from fusion of the descending mesocolon and parietal peritoneum. Blunt dissection to the midline in this plane allows complete mobilization of the descending colon. As the peritoneum and inferior mesenteric vessels are elevated and mobilized, it is important to identify the ureter; frequently, this adheres to the peritoneum and can be inadvertently reflected with the colon and its vasculature. The ureter should be identified as it passes into the pelvis in the vicinity of the apex of the root of the sigmoid mesocolon. Remember that the upper (lateral) limb of this inverted V is lateral to the ureter, whereas the lower (medial) limb is medial to the ureter.

When the left crus of the diaphragm is exposed, the inferior phrenic artery, which courses superiorly on the crus, should be identified and controlled before division of the crus. In addition, the first two lumbar arteries, which arise from the posterior aspect of the aorta, pass through or behind the diaphragmatic crura; their division, if uncontrolled, can be a source of hemorrhage that can obscure the operative field. Division of the crus is necessary because it allows control of the aorta superior to the celiac artery, which typically arises between the left and right crus just as the aorta enters the abdomen.

Renal Transplantation

Surgical Technique (Fig. 82.4)

Technical Points

After induction of general anesthesia, a central venous pressure line is placed and a Foley catheter inserted. Then, 150 to 200 mL of a 0.25% neomycin solution is instilled by gravity into the bladder, and the catheter is clamped. The abdomen is then prepped and draped. Most renal allografts are placed heterotopically, in an extraperitoneal location in the iliac fossa.

Expose the external iliac artery and vein after incising the external and internal oblique and transversus muscles and transversalis fascia (Fig. 82.4A,B). Ligate and divide the inferior epigastric vessels as well as the round ligament in women. Take care to ligate the lymphatics. Arterial, venous, and ureteral anastomoses are required.

Anatomic Points

This skin incision approximates the direction of Langer's lines and heals with comparatively minimal scarring. Incision of the superficial fascia, here typically divisible into a fatty superficial layer (Camper's fascia) and a deeper, more fibrous layer (Scarpa's fascia), follows the same line as the skin incision. Only cutaneous nerves—branches of spinal nerves T-11 through L-1—are encountered during this stage of the dissection. The major branches of these cutaneous nerves are at the interface between Camper's and Scarpa's fasciae. It is also at this level that one may encounter branches of the superficial epigastric and superficial circumflex iliac arteries and veins. These can be large enough to require electrocautery or ligation to achieve hemostasis. The incision exposes the aponeurosis of the external oblique muscle. Divide this in the direction of its fibers through the external inguinal ring. Reflect the external oblique muscle and aponeurosis to expose the internal oblique muscle. An avascular plane can be developed between the anterior surface of the peritoneal envelope and the posterior surface of the transversus abdominis muscle, immediately deep to the internal oblique muscle. The internal oblique and transversus abdominis muscles are divided across their fibers using electrocautery. Protect the peritoneal envelope with a partially open Kelly clamp or your fingers. It is important to leave an adequate margin of muscle between the inferior cut edge and the inguinal ligament to allow sufficient tissue in which to place sutures without subsequent muscle ischemia or encroachment on the inguinal ligament.

Remember that the superficial inguinal ring is located immediately superior to the pubic tubercle. As the incision through the apex of the superficial inguinal ring is made, you must be careful not to damage the ilioinguinal nerve, which is located immediately superficial to the spermatic cord as it exits through the superficial inguinal ring. This nerve provides sensation to the skin of the superior and medial thigh, the root of the penis and the root of the scrotum (in males), and the mons pubis and labium majus (in females). The other major sensory nerve that might be encountered—the iliohypogastric nerve—passes through the aponeurosis of the external oblique muscle about 2.5 cm superior to the superficial inguinal ring. This nerve provides sensation to the skin superior to the mons pubis. Other nerves of importance, such as the external spermatic branch of the genitofemoral nerve, should be spared because the incision, which is superior to their course between the internal oblique and transversus abdominis muscles, parallels their direction.

The plane deep to the transversus abdominis muscle is actually deep to the transversalis fascia. To enter this plane, one must cut and ligate the inferior epigastric arteries and veins. These vessels originate from the terminal part of the external iliac artery and pass between the transversalis fascia and peritoneum to supply the rectus abdominis muscle.

The interval between the transversalis fascia and peritoneum is truly the retroperitoneal plane, where all retroperitoneal organs are located. Thus, dissection along this plane should lead one to the urogenital and vascular structures

**FIGURE 82.4
SURGICAL TECHNIQUE**

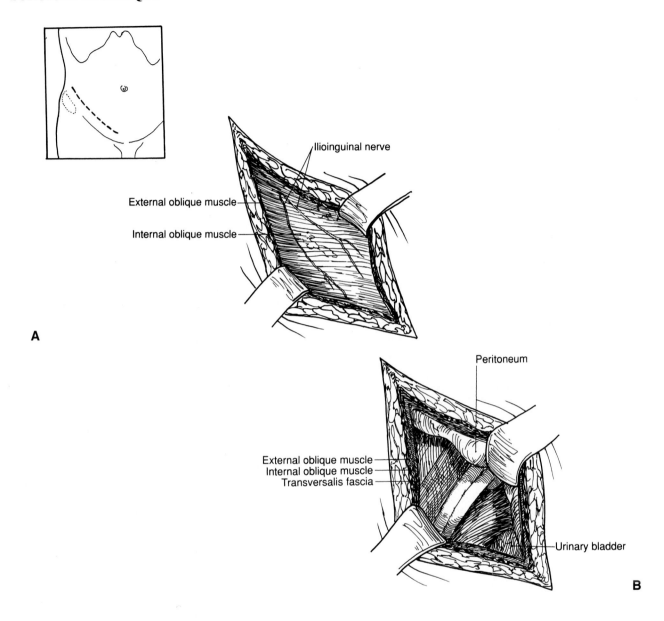

necessary to complete this procedure. As this space is developed, one will readily realize that no major nerves or vessels need be damaged, save those already mentioned.

Vascular Anastomosis (Fig. 82.5)

Technical Points

The renal artery usually is anastomosed with a cuff of aorta end to side to the external iliac artery, although it may also be sewn end to end to the internal iliac artery. In the case of multiple arteries, there are several options. If the arteries are on a cuff of aorta, it may be simplest to use a long cuff or two smaller cuffs. If a polar artery has been transected, it may be anastomosed on the back table to the side of the

main renal artery. If there are two transected vessels, they may be either implanted separately or partially anastomosed to form a single vessel that can be sutured to the iliac artery. Alternately, they can be lengthened by an arterial graft from the same donor. The latter solution also may be effective when the donor aortic cuff is atherosclerotic and the orifice of the renal artery is narrowed.

For a left kidney, the renal vein usually is anastomosed with a cuff of vena cava end to side to the external iliac vein. For a right kidney, the venous anastomosis can present some difficulty. The right renal vein can be anastomosed directly, usually with a cuff of vena cava. The vein is short on the right, however, and some surgeons prefer to increase the length. A segment of vena cava attached to the vein often is successfully

**FIGURE 82.5
VASCULAR ANASTOMOSIS**

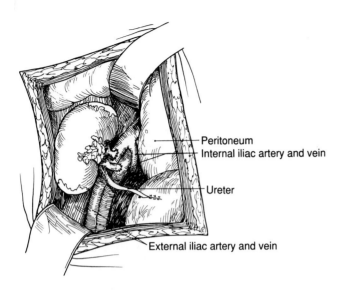

Peritoneum

Internal iliac artery and vein

Ureter

External iliac artery and vein

used. Another option is to use a transverse section of vena cava extending straight out from the renal vein. Finally, a donor iliac vein graft may be sutured end to end to the renal vein to gain length. Multiple veins tend not to be a problem; a bifurcated vein graft can be used, or one vein can be ligated.

In some arterial or venous reconstructions, a "growth factor" is used while tying, on completion of the anastomosis, to prevent stricture. For the artery and vein, continuous non-absorbable monofilament suture is used.

Anatomic Points

The shape of the pelvis, which may be classified as gynecoid, anthropoid, or android, is highly variable. In fact, some studies indicate that more than 50% of all females have an android or anthropoid pelvis, classifications supposedly characteristic of male pelves.

Reflection of the peritoneal sac reveals the common iliac vessels, which are crossed, on their peritoneal aspect, by the ureter. This occurs approximately at the point where the common iliac artery bifurcates into external and internal iliac arteries. It is also in this vicinity that the right common iliac and external iliac arterial trunk, which initially is medial to the corresponding veins, crosses the peritoneal surface of the veins to lie lateral to the vein. On the left, the arterial trunk is always lateral to the corresponding veins. In the male, the testicular artery lies on the peritoneal surface of the distal external iliac artery. Genital branches of the genitofemoral nerve will also be seen to cross the distal external iliac artery, exiting through the deep inguinal ring. The obturator artery (usually a branch of the internal iliac artery) and the obturator nerve lie medial to the external iliac vein, in the groove between the psoas major muscle and iliacus muscle. The artery can be ligated, but care should be taken not to damage this motor nerve to the hip adductors.

Ureteroneocystostomy (Fig. 82.6)

Technical Points

This part of the procedure is perhaps the most problematic and least standardized. Dozens of variations exist, although the most popular derive from three or four basic types. The extravesical ureteroneocystostomy is placed at the dome of the bladder. The bladder mucosa is exposed through a 2.5- to 3-cm incision in the muscle, and full-thickness ureter is sutured to the mucosa with interrupted or continuous absorbable sutures. A second layer of bladder wall muscle is then approximated over the first layer to create a submucosal tunnel.

In the case of ureters whose blood supply has been stripped, it may be necessary to perform a ureteroureterostomy or pyeloureterostomy to the ureter of the native kidney. In this circumstance, a native nephrectomy is required.

Double ureters can be reimplanted separately or partially anastomosed and transplanted as one. Care should be taken not to disrupt what is usually a common blood supply.

In the case of pediatric kidneys transplanted *en bloc,* the donor aorta and vena cava are used for the vascular anastomoses. It is important to ligate all the lumbar and gonadal branches on the back table (Fig. 82.6F). Separate ureteral reimplantations can be performed. Alternately, the ureters can be partially anastomosed and reimplanted together.

Ureteral reimplantation into an ileal loop is performed in one layer, anastomosing full-thickness ureter to full-thickness bowel with interrupted absorbable sutures, as demonstrated in Fig. 82.6G.

In most cases, the venous anastomosis is performed first, followed by the arterial anastomosis. As the vessels are sutured, the patient should be hydrated and given furosemide, 1 mg/kg, and mannitol, 0.2 g/kg. The systolic blood pressure should be 140 mm Hg at the time of cross-clamp release. A 500- to 1,000-mg dose of intravenous methylprednisolone is given just before the operation or just after release of the cross-clamps. The ureteral anastomosis is performed last. After hemostasis is achieved, the wound is closed in layers.

Anatomic Points

The rectovesical fascia (of Denonvilliers), located between the rectum and urinary bladder (and prostate), is significant to this part of the procedure only in the male. In females, this homologous structure is interposed between the rectum and vagina; in both sexes, it is formed by fusion of the caudalmost part of the embryonic peritoneal sac.

The blood supply of the ureter is provided by branches from the renal artery, aorta, gonadal artery, iliac (common, external, or internal) artery, and vesical artery. These arteries anastomose and lie on the ureter itself; thus, meticulous skeletonization of the ureter, with removal of the periureteral sheath and ureteric arteries, is not indicated and, in fact, can jeopardize the transplantation. Obviously, the supply from the renal artery is most important because that will serve as the sole blood supply to the donor ureter until neovascularization occurs following its anastomosis to the urinary bladder.

FIGURE 82.6
URETERONEOCYSTOSTOMY

A

B

C

D

E

Aorta

Inferior vena cava

Lumbar artery

F

Ileal loop

Ureter

G

REFERENCES

1. Dunkin BJ, Johnson LB, Kuo PC. A technical modification eliminates early ureteral complications after laparoscopic donor nephrectomy. *J Am Coll Surg* 2000;190:96–97.
2. Ko DSC, Cosimi AD. The donor and donor nephrectomy. In: Morris PJ, ed. *Kidney transplantation: principles and practice.* 5th ed. Philadelphia: WB Saunders, 2001:89–105.
3. Kuo PC, Cho ES, Flowers JL, et al. Laparoscopic living donor nephrectomy and multiple renal arteries. *Am J Surg* 1998;176:559–563.
4. Montgomery RA. The laparoscopic donor nephrectomy. In: Morris PJ, ed. *Kidney transplantation: principles and practice.* 5th ed. Philadelphia: WB Saunders, 2001:106–112.
5. Yanaga K, Podesta LG, Byoznick B, et al. Multiple organ recovery for transplantation. In: Starzl TE, Shapiro R, Simmons RI, eds. Atlas of Organ Transplantation Philadelphia: JB Lippincott, 1991:3.1–3.49.

CHAPTER 83

Hand-assisted Laparoscopic Donor Nephrectomy

Stephen C. Rayhill

Preoperative studies have confirmed that the donor is anatomically suitable for kidney donation. The donor is typed and cross-matched for two units of packed red blood cells, and preoperative antibiotics are given. The patient is liberally hydrated throughout the procedure (about 4 L).

The left kidney is commonly selected because of the greater length of renal vein. A brief section at the end of this chapter describes the modifications necessary for the right kidney. This chapter describes a vertical midline incision for this purpose; others have described the use of a Pfannenstiel incision for kidney retrieval after a completely laparoscopic operation is completed. These alternative techniques are described in the references at the end.

Incision and Placement of Trocars (Fig. 83.1)

Technical Points

Place the donor in the right lateral decubitus position (right side down) and flex the table (Fig. 83.1A). Accurately plan and mark the following trocar sites and incision lines (Fig. 83.1B). The inferior medial (camera) trocar site is placed 2 to 3 cm inferior and 5 cm to the left of the inferior margin of the umbilicus (estimate the lateral edge of the hand-assist device to be sure to be lateral to it). The lateral trocar is placed 3 cm medial and 2 cm inferior to the iliac crest.

Make a 1.5-cm incision at the medial site (being careful not to burn the skin edges) and insert a Veress needle (or Hasson port). If adhesions are suspected, make the midline hand incision first (or use a Hasson port) and then place the ports under direct vision. Insufflate the abdomen and place the 12-mm medial trocar. Insert the laparoscope and place the 12-mm lateral port under laparoscopic guidance.

Next create the midline hand-port incision. Draw a line beginning at the inferior edge of the umbilicus and extending 7 cm superiorly (depending on glove size) and make an incision just large enough to permit the hand. Insert the hand-port and subsequently use the left hand to retract the kidney atraumatically and facilitate dissection.

Anatomic Points

The inferior epigastric artery runs in the lateral aspect of the rectus sheath and should be avoided when placing the trocars.

Exposure of the Kidney (Fig. 83.2)

Technical Points

Incise the white line of Toldt laterally to the descending and sigmoid colon, beginning with the splenic attachments (Fig. 83.2A). Retract the colon medially (Mattox maneuver). Take care not to penetrate the colonic mesentery, which is often quite thin. Mobilize the spleen medially by dividing the splenorenal ligament (Fig. 83.2B). To provide maximal medial retraction of the descending colon, carefully divide the splenocolic attachments with ultrasonic dissecting shears. Open Gerota's fascia over the anterolateral aspect of the kidney and establish the plane between Gerota's fascia and the capsule (Fig. 83.2C). Open this superiorly.

Next, identify the ureter as it crosses the iliac vessels (Fig. 83.2D). Keeping the ureteral blood vessels intact by

LIST OF STRUCTURES

Left kidney	Inferior vena cava	Iliac vessels
Gerota's fascia	Left renal vein	Gonadal vessels
Ureter	Left adrenal vein	Inferior epigastric artery
Aorta	Left gonadal vein	Rectus sheath
Left renal artery	Lumbar veins	Colon
	Right kidney	White line of Toldt

FIGURE 83.1
INCISION AND PLACEMENT OF TROCARS (**A** and **B** from Cho ES, Flowers JL. Laparoscopic live-donor nephrectomy. In: Zucker KA, ed. *Surgical laparoscopy.* 2nd ed. Philadelphia: Lippincott Williams & Wilkins, 2001:657–667, with permission; **C** from Soper NJ, Halpin VJ, Meyers BF. Minimally invasive surgery: laparoscopic and thoracoscopic techniques. In: Baker RJ, Fischer JE, eds. *Mastery of surgery.* 4th ed. Philadelphia: Lippincott Williams & Wilkins, 2001:264–276, with permission.)

leaving the periureteral tissue with the ureter, dissect the ureter free from its attachments. This will allow safe dissection of Gerota's fascia inferiorly. Complete the dissection of Gerota's fascia inferiorly, laterally, and medially.

Anatomic Points

The white line of Toldt is the peritoneal thickening where the visceral peritoneum of the colon meets the parietal peritoneum of the lateral abdominal wall. This junction was formed when the descending colon became secondarily retroperitoneal in development. It is an avascular line for entrance into the retroperitoneum. Once entered, the colon can be dissected medially by dividing the alveolar tissue, securing it to the retroperitoneum.

The ureter emerges from the pelvis medial to the internal iliac vessels and crosses over the common iliac artery just superior to the junction, where it is easiest to find. Running lateral (especially in men) to the ureter are the gonadal vessels. On the left side, both are commonly attached to the posterior side of the descending colonic mesentery. Care must be taken not to transgress the colonic mesentery when dissecting these structures free (or a hernia prone defect could result). The gonadal vessels have ample collaterals and can be divided, if necessary, without consequence.

The ureter derives its blood supply from the bladder inferiorly, from the psoas muscle in its midregion, and from the renal artery superiorly. The transplanted ureter depends solely on the renal branches, which travel through the inferior pole perihilar fatty tissue, which must be preserved.

FIGURE 83.2

EXPOSURE OF THE KIDNEY (**A–C** from Cho ES, Flowers JL. Laparoscopic live-donor nephrectomy. In: Zucker KA. *Surgical laparoscopy.* 2nd ed. Philadelphia: Lippincott Williams & Wilkins, 2001:657–667, with permission; **D** from Scott-Conner CEH, Cuschieri A, Carter FJ. Colon and rectum. In: *Minimal access surgical anatomy.* Philadelphia: Lippincott Williams & Wilkins, 2000:185–210, with permission.)

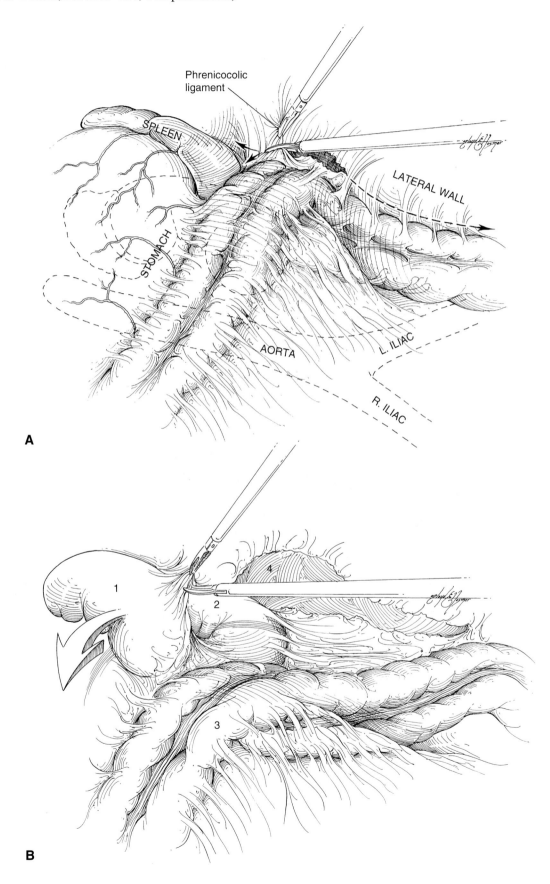

A

B

FIGURE 83.2   (Continued)

C

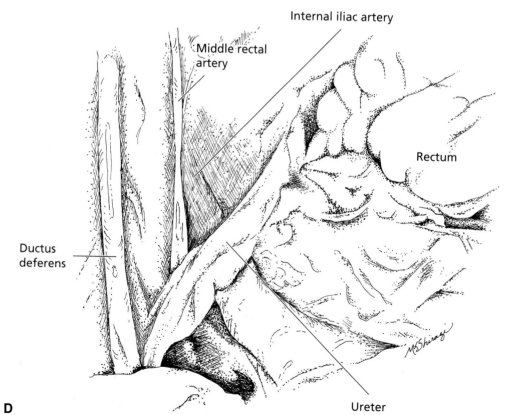

Internal iliac artery

Middle rectal artery

Rectum

Ductus deferens

Ureter

D

FIGURE 83.3
PREPARATION OF THE RENAL VEIN (**A** and **B** from Cho ES, Flowers JL. Laparoscopic live-donor nephrectomy. In: Zucker KA. *Surgical laparoscopy.* 2nd ed. Philadelphia: Lippincott Williams & Wilkins, 2001:657–667, with permission.)

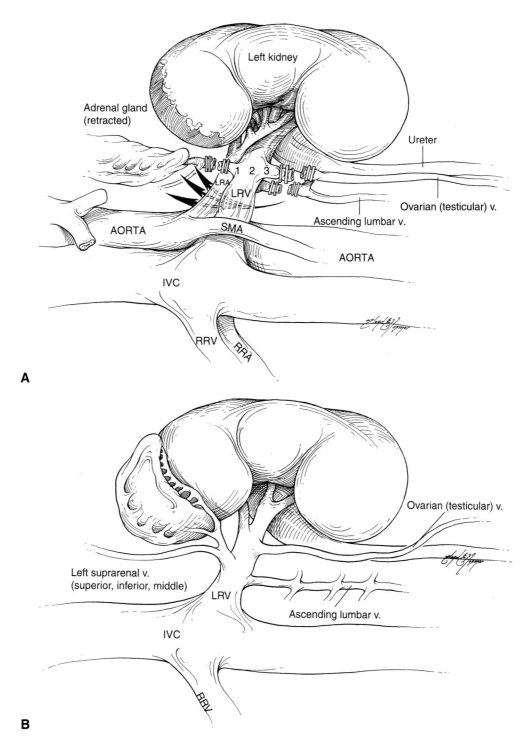

Preparation of the Renal Vein (Fig. 83.3)

Technical Points

Carefully retract the colonic mesentery to the right of the aorta. This allows for exposure of the left renal vein using gentle dissection of the anterior adventitial tissue. Identify both the left gonadal and the left adrenal veins. Carefully dissect these free and clip (using the right-angled clip applier) and divide them (Fig. 83.3A). Next, identify the lumber vein and clip (unless small) and divide it. If the lumbar vein is small and medial, divide it with the ultrasonic shears. This avoids clip placement in the vicinity of the subsequent vascular staple line. If the lumbar vein is difficult to dissect anteriorly, approach it from posterior by retracting the kidney medially. At this point, the renal vein is free.

Anatomic Points

On the left, the gonadal vein attaches to the inferior aspect of the renal vein, usually about 2 cm from the kidney (Fig. 83.3B). On the right, it attaches directly to the inferior vena cava. The gonadal artery usually originates directly from the aorta bilaterally. This may be encountered when dissecting the renal vein.

The left adrenal vein inserts onto the superior aspect of the left renal vein, usually within 1 cm distal to the insertion of the gonadal vein. The right gonadal vein drains directly into the superior vena cava, usually below the renal vein.

A lumbar vein usually drains into the renal vein posteriorly. This often substantial vein may retract into the retroperitoneal tissue when cut; hence, care must be used in clipping this vessel.

Dissection of the Renal Artery (Fig. 83.4)

Technical Points

If the renal artery is obvious anteriorly, free it of investing tissue from this vantage point. If it is not visible, elevate the kidney and retract it medially to expose the artery posteriorly. Perform this dissection far from the kidney to avoid division of early-branching lobar renal arteries. Free the artery to its junction with the aorta. In the process, dissect the adrenal gland away from the upper pole of the kidney. Perform this adrenal dissection near the gland itself to avoid injury to upper pole renal arterial branches.

Anatomic Points

The renal artery and vein are invested with a thick plexus of autonomic nerves (some are up to 2 mm thick) and a rich network of lymphatics. These are divided. The renal arteries are often multiple and do not communicate. Thus, the arteries

---

FIGURE 83.4
DISSECTION OF THE RENAL ARTERY (From Cho ES, Flowers JL. Laparoscopic live-donor nephrectomy. In: Zucker KA. *Surgical laparoscopy.* 2nd ed. Philadelphia: Lippincott Williams & Wilkins, 2001:657–667, with permission.)

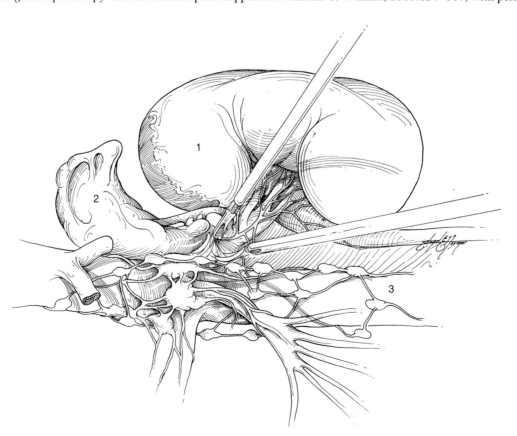

FIGURE 83.5
DIVISION OF THE DISTAL URETER, RENAL ARTERY, AND RENAL VEIN (From Cho ES, Flowers JL.
Laparoscopic live-donor nephrectomy. In: Zucker KA. *Surgical laparoscopy.* 2nd ed. Philadelphia: Lippincott Williams &
Wilkins, 2001:657–667, with permission.)

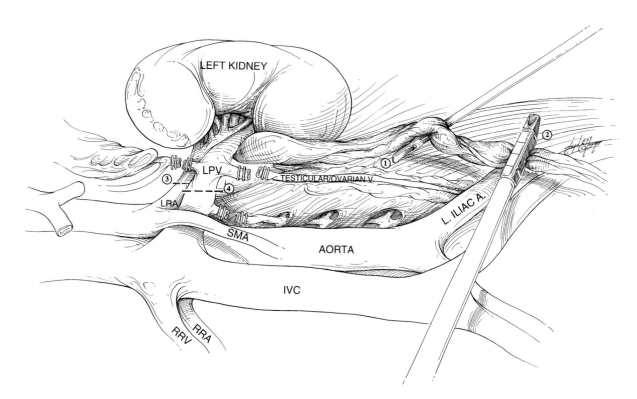

must be preserved. Small upper pole (<2 mm) arteries can
be taken with no significant consequence, but all lower pole
arteries must be preserved because they may provide blood
to the ureter. Similarly, the renal veins are often multiple;
however, unlike the arteries, the veins usually communicate.
Great care must be taken in dissecting the artery because
branches may emerge early. There are many small arterial
branches to the adrenal, which may be taken. Occasionally,
a renal artery may traverse across the inferolateral border of
the adrenal, which demands careful dissection.

*Division of the Distal Ureter, Renal Artery, and
Renal Vein (Fig. 83.5)*

Technical Points

Leaving as much periureteral tissue as possible to maintain
the ureteral blood supply, dissect the ureter free of its posterior and colonic attachments. The gonadal vein, after being
divided proximally, can be kept with the ureter or left behind.
Carry this dissection from inferior to superior, leaving more
periureteral tissue as the dissection approaches the lower pole
of the kidney. Doubly clip and divide the distal ureter. This
division of the ureter is done late to keep urine out of the
operative field during most of the dissection.

At this point, with maximal mobility of the kidney, complete the final dissection of the renal artery and vein. Topical
papaverine can be applied to the vessels, and furosemide and

mannitol may be given. Adequate amounts of fluid have ensured good urine output from both kidneys. Once brisk urine
output has been demonstrated, the kidney is ready to be removed by division of the vessels.

Doubly or triply clip the renal artery near the aorta and
divide it distally, providing an adequate cuff beyond the distal
clip (about 3 mm). Alternatively, use an endoscopic linear
stapler with a vascular cartridge. Next, apply the endoscopic
linear stapler with a vascular cartridge to the renal vein as
distally as possible and divide it.

Gently remove the kidney through the hand-port site and
flush it with cold heparinized solution. Hemostasis is ensured initially and rechecked after the intraabdominal pressure has been reduced for a minimum of 5 minutes. With excellent hemostasis ensured, close the trocar sites and midline
defect.

Postoperative management includes frequent monitoring of the hemoglobin and hematocrit levels, the vitals,
urine output, and creatinine (which may temporarily rise
slightly).

Anatomic Points

Occasionally, there is a double ureter; this must be determined
by intravenous pyelography or magnetic resonance imaging.
As mentioned earlier, the transplant ureter is totally dependent on blood supply from the renal hilum, and every effort
must be exerted to protect its blood supply.

Modification for Harvest of Right Kidney (Fig. 83.6)

Technical and Anatomic Points

The right kidney, although more difficult because of its short renal vein, can also be removed laparoscopically. Both the hand-assisted and the purely laparoscopic techniques are used. The general approach is similar to that of the laparoscopic left nephrectomy. There are two important points specific to the right nephrectomy. First, the small lumber veins that tether the vena cava posteriorly and make full dissection of the renal artery difficult must be divided, carefully, using clips or the harmonic stapler (if less than 3 mm). Second, the venous stapler must be applied in parallel to the vena cava while the kidney is retracted laterally to provide the maximum length of renal vein. A small amount of cava (pulled laterally) is usually also taken. Some centers use a nondividing stapler and cut the vein with scissors after stapling to remove the risk for bleeding if the stapler misfires.

FIGURE 83.6
MODIFICATION FOR HARVEST OF RIGHT KIDNEY (From Buell JF, Edye M, Johnson M, et al. Are concerns over right laparoscopic donor nephrectomy unwarranted? *Ann Surg* 2001;23(5):645–651, with permission.)

REFERENCES

1. Buell JF, Edye M, Johnson M, et al. Are concerns over right laparoscopic donor nephrectomy unwarranted? *Ann Surg* 2001;23(5):645–651.
2. Cho ES, Flowers JL. Laparoscopic live-donor nephrectomy. In: Zucker KA. *Surgical laparoscopy.* 2nd ed. Philadelphia: Lippincott Williams & Wilkins, 2001:657–667.
3. Philosophe B, Kuo PC, Schweitzer EJ, et al. Laparoscopic open donor nephrectomy: comparing ureteral complications in the recipients and improving the laparoscopic technique. *Transplantation* 1999;68(4):497–502.
4. Slakey DP, Wood JC, Hender D, et al. Laparoscopic living donor nephrectomy. *Transplantation* 1999;68(4):581–583.
5. Wolf JS, Marie-Blanche T, Merion RM. Hand-assisted laparoscopic live donor nephrectomy. *Urology* 1998;52:885–887.
6. Wolf JS, Merion RM, Leichtman AB, et al. Randomized controlled trial of hand-assisted laparoscopic versus open surgical live donor nephrectomy. *Transplantation* 2000;72(2):284–290.

CHAPTER 84

Abdominal Aortic Aneurysm Repair and Aortobifemoral Grafts

W. John Sharp

The anatomy of the abdominal aorta and iliac vessels is explored through the procedure of abdominal aortic aneurysm repair. The femoral region is then introduced through the closely related procedure of aortobifemoral bypass grafting.

Abdominal Aortic Aneurysm Repair

Skin Incision (Fig. 84.1)

Technical Points

Place the patient in a supine position, with a Foley catheter and appropriate monitoring devices in place. Prepare and drape the abdomen from the nipples to the knees. Cover the genitalia with a sterile towel. Secure all towels with iodophor-impregnated plastic adhesive drapes, rather than with sutures or towel clips. An antibiotic that is active against common gram-positive skin bacteria (e.g., a cephalosporin) is administered just before making the incision and for 24 hours postoperatively.

Most surgeons prefer a midline transperitoneal incision, as shown in Figs. 84.1 to 84.4. (An alternative retroperitoneal approach is presented in Figs. 84.5 and 84.6.) Extend the incision from the xiphoid to the midhypogastrium or below (Fig. 84.1A). Retract the transverse colon superiorly and divide the ligament of Treitz (suspensory muscle of the duodenum) to mobilize the duodenum to the right (Fig. 84.1B). Pack the small bowel into the right side of the abdominal cavity within a towel. Pack and retract the descending and sigmoid colon laterally and inferiorly if necessary. Self-retaining retractors such as the Omni are very helpful.

Anatomic Points

The midline incision has many anatomic advantages if a transperitoneal approach is used. In addition to providing maximal exposure of the peritoneal cavity, it affords a strong closure because several fascial and aponeurotic layers fuse as the linea alba. Retraction of the transverse colon superiorly displaces the transverse mesocolon superiorly, exposing the superior aspect of the root of the mesentery, which begins

LIST OF STRUCTURES

Aorta	Profunda femoris artery	Ureters
Left and right renal artery	Medial femoral circumflex	External oblique muscle
Left and right gonadal artery	artery	Internal oblique muscle
Inferior mesenteric artery	Lateral femoral circumflex	Transversus abdominis muscle
Lumbar arteries	artery	Anterior rectus sheath
Left and right common iliac artery	Inferior vena cava	Rectus abdominis muscle
Left and right internal iliac	Left renal vein	Inguinal ligament
(hypogastric) artery	Left and right common iliac vein	Femoral sheath
Left and right external iliac artery	Left and right internal iliac vein	Femoral triangle
Left and right common femoral	Left and right external iliac vein	Femoral nerve
artery	Femoral vein	Cutaneous branch
Superficial circumflex iliac	Profunda femoris vein	Muscular branch
artery	Hypogastric nerve plexus	Genitofemoral nerve
Superficial epigastric artery	Duodenum	Saphenous nerve
Superficial external pudendal	Ligament of Treitz (suspensory muscle	Adductor canal (of Hunter)
artery	of the duodenum)	

FIGURE 84.1
SKIN INCISION

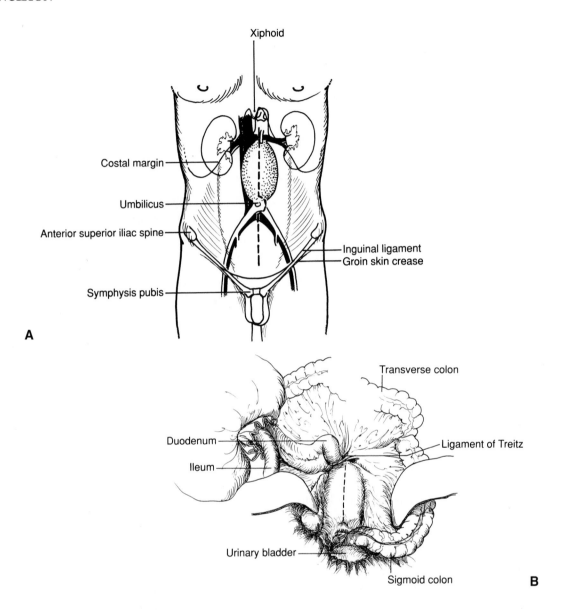

Xiphoid

Costal margin

Umbilicus

Anterior superior iliac spine

Inguinal ligament
Groin skin crease

Symphysis pubis

A

Transverse colon

Duodenum

Ileum

Ligament of Treitz

Urinary bladder

Sigmoid colon

B

at the duodenojejunal flexure. Direct visualization and palpation of the ligament of Treitz (suspensory muscle of the duodenum) is then possible. This fibromuscular band arises from the right crus of the diaphragm and then passes posterior to the pancreas and splenic veins and anterior to the left renal vasculature. It may contain numerous small vessels. Reflection of the duodenum and small bowel to the right, and of the descending and sigmoid colon to the left, exposes the aneurysm, which is covered with parietal peritoneum.

Exposure of the Infrarenal Aorta and Iliac
Arteries (Fig. 84.2)

Technical Points

Open the peritoneum over the aneurysm (Fig. 84.2A). Pre-

serve as much of the hypogastric nerve plexus as possible because sexual dysfunction frequently results if these nerves are divided or devascularized.

In more than 90% of the cases, the superior neck of the aneurysm is below the origin of the renal arteries, where the left renal vein crosses the aorta. Exercise care to avoid injury to these vessels in dissecting the neck of the aneurysm for clamping. Rather than risk tearing the left renal vein during an unusually difficult exposure, it may be intentionally divided and ligated (preferably oversewn) to the right of the gonadal and adrenal branches to provide adequate, safe exposure with preservation of collateral drainage. The left renal vein may be retroaortic and thus highly susceptible to accidental injury and subsequent massive, difficult-to-control hemorrhage.

FIGURE 84.2
EXPOSURE OF THE INFRARENAL AORTA AND ILIAC ARTERIES

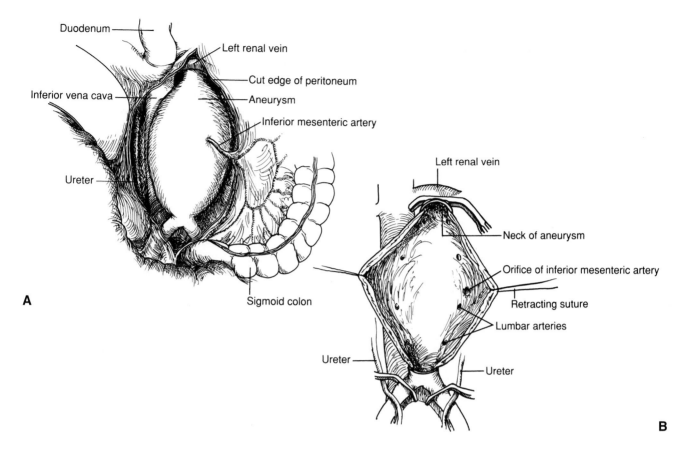

The ureters are also very near the aneurysm, and the potential for injury to these structures during dissection and retraction should be recognized. The ureters are most susceptible to injury where they cross anterior to the iliac bifurcation to enter the pelvis. The common iliac veins are closely adherent to the arteries and should be carefully separated from them only for a distance that is sufficient to allow clamping of the arteries (Fig. 84.2B).

Aspirate blood from the inferior vena cava or aorta for preclotting of knitted Dacron grafts. (Preclotting of woven, "presealed" knitted, or PTFE grafts is unnecessary.) Then have the anesthesiologist administer heparin intravenously. Clamp all vessels gently to avoid dislodging atheroma or thrombus as emboli. Open the anterior wall of the aneurysm. At the superior and inferior necks of the aneurysm, extend the incision transversely in a T pattern through the anterior half of the wall. Leave the posterior portion intact for strong purchase of sutures. Remove mural thrombus and suture-ligate bleeding lumbar arteries. Retracting sutures or a self-retaining retractor placed in the wall of the aneurysm may be helpful. Remove any debris from both necks of the aneurysm.

If the inferior mesenteric artery is backbleeding, suture-ligate it from inside the aneurysm to avoid disturbing the collateral circulation to the distal inferior mesenteric artery. If there is concern regarding the viability of the colon at the conclusion of the procedure, reimplant the inferior mesenteric artery with a cuff of aortic wall into the graft. If the inferior mesenteric artery is not reimplanted, carefully inspect the bowel for signs of ischemia before closure of the abdomen.

Anatomic Points

The hypogastric nerve plexus contains postganglionic sympathetic fibers from spinal cord segments L-1 to L-2 or L-3 and parasympathetic fibers from spinal cord segments S-2 to S-4. This plexus is located just inferior to the bifurcation of the aorta into the common iliac arteries. Fibers connecting this plexus to more superior plexuses ascend anterior to the common iliac arteries (especially on the left) and continue to predominate on the left side of the aorta. Although those parasympathetic fibers mediating erection are not endangered, whereas the sympathetic fibers controlling emission and ejaculation are, successful erection apparently demands the integrated function of both sympathetic and parasympathetic systems. For this reason, many surgeons prefer to open the aneurysm on the right side of the aorta, rather than in the midline or on the left in the male. Obviously, extensive circumferential dissection of the aorta is not only unnecessary but also is contraindicated.

The renal arteries usually arise from the aorta in the upper half of the body of vertebra L-2, slightly inferior to the origin of the superior mesenteric artery. Variations in the level of origin of the renal arteries can occur, and the displacement is usually more caudal than cranial. Moreover, supernumerary renal arteries, which typically are end arteries to kidney segments, can arise from the aorta inferior to the level of origin of the renal arteries. Should these be occluded or interrupted, a zone of renal necrosis can result.

The left renal vein, which typically crosses the peritoneal aspect of the aorta at the level of the left renal artery, is always at risk for injury. This is particularly true if the course of this vein is anomalous (eg, retroaortic). If the vein is ligated, this should be done as close as possible to its termination in the inferior vena cava. Collateral venous pathways draining the left kidney, including the left gonadal and suprarenal veins, will thus be preserved.

The gonadal arteries (spermatic or ovarian) arise from the anterolateral aspect of the aorta 2 to 5 cm caudal to the origin of the renal arteries. The collateral circulation of the testis in the male (the deferential artery, derived from the umbilical artery near the latter's origin from the internal iliac artery, and the cremasteric artery, a branch of the inferior epigastric artery) and the ovary in the female (a branch of the uterine artery) usually permits ligation of the gonadal artery with little to no morbidity.

Finally, care must be taken to avoid injury to the ureters or their blood supply. The ureters are most susceptible to trauma where they cross the peritoneal surface of the common or external iliac arteries. This is also the site where their blood supply (derived from the renal arteries, aorta, gonadal artery, common or external iliac artery, and vesical arteries) is at greatest risk.

The inferior mesenteric artery arises from the aorta about one vertebral level superior to the bifurcation of the aorta into the common iliac arteries. It is frequently completely occluded. Theoretically, it can be ligated and divided close to its origin with no ill effect; however, because the anastomoses shown in texts are not always functional, the descending and sigmoid colon should be inspected for signs of ischemia.

Construction of a Vascular Anastomosis (Fig. 84.3)

Technical and Anatomic Points

All anastomoses are made with continuous polypropylene suture. Place the first suture from the outside to the inside of the graft at the point corresponding to the junction between

FIGURE 84.3
CONSTRUCTION OF A VASCULAR ANASTOMOSIS

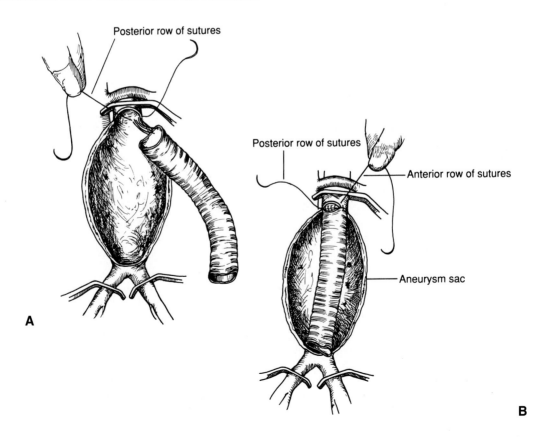

the transverse cut in the anterior wall and the intact posterior wall that is on the side opposite you. This corresponds to the 3-o'clock position as you view the open proximal aortic circumference. Continue the anastomosis in a running fashion around the face of this clock at "hourly intervals," ideally taking six bites to complete the posterior suture line to the 9-o'clock position. All sutures are placed with the same needle outside to in on the graft and inside to out on the uncut double-thickness posterior aortic wall. The posterior sutures are left loose in a parachute-like fashion and pulled tight when the posterior portion is completed (Fig. 84.3A,B).

Complete the anterior suture line using the same suture from the 9-o'clock position at the corner opposite you across the anterior wall and complete the anastomosis where it began. Make sure the suture line is taut.

After you complete the proximal anastomosis, flush and then clamp the graft distally. Inspect the anastomosis for leaks. Make the distal anastomosis in a similar fashion, either to the distal aorta if there is a neck proximal to the bifurcation or to the iliac or femoral arteries if the aneurysm involves the iliac vessels or if the patient has severe occlusive disease (see Figs. 84.7 and 84.8).

FIGURE 84.4
CLOSURE OF THE ANEURYSM WALL AND POSTERIOR PERITONEUM OVER THE GRAFT

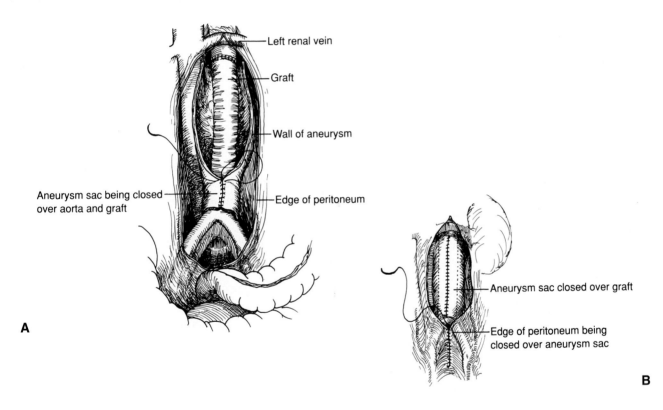

Left renal vein

Graft

Wall of aneurysm

Aneurysm sac being closed over aorta and graft

Edge of peritoneum

A

Aneurysm sac closed over graft

Edge of peritoneum being closed over aneurysm sac

B

Closure of the Aneurysm Wall and Posterior Peritoneum Over the Graft (Fig. 84.4)

Technical and Anatomic Points

Perigraft infection and aortoenteric fistulas are extremely difficult and morbid complications of aortic surgery. In addition to the use of prophylactic antibiotics, these complications are best prevented by closing the aneurysm sac over the graft and anastomosis, thus placing viable tissue between the bowel and the graft (Fig. 84.4A,B). The abdominal incision is then closed in a routine fashion. Drains are not used because of their potential for introducing contamination and initiating infection.

Retroperitoneal Approach to the Aorta (Fig. 84.5)

Technical Points

The aorta can also be well exposed by a left flank retroperitoneal approach, which is easily extended superiorly within the intercostal spaces to provide access to the suprarenal and thoracic aorta. This approach may be associated with a decreased incidence of ileus and pulmonary dysfunction as well as a shorter hospitalization.

Place the patient in a supine position with the chest in a near right lateral decubitus position and with the left arm supported on an armrest, as for a left thoracotomy. Rotate the hips 30 to 45 degrees to allow access to the groin area

FIGURE 84.5
RETROPERITONEAL APPROACH TO THE AORTA

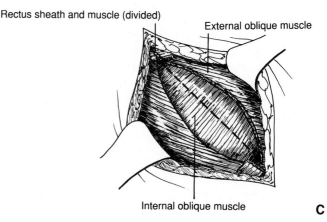

Rectus sheath and muscle (divided)

External oblique muscle

Peritoneum

Internal oblique muscle

Transversus abdominis muscle
and transversalis fascia

if needed. Position the central portion of the trunk over the table break so that flexing of the table will extend and open up the left flank. This position is easily maintained by use of a suction beanbag. The patient is then prepared and draped from the axilla to the knees. For exposure of the infrarenal and juxtarenal aorta, extend the incision from the tip of the eleventh rib or the tenth intercostal interspace laterally toward the midhypogastrium (Fig. 84.5A).

Divide the external oblique, internal oblique, and transversus abdominis muscles in the direction of the incision. Occasionally, the anterior rectus sheath and rectus abdominis muscle must be partially divided to provide adequate exposure (Fig. 84.5B,C). Avoid entering the peritoneal cavity. It is most readily avoided by entering the retroperitoneal space posteriorly. Close the peritoneum, if entered, with continuous absorbable sutures.

Anatomic Points

This incision closely approximates both Langer's lines and the course of the major trunks of the intercostal nerves, which in this region provide motor and sensory innervation to the anterior and anterolateral abdominal wall. After the external and internal oblique muscles are divided, the neurovascular layer of the abdominal wall is exposed; it is in this interval that the neurovascular bundles supplying the rectus abdominis and anterolateral muscles are located. When the rectus abdominis muscle is approached, caution is warranted to avoid injuring the inferior epigastric artery (a branch of the external iliac artery), which enters the lateral aspect of the rectus sheath

somewhat inferior to the incision. Although this artery can be ligated and divided with no ill effect owing to collaterals provided by segmental arteries and the superior epigastric artery, one should be careful not to cut it inadvertently.

Exposure of the Retroperitoneum (Fig. 84.6)

Technical Points

Enter the retroperitoneal space by blunt dissection, sweeping the left colon, ureter, and retroperitoneal tissue off the anterior surface of the retroperitoneal muscles and aorta. The lumbar branch of the left renal vein usually requires ligation and division to provide adequate exposure without tearing the vein during retraction. The suprarenal and infrarenal aorta, common iliac arteries, and left renal artery and vein are easily exposed. The internal iliac arteries, left external iliac artery, and femoral vessels are usually accessible.

The right renal artery distal to the vena cava is not easily exposed by this approach, but the need for exposure by the transabdominal approach can usually be anticipated preoperatively.

Control of the distal right external iliac artery through the left retroperitoneal approach is also problematic and may require occlusion by an intraluminal balloon catheter or a separate right lower quadrant retroperitoneal incision; however, these measures are rarely necessary.

Anatomic Points

Entering the retroperitoneal space without entering the peritoneal cavity is probably easiest by blunt dissection

FIGURE 84.6
EXPOSURE OF THE RETROPERITONEUM

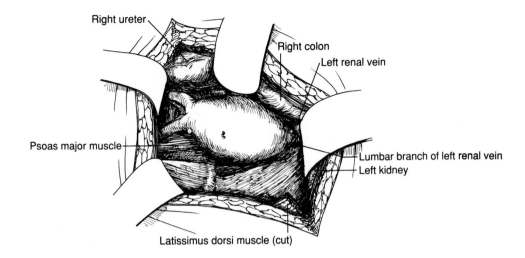

Right ureter

Right colon

Left renal vein

Psoas major muscle

Lumbar branch of left renal vein

Left kidney

Latissimus dorsi muscle (cut)

posterolaterally because, here, there is typically an accumulation of retroperitoneal fat between the transversalis fascia and the parietal peritoneum. Once the appropriate plane is entered, blunt dissection can be carried anteriorly, displacing the descending colon, lower pole of the kidneys, renal vein, left gonadal vein, and retroperitoneal tissues from the flank muscles and aorta. Any communication between the left renal vein and either a segmental lumbar vein, an ascending lumbar vein, or the beginning of the azygos vein (all of which aid in the drainage of the posterior body wall) should be identified and ligated to prevent avulsion.

This technique has several anatomic advantages, including excellent exposure of the major arteries (aorta; left common, external, and internal iliac arteries; and left renal arteries), displacement of the ureter with minimal damage to its blood supply (because the blood supply to the ureter enters from its medial aspect), and easy retraction and visualization of the left renal vein and its tributaries. The primary disadvantage of this approach is that exposure of the right common, external, and internal iliac arteries is somewhat compromised, as is exposure of the right renal artery.

Aortobifemoral Bypass Graft

Groin Incisions (Fig. 84.7)

Technical Points

If aortobifemoral bypass is planned, expose the femoral vessels before entering the abdomen. This minimizes heat and fluid loss from the peritoneal cavity.

In each groin, make an incision over the femoral pulse. Start at the level of the inguinal ligament. Make the incision about 10 cm long. The groin crease is 3 to 4 cm distal to the inguinal ligament, and the incision should extend proximal to

the crease to provide adequate exposure of the femoral artery (Fig. 84.7A). Base the incision on the bony landmarks, rather than on surface features. If femoral pulses are absent, begin the incision midway between the anterosuperior iliac spine and the pubic tubercle.

Fig. 84.7B shows the exposed femoral arteries. Injury of the femoral nerve by excessive lateral dissection or retraction will result in quadriceps weakness and sensory loss of the anterior thigh. Frequently, the femoral vein and its tributaries are relatively adherent to the arteries, especially during redo operations, and thus are susceptible to injury during dissection. The superficial circumflex iliac artery and other branches of the common femoral artery may require temporary control to expose a sufficient length of the femoral artery for clamping and arteriotomy. The profunda femoris artery frequently branches almost immediately, so that control of more than one branch may be required to carry the anastomosis down over the proximal profunda artery when necessary. (There is almost always a tributary of the femoral vein crossing inferior and lateral to the proximal profunda femoris artery; this generally requires ligation and division to facilitate exposure of the more distal profunda femoris artery.) The femoral artery usually has no branches at this level.

Next, before heparinization, make retroperitoneal tunnels for the limbs of the graft over the anterior surface of the iliac and femoral arteries. Do this by careful blunt finger dissection from the retroperitoneum and groins, being sure to keep the ureters anterior to the tunnels to avoid their obstruction between the graft and the native artery and to prevent tearing any small veins that could produce troublesome bleeding.

When the operation is being performed for occlusive disease, the surgeon has the option of complete division of the aorta with end-to-end anastomosis or, less commonly, end-to-side anastomosis to the anterior wall of the aorta (not illustrated).

FIGURE 84.7
GROIN INCISIONS

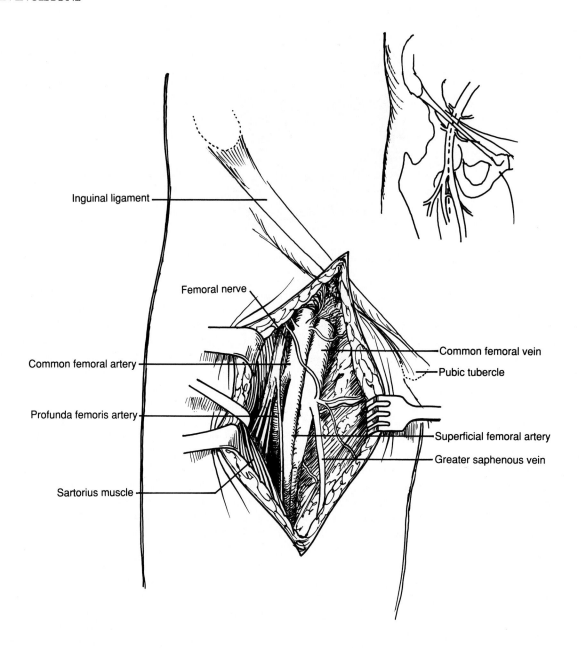

Inguinal ligament

Femoral nerve

Common femoral artery

Profunda femoris artery

Sartorius muscle

Common femoral vein

Pubic tubercle

Superficial femoral artery

Greater saphenous vein

Anatomic Points

The femoral artery lies between the femoral nerve (laterally) and the femoral vein (medially) and within the femoral triangle, approximately at the midpoint of the inguinal ligament. Hence, a vertical incision to expose the femoral artery should be located approximately halfway along the inguinal ligament, regardless of the presence or absence of a pulse in this area. Keep in mind that the inguinal groove (crease) is a cutaneous and subcutaneous reflection of the inguinal ligament. Because of the pendulous nature of these tissues, the groove is typically 3 to 4 cm distal to the inguinal ligament and may be even more distal in obese patients.

Almost immediately after passing deep to the inguinal ligament to enter the thigh, the femoral nerve branches into a variable number of cutaneous and muscular components. The cutaneous branches provide sensation to the anterior and medial thigh distal to the incision, whereas the femoral branch of the genitofemoral nerve is responsible for sensation in the territory of the incision. The genitofemoral nerve may be seen within the femoral sheath, superficial and lateral to the femoral artery. Retract the nerve laterally when exposing the artery. Two branches of the femoral nerve (the saphenous nerve, which provides sensation to the medial leg and posteromedial foot, and the nerve to the vastus medialis muscle) may be injured in skeletonizing the femoral artery. These nerves are also within the femoral sheath and lie lateral to the femoral artery in the area of dissection. The saphenous nerve crosses the femoral artery within the adductor canal (of Hunter). Other important branches of the femoral nerve provide innervation to the anterior thigh muscles. Again, these nerves remain lateral to the artery, so that they are endangered by excessive lateral dissection or retraction.

Typically, three superficial branches of the femoral artery—the superficial epigastric, superficial circumflex iliac, and superficial external pudendal arteries—originate just distal to the inguinal ligament. Although these all anastomose with other arteries and thus can be sacrificed, a reasonable effort should be made to preserve them for their potential contribution to collateral circulation. The branches of the profunda femoris artery that may create problems are the medial and lateral femoral circumflex arteries. Either or both of these arteries can arise independently from the femoral artery instead of from the profunda femoris artery, or they may be so near the origin of the profunda femoris artery as to necessitate their independent control. The profunda femoris vein lies anterior to the profunda femoris artery and posterior to the femoral artery and often must be sacrificed to expose the profunda femoris artery.

FIGURE 84.8
FEMORAL ANASTOMOSES

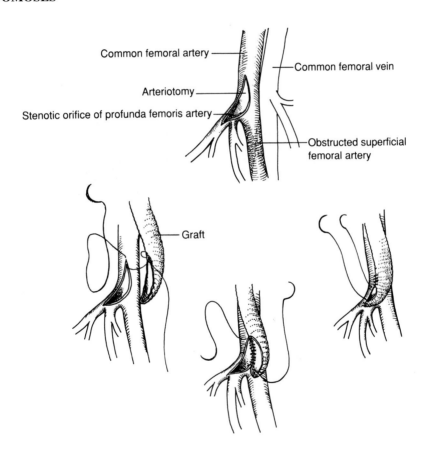

Aortobifemoral Graft

Femoral Anastomoses (Fig. 84.8)

Technical and Anatomic Points

The common, superficial, and profunda femoris arteries are all clamped. Plan the orientations of these clamps so that they are as atraumatic as possible. When plaque is present, it frequently is not circumferential, and the clamp should be placed in such a manner as to avoid fracturing the plaque. Begin the arteriotomy proximal, in the anterior wall of the common femoral artery. Because of the high incidence of femoral occlusion and stenosis of the profunda femoris orifice, extension of the arteriotomy and anastomosis into the proximal profunda femoris to direct flow into it may be necessary. The type of femoral anastomosis otherwise varies and depends on the peculiarities of the individual disease pattern. An overriding principle is always to make sure that the profunda femoris is well perfused (Fig. 84.8). When the common femoral artery and its branches are free of disease, it is acceptable to place the anastomosis to the common femoral artery. It often overrides the origin of the superficial femoral artery.

Cut the femoral limbs of the graft obliquely, making them an appropriate length to provide tension-free anastomosis without redundant graft. This anastomosis, too, is made with continuous polypropylene suture. I prefer to parachute this anastomosis beginning outside to in on the graft two bites away from the heel on the side away. This is continued toward the operator for two bites around the heel and then pulled down. The anastomosis is continued with the same needle toward the toe of the graft and completed

where it was begun. This method allows the heel and toe of the anastomosis (the critical portion) to be done open under direct vision and minimizes needle and suture changing (Fig. 84.8C,D). Allow the arteries to backbleed. Flush the graft before completing the anastomosis and removing all clamps.

In vascular surgery, the groin is the most common site for wound separation and infection. To provide maximum tissue coverage over the grafts, close the wound in three layers.

REFERENCES

1. Bietz D, Merendino KA. Abdominal aortic aneurysm and horseshoe kidney. *Ann Surg* 1975;181:333. (Discusses considerations in management of a horseshoe kidney.)
2. Brener BJ, Darling RC, Frederick PL, et al. Major venous anomalies complicating abdominal aortic surgery. *Arch Surg* 1974;108:159.
3. Couch NP, Clowes AW, Whittemore AD, et al. The iliac-origin arterial graft: a useful alternative for iliac occlusive disease. *Surgery* 1985;97:83.
4. Crawford ES. Thoraco-abdominal and abdominal aortic aneurysms involving renal, superior mesenteric, and celiac arteries. *Ann Surg* 1974;179:763.
5. Darling RC, Brewster DC, Hallett JW Jr, et al. Aorto-iliac reconstruction. *Surg Clin North Am* 1979;59:565.
6. Diehl JT, Cali RF, Hertzer NR, et al. Complications of abdominal aortic reconstruction: an analysis of perioperative risk factors in 557 patients. *Ann Surg* 1983;197:49.
7. Ferguson LRJ, Bergan JJ, Conn J Jr, et al. Spinal ischemia following abdominal aortic surgery. *Ann Surg* 1975;181:267.
8. Giordano JM, Trout HH III. Anomalies of the inferior vena cava. *J Vasc Surg* 1986;3:924. (Presents good review of embryogenesis and anomalies of the inferior vena cava.)
9. Imparato AM, Berman IR, Bracco A, et al. Avoidance of shock and peripheral embolism during surgery of the abdominal aorta. *Surgery* 1973;73:68.
10. Inahara T. Eversion endarterectomy for aortoiliofemoral occlusive disease: a 16-year experience. *Am J Surg* 1979;138:196.
11. Peck JJ, McReynolds DG, Baker DH, et al. Extraperitoneal approach for aortoiliac reconstruction of the abdominal aorta. *Am J Surg* 1986;151:620.
12. Shepard AD, Scott GR, Mackey WC, et al. Retroperitoneal approach to high-risk abdominal aortic aneurysms. *Arch Surg* 1986;121:444.
13. Sicard GA, Allen BT, Munn JS, et al. Retroperitoneal versus transperitoneal approach for repair of abdominal aortic aneurysms. *Surg Clin North Am* 1989;69:795.
14. Szilagyi DE, Elliott JP, Smith RF, et al. A thirty-year survey of the reconstructive surgical treatment of aortoiliac occlusive disease. *J Vasc Surg* 1986;3:421.
15. Thompson JE, Hollier LH, Patman RD, et al. Surgical management of abdominal aortic aneurysms: factors influencing mortality and morbidity: a 20-year experience. *Ann Surg* 1975;181:654.
16. Veith FJ, Gupta S, Daly V. Technique for occluding the supraceliac aorta through the abdomen. *Surg Gynecol Obstet* 1980;151:426. (Provides clear description of emergency exposure and control of the aorta at the hiatus.)

CHAPTER 85

Lumbar Sympathectomy

Sympathectomy is performed for causalgia. Lumbar sympathectomy is sometimes performed in patients with symptomatic ischemia of a lower extremity who are not candidates for a bypass procedure. Results are unpredictable; thus, the operation is presently reserved for a very limited subset of patients who have failed, or who are not candidates for, other medical or surgical treatment modalities.

Incision and Exposure of the Peritoneum (Fig. 85.1)

Technical Points

Position the patient supine on the operating table. Elevate the side to be operated on slightly if the patient is obese. Plan a transverse skin incision that begins at a point on the midaxillary line that is halfway between the costal margin and the anterosuperior iliac spine. Progress medially to the lateral border of the rectus muscle. Deepen the incision until the fascia of the external oblique muscle is encountered. Split this muscular and aponeurotic layer in the direction of its fibers to expose the underlying internal oblique muscle. This split should run from the tip of the eleventh rib laterally to the edge of the rectus sheath medially. Widely undermine each muscle layer as you proceed. Split the fibers of the internal oblique muscle in a similar fashion. Identify the underlying transversus abdominis muscle. Split its fibers and open the transversalis fascia, sweeping away a variable amount of preperitoneal fat to expose the peritoneum.

LIST OF STRUCTURES

External oblique muscle
Internal oblique muscle
Transversus abdominis muscle
Transversalis fascia
Iliac fascia
Peritoneum
Lumbar sympathetic chain
   Ganglia
   Rami communicantes
   Preganglionic fibers
   Postganglionic fibers
Aorta
Inferior vena cava
Kidney
Ureter

Anatomic Points

The skin incision should follow Langer's lines, which in this region are almost transverse. This approach provides the best cosmetic results and also minimizes the risk for skin denervation. Although dermatome patterns are somewhat oblique, their overlapping nature prevents total denervation. Remember that the plane between the internal oblique and transversus abdominis muscle is the neurovascular plane in which lie the main segmental vessels and nerves.

Exposure of the Sympathetic Chain (Fig. 85.2)

Technical Points

The peritoneum, to which the ureter adheres, enfolds the viscera like a sac. To expose the sympathetic chain, it must be rolled medially off of the underlying muscles.

Identify the peritoneal sac as a smooth, fatty layer. Develop planes superficial to this layer both superiorly and inferiorly. Place retractors in the wound. Gently elevate the peritoneal sac from the underlying muscles. Identify the layer of psoas major muscle, and continue to elevate the peritoneum until you feel the lumbar spine.

If you make a hole in the peritoneum, repair it with a running absorbable suture, such as 3-0 Vicryl. Be careful not to injure nearby structures, such as the bowel or ureter, when placing this suture.

The sympathetic chain lies lateral to the lumbar spine and can be identified by its characteristic location and feel. The chain feels like a long, taut banjo string; it is anchored to the paravertebral tissues and interrupted by multiple fusiform swellings (ganglia). The number of ganglia varies from one to four; generally, three to four ganglia will be encountered in the field of dissection.

Inexperienced surgeons have mistaken both ureter and genitofemoral nerve for the sympathetic chain. Remember that the sympathetic chain can be differentiated from these structures by its firm feeling, periodic swellings, and lack of mobility.

Anatomic Points

Because the major goal of this part of the dissection is to expose the sympathetic chain and yet remain extraperitoneal, one must keep the relationships of the retroperitoneal

ORIENTATION

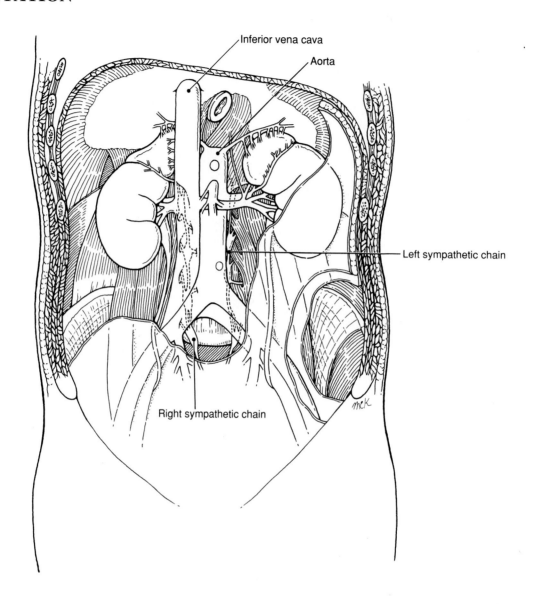

structures in mind. The gastrointestinal tract and its blood supply can be gently mobilized anteromedially, as can the ureter. When this is done, the belly of the psoas major muscle can be visualized, and muscle fibers can be followed to their origins on the transverse processes and bodies of the lumbar vertebrae. The lumbar sympathetic chain lies immediately anterior to the vertebral origin of this muscle and deep to the psoas fascia. As a consequence, to visualize the sympathetic chain adequately, the iliac fascia (a continuation of the transversalis fascia) must be reflected from the origin of the psoas muscle. One must remember that, on the left, the aorta is usually medial to the chain, but on the right, it is typically posterior to the inferior vena cava. As a consequence, adequate exposure on the right may require ligation and division of one or more lumbar veins.

Excision of the Sympathetic Chain (Fig. 85.3)

Technical Points

Identify the highest sympathetic ganglion, which lies just below the crus of the diaphragm. This ganglion is easy to identify because it is Y shaped. Clip the preganglionic fibers above this ganglion with a hemoclip and divide the chain. Elevate the sympathetic chain by grasping it with a long hemostat and pull downward. Clip any lumbar veins crossing over the sympathetic chain. Clip and divide fibers tethering the ganglia laterally. Terminate the dissection at the level of the iliac vein. Obtain frozen-section confirmation of autonomic nervous tissue.

Irrigate the field, check hemostasis, and close the muscles in layers.

FIGURE 85.1
INCISION AND EXPOSURE OF THE PERITONEUM

Internal oblique muscle

FIGURE 85.2
EXPOSURE OF THE SYMPATHETIC CHAIN

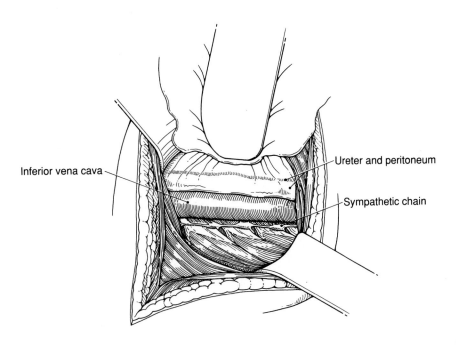

Inferior vena cava

Ureter and peritoneum

Sympathetic chain

FIGURE 85.3
EXCISION OF THE SYMPATHETIC CHAIN

Anatomic Points

The most superior ganglion that is usually accessible to the surgeon is that which is located on the second lumbar vertebra. This is the most constant of the lumbar ganglia in terms of location, and the largest.

The sympathetic chain itself is composed of preganglionic fibers. The higher ganglia (L-1, L-2, and possibly L-3) will also have white (preganglionic) and gray (postganglionic) rami communicantes attached to the segmental nerve, whereas those that are more inferior will have only gray rami.

Inferior dissection is typically limited by the common iliac vessels and thus does not usually include the fifth lumbar ganglion. Dissection typically removes three ganglia and the preganglionic fibers connecting these ganglia.

REFERENCES

1. Holiday FA, Barendregt WB, Slappendel R, et al. Lumbar sympathectomy in critical limb ischaemia: surgical, chemical or not at all? *Cardiovasc Surg* 1999;7:200–202.
2. Kim GE, Ibrahim IM, Imparato AM. Lumbar sympathectomy in end-stage arterial occlusive disease. *Ann Surg* 1976;183:157.
3. Wronski J. Lumbar sympathectomy performed by means of videoscopy. *Cardiovasc Surg* 1998;6:453–456.

THE INGUINAL REGION

This anatomically complex region has been the subject of many books. In this part, inguinal and femoral hernia repair (Chapters 86 and 87) by various methods is illustrated. Inguinal lymph node dissection (Chapter 88) and sentinel node biopsy for melanoma of the trunk (Chapter 89) conclude the part, which serves as a transition to the next two sections: *The Sacral Region and Perineum* (Chapters 90 to 94) and *The Lower Extremity* (Chapters 95 to 101).

CHAPTER 86

Repair of Inguinal and Femoral Hernias

The muscular and aponeurotic layers of the abdominal wall form a strong continuous barrier that supports and contains the intraabdominal viscera. This continuous barrier is breached in the groin by the inguinal canal, an oblique passage from the abdomen to the scrotum (in the male) or to the labium majus (in the female). This anatomically complex area is a frequent site of hernia formation.

Three types of groin hernias are distinguishable clinically: indirect inguinal, direct inguinal, and femoral. An individual may have one, two, or (occasionally) all three hernias within the same groin.

Indirect inguinal hernia is the most common hernia in both males and females. In the male, indirect inguinal hernia is associated with persistent patency of the processus vaginalis. Communicating hydroceles are closely related. The spermatic cord traverses the abdominal wall as it passes from the internal to the external ring to supply the testis. This produces an area of natural weakness in the male. In the female, the round ligament exits the abdomen to anchor in the labia majora and mons pubis. Indirect hernias in females form in much the same way as do those seen in males.

Direct hernias are generally acquired as a result of weakness in the floor of the inguinal canal that allows intra-abdominal pressure to produce a bulge through the thinned-out transversalis fascia. Indirect hernias occur lateral to the inferior epigastric vessels, whereas direct hernias project straight through the floor of the canal in the region of Hesselbach's triangle, medial to the inferior epigastric vessels.

The femoral canal is inferior to the inguinal ligament. A *femoral hernia* occurs when weakness in the femoral canal allows herniation of peritoneum, followed by intraabdominal viscera, into the canal. Femoral hernias are seen most commonly in elderly patients. Small, incarcerated femoral hernias may feel exactly like enlarged lymph nodes. The combination of small bowel obstruction and palpable adenopathy in one groin should lead one to suspect an incarcerated femoral hernia.

In this chapter, four types of inguinal hernia repair—the Bassini, McVay, Shouldice, and plug-and-patch methods—are described. Femoral hernia repair from both below and above is described. References at the end of the chapter give details of other techniques, and laparoscopic herniorrhaphy is described in Chapter 87.

Descriptions of the anatomy of the inguinal region are confusing, in part because the standard texts of anatomy are based on dissection of the embalmed cadaver (in which tissue planes

LIST OF STRUCTURES

Inguinal region
Processus vaginalis
External (superficial) inguinal ring
    Medial and lateral crus
    Intercrural fibers
Internal (deep) inguinal ring
Hesselbach's triangle
Inferior epigastric artery and vein
    Pubic branch of artery (accessory
        obturator artery)
    Obturator artery
Superficial (Camper's and Scarpa's)
    fascia
Innominate fascia
External oblique muscle and
    aponeurosis
Internal oblique muscle and
    aponeurosis

Transversus abdominis muscle
Transversalis fascia
    Iliopubic tract
    Transversalis fascial sling
Preperitoneal tissue
Peritoneum
Pubic tubercle
Inguinal ligament
Pectinal (Cooper's) ligament
Lacunar ligament
Conjoined tendon
Interfoveolar ligament
Ilioinguinal nerve
Iliohypogastric nerve
Genitofemoral nerve
    Genital branch
Femoral canal

Femoral sheath
Femoral artery and vein
    Greater saphenous vein
Saphenous hiatus
Fascia lata
Male
    Spermatic cord
    External spermatic fascia
    Cremasteric muscle and fascia
    Internal spermatic fascia
    Vas deferens
    Scrotum
    Testis
    Testicular vessels
Female
    Round ligament
    Labium majus

ORIENTATION

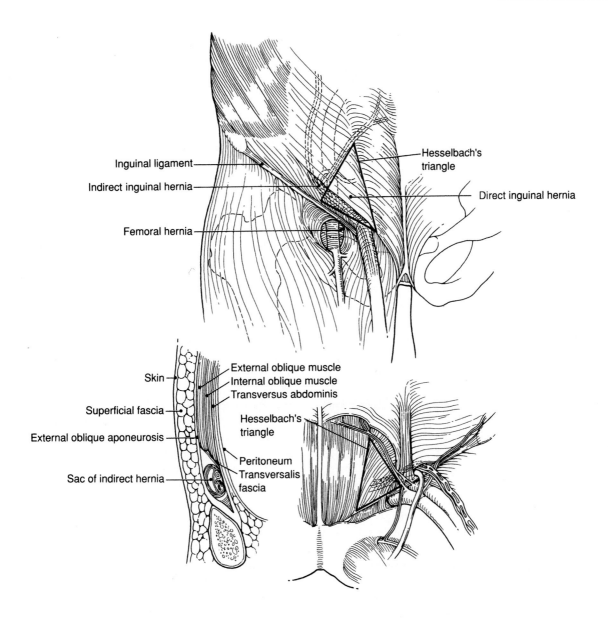

are not nearly as definable as in fresh tissues) and in part because of the plethora of synonyms applied to structures in this region. Here, the terminology commonly used by surgeons is presented. (Because of the inherent complexity, a long orientation section is given here.)

The abdominal wall is multilayered. These layers can be classified as either superficial or deep, and they are mirror images of each other, with the reflecting plane being the internal oblique muscle. Thus, from superficial to deep, the following layers are encountered:

1. Skin
2. Superficial (Camper's and Scarpa's) fascia

3. "Outer" investing (innominate) fascia
4. External oblique muscle and aponeurosis
5. Internal oblique muscle and aponeurosis (Note: in the inguinal canal, the spermatic cord or round ligament of the uterus substitutes for this layer.)
6. Transversus abdominis muscle and aponeurosis
7. "Inner" investing or endoabdominal (transversalis) fascia
8. Preperitoneal tissue
9. Peritoneum

The inguinal canal is a triangular passageway through the body wall in which lies the spermatic cord or its female homologue, the round ligament of the uterus. Its entrance is the internal inguinal ring, which is associated with the transversalis fascia and which is located immediately superior to the middle of the inguinal ligament and lateral to the inferior epigastric vessels. Its exit is the external inguinal ring, which is associated with the external oblique muscle and innominate fascia and which is located immediately superior to the medial end of the inguinal ligament at the pubic tubercle. Its anterior wall is the external oblique aponeurosis, its posterior wall is the transversus abdominis aponeurosis fused with transversalis fascia, and its base is the inguinal ligament.

The inguinal ligament is the somewhat thickened and inrolled free edge of the external oblique aponeurosis that forms the inferior "shelving edge" of the inguinal canal. Laterally, it is attached to the anterosuperior iliac spine and the adjacent iliac fascia. Medially, it attaches to the pubic tubercle and adjacent pectineal ligament (of Cooper). The parallel fibers of the inguinal ligament that fan out to attach to the pubic tubercle and adjacent pectineal ligament form the lacunar ligament. It should be noted that the free edge of the lacunar ligament does not extend far enough laterally to participate in the formation of the normal femoral canal. The lacunar ligament does, however, lie inferior to (and thus supports) the spermatic cord in the medial part of the inguinal canal.

Immediately superior and lateral to the pubic tubercle, the aponeurotic fibers of the external oblique muscle diverge to attach to the body of the pubis superomedially (medial crus) and to the pubic tubercle inferolaterally (lateral crus). The triangular interval between the two crura, through which the spermatic cord or round ligament of the uterus passes, is the superficial or external inguinal ring. Intercrural fibers, which are derived from innominate fascia, are oriented at right angles to the external oblique fibers, convert the triangular hiatus into an oval, and usually prevent spreading of the crura. External spermatic fascia, the outer covering of the spermatic cord, is also derived from innominate fascia.

When fibers of the external oblique aponeurosis are split superolaterally from the superficial inguinal ring, the inguinal canal is opened. The somewhat transversely oriented muscular fibers of the internal oblique muscle can then be seen arching over the spermatic cord. The cremasteric muscle and fascia, which constitute the middle covering of the spermatic cord, are in continuity with the internal oblique muscle and its investing fascia. Internal oblique fibers in this region originate from iliac fascia, pass superficial to the spermatic cord and deep (internal) inguinal ring, and attach to the rectus sheath and adjacent body of the pubis. Rarely (3% of cases), the lowest internal oblique fibers are aponeurotic, join aponeurotic fibers of the transversus abdominis muscle, and insert into the pubic tubercle and pectineal ligament (of Cooper) as a conjoint tendon. However, typically, the lowest fibers are muscular and do not extend below the arch formed by the deeper transversus abdominis muscle. Because the internal oblique is primarily muscular in the inguinal region, it is of little importance in the surgical repair of groin hernias.

The third musculoaponeurotic layer is composed of the transversus abdominis muscle and aponeurosis and its investing fascia, the inner layer of which is transversalis fascia. By itself, transversalis fascia, which is intimately attached to the transversus abdominis muscle, has little intrinsic strength. Thus, it is considered with the muscle layer rather than as a separate, distinct entity.

Lower muscular or aponeurotic fibers of the transversus abdominis form a distinct arch extending from their lateral attachment (iliac fascia) to their medial attachment on the superior pubic ramus, lateral to the rectus abdominis muscle. As transversus abdominis fibers arch over spermatic cord structures laterally, they define the superior margin of the deep inguinal ring. Medial to the deep inguinal ring, the distinct arch is the superior limit of most direct inguinal hernia defects. Inferior to this arch, aponeurotic fibers of the transversus abdominis are present but are significantly reduced in number; these fibers diverge from each other, and the transversalis fascia fills the intervening gaps. It is this area—the posterior wall of the inguinal canal—through which a direct hernia occurs. Still more inferiorly, a collection of aponeurotic transversus and transversalis fascia fibers form the important iliopubic tract. Laterally, iliopubic tract fibers attach to the iliac fascia. From this attachment, which is overlapped by the inguinal ligament, fibers pass medially and deeply, diverging from the inguinal ligament. Fibers of the iliopubic tract define the lower border of the deep inguinal ring, cross the external iliac and femoral vessels and femoral canal as the anterior wall of the femoral sheath, and then fan out to attach to the pectineal ligament (of Cooper). Medial to the femoral canal, some fibers recurve inferolaterally, forming the medial wall of the femoral sheath. Thus, it is the iliopubic tract, not the more superficial and medial lacunar ligament, that forms the medial border of the femoral canal. Further, it should be noted that the iliopubic tract is often confused with the inguinal ligament because it more or less parallels the course of this ligament.

Although the transversus abdominis and transversalis fascia are considered as a unit, some attention must be paid to regional expressions that are unique to transversalis fascia only. One of these regional expressions is the transversalis fascial sling and its reinforcement by the interfoveolar ligament, which together form the medial boundary of the deep inguinal ring. The transversalis fascial sling results from the obliquity of the inguinal canal with respect to the plane of the deep inguinal ring. Abdominopelvic structures destined to become spermatic cord structures are located in preperitoneal tissue. When these evaginate the transversalis fascia covering the deep inguinal ring (creating the internal spermatic fascia) to enter the inguinal canal, the axis of this tubular prolongation creates a redundancy of transversalis fascia at the medial side of the deep inguinal ring. This sling, which is intimately attached to the transversus abdominis muscle, is mobile and probably represents the so-called shutter mechanism thought to operate at the deep inguinal ring when lateral abdominal muscles contract.

Remember that, during the embryologic descent of the testes, the first structure to pass out the deep inguinal ring into the inguinal canal, and finally out the superficial ring into the incipient scrotum, is the processus vaginalis, a tubular evagination of the peritoneal sac. Failure of fusion and subsequent fibrosis of this evagination provide a route for indirect hernias.

The femoral sheath and canal are located inferior to the inguinal ligament. The femoral sheath is a continuation of the transversalis fascia into the thigh. Lateral to medial, it contains the femoral artery, femoral vein, and femoral canal. The femoral canal contains areolar tissue and lymphatic structures. The internal mouth of this canal—the *femoral ring*—is bounded anteriorly and medially by the iliopubic tract, laterally by periadventitial tissue medial to the femoral vein, and posteriorly by the pectineal ligament (of Cooper).

In summary, it is the transversus abdominis and transversalis fascia layer that normally prevents inguinal and femoral hernias. Variations or defects in this layer allow groin hernias to occur.

FIGURE 86.1
INCISION AND EXPOSURE OF THE SPERMATIC CORD

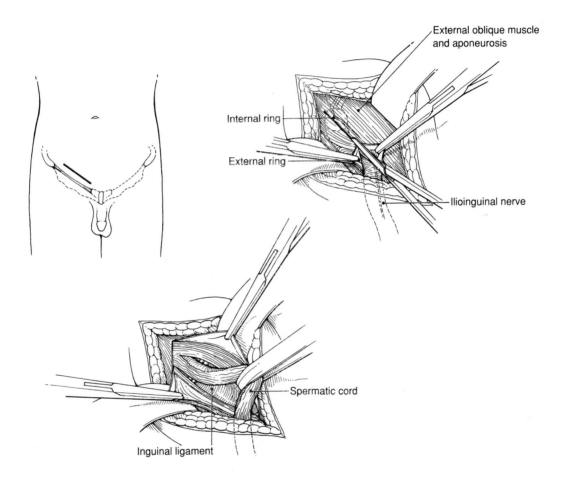

External oblique muscle and aponeurosis

Internal ring

External ring

Ilioinguinal nerve

Spermatic cord

Inguinal ligament

Inguinal Hernia Repair

Incision and Exposure of the Spermatic Cord (Fig. 86.1)

Technical Points

The traditional hernia incision lies in a straight line from the anterosuperior iliac spine to the pubic tubercle. A more cosmetic incision can be made in a skin crease. The most important consideration is to make the incision directly over the pubic tubercle so that exposure in this area is good.

Often, the incision can be completely hidden within the hair-bearing area of the pubis. Deepen the incision until the external oblique aponeurosis is identified.

Palpate the external ring. Verify the position of the external ring by passing your finger through it. Use Metzenbaum scissors to extend the incision of the external oblique aponeurosis in its midportion in the direction of its fibers through the external ring. Place hemostats on the two leaves of the external oblique aponeurosis and lift up. Look underneath and be careful to identify and protect from injury the ilioinguinal nerve. This nerve generally lies just under the external oblique muscle but is somewhat variable in its location.

By sharp and blunt dissection, separate the spermatic cord from the underside of the external oblique aponeurosis. Inferiorly, the inguinal ligament should come into view. Free the spermatic cord circumferentially at the pubic tubercle. Dissection is easiest here because the bony pubic tubercle protects the floor of the canal from injury and provides a constant deep reference point. Pass a Penrose drain around the spermatic cord and lift up. Free the cord to the level of the internal ring. Place a self-retaining retractor within the leaves of the external oblique aponeurosis to hold the canal open.

Anatomic Points

The aponeuroses and ligaments involved in the inguinal canal converge on bone at the pubic tubercle, making this end of the canal relatively fixed. Superficial circumflex iliac vessels coursing superolaterally near the lateral end of the incision, as well as superficial external pudendal vessels crossing anterior to the superficial ring and spermatic cord, probably will be encountered in this stage of the dissection.

After the skin incision is made, fascial layers are encountered. The superficial fascia here is divisible into the more superficial, fatty Camper's fascia and the deeper, fibrous Scarpa's fascia. Deep to Scarpa's fascia is innominate fascia, the deep fascia of the abdomen. The thickness and complexity of the superficial fascia is dependent on the body habitus of the patient. In the obese patient, the fat lobules of Camper's fascia are large and irregular. A fat layer can occur deep to Scarpa's fascia, but here, the fat lobules are smaller. No fat is present deep to the innominate fascia, through which the fibers of the external oblique aponeurosis are visible. In the dissection through superficial fascia, named vessels that will be encountered include the superficial epigastrics coursing superomedially from the vicinity of the deep inguinal ring, the superficial circumflex iliacs coursing superolaterally near the lateral end of the incision, and the superficial external pudendals running medially anterior to the superficial ring or spermatic cord.

The external ring is immediately superolateral to the pubic tubercle. The outer covering of the cord—the external spermatic fascia—is continuous with innominate fascia and must be incised when the external ring is opened. Exercise caution in this, though, for just deep to the external oblique aponeurosis, typically on the anterior side of the spermatic cord, the ilioinguinal nerve (L-1) exits the external ring to lie immediately deep to the external spermatic fascia. The iliohypogastric nerve (L-1 and sometimes T-12) does not pass through the external ring but instead is usually slightly superior to this landmark.

As the spermatic cord is mobilized, the inguinal ligament and its medial expansion (lacunar ligament) will be visible. At this point in the dissection, vascular structures should not be encountered because these are deep to transversalis fascia or its spermatic cord continuity.

Inspection of the Spermatic Cord and Identification and Ligation of the Indirect Hernia Sac (Fig. 86.2)

Technical Points

Stretch the spermatic cord slightly and use forceps to pick up on the longitudinally running cremasteric fibers. Incise these in the direction of their fibers for a distance of several centimeters. Place hemostats on the two leaves of the cremaster muscle. Gently shell the cord from its surrounding cremasteric fibers. Try to keep intact the internal spermatic fascia because this will help to protect the cord and cord structures from injury. The cord should "shell out" cleanly, surrounded by its enveloping fascia. Palpate the vas deferens, which will feel like a piece of whipcord running within the structures of the cord. Place the Penrose drain around the cord, excluding the cremaster muscle.

Often, the cremasteric layer is quite fatty and bulky. If this is the case, it is advisable to excise it in order to skeletonize the cord sufficiently to attain a good repair. Skeletonizing the cord will interfere with the ability of the testis to retract into the scrotum and may be objectionable to some men. It should be done only when necessary to achieve a sound repair. To skeletonize the cord, divide the leaves of cremasteric fibers into two or three pedicles that can then be clamped above and below and excised. Ligate these with 2-0 silk. The proximal pedicle will generally disappear into the peritoneal cavity when the tension on the cord is relaxed. The object is to thin the cord out sufficiently at the level of the internal ring to allow a sound repair to be performed. Spread out the cord and its contents over your finger and look for a hernia sac. This will be visible as a whitish, moon-shaped structure protruding from the internal ring. A sac that extends all the way down into the scrotum will be a cylindrical structure, the termination of which will not be able to be identified. If you do not see a sac, place traction on the cord until a lappet of peritoneum is pulled up into the cord. The appearance of this peritoneal lappet confirms that there is no sac.

If a sac is identified within the cord, place hemostats on the sac and separate it from other cord structures by sharp and blunt dissection. A sac that continues all the way into the scrotum can be transected and a small amount of distal sac left *in situ*. Divide the sac with electrocautery. Take care to secure hemostasis. Leave the sac open. Dissect the proximal sac circumferentially all the way to the internal ring. The vas deferens at the internal ring will often be quite adherent and close to the sac; therefore, you must be especially careful to avoid injuring it.

Place strong traction on the cord so that a good high ligation of the sac can be performed. Open the sac and inspect it to be sure that it is empty. Reduce any contained viscera or omentum. Twist the sac to milk its contents down out of the way and transfix it with a suture ligature of 2-0 silk. Amputate the sac and allow it to retract. Alternatively, place a pursestring suture in the neck of the sac with the sac open. This approach has the advantage of being done under direct vision and may be most suitable for large sacs.

FIGURE 86.2
INSPECTION OF THE SPERMATIC CORD AND IDENTIFICATION AND LIGATION OF THE INDIRECT HERNIA SAC

A sliding hernia is one in which part of the wall of the sac is composed of one of the viscera, generally, the bladder, sigmoid colon, or cecum. Do not attempt to dissect the sac from the viscus in such cases. Rather, amputate the sac just above the attachment of the viscus and close it just above the attachment. Separate the sac fully from the cord and reduce the viscus and sac into the abdomen. This will prevent any remaining finger of peritoneum from acting as a lead point for recurrent hernia.

Check hemostasis in the cord and the floor of the canal. Secure small bleeding veins on the cord by suture ligature with fine silk or with ties. If a tight repair is done, swelling in the immediate postoperative period may create a "venous tourniquet" effect, causing otherwise insignificant vessels to bleed. A painful scrotal hematoma may result.

Anatomic Points

The cremasteric muscle and fascia are continuous with the internal oblique muscle and its investing fascia. Deep to this layer, and on the posterior side of the spermatic cord, is the genital branch of the genitofemoral nerve (L-1, L-2). This nerve supplies the cremaster muscle. Severance of the nerve can best be avoided by separation, rather than division, of cremasteric fibers. If you must divide cremaster fibers, be careful not to entrap the nerve.

In indirect inguinal hernias, a hernia sac passes through the deep inguinal ring, following the route of testicular descent. As a consequence, the indirect inguinal hernia sac becomes a cord constituent and is covered by external spermatic fascia, cremasteric fascia, and internal spermatic fascia (continuous with the transversalis fascia). By contrast, a direct inguinal hernia, although covered by attenuated transversalis fascia of the posterior wall of the inguinal canal, lies adjacent to the spermatic cord, not within it. If it progresses to the point of exiting the external ring, it will be covered by external spermatic fascia, but it will remain outside the cremasteric fascia.

FIGURE 86.3
BASSINI REPAIR

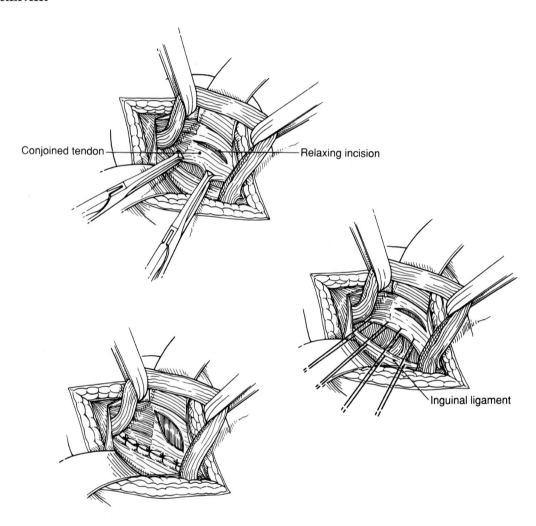

Bassini Repair (Fig. 86.3)

Technical Points

Assess the strength of the floor of the canal. High ligation of the sac is all that is required for a simple indirect hernia in a young male. Often, the presence of the hernia has dilated the internal ring and may have partially weakened the floor. The floor is basically sound, but the anatomy may have been distorted by the hernia sliding through the internal ring. In this case, a Bassini repair is a good option because it does not require opening of the floor of the canal and does not risk weakening what is basically already a strong structure.

A Bassini repair is performed by suturing conjoint tendon to inguinal ligament. Elevate the upper flap of the external oblique muscle. Make a relaxing incision in the medial superior aspect of the conjoined tendon using electrocautery. Be careful to check hemostasis in this incision. Place Allis clamps on the conjoined tendon, seen here as a muscular and aponeurotic arc spanning the superior aspect of the floor of the canal. Test the mobility of the conjoined tendon by pulling it down to the inguinal ligament. It should pull down easily with minimal tension as the relaxing incision opens up. Extend the relaxing incision superiorly if necessary. Suture the conjoined tendon to the inguinal ligament with interrupted heavy sutures; 0-0 silk on a Mayo needle is particularly convenient for this purpose. Place the sutures no more than 3 to 4 mm apart. Tie the sutures snugly, but not so tightly as to necrose tissue. Tighten the internal ring so that it will no longer accept the tip of your finger. A Kelly clamp should slide easily down along the cord. Recheck hemostasis.

Anatomic Points

Although a true conjoined tendon is seldom seen, there is nevertheless a continuous musculoaponeurotic arch formed by the lower fibers of the transversus abdominis muscle. Relaxing incisions medial to the conjoined tendon area are necessary because aponeurotic fibers of the internal oblique

and transversus abdominis muscles continue to the midline as part of the anterior rectus sheath. As the Bassini repair does not require violation of the transversalis fascia layer, no named vessels should be encountered. Hemostasis can be achieved using electrocautery only.

As the internal ring is approached and as it is tightened, remember that the inferior epigastric vessels lie deep to the transversalis fascia, immediately medial to the internal ring. Care should be taken to avoid these vessels when placing sutures near the internal ring.

FIGURE 86.4
McVAY REPAIR

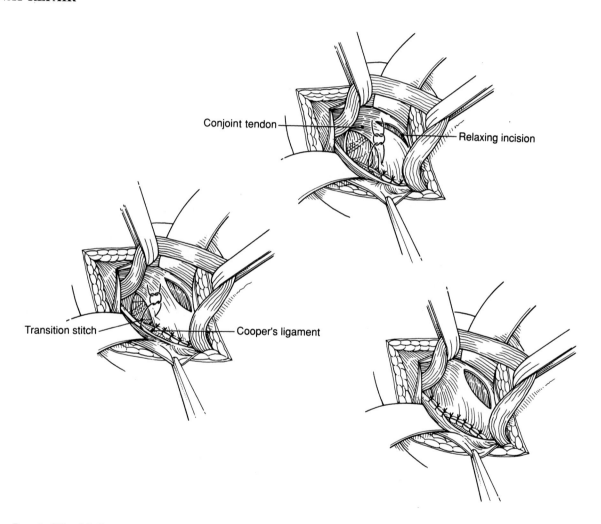

McVay Repair (Fig. 86.4)

Technical Points

When the floor of the canal is weak, a McVay repair may be preferred over a Bassini repair. Use the McVay repair when a good conjoined tendon that is strong and largely aponeurotic is identified in the floor of the canal. The McVay repair involves suturing conjoined tendon to the pectineal ligament (of Cooper), which is a fixed and unyielding structure. An

adequate relaxing incision is necessary to allow the conjoined tendon sufficient mobility to extend down to Cooper's ligament without tension. Make this relaxing incision as described previously.

Beginning at the pubic tubercle, break through the floor of the canal, which generally will be thin and tenuous. Just deep to the inguinal ligament, identify Cooper's ligament, a whitish, shining structure. Push fatty and areolar tissue away from Cooper's ligament and clean it laterally. Identify the sheath of the femoral vein in the lateral region of the dissection, taking care not to damage the vein. Place Allis clamps on the conjoined tendon and pull it down to determine whether adequate mobility has been achieved to bring it to Cooper's ligament without tension.

Suture the conjoined tendon to Cooper's ligament with multiple interrupted sutures; 0-0 Nuralon on a Mayo needle is particularly convenient for this. The heavy Mayo needle is especially important for a Cooper's ligament repair because the tip will not be damaged or bent by the tough periosteum underlying Cooper's ligament. Begin at the pubic tubercle and commence laterally. As the femoral vein is approached and the repair progresses from the deep plane of Cooper's ligament to the more superficial plane of the inguinal ligament, place a transition stitch midway between Cooper's ligament and the inguinal ligament. Take care not to injure the vein or to constrict it. Place the last suture between the conjoined tendon and the inguinal ligament at the level of the internal ring. Tie all sutures and test the strength of the repair and the size of the internal ring. Close the canal as previously described.

Anatomic Points

The McVay repair demands that the pectineal ligament (of Cooper) be visualized. To visualize this ligament, the transversus aponeurosis and transversalis fascia layer must be violated because Cooper's ligament is on a deeper plane than the inguinal ligament and pubic tubercle. Once Cooper's ligament is exposed, be aware of the potential for comparatively large vessels, such as the pubic branch of the inferior

FIGURE 86.5
SHOULDICE REPAIR

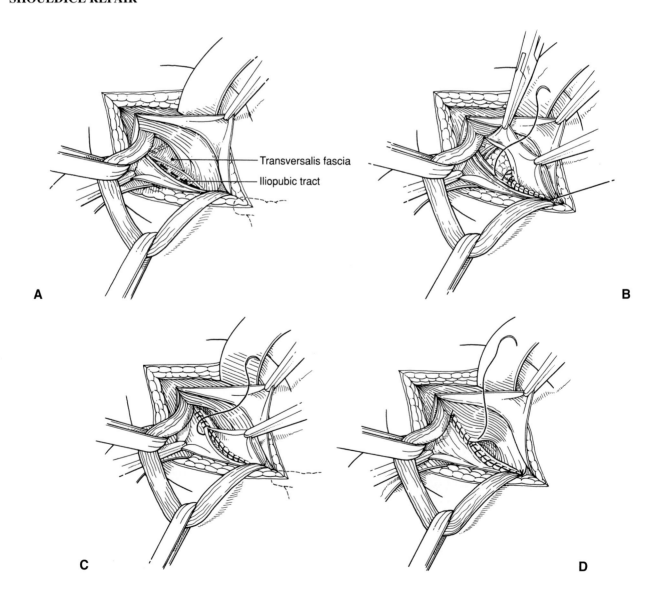

epigastric artery, to be present in this area. This artery lies on the iliopubic tract, runs inferiorly across Cooper's ligament, and ultimately joins the obturator artery; a branch of this courses medially on Cooper's ligament. In about 25% of patients, the pubic branch is 2 to 3 mm in diameter and is referred to as an *accessory obturator artery.*

Shouldice Repair (Fig. 86.5)

Technical Points

When the floor is significantly weakened but some transversalis fascia is identifiable, especially within the iliopubic tract, a Shouldice repair is a good option. Carefully clean the floor of the canal, but do not break through it. Identify the iliopubic tract, which is a thickening of the transversalis fascia adjacent to and adherent to the inguinal ligament. Generally, it is about 2 to 3 mm wide and is identifiable as a slightly whitish, glistening, fibrous band. Incise the transversalis fascia next to the iliopubic tract from the internal ring to the pubic tubercle. Take care not to injure the inferior epigastric vessels at the internal ring or a small branching vessel that is occasionally encountered at the pubic tubercle. Place hemostats on a superior leaf of transversalis fascia and elevate it. By sharp and blunt dissection, separate the underlying preperitoneal fat from the transversalis fascia. The arch of the transversus abdominis aponeurosis should be readily visible as a shiny, white area of thickening on the underside of this tissue layer.

Place a sponge stick in the floor of the canal to hold the contents of the floor out of your way as you proceed with the repair. Use 2-0 or 3-0 monofilament suture; Prolene is a good choice for this suture. Begin your suture line at the pubic tubercle and sew the underside of the arch of the transversus abdominis aponeurosis to the free edge of the iliopubic tract. The suture line runs from the pubic tubercle to the internal ring. Do not try to tighten the internal ring. Four overlapping suture lines will progressively tighten, and it will be quite snug by the end of the repair. At this point, it should be loose.

At the internal ring, bring your suture up through the free edge of the upper leaf of transversalis fascia and commence suturing it to the inguinal ligament with a running suture. This suture line continues from the internal ring laterally to the pubic tubercle medially and is tied to itself. This concludes the first and second suture lines. At the conclusion of this, the floor should be closed, and the internal ring should be approximated, but not tight.

The third and fourth suture lines bring conjoined tendon to inguinal ligament. Begin a suture at the internal ring and bring conjoined tendon down to the inguinal ligament using a running suture from the internal ring to the pubic tubercle. At the pubic tubercle, turn the suture line around and reinforce it by crisscrossing over the previous suture. At the internal ring, check the snugness of the fit around the cord. It should be possible to place a Kelly clamp down through the internal ring next to the cord, but it should not be possible to pass the

tip of your finger down next to the cord. Tie the suture. Check hemostasis in the floor.

Anatomic Points

The deepest fibrous tissue immediately adjacent to the inguinal ligament is often loosely considered to be part of the inguinal ligament. This is the iliopubic tract, an expression of the transversus abdominis aponeurosis and transversalis fascia. This relatively flimsy structure is used for the first suture line of the Shouldice repair because it is mobile, allowing the relatively high arch of the transversus abdominis aponeurosis to be sutured without tension.

Closure of the Canal (Fig. 86.6)

Technical and Anatomic Points

Close the canal by suturing the external oblique aponeurosis together using a running suture of 3-0 Vicryl. Reapproximate the external ring if possible. Place a few sutures of 3-0 Vicryl in the subcutaneous tissue and close the skin with a running subcuticular absorbable suture. Place a dressing on the incision and remove the drapes.

At the conclusion of the operation, it is important to palpate the testis in the scrotum and to pull it back down into the scrotum. Generally, traction on the cord will have elevated the testis almost to the level of the external ring during the course of the dissection. If it is allowed to remain in this position, scar tissue may tether it permanently at the external ring, producing an undesirable cosmetic and functional result.

FIGURE 86.6
CLOSURE OF THE CANAL

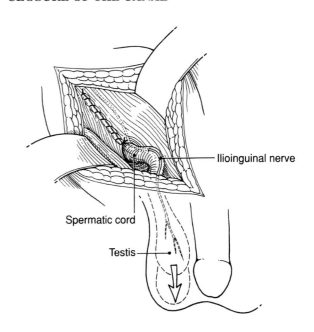

Ilioinguinal nerve

Spermatic cord

Testis

FIGURE 86.7
PLUG-AND-PATCH REPAIR

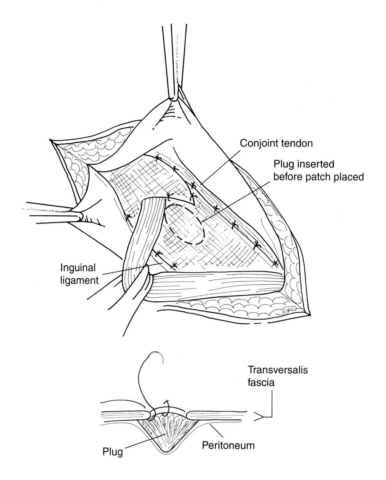

Plug-and-Patch Repair (Fig. 86.7)

Technical and Anatomic Points

Identify, dissect, and perform high ligation of the sac of any indirect hernia present. Define the edges of the any defect in the transversalis fascia. Circumferentially excise it, exposing the preperitoneal fat. Place a preformed plug into this defect in such a manner that the leaflets of the plug expand underneath the transversalis fascia. Tack it in place with one or two sutures of 3-0 Vicryl.

Take the patch and place it around the spermatic cord. Suture it to conjoined tendon superiorly and inguinal ligament inferiorly.

Femoral Hernia Repair

Femoral Hernia Repair from Below (Fig. 86.8)

Technical Points

Repair of the femoral hernia from below does not allow a good anatomic repair. However, this procedure can be done under local anesthesia and is sometimes performed in extremely frail, elderly or debilitated patients.

Make an incision directly over the femoral hernia. This incision should be parallel to the inguinal ligament and will generally lie about 2 cm below it. Identify the sac of the hernia and, by sharp and blunt dissection, free it from the surrounding soft tissues. Open the sac, and reduce any contents into the abdominal cavity. It may be necessary to incise the inguinal ligament vertically, retracting the spermatic cord upward, to enlarge the canal sufficiently to reduce the contents of the sac. Twist the sac and ligate it with a suture ligature. Amputate the sac, and reduce the stump into the abdomen.

Closure of the femoral canal from below is best achieved by inserting a patch of prosthetic material, such as Marlex. Roll the Marlex patch up into a small ball and place it in the femoral canal, suturing it in place. Take care not to injure or impinge on the femoral vein. Close subcutaneous tissues with interrupted Vicryl sutures and close the skin.

Anatomic Points

Repair of a femoral hernia from below necessitates ligation and division of several veins that either join the upper end of the saphenous vein or run through the saphenous hiatus of the femoral sheath and fascia lata to drain directly into the

FIGURE 86.8
FEMORAL HERNIA REPAIR FROM BELOW

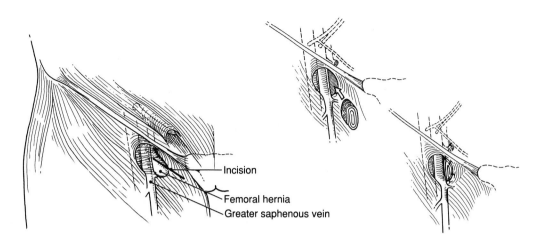

Incision
Femoral hernia
Greater saphenous vein

femoral vein. The anatomic key to repair from below is to remember that the femoral ring is bounded by the iliopubic tract anteriorly and medially, by Cooper's ligament posteriorly, and by venous periadventitial tissue laterally. It is to these structures that the prosthetic material is sutured. Of these boundaries, the lateral wall of periadventitial tissue is the least fixed. Therefore, compression of the femoral vein is easily possible, as is needle trauma to the vein if sutures are placed too deeply.

The entrance to the femoral canal is about 1 cm deep to the external opening of the canal, through which the hernia protrudes. Adequate closure of the opening of this canal is difficult from below; for this reason, closure with a plug of mesh may be simpler than attempting suture closure.

FIGURE 86.9
FEMORAL HERNIA REPAIR FROM ABOVE

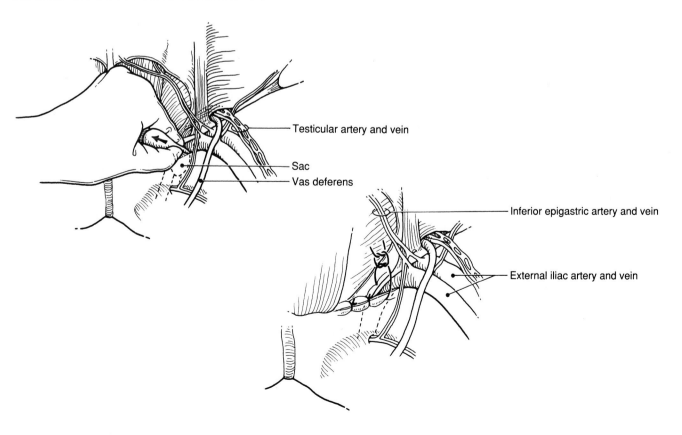

Testicular artery and vein
Sac
Vas deferens
Inferior epigastric artery and vein
External iliac artery and vein

Femoral Hernia Repair from Above (Fig. 86.9)

Technical Points

Repair of the femoral hernia through the floor of the inguinal canal not only is more anatomically appropriate but also permits controlled reduction of incarcerated sac contents as well as resection of infarcted bowel, if necessary. This approach involves dissection through an otherwise intact inguinal floor. Despite this single disadvantage, this method is generally the preferred approach for most femoral hernias.

Open the inguinal canal in the manner described for inguinal hernias. Open the floor of the canal by sharp and blunt dissection to identify Cooper's ligament. The repair of the floor that will be done is the McVay repair. The neck of the femoral hernia sac will be identifiable as a diverticulum of peritoneum extending down from the abdomen through the femoral canal, a space medial to the femoral vein. Open the femoral hernia sac and reduce its contents. It may be necessary to cut the inguinal ligament to do this. Note that a vessel—the so-called artery of death—frequently runs along the underside of the inguinal ligament; this must be identified and ligated before division of the inguinal ligament. Ligate and divide the sac of the femoral hernia.

Close the floor of the canal in the McVay fashion, obliterating the femoral canal and excluding it from the abdomen. Take care not to impinge on the femoral vein.

Anatomic Points

This is a classic Cooper's ligament repair. The only anatomic point that has not been previously covered is the artery of death. This artery arises from the pubic branch of the inferior epigastric artery and, if left uncontrolled, can cause serious morbidity. The vessel is at greatest risk when a femoral hernia is repaired from below. From that approach, it is invisible, and injury to it during division of the inguinal ligament may not be immediately obvious, resulting in delayed, possibly occult, retroperitoneal bleeding.

REFERENCES

1. Condon RE. The anatomy of the inguinal region and its relation to groin hernia. In: Nyhus LM, Condon RE, eds. *Hernia.* 3rd ed. Philadelphia: JB Lippincott, 1989:18.
2. Condon RE. Surgical anatomy of the transversus abdominis and transversalis fascia. *Ann Surg* 1971;173:1.
3. DeBord JR. The historical development of prosthetics in hernia surgery. *Surg Clin North Am* 1998;78:973–1006.
4. Heise CP, Starling JR. Mesh inguinodynia: a new clinical syndrome after inguinal herniorrhaphy? *J Am Coll Surg* 1998;187:514–518.
5. Henry AK. Operation for femoral hernia: by a midline extraperitoneal approach. *Lancet* 1936;230:531.
6. Lichtenstein IL. Herniorrhaphy: a personal experience with 6321 cases. *Am J Surg* 1987;153:53.
7. Lichtenstein IL, Shore JM. Simplified repair of femoral and recurrent inguinal hernias by a "plug" technique. *Am J Surg* 1974;128:439.
8. Lichtenstein IL, Shulman AG, Amid PK, et al. The tension-free hernioplasty. *Am J Surg* 1989;157:188. (Describes mesh inguinal hernioplasty.)
9. Madden JL, Agorogiannis AB. The anatomy and repair of inguinal hernias. *Surg Clin North Am* 1971;51:1269.
10. McKernan JB, Laws HL. Laparoscopic preperitoneal prosthetic repair of inguinal hernias. *Surg Rounds* 1992:597. (Provides clear description, with color photographs, of an evolving technique.)
11. McVay CB. The anatomic basis for inguinal and femoral hernioplasty. *Surg Gynecol Obstet* 1974;139:931.
12. McVay CB. The normal and pathologic anatomy of the transversus abdominis muscle in inguinal and femoral hernia. *Surg Clin North Am* 1971;51:1251.
13. Mizrachy B, Kark AE. The anatomy and repair of the posterior inguinal wall. *Surg Gynecol Obstet* 1973;137:253. (Describes Shouldice technique.)
14. Moran RM, Blick M, Collura M. Double layer of transversalis fascia for repair of inguinal hernia: results in 104 cases. *Surgery* 1968;63:423.
15. Nyhus LM. An anatomic reappraisal of the posterior inguinal wall: special consideration of the iliopubic tract and its relation to groin hernias. *Surg Clin North Am* 1964;44:1305.
16. Ponka JL. Seven steps to local anesthesia for inguinofemoral hernia repair. *Surg Gynecol Obstet* 1963;117:115.
17. Pritchard TJ, Bloom AD, Zollinger RM. Pitfalls in ambulatory treatment of inguinal hernias in adults. *Surg Clin North Am* 1991;71:1353.
18. Robbins AW, Rutkow IM. The mesh-plug hernioplasty. *Surg Clin North Am* 1993;73:501–512.
19. Rutkow IM, Robbins AW. Classification systems and groin hernias. *Surg Clin North Am* 1998;78:1117–1127. (Presents the case for a new classification system.)
20. Shearburn EW, Myers RN. Shouldice repair for inguinal hernia. *Surgery* 1969;66:450.
21. Sorg J, Skandalakis JE, Gray SW. The emperor's new clothes or the myth of the conjoined tendon. *Am Surg* 1979;45:588.
22. Spaw AL. Laparoscopic hernia repair: the anatomic basis. *J Laparoendosc Surg* 1991;1:269. (Presents good review of anatomy.)
23. Starling JR, Harms BA, Schroeder ME, et al. Diagnosis and treatment of genitofemoral and ilioinguinal entrapment neuralgia. *Surgery* 1987;102:581. (Provides good review of presenting symptoms, possible causes, and management.)

CHAPTER 87

Laparoscopic Inguinal Hernia Repair

Laparoscopic inguinal hernia repair takes a totally different approach from open repair. It is most nearly analogous to a preperitoneal open repair, sometimes termed the *Nyhus repair,* performed with mesh. The logic is similar to that employed during laparoscopic ventral herniorraphy: because the problem is a weakness in the transversalis fascia (or a persistently patent processus vaginalis), approach the defect from inside. Peritoneum is stripped from the region, and the defect is repaired with a large sheet of prosthetic mesh. Intraabdominal pressure holds the mesh buttressed against the muscular and aponeurotic layers of the abdominal wall, which are not dissected. Tacks are placed to secure the mesh in place. The anatomy that is stressed for this repair is very different than that stressed in Chapter 86. There is little emphasis on the muscular and aponeurotic layers of the abdominal wall. Avoiding complications during these procedures requires intimate knowledge of the anatomy of crucial nerves and blood vessels that must be avoided when the mesh is secured. Major complications of the procedure include vascular injury and neuropraxia. The procedure may be done transabdominal preperitoneal (TAPP) or totally extraperitoneal (TEP). In this chapter, the transabdominal approach is shown first, followed by the modification employed for TEP.

The muscular and aponeurotic structures of the anterior abdominal wall appear different when viewed from inside with the peritoneum removed (see part A of the orientation figure). Note how the ductus (or vas) deferens enters through the deep inguinal ring and then passes inferiorly and medially

to join the seminal vesicles in the region of the base of the bladder. The internal spermatic vessels pass from lateral to medial and ascend to pass through the deep inguinal ring. The inferior epigastric vessels ascend and pass medially, defining the lateral border of Hesselbach's triangle. The medial umbilical ligaments, the obliterated remnants of the umbilical arteries, form useful visual landmarks. The median umbilical landmark is rarely seen. Part B of the orientation figure shows peritoneum intact on the right side, demonstrating the peritoneal folds and visual landmarks with peritoneum intact. On the left side, the peritoneum has been removed to reveal underlying structures of significance. Note the iliopubic tract, the femoral canal, Cooper's ligament, and the arch of the aponeurosis of the transversus abdominis. Contrast this view with the anterior and posterior views shown in the orientation figure for Chapter 86.

Multiple nerves and vessels, most never encountered during open inguinal or femoral herniorrhaphy, are at risk during laparoscopic repair. Nerves include the lateral femoral cutaneous nerve, the anterior femoral cutaneous nerve, the femoral nerve, the femoral branch of the genitofemoral nerve, and the genital branch of the genitofemoral nerve. The vascular structures at risk include the external iliac artery and vein and aberrant obturator arteries. The latter, also termed the "artery of death," is a potential pitfall when a femoral hernia is repaired from above (see Fig. 86.8 in Chapter 86).

Two triangles, which lie together to form a rough trapezoid, encompass the majority of these structures and form a

LIST OF STRUCTURES

Peritoneum
Transversalis fascia
Patent processus vaginalis
Ductus deferens
Seminal vesicles
Round ligament of uterus
Bladder
Deep (internal) inguinal ring
Medial umbilical ligament (fold)
    Urachus
Median umbilical ligaments (folds)
    Obliterated umbilical artery

Lateral umbilical ligaments (folds)
    Inferior epigastric artery and vein
Supravesical fossa
Medial umbilical fossa
Lateral umbilical fossa
Hesselbach's triangle
Iliopubic tract
Femoral canal
Cooper's ligament
Conjoint tendon
Arch of aponeurosis of transversus
    abdominis
Lateral femoral cutaneous nerve

Anterior femoral cutaneous nerve
Femoral nerve
Genitofemoral nerve
    Femoral branch
    Genital branch
Ilioinguinal nerve
Iliohypogastric nerve
External iliac artery and vein
Femoral artery and vein
Internal iliac artery and vein
Obturator artery
    Aberrant obturator artery
Prevesical space (of Retzius)

(**A** from Wind GG. The inguinal region. In: *Applied laparoscopic anatomy: abdomen and pelvis.* Baltimore: Williams & Wilkins, 1997:85–140, with permission; **B** from Colborn GL, Skandalakis JE. Laparoscopic cadaveric anatomy of the inguinal area. *Probl Gen Surg* 1995;12:13–20, with permission.

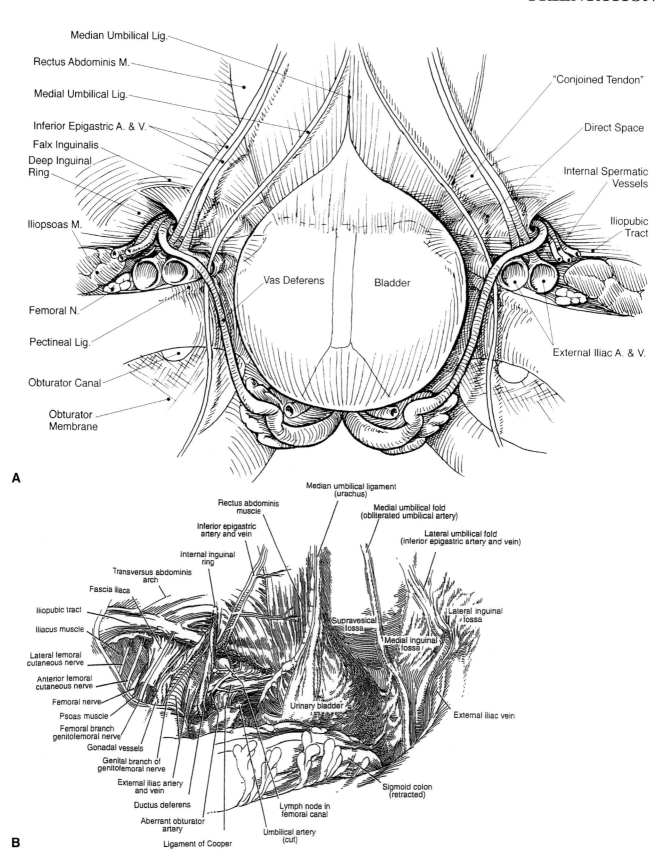

C from Colborn GL, Brick WG. Inguinal region. In: Scott-Conner CEH, Cuschieri A, Carter FJ, eds. *Minimal access surgical anatomy.* Philadelphia: Lippincott Williams & Wilkins, 2000:239–266, with permission.)

ORIENTATION (Continued)

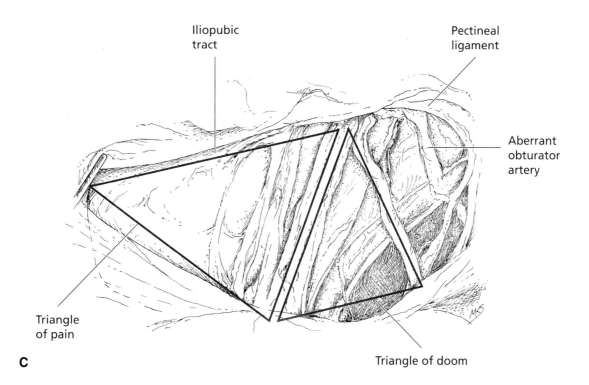

Iliopubic tract

Pectineal ligament

Aberrant obturator artery

Triangle of pain

C

Triangle of doom

useful mnemonic device (see part C of the orientation figure). The "triangle of pain" is bounded by the iliopubic tract superiorly, the testicular vessels medially, and the cut edge of the peritoneum inferiorly. It contains most of the nerves previously mentioned. The "triangle of doom," bounded by the testicular vessels laterally, the ductus deferens medially, and the cut peritoneal edge inferiorly, contains the vessels. Extreme care must be exercised while dissecting in these triangles, and no staples or other fixation devices should be placed in these regions.

TAPP—Orientation and Initial View of Male and Female Pelvis (Fig. 87.1)

Technical Points

Position the patient supine. Place three ports as shown (Fig. 87.1A). Use an angled (30- or 45-degree) laparoscope for better visualization of the inguinal region. Note that in the male, the ductus deferens and inferior spermatic vessels form the apex of a triangle that points to the internal inguinal ring (Fig. 87.1B). Normally, the peritoneum over this region is smooth, or, at most, a tiny dimple or crescentic fold will be seen at the internal ring. In the female, the round ligament is seen to terminate in the internal ring (Fig. 87.1C). Confirm the presence of a hernia or of multiple defects by noting outpouchings in the peritoneum either medial (direct) or lateral (indirect) to the inferior epigastric vessels (Fig. 87.1D,E).

Anatomic Points

As the parietal peritoneum covers the undersurface of the anterior abdominal wall and pelvis, underlying structures tent it up, creating five peritoneal folds. These form visual landmarks useful to the laparoscopic surgeon.

In the midline, the remnant of the obliterated urachus links the umbilicus with the dome of the bladder. Although this median umbilical fold is shown in parts A and B of the orientation figure, it is rarely actually visible to the laparoscopic surgeon, perhaps because it is so close to the umbilically placed laparoscope. The space above the bladder is termed the *supravesical fossa.*

The paired medial umbilical ligaments are much more obvious. These contain the obliterated remnants of the umbilical arteries. They lead from the umbilicus to the internal iliac arteries bilaterally. The region of interest to the laparoscopic hernia surgeon lies just lateral to the medial umbilical ligaments.

In the male, a very obvious triangle marks the convergence of the testicular vessels and ductus deferens on the internal (deep) inguinal ring. In the female, the corresponding gonadal (ovarian) vessels do not traverse the internal inguinal ring; thus, the triangle is incomplete, and only the round ligament points the way to the internal ring.

Of the landmarks that delineate Hesselbach's triangle, only the inferior epigastric vessels (contained in the lateral umbilical folds) are visible. The space between the medial and

FIGURE 87.1
TAPP—ORIENTATION AND INITIAL VIEW OF MALE AND FEMALE PELVIS (B, D, and **E** from Colborn GL, Brick WG. Inguinal region. In: Scott-Conner CEH, Cuschieri A, Carter FJ, eds. *Minimal access surgical anatomy.* Philadelphia: Lippincott Williams & Wilkins, 2000:239–266, with permission; **C** from Hedican SP. Pelvis. In: Scott-Conner CEH, Cuschieri A, Carter FJ, eds. *Minimal access surgical anatomy.* Philadelphia: Lippincott Williams & Wilkins, 2000:211–238, with permission.)

FIGURE 87.1 (Continued)

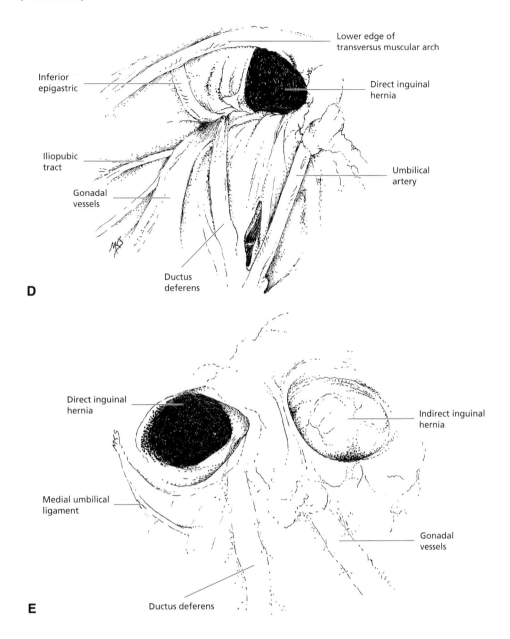

lateral umbilical folds is termed the *medial umbilical fossa.* Similarly, the region lateral to the lateral umbilical folds (ie, lateral to the inferior epigastric vessels), is the *lateral umbilical fossa.*

TAPP—Peritoneal Incision (Fig. 87.2)

Technical Points

Identify the medial umbilical ligament visually and the anterosuperior iliac spine (by palpation on the outside of the abdomen, if necessary). Make an incision in the peritoneum (Fig. 87.2A) from the level of the median umbilical ligament to the anterosuperior iliac spine about 2 cm cephalad to the upper edge of the hernia. Develop flaps in the superior and inferior direction. In particular, carefully reflect the inferior flap of peritoneum to expose the muscular and aponeurotic structures of the inguinal region from within (Fig. 87.2B).

Anatomic Points

In contrast to open hernia repair, in which muscular and aponeurotic structures are divided from superficial to deep, only the deepest structures are seen during laparoscopic surgery, and none of these are actually divided (Fig. 87.2C). The iliopubic tract, a condensation of the transversalis fascia, may be seen, indicating the position of the (unseen) inguinal ligament. The arch of the aponeurosis of the transversus

FIGURE 87.2

TAPP—PERITONEAL INCISION (A–C from Colborn GL, Skandalakis JE. Laparoscopic cadaveric anatomy of the inguinal area. *Probl Gen Surg* 1995;12:13–20, with permission.)

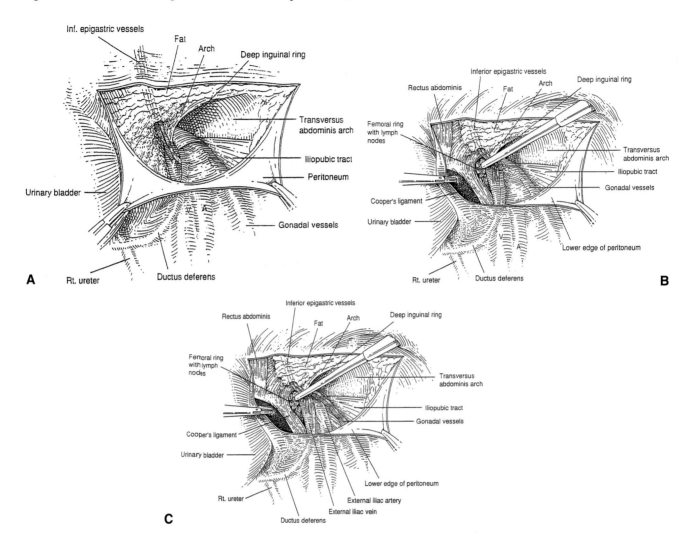

abdominis muscle can be seen passing from lateral to medial as the muscular fibers of the transversus abdominis give way to aponeurosis. This aponeurosis contributes to the formation of the conjoint tendon and blends with the linea alba medially. Medially, the rectus abdominis muscle may be seen.

TAPP—Reducing Sac of Hernia and Defining Anatomy (Fig. 87.3)

Technical Points

Gently tease fat and peritoneum from the region of Hessel-bach's triangle and the iliopubic tract (Fig. 87.3A). The sac of a direct hernia will generally reduce as the peritoneal flap is developed (Fig. 87.3B). An indirect sac must be reduced from within the spermatic cord (if the sac is not very long) or amputated and allowed to remain (if a large sac). To amputate a large sac, begin dissection on the side opposite the cord structures and work toward the cord (Fig. 87.3C). Only

when the cord structures are seen to be separate from the sac should it be amputated.

Anatomic Points

The entire region of interest should now be exposed. Identify the pubic tubercle, Cooper's ligament, the iliac artery and vein, and the inferior epigastric vessels (Fig. 87.2C).

TAPP—Placement of Mesh (Fig. 87.4)

Technical Points

Carefully check the region for hemostasis because access will be lost once the mesh is placed. The field should resemble Fig. 87.4A. Tailor a large piece of mesh (at least 11 by 6 cm) to cover the internal ring completely, including direct, indirect, and femoral hernial orifices. Roll the mesh into a narrow cylinder and introduce it into the peritoneal cavity.

FIGURE 87.3
TAPP—REDUCING SAC OF HERNIA AND DEFINING ANATOMY (A–C from Wind GG. The inguinal region. In: *Applied laparoscopic anatomy: abdomen and pelvis.* Baltimore: Williams & Wilkins, 1997:85–140, with permission.)

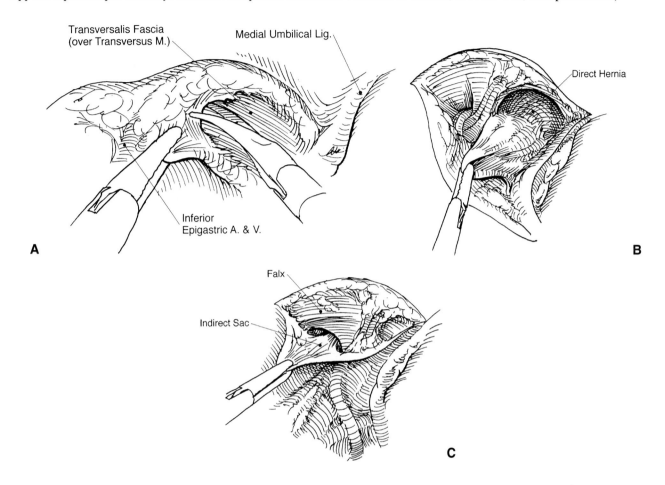

Unroll it and place it under the peritoneal flaps. Position it with care so that the area of potential and actual weakness is covered with good overlap.

Place staples along the upper edge of the mesh (Fig. 87.4B) and along the iliopubic tract medially. Never place staples in the triangle of doom or pain (see part C of the orientation figure).

Anatomic Points

A large number of nerves and vessels are vulnerable during this dissection. Although the nerves are primarily encountered in the triangle of pain and the vessels in the triangle of doom, the entire area inferior to the iliopubic tract and lateral to the ductus deferens should be considered to be "off limits" for staples, tacks, or overly vigorous dissection (Fig. 87.4C).

The femoral nerve, the single largest branch of the lumbar plexus, emerges from the lateral border of the psoas major muscle about 6 cm above the iliopubic tract. It then passes behind the inguinal ligament to enter the thigh. Pain and weakness of the anterior thigh result from injury.

The anterior cutaneous branch of the femoral nerve (Fig. 87.4D) arises early and may be encountered near or beneath the iliopubic tract just lateral to the external iliac vessels.

The lateral femoral cutaneous nerve is one of the two nerves most commonly injured during laparoscopic herniorrhaphy. It emerges from the lateral border of the psoas major muscle and exits the pelvis by passing beneath the inguinal ligament, usually within 1 cm of the anterosuperior iliac spine.

The genitofemoral nerve passes down along the psoas major muscle, crosses behind the ureter, and divides into the genital and femoral branches. The exact site of bifurcation varies. In one common variant, the genital branch of the genitofemoral nerve passes below the iliopubic tract to enter the inguinal canal from below, placing it at risk during laparoscopic herniorrhaphy (Fig. 87.4D). Burning pain and numbness in the labium or scrotum and medial thigh result from injury.

The ilioinguinal and iliohypogastric nerves lie in a plane superficial to the plane in which laparoscopic hernia surgery is performed. These nerves are not seen but can be injured if counterpressure (with one hand from outside the abdomen) is used to facilitate placement of deep staples or tacks in the vicinity of the iliopubic tract, particularly lateral to the internal ring.

The actual distribution of the individual nerves varies, and these nerves are generally not visualized during laparoscopic herniorrhaphy.

The obvious vascular structures at peril include the external iliac artery and vein, exiting below the inguinal ligament to become the femoral vessels, and the inferior epigastric and testicular vessels. Less obvious is the potential for an aberrant obturator artery to be injured. These common anomalous vessels link the internal iliac artery with the obturator artery.

These numerous vascular and neural structures must be protected from rough dissection or placement of tacks or staples. A simple rule articulated by Seid and Amos (see

---

FIGURE 87.4

TAPP—PLACEMENT OF MESH (A, C, and **D** from Colborn GL, Brick WG. Inguinal region. In: Scott-Conner CEH, Cuschieri A, Carter FJ, eds. *Minimal access surgical anatomy.* Philadelphia: Lippincott Williams & Wilkins, 2000:239–266, with permission; **B** from Wind GG. The inguinal region. In: *Applied laparoscopic anatomy: abdomen and pelvis.* Baltimore: Williams & Wilkins, 1997:85–140, with permission.)

FIGURE 87.4   (Continued)

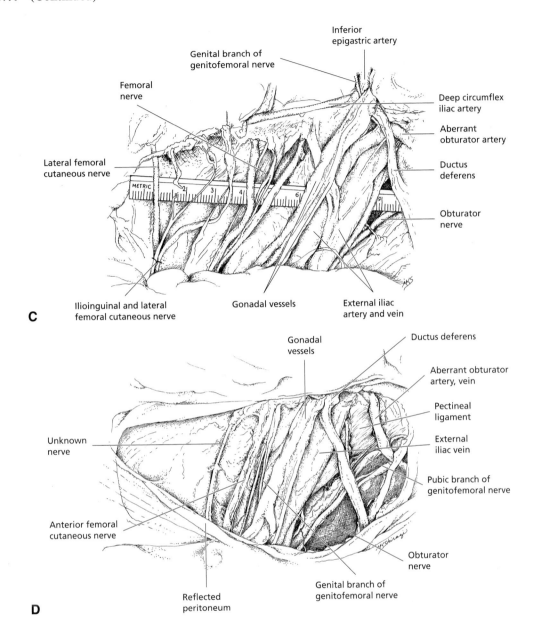

C

D

references) is never to place a staple below the iliopubic tract anywhere lateral to the ductus (all the way to the anterosuperior iliac spine).

TAPP—Peritoneal Closure (Fig. 87.5)

Technical and Anatomic Points

Close the peritoneal flap to cover the mesh completely. Do this by apposing the two peritoneal edges at the point where tension is least and then progressing along the incision until full closure has been obtained. Staples may be used for this purpose (Fig. 87.5A). Take care to place these sufficiently close that gaps do not occur. Clips are used by some surgeons (Fig. 87.5B) to diminish this problem by providing greater peritoneal overlap (Fig. 87.5C,D).

Desufflate the abdomen, check hemostasis, and close the trocar sites in the usual fashion.

TEP—Trocar Placement and Development of Dissection Plane (Fig. 87.6)

Technical Points

The crucial maneuver is developing a plane in the proper extraperitoneal space at the beginning of the dissection. If this is done properly, the rest of the repair is similar to that previously described. If the wrong plane is entered or if a hole is made in the peritoneum, dissection may be more difficult.

Make initial entry into the preperitoneal space with an open technique. After incising the fascia, visualize the fat of the preperitoneal space. Use blunt dissection with a finger to

FIGURE 87.5
TAPP—PERITONEAL CLOSURE (A–D from Wind GG. The inguinal region. In: *Applied laparoscopic anatomy: abdomen and pelvis.* Baltimore:Williams & Wilkins, 1997:85–140, with permission.)

establish an initial plane progressing toward the pubic symphysis. Introduce a dissecting balloon and pass it to the pubic symphysis (Fig. 87.6A), expanding the balloon to develop a working space. Note that the bladder is mobilized downward (Fig. 87.6B). Do not attempt this dissection in a patient who has had previous surgery in the space of Retzius because the plane may be obliterated.

Place additional trocars as shown (Fig. 87.6C). As during

TAPP, a direct sac will generally reduce as dissection progresses laterally. An indirect sac may cause difficulty. Carefully separate the sac from the ductus deferens medially and testicular vessels laterally (Fig. 87.6D). If necessary, divide the sac, taking extreme care not to include ductus deferens, testicular vessels, or intraperitoneal structures (Fig. 87.6E).

Identification of structures and placement of mesh proceeds exactly as described earlier. At the end of the procedure,

FIGURE 87.6
TEP—TROCAR PLACEMENT AND DEVELOPMENT OF DISSECTION PLANE (**A** and **C** from Crawford DL, Phillips EH. Totally extraperitoneal laparoscopic herniorraphy. In: Zucker KA, ed. *Surgical laparoscopy.* 2nd ed. Philadelphia: Lippincott Williams & Wilkins, 2001:571–584, with permission; **B, D,** and **E** from Wind GG. The inguinal region. In: *Applied laparoscopic anatomy: abdomen and pelvis.* Baltimore: Williams & Wilkins, 1997:85–140, with permission.)

the peritoneum simply falls back against the mesh, and there is no peritoneal incision to repair.

Anatomic Points

The prevesical space of Retzius gives free entry, through loose fatty areolar tissue, to the extraperitoneal anterior bladder and ultimately to the prostate. This space is accessed during retropubic prostatectomy and hence becomes obliterated with scar tissue. The only significant structures that should be encountered are the pubic symphysis, visible as a large white transversely oriented structure, and the urinary bladder. The bladder is displaced posteriorly as dissection progresses and is not seen.

REFERENCES

1. Annibali RG, Fitzgibbons RJ Jr, Filipi CJ, et al. Laparoscopic inguinal hernia repair. In: Greene FL, Ponsky JL, eds. *Endoscopic surgery.* Philadelphia: WB Saunders, 1994:352–386.
2. Brick WG, Colborn GL, Gadacz TR, et al. Crucial anatomic lessons for laparoscopic herniorrhaphy. *Am Surg* 1995;61:172–177.
3. Broin EO, Horner C, Mealy K, et al. Meralgia paraesthetica following laparoscopic inguinal hernia repair: an anatomical analysis. *Surg Endosc* 1995;9:76–78.
4. Chapman WHH, Crombie CH, Cox SS, et al. Laparoscopic inguinal hernia repair. *Curr Surg* 1996;53:477–485.
5. Colborn GL, Brick WG. Inguinal region. In: Scott-Conner CEH, Cuschieri A, Carter FJ, eds. *Minimal access surgical anatomy.* Philadelphia: Lippincott Williams & Wilkins, 2000:239–266. (Gives more details of anatomy and is accompanied by color photographs.)
6. Colborn GL, Brick WG, Gadacz TR, et al. Inguinal anatomy for laparoscopic herniorrhaphy. I. The normal anatomy. *Surg Rounds* 1995;189–198.
7. Colborn GL, Brick WG, Gadacz TR, et al. Inguinal anatomy for laparoscopic herniorrhaphy. II. Altered inguinal anatomy and variations. *Surg Rounds* 1995;223–232.
8. Colborn GL, Skandalakis JE. Laparoscopic cadaveric anatomy of the inguinal area. *Probl Gen Surg* 1995;12:13–20.
9. Crawford DL, Phillips EH. Laparoscopic repair and groin hernia surgery. *Surg Clin North Am* 1998;78:1047–1062.
10. Crawford DL, Phillips EH. Totally extraperitoneal laparoscopic herniorrhaphy. In: Zucker KA, ed. *Surgical laparoscopy.* 2nd ed. Philadelphia: Lippincott Williams & Wilkins, 2001:571–584. (Provides excellent detailed description.)
11. Dibenedetto LM, Lei Q, Gilroy AM, et al. Variations in the inferior pelvic pathway of the lateral femoral cutaneous nerve: implications for laparoscopic hernia repair. *Clin Anat* 1996;9:232–236.
12. Eubanks S, Newman L 3rd, Goehring L, et al. Meralgia paresthetica: a complication of laparoscopic herniorrhaphy. *Surg Laparosc Endosc* 1993;3:381–385.
13. Keating JP, Morgan A. Femoral nerve palsy following laparoscopic inguinal herniorrhaphy. *J Laparoendosc Surg* 1993;3:557–559.
14. Kraus MA. Nerve injury during laparoscopic inguinal hernia repair. *Surg Laparosc Endosc* 1993;3:342–345.
15. Ramshaw BJ, Tucker JG, Duncan TD, et al. Technical considerations of the different approaches to laparoscopic herniorrhaphy: an analysis of 500 cases. *Am Surg* 1996;62:69–72.
16. Sampath P, Yeo CJ, Campbell JN. Nerve injury associated with laparoscopic inguinal herniorrhaphy. *Surgery* 1995;118:829–833.
17. Seid AS, Amos E. Entrapment neuropathy in laparoscopic herniorrhaphy. *Surg Endosc* 1994;8:1050–1053.
18. Skandalakis JE, Colborn GL, Androulakis JA, et al. Embryologic and anatomic basis of inguinal herniorrhaphy. *Surg Clin North Am* 1993;73:799–836.
19. Voeller GR, Mangiante EC Jr, Wilson C. Totally preperitoneal laparoscopic inguinal herniorrhaphy using balloon dissection. *Surg Rounds* 1995;208:107–112.
20. Woods S, Polglase A. Ilioinguinal nerve entrapment from laparoscopic hernia repair. *Aust N Z J Surg* 1993;63:823–824.

CHAPTER 88

Superficial Groin Dissection

Peter R. Jochimsen

Superficial groin dissection removes the lymph node–bearing tissue anterior and above the fascia lata of the groin and the external oblique musculature of the lower abdominal wall. The dissection is most often required to eradicate metastatic disease arising from tumors of the skin of the lower extremity or lower abdomen and flank, squamous cell carcinoma of the anus and anal canal, vulvar cancers involving these nodes, as well as metastases from penile, distal urethral, and scrotal tumors.

The increasing use of "sentinel node" technology (see Chapter 89) has generally rendered the distinction between therapeutic and prophylactic node dissection moot. In patients presenting with palpable inguinal adenopathy or with demonstrated metastatic disease on fine-needle aspiration of an inguinal node, or when sentinel node biopsy is positive and no additional metastatic disease is identified, inguinal node dissection is indicated. In some circumstances, even in the face of wider spread of disease, local control may be obtained by removal of involved nodes.

There is significant morbidity associated with this dissection. More than 20% of patients suffer wound complications, including wound infection; more commonly, patients develop chronic swelling (lymphedema) of the lower extremity following removal of the regional inguinal nodes. A variety of incisions have been advocated to decrease wound complications and edema. Preservation of the saphenous vein, rather than its division at the saphenofemoral junction (as shown here), has been advocated by some to decrease further the incidence of lymphedema. There remains, however, concern that preservation of this structure may compromise the ability of the surgeon to obtain complete lymphatic clearance of the groin.

LIST OF STRUCTURES

Inguinal lymph nodes
    Superficial inguinal lymph nodes
    Deep inguinal lymph nodes
    Node of Cloquet
External iliac lymph nodes
Pelvic lymph nodes
Anterosuperior iliac spine

Pubic tubercle
Inguinal ligament
External oblique aponeurosis
External inguinal ring
Spermatic cord
Labium majorum
Fascia lata

Femoral nerve
Femoral artery
Femoral vein
    Saphenous vein
    Saphenofemoral junction
Pectineus muscle
Sartorius muscle

605

FIGURE 88.1
INCISION

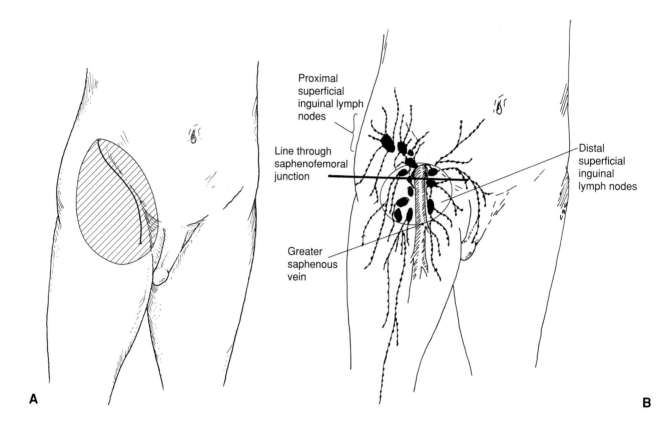

A
B

Incision (Fig. 88.1)

Technical Points

In an attempt to decrease the wound infection rate, prophylactic antibiotics are given on call to the operating room. After the induction of anesthesia, position the patient supine. Place a Foley catheter. External rotation of the hip and flexion of the knee will improve exposure in obese individuals.

Make a sigmoidal incision from just over the anterosuperior iliac spine down to the inguinal ligament, continuing parallel to the inguinal ligament and then downward on the medial thigh (Fig. 88.1A). Flaps are then developed superiorly and inferiorly, as indicated by the shaded area.

Use rake retractors to elevate the superior flap. With cutting electrocautery, elevate this flap onto the external oblique aponeurosis for the full extent of the incision from the anterosuperior iliac spine to the pubic tubercle. Once onto the external oblique aponeurosis, retract all of the soft tissue inferiorly. Take care at the external ring in the male so as not to compromise the spermatic cord. Such care is not needed in the female; rather, avoid entering the soft tissues of the labia, where bleeding may become a problem.

Next, create the inferior flap, again using rakes to elevate the skin and the most superficial subcutaneous tissue, leaving deep subcutaneous tissue behind. Begin laterally, bringing the upper soft tissue mass that has been dissected free superiorly

laterally, and working medial to the first important structure, the femoral nerve. The lateral-most extent of the dissection in the leg is the sartorius muscle. Divide the fascia lata anterior to this structure.

Anatomic Points

The fascia lata is the deep fascia of the thigh. Proximally, it is continuous with the aponeuroses of the external oblique muscles and the thoracolumbar fascia. It is adherent at the pelvic bones and inguinal ligament. Inferiorly, it is continuous with the deep fascia of the leg. Laterally, this fascia forms a strong aponeurosis, which is sometimes harvested for fascial grafts. Medially, in the region of this dissection, it becomes thinner.

The area of interest here is the femoral triangle. The sartorius muscle, the first muscular landmark encountered during this dissection, forms its lateral boundary. Covered with fascia lata, the sartorius is the longest muscle in the body. This slender strap of a muscle runs obliquely from its origin on the anterosuperior iliac spine to terminate on the proximal medial tibia. The innervation is segmental, usually dual. The sartorius is occasionally absent.

The upper border of the femoral triangle is formed by the inguinal ligament, and the lateral border by the adductor longus muscle (not seen at this point). Contents of significance within this triangle are, from lateral to medial, the femoral nerve, artery, vein, and lymphatics (see Fig. 100.1B in Chapter 100).

The superficial inguinal lymph nodes, removed during this dissection, are divided into a proximal and distal group by a line drawn through the saphenofemoral junction (Fig. 88.1B). The proximal group, usually five or six in number, lie below the inguinal ligament and parallel to it. The distal group (four or five) are encountered on both sides of the greater saphenous vein.

Medial to the femoral vein, the deep inguinal nodes (two or three in number) communicate through the femoral canal with the external iliac nodes (see part B of orientation figure in Chapter 87). Typically, there is one node below the femoral canal and two or three above it. A large node encountered in this region is often termed *Cloquet's node*. Because the next nodal group, the external iliac nodes, lie within the pelvis, pathologic involvement of Cloquet's node may signify nodal involvement outside the boundary of the dissection shown here.

Lymph nodes in this region receive afferent lymphatics from the trunk (see also Fig. 89.1D in Chapter 89), the external genitalia, the lower part of the anal canal and perianal region, and the lower extremity.

Division of Saphenous Vein at Saphenofemoral Junction (Fig. 88.2)

Technical Points

Progressing medially, elevate fascia lata and soft tissue from the femoral nerve onto the femoral artery and more medially the femoral vein. Identify the saphenofemoral junction. Doubly clamp the saphenous vein at the saphenofemoral junction; divide and suture-ligate it. If damage occurs to the saphenofemoral junction or the femoral vein, and if vigorous bleeding results, immediately place the patient in the reverse Trendelenburg position to avoid the possibility of air embolism. Repair the damaged vein with fine vascular suture.

Anatomic Points

The femoral nerve is the largest branch of the lumbar plexus. It descends through the retroperitoneum in company with the psoas major muscle, emerging from that muscle in its lower third. The nerve then passes under the ligament (see part A of orientation figure in Chapter 87) to emerge into the thigh, where it is encountered during this dissection. A small tongue of psoas major muscle separates the femoral nerve from the next structure encountered as the dissection progresses medially—the femoral artery.

The femoral artery is the direct continuation of the external iliac artery, which, like the femoral nerve, emerges from the pelvis by passing under the inguinal ligament (see Fig. 30.4 in Chapter 30, Fig. 100.1 in Chapter 100, and part A of the orientation figure in Chapter 87). The first 3 to 4 cm of femoral artery and femoral vein are encased together in the femoral sheath, a prolongation of the transversalis fascia.

The femoral vein is the next most medial structure. A space medial to the vein, the femoral canal, is a frequent site of hernia formation. It is filled with fatty areolar tissue and lymphatics.

FIGURE 88.2
DIVISION OF SAPHENOUS VEIN AT SAPHENOFEMORAL JUNCTION

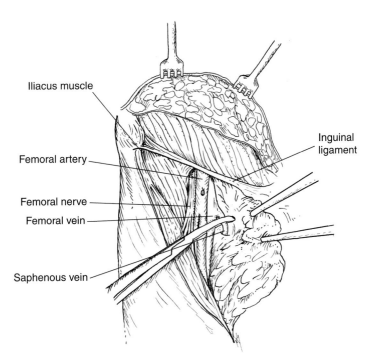

The greater saphenous vein terminates on the anterior surface of the femoral vein at the saphenofemoral junction. Several smaller veins (the superficial circumflex iliac, superficial epigastric, and superficial external pudendal veins) also terminate in a highly variable manner at or near this junction.

The fossa ovalis, or saphenous hiatus, is the opening in the fascia lata that allows the saphenous vein to penetrate the deep fascia and access the femoral vein. It is found about 2.5 to 3.5 cm below and lateral to the pubic tubercle (see Fig. 86.8 in Chapter 86).

Second Division of Saphenous Vein (Fig. 88.3)

Technical Points

Continue medially onto the pectineus muscle. Always remain superficial to vessels and nerve. Medially divide the fascia lata and excise it from the inguinal ligament. Place a moist laparotomy pad on the soft tissue mass and continue the dissection inferiorly. As the dissection nears completion, the saphenous vein will again be encountered in the soft tissue. Because this vein has been ligated at the saphenofemoral junction, there will be considerable pressure in the vein. Take care to identify and dissect it gently before transecting it. Often, two vessels rather than a single trunk are encountered

at this level. In this case, both branches will need to be identified and individually ligated.

Anatomic Points

As the saphenous vein ascends in the upper thigh, it is joined by several major tributaries. One fairly constant branch, the anterior femoral cutaneous vein, crosses the apex of the femoral triangle to enter the greater saphenous vein in the upper thigh.

The pectineus muscle is a flat, quadrilateral-shaped muscle that forms part of the floor of the femoral triangle. Its fibers run from the pubis toward the lesser trochanter and linea aspera of the femur, almost perpendicular in direction to those of the sartorius.

Completion of Lymphadenectomy (Fig. 88.4)

Technical Points

Identify and divide the remaining attachments by blunt and sharp dissection. Because the lymphatics connect through the femoral canal with pelvic lymphatics, carefully ligate any major attachments to decrease seroma formation. Tumor at this location may indicate spread to the pelvic nodes, and consideration for proceeding with a deep dissection must be individualized (see references).

FIGURE 88.3
SECOND DIVISION OF SAPHENOUS VEIN

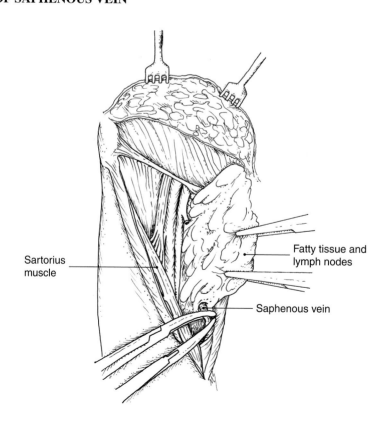

Sartorius muscle

Fatty tissue and lymph nodes

Saphenous vein

FIGURE 88.4
COMPLETION OF LYMPHADENECTOMY

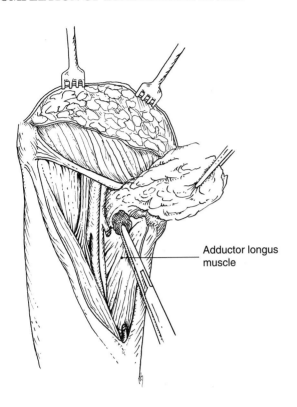

Adductor longus muscle

Check the field carefully for hemostasis or leakage of lymph.

Anatomic Points

The superficial and deep inguinal nodes communicate, through the femoral canal, with the external iliac nodes and thence up to the common iliac and paraaortic nodes. Access to the external iliac nodes requires division of the inguinal ligament.

Transposition of Sartorius Muscle (Fig. 88.5)

Technical Points

The field shown in Fig. 88.4 has exposed major vessels and a crevice from which soft tissue has been removed. To provide viable coverage for the vessels (important if wound breakdown should occur) and to close any dead space, transpose the sartorius muscle.

Detach the muscle from its insertion on the anterosuperior iliac spine and mobilize it sufficiently to move it medially to cover the femoral nerve, artery, and vein (Fig. 88.5A). Suture it in place with interrupted absorbable suture (Fig. 88.5B).

Bring a large, closed-suction drain through a separate stab wound on the inferior medial thigh and position it medial and parallel to the sartorius muscle. Approximate the flaps with interrupted absorbable suture on the subcutaneous tissue. Close the skin with a running nylon suture.

FIGURE 88.5
TRANSPOSITION OF SARTORIUS MUSCLE

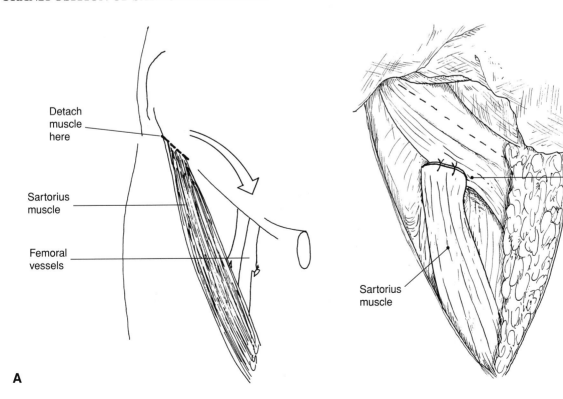

Detach muscle here

Sartorius muscle

Femoral vessels

Inguinal ligament

Sartorius muscle

A

B

Apply an antibiotic pressure dressing. Wrap the leg with Ace wraps to encourage deep venous circulation and prevent edema. Keep the patient on bed rest and maintain the Foley catheter until postoperative day 2 or 3, when ambulation is reinstituted.

Pull the drain when drainage has decreased to 25 to 40 mL in 24 hours. Lymphocele or seroma formation is common. Sterilely aspirate these with syringe or vacuum bottle if very large.

Anatomic Points

Because the blood supply and innervation of the sartorius muscle come segmentally from deep to this muscle, it is easily detached and transposed without interfering with its neuromuscular pedicles. Transposition medially puts the muscle in a less oblique relationship with its termination on the medial aspect of the tibia and allows the muscle to be sutured in a relaxed position, with the bulk of the muscle filling the depression created by the dissection.

REFERENCES

1. Karakousis CP. Therapeutic node dissections in malignant melanoma. *Ann Surg Oncol* 1998;5:473.
2. Pearlman NW, Robinson WA, Dreiling LK, et al. Modified ilioinguinal node dissection for metastatic melanoma. *Am J Surg* 1995; 170:647. (Provides details of alternative incision, sparing saphenous vein.)
3. Scott-Conner CEH. Inguinal and pelvic lymphadenectomy. In: *Chassin's operative strategy in general surgery.* 3rd ed. New York: Springer-Verlag, 2002:873–879. (Describes deep dissection.)

CHAPTER 89

Sentinel Node Biopsy for Melanoma of Trunk; Wide Local Excision

Peter R. Jochimsen

Sentinel lymph node determination in patients with truncal melanoma presents its own peculiar problems owing to the often ambiguous drainage of the truncal lymphatics. Although extremity melanomas generally go to the predictable regional nodes, the lymphatics of lesions of the trunk can unpredictably travel to unsuspected sites.

Sentinel node identification and removal is generally recommended for patients whose lesions measure 1 to 4 mm in thickness. Patients with lesions thinner than that generally do not have metastases. Those with lesions greater than 4 mm have, it is thought, advanced disease, and in the absence of palpable adenopathy, search for regional nodes is ill advised.

The reasons for identifying nodal involvement include the associated prognostic information, fulfilling a desire to identify spread of disease early, and consideration of adjuvant therapy with a drug of proven efficacy (ie, interferon-α_{2b}).

Sentinel Node Biopsy (Fig. 89.1)

Technical Points

Because it takes 3 to 4 hours to optimize the distribution of the isotope, the patient is injected with about 0.5 mCi of technetium-99 sulfur colloid the morning of surgery, several hours before operation. This is done in the nuclear medicine suite, usually by the nuclear medicine physician.

If the primary lesion has had incisional or punch biopsy, injection should be done at four quadrants around the lesion. If the lesion has been completely excised, the midpoint of the incision is assumed to represent the region closest to the lesion, and the injection is done above and below that site. Intradermal injection is done essentially circumferentially around the site of the lesion (Fig. 89.1A).

LIST OF STRUCTURES

Axillary lymph nodes
Inguinal lymph nodes
Umbilicus

Lymphoscintigraphy is obtained almost immediately and repeated at irregular intervals. Whole-body imaging is required for truncal lesions to ensure that ambiguous drainage or drainage to more than one nodal area is identified. An example is shown in Fig. 89.1B, which depicts drainage to an axillary node from a lesion near the umbilicus. Occasionally, drainage to two nodal basins is identified (Fig. 89.1C) and must be investigated surgically. The nuclear medicine physician marks the skin overlying the identified nodes.

In the operating room, under general or, if appropriate, regional anesthesia, the patient is prepped and draped. Inject 1 to 3 mL of isosulfan blue (Lymphazurin dye) intradermally at the site of the primary lesion using a 25-gauge or smaller needle. Place the dye circumferentially around the lesion or biopsy scar. Massage the area gently for a few minutes.

Use the handheld gamma detector (see Figs. 18.2 and 18.3) to identify the node and make an incision over that spot. Orient the incision in such a fashion that it can be excised with the soft tissue of the regional nodal basin, should completion lymphadenectomy be required.

It is our practice to take and record emissions for 10 seconds over the node before the skin is incised and again after the incision is made, and then to count the emissions in the node as it rests on the detector head after excision. The bed of the node is also counted, and if any residual counts remain, further search is made to ascertain that no significant node has been overlooked.

Before removing the node, inspect it to see whether it has taken up the blue dye. Identify any blue lymphatic channels and pursue these to other nodes that may be involved. Remove any grossly abnormal nodes that are encountered.

Unless the lymph node appears to be grossly involved with metastatic disease, defer the decision for regional lymphadenectomy until the permanent sections are read. Close the sentinel node biopsy site with absorbable suture.

Anatomic Points

Although the general pattern of lymphatic drainage of the trunk, based on careful anatomic studies, follows the logical pattern shown in Fig. 89.1D, numerous exceptions exist.

FIGURE 89.1
SENTINEL NODE BIOPSY

Lymphatics above the L-2 dermatome (sometimes termed *Sappey's line*) drain to axillary nodes, and those below L-2 drain to inguinal nodes, with the midline determining the laterality of drainage. Zones of uncertainty exist where territories abut each other. The exceptions to the rule become significant when therapeutic decisions are made in individual cases. In the lymphoscintogram shown in Fig. 89.1B, the primary site is near the umbilicus and hence falls in a region of anatomically ambiguous drainage, and only the nuclear medicine study shows which territory this lesion occupies. Fig. 89.1C illustrates a case in which drainage crosses not only Sappey's line but also the midline.

FIGURE 89.2
WIDE EXCISION OF PRIMARY SITE

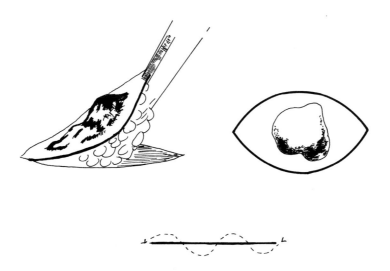

Wide Excision of Primary Site (Fig. 89.2)

Technical and Anatomic Points

The margins of the wide excision depend on the thickness of the primary site. For *in situ* and other thin lesions, 0.5- to 1-cm margins are sufficient. For thicker lesions, 1- to 2-cm margins are appropriate. The location of the primary site will often predict the extent of reasonable margins. Generally, the site can be closed primarily, by elevating flaps or developing simple rotation flaps. Skin grafts are rarely required.

REFERENCES

1. Gershenwald JE, Tseng CH, Thompson W, et al. Improved sentinel lymph node localization in patients with primary melanoma with the use of radiolabeled colloid. *Surgery* 1998;124:203–210.
2. Porter GA, Ross MI, Berman RS, et al. Significance of multiple nodal basin drainage in truncal melanoma patients undergoing sentinel lymph node biopsy. *Ann Surg Oncol* 2000;7:256–261.
3. Reintgen DS, Rapaport DP, Tanabe KK, et al. Lymphatic mapping and sentinel lymphadenectomy. In: Balch CM. Houghton AN, Sober AJ, et al, eds. *Cutaneous melanoma.* 3rd ed. St Louis: Quality Medical Publishing, 1998:227–244.
4. Sugarbaker EV, McBride CM. Melanoma of the trunk: the results of surgical excision and anatomic guidelines for predicting nodal metastasis. *Surgery* 1976;80:22–30. (Reviews anatomic studies done in the 1800s by Sappey and shows that they are a good general guideline but that exceptions exist.)

SECTION V

The Sacral Region and Perineum

The sacral region and perineum, already introduced in Chapter 75, are presented in greater detail in this section. First, the simple operation of pilonidal cystectomy (Chapter 90) is described as a means of illustrating the anatomy of the sacrum and the presacral region. This is often one of the first operations performed by the beginning surgeon, yet results are often less than perfect, and numerous modifications of the operation—described in the references—exist.

The anorectum is then described through the procedure of hemorrhoidectomy (Chapter 91) and other minor rectal procedures (Chapter 92). Although these are considered to be minor procedures, surgery in this area can cause considerable pain and disability; hence, careful attention to operative technique is important.

The transsacral approach to rectal lesions is described in Chapter 93. This uncommon approach provides excellent exposure of the lower rectum and is useful in a variety of situations. Finally, rigid sigmoidoscopy is described in Chapter 94.

CHAPTER 90

Pilonidal Cystectomy

Whether pilonidal cysts are congenital or acquired lesions remains a topic of debate. The frequent appearance of an epithelialized tract in the midline, leading to a cyst that may or may not contain hair, suggests a congenital origin. A pilonidal cyst (or sinus) characteristically occurs in the posterior midline skin overlying the sacrum. Secondary infection within the cyst or sinus causes pain, drawing attention to the cyst. Incision and drainage may be needed but are not definitive treatment, and recurrent bouts of infection are typical. Definitive treatment involves either marsupialization or excision of the cyst.

The variety of techniques that are available for dealing with pilonidal cysts indicates that complications have occurred with all approaches. Marsupialization, the simplest procedure, is described in this chapter. More complex procedures involving construction of flaps may be indicated in some complicated cases. Consult the references at the end for a description of these alternative approaches.

Positioning the Patient (Fig. 90.1)

Technical Points

Place the patient in a prone jackknife position. Use tincture of benzoin on the lateral buttocks to prepare the skin. Place tape on the lateral buttocks and use this tape to pull laterally, spreading the gluteal cleft. Shave the region of the cyst and the gluteal region.

Anatomic Points

The prominent and important structures in this area are all musculoskeletal. The bony sacrum forms the posterior part of the bony pelvic ring and is the distal continuation of the vertebral column. Formed by the fusion of the five sacral vertebrae

(the number of vertebrae that fuse to form the sacrum varies from four to six, but is commonly five), the sacrum is a complexly curved and heavy bone that is shield shaped when viewed from behind. The posterior surface is roughened and has two paramedian crests—the lateral sacral and intermediate crest—which, with the prominent midline middle sacral crest, form points of attachment for fascial and aponeurotic structures. Four broad posterior sacral foramina between the five fused vertebrae are points of ingress and egress for the dorsal rami of the sacral spinal nerves. Viewed from the side, a prominent anterior concavity, commonly termed the *hollow of the sacrum,* is obvious. This forms a space in which lie the rectum, muscles of the pelvic diaphragm, neurovascular structures, and a variable amount of fat. At the top of this concavity, the sacral promontory (located at the point of articulation of the body of the lowest lumbar vertebra with the sacrum) forms an easily palpable bony landmark for the surgeon operating within the pelvis. The sacrum is shorter and wider in the female pelvis than in the male pelvis, contributing to the wider, rounder gynecoid shape that is designed to accommodate the head of a full-term infant at the time of delivery.

The coccyx is composed of three to five remaining vertebrae (commonly, four). These small, nubbin-like, rudimentary vertebrae articulate with the sacrum. Only the first coccygeal vertebra possesses identifiable transverse processes and homologues of pedicles (coccygeal cornua). No vertebral canal is present. The mobility of the coccygeal vertebrae varies considerably from individual to individual, and the terminal three coccygeal vertebrae are commonly fused.

Recall that the perineum is diamond shaped, bounded anteriorly by the pubic symphysis, laterally by the two ischial tuberosities, and posteriorly by the tip of the coccyx. It may be

LIST OF STRUCTURES

Sacrum
    Lateral sacral crest
    Intermediate sacral crest
    Middle sacral crest
    Posterior sacral foramina
    Sacral promontory
Ilium
Sacroiliac joint

Coccyx
Lumbodorsal fascia
Gluteus maximus muscle
Gluteus medius muscle
Gluteus minimus muscle
Gluteal cleft
Gluteal aponeurosis
Sacral nerves

Posterior femoral cutaneous nerve
    Gluteal branches
Anus
Rectum
Anococcygeal raphe
Levator ani muscles

FIGURE 90.1
POSITIONING THE PATIENT

divided into two triangles—the anterior or urogenital triangle and the posterior or anal triangle—by drawing a transverse line that passes just anterior to the anus and connects the ischial tuberosities. Thus, the tip of the coccyx marks the end of the gluteal region and the beginning of the perineal (anal triangle) region. This is an important distinction because of the differences in the pathologic processes found in each region. The tip of the coccyx, therefore, is a critical, easily palpated landmark for the surgeon. The anococcygeal raphe extends from the tip of the coccyx to the anus. This fibrous band is formed by the decussation of fibers of the two levator ani muscles, two broad flat muscles that form the main part of the pelvic diaphragm.

The gluteus maximus is a large muscle that plays an important role in extension of the hip; it is inactive in standing. It originates primarily from the sacrum, along a roughly diagonal line extending from the tip of the coccyx to the iliac crest, although it also takes its origin from the aponeurosis of the sacrospinous and sacrotuberous ligaments. The gluteal aponeurosis, which is the fascia covering the gluteus medius, from which the most cephalad part of this muscle, the gluteus maximus, arises, extends from the region of the sacroiliac joint anteriorly, along the crest of the ilium. The gluteus medius lies lateral, deep to the gluteal aponeurosis and gluteus maximus. Whereas the gluteus maximus extends and laterally rotates the thigh, the gluteus medius abducts and medially rotates it; its primary function is to prevent pelvic sag on the unsupported side during walking. The gluteus minimus, which lies deep to the gluteus medius, has similar functions.

The midline gluteal cleft is formed by the infolding of skin and fatty tissue enveloping the gluteal muscles. It extends from the midsacral level to the anus, blending imperceptibly with the perineum in the region of the anus. The skin of this region is thick (although thinner than the skin of the back or buttocks) and is covered with a variable amount of hair. Abnormalities of the skin of the gluteal cleft may provide a clue

FIGURE 90.2
DELINEATION OF THE CYST AND INCISION OF TRACTS

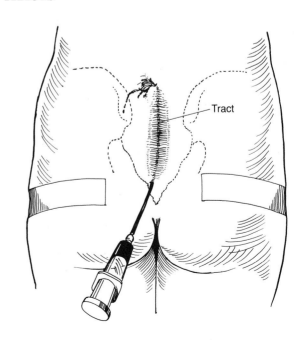

to underlying sacral anomalies, which are relatively common. Particularly in hirsute individuals, an increased amount of hair may be present in the gluteal cleft normally, which may account for the formation of pilonidal cysts in this area. Moreover, a localized patch of hair, a dimple, or a lipoma-like mass may be the only external clue to an underlying spina bifida occulta, which is an asymptomatic anomaly of fusion of the lower vertebral column.

Sensory innervation in the region of the gluteal cleft is derived from branches of the sacral and coccygeal nerves. The skin overlying the lower and lateral portions of the gluteal muscles is innervated by gluteal branches of the posterior femoral cutaneous nerve.

Delineation of the Cyst and Incision of Tracts (Fig. 90.2)

Technical Points

Look for an external opening of the tract. This is most likely to be found in the midline. Cannulate this opening with a blunt-tipped needle and gently inject a mixture of 50% hydrogen peroxide and 50% methylene blue. This will help to define the tracts and stain the tissues involved by the burrowing process. Several lateral openings may be identified as the methylene blue exits the tissues. These are often visible externally as small, inflamed openings.

Insert a probe into the external opening and define the main tract. Generally, this will track in the midline superiorly or

FIGURE 90.3
EXCISION OF OVERLYING SKIN AND MARSUPIALIZATION OF TRACTS

A

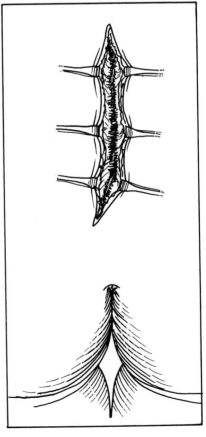

B

inferiorly. Take care not to go below the coccyx. Extension into the perianal region is extremely unusual and is usually indicative of other pathology. Place a grooved director over the probe and incise the tissue overlying the tract with electrocautery. Look for and cannulate any lateral satellite extensions of the tract, opening these in continuity with the primary tract.

Anatomic Points

The sacral nerves that provide sensory innervation to the skin of the gluteal cleft emerge from the laterally placed posterior sacral foramina and turn medially and downward. In the midline, no nerves are cut, and no significant structures occupy the space between the skin of the gluteal cleft and the underlying fascia. Although a network of superficial veins exists here, as elsewhere in the body, it is rare to encounter even small veins in the midline. Hence, dissection can proceed swiftly and is attended by little risk.

The fascia overlying the sacrum is a continuation of the lumbodorsal fascia and lies relatively deep to the skin, under a variable amount of fatty connective tissue. Although the fatty layer is typically less than that encountered laterally over the gluteal muscles, it may be several centimeters thick in obese individuals. Pilonidal sinuses are located relatively superficially (typically within 1 to 1.5 cm of the skin) in this region.

Excision of Overlying Skin and Marsupialization of Tracts (Fig. 90.3)

Technical and Anatomic Points

After all of the tracts have been incised, place Allis clamps on the edges of the overhanging skin and excise the excess skin. The objective here is to convert the incision into a wide, flat depression. Curet the base of the cyst to remove gelatinous material, granulation tissue, and hair. Do not disrupt the posterior wall of the cyst.

FIGURE 90.4
CONCLUSION OF MARSUPIALIZATION

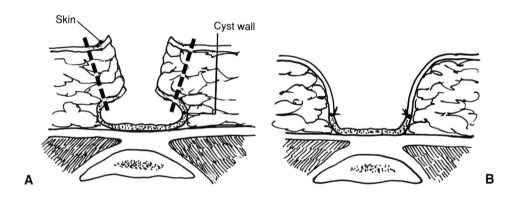

A   B

Conclusion of Marsupialization (Fig. 90.4)

Technical and Anatomic Points

Place interrupted sutures of 2-0 Vicryl from the dermal layer of the skin down to the back wall of the cyst in such a way as to cover the intervening subcutaneous fat. The objective is to bring the skin down to the back wall of the cyst. At the conclusion of the procedure, a narrow, open area, consisting of the back wall of the cyst, should still be visible. This small area is left to heal by secondary intention.

Check hemostasis and pack the incision with dry, sterile gauze.

REFERENCES

1. Allen-Mersh TG. Pilonidal sinus: finding the right track for treatment. *Br J Surg* 1990;77:123–132. (Presents excellent review of alternatives.)
2. Farringer JL, Pickens DR. Pilonidal cyst: an operative approach. *Am J Surg* 1978;135:262.
3. Fishbein RH, Handelsman JC. A method for primary reconstruction following radical excision of sacrococcygeal pilonidal disease. *Ann Surg* 1979;190:231.
4. Senapati A, Cripps NPJ, Thompson MR. Bascom's operation in the day-surgical management of symptomatic pilonidal sinus. *Br J Surg* 2000;87:1067–1070. (Describes lateral incision and closure.)
5. Surrell JA. Pilonidal disease. *Surg Clin North Am* 1994;74:1309–1315.
6. Zimmerman CE. Outpatient excision and primary closure of pilonidal cysts and sinuses. *Am J Surg* 1978;136:640. (Describes primary closure for simple cases.)

CHAPTER 91

Hemorrhoidectomy

Hemorrhoids are dilated venous cushions that lie just inside the anal verge. Almost universally present in adults in Western cultures, their etiology is still a matter of speculation. Chronic constipation with accompanying straining at stool and pregnancy are commonly identified as predisposing factors. An associated arteriovenous communication may be present. Large bleeding hemorrhoids are sometimes seen in patients with cirrhosis and portal hypertension; the hemorrhoidal (rectal) plexus becomes an outflow tract and a site of spontaneous portosystemic collateral formation in these patients. Symptomatic hemorrhoids cause various problems ranging from itching and pain to bleeding and prolapse.

A grading scale is used to classify hemorrhoids. Grade I hemorrhoids become congested during defecation but do not prolapse through the anal canal. Grade II hemorrhoids protrude during straining, but spontaneously reduce upon relaxation. Grade III hemorrhoids require manual reduction, which is usually easily accomplished. Grade IV hemorrhoids are irreducible protrusions and are sometimes confused with a true rectal prolapse. If grade II or III hemorrhoids do not reduce, edema rapidly occurs because the anal sphincter acts as a tourniquet. Swelling and pain prevent reduction, and an acute prolapse is said to have occurred. Grade IV hemorrhoids, which are chronically prolapsing, are often associated with a lax anal sphincter that is unable to retain the hemorrhoids in a reduced position.

Hemorrhoidectomy is generally performed for large, mixed, external and internal hemorrhoids (grades II through IV) that require surgical treatment. Alternative treatment methods (rubber-band ligation, cryotherapy, or laser treatment) may be appropriate for internal hemorrhoids and may be especially useful for grade I and II hemorrhoids that are associated with bleeding. These modalities are not applicable for large, mixed hemorrhoids, however.

Generally, sigmoidoscopy is performed before hemorrhoidectomy if it has not been performed in an office setting. Although the procedure may be performed using local anesthesia, it is more commonly performed with administration of general, spinal, or caudal anesthesia. The references at the end describe alternative methods for the treatment of internal hemorrhoids as well as the specific technique for administering local anesthesia before minor rectal surgery.

Position of Patient and Dilatation of Anus (Fig. 91.1)

Technical Points

The procedure may be performed in the prone jackknife or lithotomy position. The prone jackknife position is more convenient for the surgeon. The lithotomy position is preferred by some because it provides better control of the airway. If the procedure is done using general anesthesia, the lithotomy position may be somewhat safer. It is the position most commonly employed by British-trained surgeons; by contrast, most surgeons trained in the United States use the prone position.

After adequate anesthesia has been induced, the anus is carefully dilated until four fingers can be introduced. Use povidone-iodine solution (Betadine) to lubricate your fingers, rather than water-soluble lubricant, because the latter makes the operative field slippery and thus makes it more difficult to do the procedure.

Anatomic Points

The perineum is a diamond-shaped region bounded by the pubic symphysis anteriorly, the coccyx posteriorly, and the

LIST OF STRUCTURES

Perineum	Anal verge	Superior rectal (hemorrhoidal) vein
Anterior or urogenital triangle	Dentate line (pectinate line)	Internal iliac vein
Posterior or anal triangle	Anal crypts	Middle rectal (hemorrhoidal) vein
Pelvic ring	Anal columns (of Morgagni)	Rectal (hemorrhoidal) plexus of veins
Symphysis pubis	Internal pudendal arteries	Internal anal sphincter
Ischial tuberosities	Inferior rectal (hemorrhoidal)	External anal sphincter
Coccyx	arteries	Intersphincteric groove
Anus	Inferior mesenteric vein	

FIGURE 91.1
POSITION OF PATIENT AND DILATATION OF ANUS

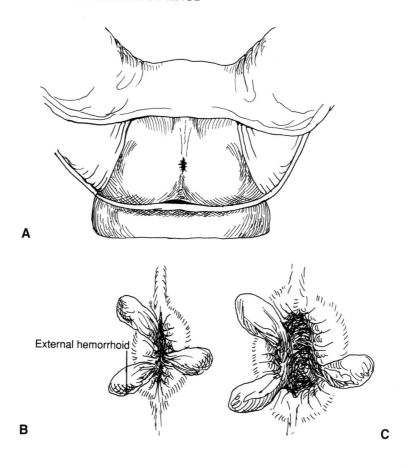

two ischial tuberosities laterally. A transverse line connecting the anterior edge of the ischial tuberosities and passing just anterior to the anus divides the region into two triangles, an anterior urogenital triangle and a posterior anal triangle. The detailed anatomy of the perineum is discussed in Chapter 75 and hence is only briefly be reviewed here. The anterior triangle contains the urogenital structures, associated musculature, and neurovascular structures in both sexes. The posterior triangle contains the anus and associated musculature as well as neurovascular structures.

The anus is the terminal part of the gastrointestinal tract. In the anal canal, the mucosa of the rectum becomes squamous epithelium and blends, finally, with the squamous epithelium of the skin of the perianal region. The dentate line or pectinate line is an important landmark. Above the dentate line, venous and lymphatic drainage is predominantly upward, with the drainage of the lower rectum. Venous drainage predominantly enters the portal system. Sensation above the dentate is poorly localized and pain is of a diffuse, visceral type, presumably mediated by the autonomic nervous system. Mucosa forms the epithelial lining. Internal hemorrhoids, predominantly dilatations of the superior

and middle rectal (hemorrhoidal) venous plexus, are found in this region.

Below the dentate line, venous and lymphatic drainage is superficial. Venous drainage is through the inferior rectal (hemorrhoidal) veins, which drain into the internal pudendal veins and thence into the internal iliac veins (caval system). Lymphatics of the region drain into the inguinal lymph nodes. Here, sensation, mediated by somatic sensory neurons, is precise, and pain is extremely well localized. The anal region has been described by some surgeons as the second most sensitive structure in the body, with the eye rated the most sensitive. The sensory nerves in this region are inferior rectal (hemorrhoidal) branches of the pudendal nerves. Hemorrhoids in this region are external hemorrhoids. The distinction between internal hemorrhoids and external hemorrhoids is important for both patient and surgeon. Pain in the region of internal hemorrhoids is dull and poorly localized. Because of this relatively poor sensory innervation, internal hemorrhoids may be treated in the office by rubber-band ligation, injection, freezing, or laser therapy, with little or no need for anesthesia. By contrast, external hemorrhoids are exquisitely sensitive, and manipulations are not tolerated without anesthesia.

FIGURE 91.2
DEFINITION OF HEMORRHOIDAL PEDICLES

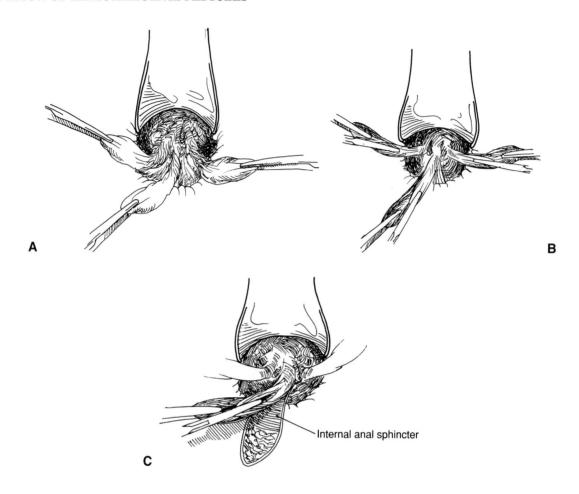

Internal anal sphincter

Definition of Hemorrhoidal Pedicles (Fig. 91.2)

Technical Points

Generally, three hemorrhoidal pedicles can be delineated: the left lateral, right anterior, and right posterior pedicles. Place Kelly clamps on each of the three pedicles and pull laterally to define a triangle. Place a second pair of Kelly clamps on each pedicle near the dentate line to pull internal hemorrhoidal tissue further out of the anus. If the anus has been dilated adequately, it is often not necessary to place a retractor to define the hemorrhoids.

If the procedure is being done in the lithotomy position, excise the posterior hemorrhoid first. In this fashion, blood from this hemorrhoidectomy will not drip into the operative field when the second and third hemorrhoids are excised. Each hemorrhoid is excised in a similar fashion; thus, only one will be described.

Anatomic Points

The common pattern of three hemorrhoidal pedicles has been postulated to result from the typical pattern of termination of the superior rectal (hemorrhoidal) arteries. The right superior rectal (hemorrhoidal) artery generally splits into an anterior and posterior division, whereas the left superior rectal (hemorrhoidal) artery remains single. Arteriovenous communication has been demonstrated, and the common observation of arterial bleeding at a hemorrhoidectomy site supports this etiology. When more than three hemorrhoidal pedicles are present, the surgeon may still be able to define three major groups, obliterating smaller hemorrhoids through the three major incisions.

The hemorrhoidal plexus may serve a physiologic role by forming a cushion that distends with blood at the time of defecation. This cushion then acts as a seal to prevent further leakage of stool when defecation ends. Minor degrees of fecal soilage may occur after hemorrhoidectomy, particularly if too much tissue has been removed.

Hemorrhoidectomy (Fig. 91.3)

Technical and Anatomic Points

The object of hemorrhoidectomy is to preserve the squamous epithelium of the anal canal (to prevent postoperative

FIGURE 91.3
HEMORRHOIDECTOMY

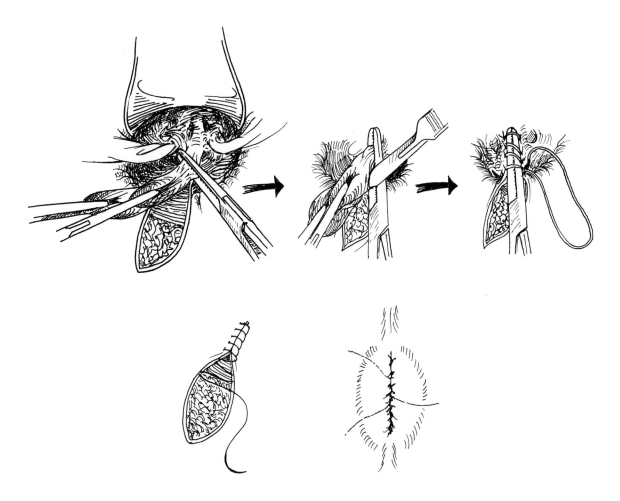

stricture) while excising all the subcutaneous venous tissue, ligating the hemorrhoidal pedicles, and restoring near-normal anatomy. Make an elliptical skin incision over the hemorrhoid, excising as little skin as possible. If large, external hemorrhoids have been present, there will be redundant skin, and the skin incision can then be more generous. Take special care not to excise skin unnecessarily from the anal canal because an anal stricture may result. Develop flaps laterally just under the skin and mucosa.

Use Metzenbaum scissors to shell out a mass of dilated veins from the underlying sphincter muscle (which should be clearly visible). The hemorrhoidal pedicle will come down to a small base, which can be secured with a Kelly clamp. Place a Kelly clamp in a radial fashion along this pedicle. Amputate the hemorrhoid and oversew the pedicle with a running lock-stitch of 2-0 Vicryl. Leave this suture long and tag it with a hemostat. Check hemostasis in the base of the pedicle. Secure small bleeders with electrocautery or with suture-ligature of 3-0 Vicryl. When hemostasis has been achieved, close the skin and mucosa.

Assess the external skin wound, excising any redundant tissue to avoid large "dog ears" or skin tags. Minor redundancies will generally smooth out and can be ignored. Then, begin wound closure at the inner apex of the suture line using a running lock-stitch of 3-0 Vicryl. Use traction on the previously tagged 2-0 Vicryl suture to expose the apex. Cut this deep suture once the mucosal suture line is well established. From the apex, proceed out toward the anoderm. As the squamous mucosa of the anal canal is encountered, convert the lock-stitch to a running subcuticular suture. This should completely close the small incision.

The two remaining hemorrhoids should be dealt with in a similar fashion. At the conclusion of the procedure, there will be three linear radial suture lines. Check hemostasis. If hemostasis is good, no pack is required. Some surgeons place a small pack of Gelfoam in the anal canal to ensure hemostasis. This is not, however, a substitute for surgical hemostasis.

Inject the anal canal with bupivacaine hydrochloride (Marcaine), if desired, to provide long-acting analgesia.

REFERENCES

1. Buls JG, Goldberg SM. Modern management of hemorrhoids. *Surg Clin North Am* 1978;58:469.
2. Corman ML. Rubber band ligation of hemorrhoids. *Arch Surg* 1977;112:1257.
3. Corman ML, Veidenheimer MC, Coller JA. Anoplasty for anal stricture. *Surg Clin North Am* 1976;56:727.
4. Ferguson JA, Mazier WP, Ganchrow MI, et al. The closed technique of hemorrhoidectomy. *Surgery* 1971;70:480.
5. Goligher JC. Haemorrhoids or piles. In: *Surgery of the anus, rectum, and colon.* 4th ed. London: Bailliere Tindall, 1980:113. (Provides detailed description of multiple techniques, advantages, and disadvantages. The new edition of this book is not as detailed.)
6. Khubchandani IT. Operative hemorrhoidectomy. *Surg Clin North Am* 1988;68:1411.
7. Kratzer GL. Improved local anesthesia in anorectal surgery. *Am Surg* 1974;40:609.
8. Lee HH, Spencer RJ, Beart RW Jr. Multiple hemorrhoidal bandings in a single session. *Dis Colon Rectum* 1994;37:37–41.
9. Lord PH. Approach to the treatment of anorectal disease, with special reference to hemorrhoids. *Surg Annu* 1977;9:195.
10. Mazier WP. Hemorrhoids, fissures, and pruritus ani. *Surg Clin North Am* 1994;74:6. (Provides excellent review of management alternatives.)
11. Nesselrod JP. Anatomy, pathogenesis and treatment of hemorrhoids and related anorectal conditions. *Rev Surg* 1966:23:229.
12. Nivatvongs S. An improved technique of local anesthesia for anorectal surgery. *Dis Colon Rectum* 1982;25:259.
13. Nivatvongs S, Goldberg SM. An improved technique of rubber band ligation of hemorrhoids. *Am J Surg* 1982;144:379.
14. Nivatvongs S, Stern HS, Fryd DS. The length of the anal canal. *Dis Colon Rectum* 1981;24:600.
15. Rand AA. Whitehead's radical circumferential hemorrhoidectomy: modified by sliding skin-flap grafts. *Surg Clin North Am* 1972;52:1031. (Describes radical procedure, generally not necessary.)
16. Sohn N, Weinstein MA, Robbins RD. Anorectal disorders. *Curr Probl Surg* 1983;20:1. (Presents good review of multiple problems, including hemorrhoids.)
17. Thomson WHF. The nature of haemorrhoids. *Br J Surg* 1975;62:542. (Presents good review.)
18. Wantz GE. A rubberband ligation for internal hemorrhoids. *Surg Rounds* 1978;59.

CHAPTER 92

Drainage of Perirectal Abscesses, Surgery For Anal Fistulas, and Lateral Internal Sphincterotomy

Perirectal abscesses begin as infections in the anal glands, which empty into the anal crypts. From the anal crypt, infection spreads laterally into the soft tissues of the ischiorectal fossa. The abscess commonly presents as a painful swelling visible in the external aspect of the buttock. Occasionally, infection will track above the levator sling, causing pain and a mass that is palpable on rectal examination. Drainage of a perirectal abscess often results in a chronic anal fistula, a communication from the inside of the anorectum to the skin of the outside. Perirectal abscesses and anal fistulas will be considered together because of their common pathogenesis.

A separate minor rectal operation—lateral internal sphincterotomy—is performed for chronic sphincter spasm associated with anal fissures. Pain from the fissure causes a vicious cycle of sphincter spasm, pain with defecation, trauma to the mucosa, and development of a chronic ulcer. Division of the internal sphincter breaks the cycle and allows the fissure to heal. In this chapter, the anatomy of the anal sphincter mechanism is presented through the operations for perirectal abscess and anal fistula as well as through the discussion of lateral internal sphincterotomy.

Drainage of a Perirectal Abscess (Fig. 92.1)

Technical Points

Abscesses and fistulas are commonly classified according to the path taken by the burrowing infection relative to the levator sling and the external anal sphincter (Fig. 92.1A). The most common type of abscess is the perianal abscess, which results from infection tracking down the intersphincteric plane to the perianal skin. These small, relatively superficial abscesses are very close to the anal verge and usually

can be drained in the office; any resulting fistula will traverse part of the internal sphincter and can be opened without fear of incontinence. When the infection tracks laterally across the internal and external sphincters into the ischiorectal fat, an ischiorectal abscess results. Less commonly, infection tracks cephalad, and pus accumulates above the levator sling.

Drainage of a perirectal abscess is generally performed with the patient in the lithotomy position. After administration of general anesthesia, a careful rectal examination is performed. Feel the tissues lateral to the rectum between your thumb (outside the anal canal) and forefinger (within the anal canal) to determine their thickness. Often, even though a mass is not palpable, a thickening in one area may be apparent on careful examination. Prep the area with povidone-iodine solution (Betadine). Perform a proctoscopy if you have not already done so as part of the initial evaluation. Make an incision through the skin over the abscess, as close as possible to the anal verge. (This will help to ensure that, if a fistula results, the tract will be short.) If you are unsure where the abscess is located, aspirate with an 18-gauge needle and syringe before drainage and confirm the presence of pus. Deepen the incision using a hemostat until the cavity of the abscess is encountered. Carefully insert a finger and break up all loculations to drain all of the cavity well (Fig. 92.1B). Irrigate the cavity and pack it with clean packing. If necessary, excise some of the skin edges to provide easier access to a deep cavity.

Submucous abscesses should then be drained into the rectum, rather than externally. To do this, place a retractor in the anal canal, dilating the anus to expose the abscess. Confirm its location by aspiration with a needle and syringe. Incise the mucosa overlying the abscess and allow it to drain into

LIST OF STRUCTURES

Anus	Levator ani muscles	Gluteus maximus muscles
Anal canal	Pubococcygeus muscle	Superficial transverse perineal muscle
Dentate line (pectinate line)	Puborectalis muscle	Obturator fascia
Internal sphincter	Iliococcygeus muscle	Hemorrhoidal venous plexus
External sphincter	Coccygeus muscles	Ischiorectal fossa

FIGURE 92.1
DRAINAGE OF A PERIRECTAL ABSCESS

Types of Abscesses

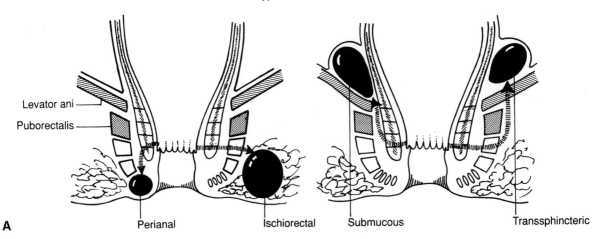

Levator ani

Puborectalis

A

Perianal   Ischiorectal   Submucous   Transsphincteric

B

Puborectalis

Deep part of external anal sphincter

C   Superficial part of external anal sphincter

the rectum. If the cavity is large, place a Penrose drain in the abscess cavity to keep it open. Generally, such a drain will be passed within 1 to 2 days.

Anatomic Points

The internal anal sphincter is composed of circular smooth muscle and is continuous with the circular smooth muscle layer of the rectum. In the region of the internal sphincter, this muscle layer becomes considerably thickened, forming a visible and palpable band around the anus. It is first surrounded by longitudinal muscle fibers that are continuous with longitudinal muscle fibers of the rectum and the pubococcygeus (a part of the levator ani). This complex is then encircled by a ring of skeletal muscle, the external anal sphincter. This sphincter is continuous superiorly with the puborectalis part of the levator ani.

The paired levator ani muscles arise from the spine of the ischium, the obturator fascia, and the inner surface of the body of the pubic ramus. Together with the coccygeus muscles and associated fascia, they form a hammock-like structure, the so-called floor of the pelvic cavity or pelvic diaphragm. The pubococcygeus muscle, whose most medial and deepest fibers constitute the puborectalis muscle, is the portion of the levator ani that arises from the dorsal surface of the pubis and the anterior part of the obturator fascia. The iliococcygeus arises from the posterior part of the obturator fascia and ischial spine. Sometimes, a clear separation between these two components is visible, although more often, they appear to blend into a single muscle. The levator ani muscles are innervated by a branch of the fourth sacral spinal nerve (which enters the pelvic aspect of the muscle) and branches of the pudendal nerves, which enter the perineal aspect of the muscle. Many consider the levator ani muscles to be part of the external sphincter.

The *triple sling* is a term applied to three muscle loops formed by the levator ani and external sphincter muscle complex when viewed from the side (Fig. 92.1C). These three loops enhance continence by compressing and angulating the anorectum. The deepest loop, and probably the most important, is the puborectalis portion of the levator ani. This pulls the rectum anteriorly. The intermediate loop is the portion of the external sphincter that arises from and inserts onto the coccyx after looping around the rectum. Contraction of this muscle loop pulls the anorectum toward the coccyx. The most superficial loop is the subcutaneous portion of the external sphincter, which surrounds the anus and is attached to perineal skin and the perineal body anteriorly. The external anal sphincter, with its triple-sling mechanism, is critical for maintenance of continence; if it is intact, division of the internal sphincter will not result in incontinence.

The ischiorectal fossa, which is bounded by the levator ani muscles superiorly and medially and the obturator internus muscle laterally, contains predominantly fat. The internal pudendal neurovascular structures cling to the lateral wall and supply the contents of the ischiorectal fossa. Medially, the anococcygeal raphe divides the left from the right ischiorectal space. Anteriorly and posteriorly, two narrow but potentially deep extensions of this space are found. The posterior extension lies deep to the gluteus maximus, whereas the anterior extension lies deep to the urogenital diaphragm.

FIGURE 92.2
SURGERY FOR ANAL FISTULA

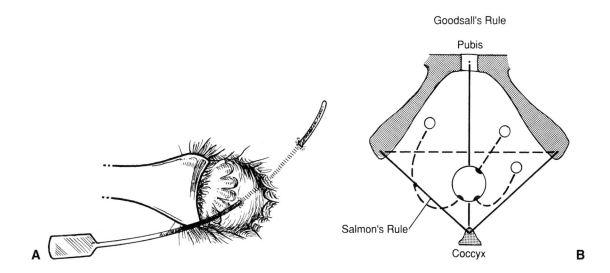

Surgery for Anal Fistula (Fig. 92.2)

Technical Points

Position the patient either prone or in the lithotomy position, according to individual preference. Identify the external openings of the fistula, which may be multiple. Gently dilate the anus until a Hill-Ferguson retractor can be inserted. The internal opening of the fistula is often visible as a hypertrophied anal papilla. Use a crypt hook to explore the crypts gently, searching for the internal opening. Cannulate the internal opening and gently probe from the internal opening toward the fistulous tract. Try to pass a probe from the internal opening through the tract and out the external opening (Fig. 92.2A).

The tract may not be straight, particularly if the external opening is at some distance from the anus. It may be necessary to open the tract in stages or to use a flexible or malleable probe to follow the tract. Be careful to avoid making a false passage. The tract will generally pass outside the internal sphincter but inside the external sphincters. Several rules are useful in predicting the location and tract of the fistula from the location of the external orifice. Goodsall's rule is the simplest; it states that if the external orifice lies anterior to a line drawn between the two ischial tuberosities, the tract will run directly to an internal opening, which will also be anterior. Fistulas with an external opening posterior to this line have curved tracts that enter the anus in the posterior midline (Fig. 92.2B). As an extension of this, Salmon's rule states that when the primary external opening lies more than 1.5 inches from the anal verge and is anterior, the tract will curve and enter from a posterior position.

Divide the soft tissues overlying the tract using electrocautery and excise part of the margin to convert the deep slitlike defect into a V-shaped defect. Send a portion of the margin of the tract for biopsy. Obtain a biopsy specimen from any suspicious-looking areas. Make sure that all tracts are fully opened. Achieve hemostasis by electrocautery.

If there are multiple tracts, or if the tracts are complicated or traverse a large portion of the sphincter mechanism, it may be necessary to pass Penrose drains through them or to use a seton in an effort to avoid dividing the sphincters. Multiple tracts draining to the outside can be drained with multiple incisions and Penrose drains, which can then be withdrawn slowly. When the fistula passes deep to the sphincter mechanism, it may be prudent to pass a seton through the fistulous tract and tie it loosely. This heavy suture produces fibrosis and tissue reaction, scarring the sphincter in the region where it is to be divided. Several weeks or months later, the sphincter can then be divided without having the muscle tissue gape open, thus minimizing the risk for subsequent incontinence.

Anatomic Points

The anal canal is the terminal portion of the gastrointestinal tract. Among the significant internal anatomic structures of this narrow intersphincteric region of the bowel is the pectinate line, which is continuous with the more proximal anal (rectal) columns (of Morgagni). These permanent longitudinal folds and the mucosa between them appear dark because of the presence of the rectal (hemorrhoidal) venous plexus, the origin of the internal hemorrhoids. At their distal ends, the anal (rectal) columns are connected by thin folds of mucosa, forming the anal (or rectal) valves. Behind these valves are the anal sinuses (of Morgagni), into which the anal glands open. Most anal fistulas and perirectal abscesses begin in these sinuses. Finally, the intersphincteric groove, between the internal (smooth muscle) and external (striated muscle) anal sphincters, can be palpated but not seen.

FIGURE 92.3
LATERAL INTERNAL SPHINCTEROTOMY

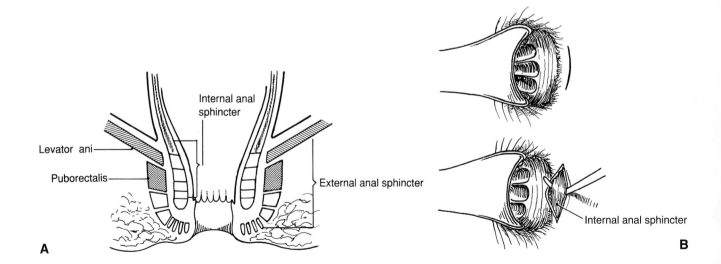

A

B

Lateral Internal Sphincterotomy (Fig. 92.3)

Technical Points

Position the patient in the lithotomy position. Gently dilate the anus and place a retractor. Identify the fissure and curet the base. Make an incision in the intersphincteric groove at 3 o'clock or 9 o'clock. This incision should be about 4 to 5 mm long and should parallel the intersphincteric groove. Using a hemostat, gently dissect down until the internal sphincter is identified. Use a right-angled clamp to hook up and elevate fibers of the internal sphincter into the incision and divide them with electrocautery (Fig. 92.3A). Do this until palpation confirms that the internal sphincter has been divided.

Alternatively, with an index finger in the anal canal, pass a number 11 blade down parallel to the internal sphincter in the intersphincteric groove. Turn the blade so that it points toward the anal canal and divide the sphincter carefully. You will know when the sphincter is completely divided when there is a sensation of the last fibers giving way as they are cut. The sphincter will then seem much more open. Apply pressure to this area from within the anal canal for a couple of minutes to ensure hemostasis. The incision can then be dosed with single chromic suture.

Anatomic Points

The internal sphincter lies like a cylinder within the spout of the funnel-shaped external sphincter–levator ani complex (Fig. 92.3B). The intersphincteric groove is palpable and, in some individuals, visible, as a groove that lies about 2 cm into the anal canal. The external sphincter and, in particular, the angulation of the anal canal produced by the triple-sling mechanism, are critical for the maintenance of normal continence. This is not altered in any way by division of the internal sphincter.

REFERENCES

1. Abcarian H. Lateral internal sphincterotomy: a new technique for treatment of chronic fissure-in-ano. *Surg Clin North Am* 1975;55:143.
2. Abcarian H. Surgical correction of chronic anal fissure: results of lateral internal sphincterotomy versus fissurectomy-midline sphincterotomy. *Dis Colon Rectum* 1980;23:31.
3. Bell GA. Lateral internal sphincterotomy in chronic anal fissure: a surgical technique. *Am Surg* 1980;46:572.
4. Christensen MA, Pitsch RM, Cali RI, et al. "House" advancement pedicle flap for anal stenosis. *Dis Colon Rectum* 1992;35:201–203. (Describes technique for managing anal stenosis.)
5. Garcia-Aguilar J, Belmonte C, Wong WD, et al. Anal fistula surgery: factors associated with recurrence and incontinence. *Dis Colon Rectum* 1996;39:723–729.
6. Goligher JC, Leacock AG, Brossy JJ. The surgical anatomy of the anal canal. *Br J Surg* 1955;43:51.
7. Hanley PH. Anorectal supralevator abscess-fistula in ano. *Surg Gynecol Obstet* 1979;148:899.
8. Janicke DM, Pundt MR. Anorectal disorders. *Emerg Med Clin North Am* 1996;14:757–788.
9. Khubchandani IT. Anal stenosis. *Surg Clin North Am* 1994;74:1353–1360.
10. Marks CG, Ritchie JK. Anal fistulas at St. Mark's Hospital. *Br J Surg* 1977;64:84. (This classic reference describes the anatomy of various fistulas and their management.)
11. Mazier WP, De Moraes RT, Dignan RD. Anal fissure and anal ulcers. *Surg Clin North Am* 1978;58:479.
12. McCourtney JS, Finlay IG. Setons in the surgical management of fistula in ano. *Br J Surg* 1995;82:448–452. (Presents excellent review of indications and technique.)
13. Notaras MJ. Anal fissure and stenosis. *Surg Clin North Am* 1988;68:1427.
14. Parks AG, Gordon PH, Hardcastle JD. A classification of fistula-in-ano. *Br J Surg* 1976;63:1. (Provides description of and nomenclature for different fistulas.)
15. Rosen L. Anorectal abscess-fistulae. *Surg Clin North Am* 1994;74:1293–1308.
16. Ross ST. Fistula in ano. *Surg Clin North Am* 1988;68:1417.
17. Siddarth P, Ravo B. Colorectal neurovasculature and anal sphincter. *Surg Clin North Am* 1988;68:1185.
18. Sohn N, Weinstein MA. Acute anal fissure: treatment by lateral subcutaneous internal anal sphincterotomy. *Am J Surg* 1978;136:277.

CHAPTER 93

Transsacral Approach to Rectal Lesions

The transsacral approach is most commonly used for resection of benign retrorectal tumors, or for removal of sessile polyps that cannot be reached by other approaches to the rectum. It is a useful approach to the retrorectal space. It has also been described as a means of access for low anastomosis, but use of the circular stapling device has largely superseded this approach.

Incision and Exposure of the Retrorectal Space (Fig. 93.1)

Technical Points

A combined abdominal and transsacral approach is recommended for removal of large retrorectal tumors. In this case, the patient should be prepped with both the abdominal and sacral regions exposed. The retrorectal or presacral area is approached transabdominally by the same approach that is used for abdominoperineal resection (see Chapter 53). The sacral portion of the operation is described here. Small tumors may be approached transsacrally, without entering the abdomen. The combined approach provides adequate exposure for complete and adequate excision. This is especially important with tumors that extend up into the pelvis, and this approach allows excellent hemostatic control.

Place the patient in the right lateral decubitus position. Make a transverse incision, about 10 cm in length, over the sacrococcygeal joint. Confirm the position of the sacrococcygeal joint by palpation with an index finger within the anal canal if necessary. Deepen this incision until the periosteum of the bone is encountered. Divide the sacrococcygeal joint with heavy scissors. The coccyx may be removed with the specimen. Enter the retrorectal space by sharp and blunt dissection. It will be necessary to divide the periosteum and ligamentous attachments at the sacrococcygeal joint to do this. The next large structure that will be encountered is the muscular wall of the rectum, which can easily be surrounded and dissected free. Many tumors are attached to the coccyx or lower segments of the sacrum. Up to the third segment of the sacrum may be removed at the time of tumor resection without functional impairment. Removal of the sacral nerve roots up to S-1 or S-2 has been relatively well tolerated and is preferable to tumor recurrence.

A retrorectal tumor may be dissected free out of the presacral space by sharp and blunt dissection. It should be removed in its entirety because even benign tumors in this location are prone to recur after inadequate excision.

Anatomic Points

The wedge-shaped sacrum is typically composed of five fused sacral vertebrae, the gross size of which decreases dramatically from the first sacral to the last (fifth) sacral elements. With the exception of the last sacral element, essentially all components of typical vertebrae are represented within each of the five sacral elements. The concave pelvic surface of the sacrum is marked centrally by four transverse ridges that correspond to the planes of separation between the vertebral bodies. Lateral to each of these ridges are paired ventral sacral foramina through which pass the ventral (anterior) primary divisions of spinal nerves S-1 to S-4. Lateral to these foramina are expanded and fused costal elements. From this surface, most of the piriformis and a small part of the iliacus muscles arise; the most cranial fibers of the coccygeus insert distally. The anterior primary divisions of the sacral

LIST OF STRUCTURES

Sacrum
Coccyx
Sacrococcygeal joint
Presacral fascia
Piriformis muscle
Iliacus muscle
Coccygeus muscle
Multifidus muscles
Gluteus maximus muscle
Levator ani muscle

Anococcygeal ligament
Presacral venous plexus
Rectum
Anal canal
Internal anal sphincter
External anal sphincter
Intersphincteric groove
Pectinate line
Puborectalis muscle
Inferior mesenteric artery

Superior rectal (hemorrhoidal) artery
Common iliac artery and vein
Internal iliac artery and vein
Middle rectal (hemorrhoidal) artery and vein
Internal pudendal artery and vein
External iliac artery and vein
Inferior rectal (hemorrhoidal) artery and vein

ORIENTATION

Tumor

nerves and muscles and the caudal-most extent of the external vertebral venous plexus (part of Batson's plexus) are posterior to the pelvic or internal investing fascia (continuous with transversalis fascia), whereas the superior rectal (hemorrhoidal) artery, middle rectal (hemorrhoidal) artery,

internal iliac arteries and branches, and corresponding veins lie anterior to this fascia.

The convex posterior surface of the sacrum presents five prominent longitudinal ridges or crests. The middle sacral crest is formed by the fused spinous processes of the first four

FIGURE 93.1
INCISION AND EXPOSURE OF THE RETRORECTAL SPACE

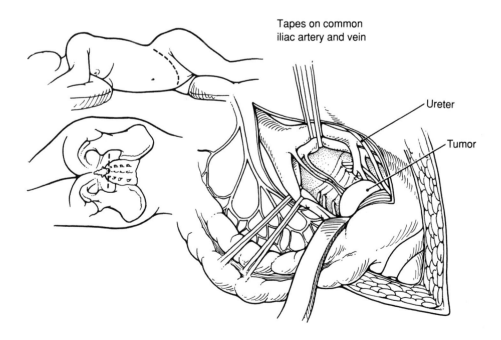

Tapes on common
iliac artery and vein

Ureter

Tumor

(sometimes, three) sacral spinous processes. Lateral to this is a shallow sacral groove, representing fused sacral laminae; the lateral limit of this groove is the intermediate sacral crest. The laminae of the caudal-most one or two sacral elements do not fuse, thereby creating the sacral hiatus flanked by the sacral cornua. The sacral extension of the multifidus muscles (a part of the transversospinalis group of intrinsic back muscles) and parts of the erector spinae muscles are attached to this surface of the sacrum. Lateral to this is the lateral sacral crest, which is lateral to the posterior sacral foramina. In addition, fibers of the gluteus maximus also arise from the inferolateral corner of the dorsal surface of the sacrum.

The coccyx typically is composed of four rudimentary vertebrae. The first coccygeal vertebra (Co-1) forms its base. This element has paired coccygeal cornua, which represent paired rudimentary pedicles and superior articular processes. In addition, it possesses rudimentary transverse processes, which may articulate or fuse with the inferolateral sacral angle, completing a foramen for S-5. The remaining coccygeal vertebrae, which present as bony nodules, represent the bodies of the last vertebrae. The coccygeus muscle inserts on the pelvic surface of the coccyx, whereas fibers of the gluteus maximus arise from its dorsal surface. In addition, fibers of the levator ani, external anal sphincter, and anococcygeal ligament (the midline raphe to which components of the pelvic diaphragm attach) all attach to the tip of the coccyx.

Several ligaments are involved in the sacrococcygeal joint. Between the bodies of S-5 and Co-1 is a thin intervertebral disk composed of fibrocartilage. The ventral sacrococcygeal ligament, located on the pelvic surface of the sacrum and coccyx, is an extension of the anterior longitudinal ligament. The deep dorsal sacrococcygeal ligament corresponds to the posterior longitudinal ligament. The flat superficial dorsal sacrococcygeal ligament is attached to the margin of the sacral hiatus and the dorsal coccygeal surface, forming a roof for the lower sacral canal. The lateral sacrococcygeal ligaments correspond to intertransverse ligaments; if the coccygeal transverse processes of the coccyx do not fuse with the sacrum, these complete the S-5 foramina. Paired intercornual ligaments connect the sacral and coccygeal cornua.

The sacral hiatus, which is continuous with the terminal vertebral canal, permits passage of the last two pairs of spinal nerves (S-5 and Co-1) and the filum terminale. The last pair of sacral nerves (S-5) passes laterally, immediately inferior to the sacral cornua, and deep to the superficial dorsal sacrococcygeal ligament, to provide sensory innervation to the adjacent skin. The coccygeal nerves (Co-1), which have a similar function, pass laterally immediately inferior to the coccygeal cornua. The filum terminale stays in the midline and attaches to the proximal coccyx. These nerves (S-5 and Co-1) can be sacrificed with no loss of muscular function. When necessary, S-4 can also be sacrificed without compromising anorectal function because the inferior rectal branches of the pudendal nerve carry fibers from spinal cord levels S-2 to S-4.

Disarticulation of the sacrococcygeal joint and removal of the coccyx involve removal of the periosteum and division of the fibers of those muscles and ligaments that attach to the coccyx. When this is done, a presacral venous plexus, the caudal part of Batson's vertebral venous plexus, will be encountered. This should lie between the periosteum and the presacral fascia (an extension of transversalis fascia). For the rectum to be visible, the presacral fascia, which is complicated by its separation into a sacral layer and a rectal layer (Waldeyer's fascia), must be divided.

Posterior Approach for Small Retrorectal Tumors (Fig. 93.2)

Technical Points

Position the patient in the prone jackknife position. Make a transverse incision over the sacrococcygeal joint. Divide the sacrococcygeal joint as described in Fig. 93.1. By sharp and blunt dissection, delineate the muscular wall of the rectum. Use traction on the coccyx (which should generally be resected with the specimen) or tumor to define the plane between posterior rectal wall and tumor. Sharply dissect the tumor from the rectal wall. Check hemostasis and close the sacral incision with interrupted Dexon sutures. It is not necessary to drain the space.

A sessile mucosal lesion, such as a villous adenoma, may be resected by the same approach. In this case, expose the rectum as previously described and perform a posterior proctotomy. Place two stay sutures of 2-0 silk in the posterior wall of the rectum and make a longitudinal incision through the wall of the rectum. Identify the lesion by inspection or palpation and place retractors to expose it. Place stay sutures of 2-0 silk on each side of the lesion and elevate it into the field. Excise the lesion in its entirety, removing a disk of mucosa with the lesion. Take care to obtain a clear margin around the lesion on all sides. Mobilize the mucosa and close it with a running lock-stitch of 2-0 Dexon. Close the proctotomy in layers using running Dexon sutures on the inner layer and interrupted silk sutures on the outer layer. Close the sacral incision with interrupted Dexon sutures. It is not necessary to drain the space.

Anatomic Points

The posterior approach provides an excellent view of the abrupt narrowing of the terminal rectum as it becomes the anal canal. The deeper parts of the external anal sphincter, which is continuous with fibers of the puborectalis part of the levator ani, are easily seen. The external anal sphincter encircles the smooth muscle fibers of the terminal rectum and anal canal. The outer smooth muscle fibers are longitudinal, whereas the inner muscle fibers are circular. The terminal extent of the circular muscle layer is thickened and forms the internal anal sphincter. The internal anal sphincter ends more proximally than does the external anal sphincter, so that an intersphincteric groove may be palpated transanally.

The mucosa of the proximal anal canal is morphologically and functionally similar to that of the rectum. At the pectinate line, the mucosa changes rather abruptly to become stratified

FIGURE 93.2
POSTERIOR APPROACH FOR SMALL RETRORECTAL TUMORS

squamous epithelium. The pectinate line is located approximately at the middle of the internal anal sphincter and is commonly thought to represent the site of the embryologic anal membrane.

Recall the pattern of blood supply to the terminal rectum and anus. Proximally, the superior rectal (hemorrhoidal) artery divides into left and right branches approximately at the end of the sigmoid colon (vertebral level S-3). Typically, the right branch then divides into an anterior and posterior branch, so that there are three comparatively large arterial branches derived from the inferior mesenteric artery. Laterally, the middle rectal (hemorrhoidal) arteries, which ultimately are derived from the internal iliac artery, should be located anterior to the paired lateral "rectal stalks." The arterial supply of the terminal anal canal is provided by the inferior rectal (hemorrhoidal) arteries, which are perineal branches of the internal pudendal arteries. As usual, venous drainage parallels the arterial supply. Lymphatic drainage of the rectum and proximal anal canal (above the pectinate line) is to the pelvic and preaortic nodes, whereas drainage of the distal anal canal is to the inguinal nodes. Sensory innervation of the rectum and proximal anal canal is autonomic and is closely associated with the anterior divisions of S-2 to S-4, which emerge through the anterior sacral foramina into the piriformis muscle. The autonomic fibers join the inferior hypogastric plexus, which is located in the extraperitoneal connective tissue that lies lateral to the rectum, seminal vesicles, and prostate (in males), or rectum, uterine cervix, and vaginal fornices (in females). Innervation of the distal anal canal is somatic, carried by the inferior rectal branches of the pudendal nerves, which have the same level of spinal cord origin as the autonomic fibers.

REFERENCES

1. Bailey HR, Huval WV, Max E, et al. Local excision of carcinoma of the rectum for cure. *Surgery* 1992;111:555. (Provides excellent description of the technique for local, transanal excision, which is applicable to sessile polyps or other lesions.)

2. Hargrove WC III, Gertner MH, Fitts WT. The Kraske operation for carcinoma of the rectum. *Surg Gynecol Obstet* 1979;148:931.

3. Hawkins FE Jr, Marks C. The parasacral approach to the rectum. *Am*

Surg 1984;50:623–627. (Describes York Mason modification of Kraske procedure.)

4. Localio SA, Eng K, Ranson JHC. Abdominosacral approach for retrorectal tumors. *Ann Surg* 1980;191:555.

5. Localio SA, Francis KC, Rossano PG. Abdominosacral resection of sacrococcygeal chordoma. *Ann Surg* 1967;166:394.

6. Mason AY. Transsphincteric approach to rectal lesions. *Surg Annu* 1977;9:171.

7. Muldoon JP. Exposure and manipulation of rectal lesions. *Surg Clin North Am* 1978;58:555. (Provides excellent description of various methods.)

8. O'Brien PH. Kraske's posterior approach to the rectum. *Surg Gynecol Obstet* 1976;142:413.

9. Tani T, Endo Y, Kodama M. Abdomino-sacral approach for coloanal anastomosis for lower rectal cancer. *Am J Surg* 1999;178:423–425.

10. Wanebo HJ, Marcove RC. Abdominal sacral resection of locally recurrent rectal cancer. *Ann Surg* 1981;194:458.

11. Watanabe Y, Sato M, Tokui K, et al. A minimally invasive approach to rectal cancer: sacrolaparoscopic approach. *Hepatogastroenterology* 1999;46:909–913. (Discusses application of transsacral approach to minimally invasive surgery.)

12. Westbrook KC, Lang NP, Broadwater JR, et al. Posterior surgical approaches to the rectum. *Ann Surg* 1982;195:677.

CHAPTER 94

Sigmoidoscopy

This chapter deals with the performance of rigid sigmoidoscopy. Flexible fiberoptic sigmoidoscopy is performed essentially as detailed in Chapter 70, except that the distance to be traversed is not as great. Rigid sigmoidoscopy is indicated in patients who have poorly prepped colons or who are being examined for foreign bodies or massive lower gastrointestinal bleeding. In these cases, the fiberoptic scope may not permit an adequate examination. The following figures detail the sequence of maneuvers necessary to pass the rigid sigmoidoscope and to examine the rectosigmoid colon thoroughly.

Positioning of the Patient and Insertion of the Scope (Fig. 94.1)

Technical Points

Place the patient on a proctoscopy table in the knee–chest position. If such a table is not available, the left lateral decubitus or Sims position is a useful alternative. If the patient is in the Sims position, make sure that the buttocks extend over the edge of the table. This will allow you to maneuver the scope fully and to move your head around as needed to get a good view of the entire lower bowel.

First, perform a digital rectal examination to confirm that there is no pathologic lesion within the immediate anorectal area and to determine the angle of the rectal canal. Place the obturator within the sigmoidoscope and introduce the sigmoidoscope by gentle pressure.

The anal canal first passes anteriorly and then angles sharply back toward the hollow of the sacrum. Therefore, the scope must initially be passed in a direction pointing toward the patient's umbilicus, and then almost immediately angled back toward the small of the back once the sphincter mechanism has been traversed. As soon as you feel the scope traverse the sphincter mechanism, remove the obturator and pass the scope under direct vision. On the way in,

concentrate on passing the scope safely and atraumatically. On the way out, concentrate on visualizing and examining the entire rectosigmoid colon for any signs of pathology.

The first few centimeters of the scope in the lower rectum should take you straight back toward the hollow of the sacrum. It will then be necessary to pass the scope more anteriorly. Insufflate air as you proceed in order to open up the bowel enough to see where you are headed. Angle the scope from side to side to traverse the rectal valves (of Houston), of which there are generally three. When you have inserted the scope to a depth of about 15 cm, you will have reached the peritoneal reflection and the bowel will angle sharply, usually to the left. At this point, you must angle the tip of the scope sharply to pass by it. Often, it is not possible to pass the scope deeper than 15 to 18 cm. If you cannot advance it safely under direct vision, do not attempt to do so.

Anatomic Points

The embryology of the terminal gastrointestinal tract helps to explain the anatomy of this region. Initially, the terminal hindgut or cloaca, an endodermally lined cavity, is common to the reproductive, excretory, and digestive systems. The ventral aspect of the cloaca is continuous with the allantois, a small cloacal diverticulum that is the forerunner of the urachus. Distally, at the cloacal membrane, cloacal endoderm, and surface ectoderm are in contact. Externally, the cloacal membrane is located in the proctodeum (anal pit), a caudal depression that results from the proliferation of mesoderm surrounding the cloacal membrane. (Because there is no mesoderm in the cloacal membrane, there is no mesodermal proliferation.) Relatively early, a coronally oriented wedge of mesenchyme—the urorectal septum—develops in the interval between the posterior hindgut and the ventrally located allantois, growing caudally until it makes contact with the cloacal membrane. This divides the cloaca into a posterior terminal gastrointestinal tract and a ventral urogenital sinus. The point of contact between the urorectal septum and the cloacal membrane becomes the central perineal tendon (perineal body). During this time, the cloacal membrane, both anterior and posterior to the central perineal tendon, degenerates and ruptures, establishing communication of the terminal gastrointestinal tract and urogenital system with the environment (at this time, the amniotic cavity).

LIST OF STRUCTURES

Anal canal
Rectum
Sigmoid colon
Peritoneal reflection
Rectal valves (of Houston)

FIGURE 94.1
POSITIONING OF THE PATIENT AND INSERTION OF THE SCOPE

Sims position

Knee-chest position

The events just described, which result in the formation of the anal canal, explain many peculiarities of the anal canal. The location of the cloacal membrane is approximately indicated by the pectinate line. Proximal to this line, the epithelium of the anal canal is derived from hindgut, whereas distal to this line, it is derived from surface ectoderm. Superior to the pectinate line, the predominant blood supply stems from the superior rectal (hemorrhoidal) artery, the terminal branch of the inferior mesenteric artery, which supplies the hindgut structures. Inferior to this line, the blood supply is provided by the middle and inferior rectal (hemorrhoidal) arteries, which ultimately are branches of the internal iliac (hypogastric) artery, basically a parietal artery. Venous drainage of the anal canal proximal to the pectinate line is accomplished by the superior rectal (hemorrhoidal) vein, a tributary of the portal system, whereas distally, venous drainage is a function of the middle and inferior rectal (hemorrhoidal) veins, which are tributaries of the caval system. The lymphatic drainage of the anal canal is indicative of its dual origin: proximal to the pectinate line, the lymphatics tend to drain to the preaortic and paraaortic nodes, whereas distal to this line, the lymphatics drain to the inguinal nodes. Proximal to the pectinate line, sensory innervation is provided by visceral nerves, whereas distally, sensory innervation is a function of somatic nerves. Finally, although there is spatial overlap, the more proximal internal anal sphincter is in continuity with the smooth muscle of the gut (innervated by parasympathetic fibers), whereas the external anal sphincter is in continuity with striated muscle fibers of the levator ani (somatic motor innervation).

With respect to the surgical anatomy relating to rigid proctoscopy, the most important thing to remember is the almost right-angled bend between the lumen of the anal canal and that of the rectum. This severe angle dictates that the proctoscope must first be directed toward the umbilicus for a distance of 4 to 5 cm, then superoposteriorly toward the lumbar vertebrae. The angle between the anal canal and rectum is maintained by the puborectalis muscle, the thickest and most medial part of the levator ani. Its fibers arise from the inner surface of the body of the pubis and blend with the deep fibers of the external anal sphincter posterior to the anal canal. This voluntary muscle is essential to anal continence.

FIGURE 94.2
EXAMINATION OF THE RECTOSIGMOID COLON

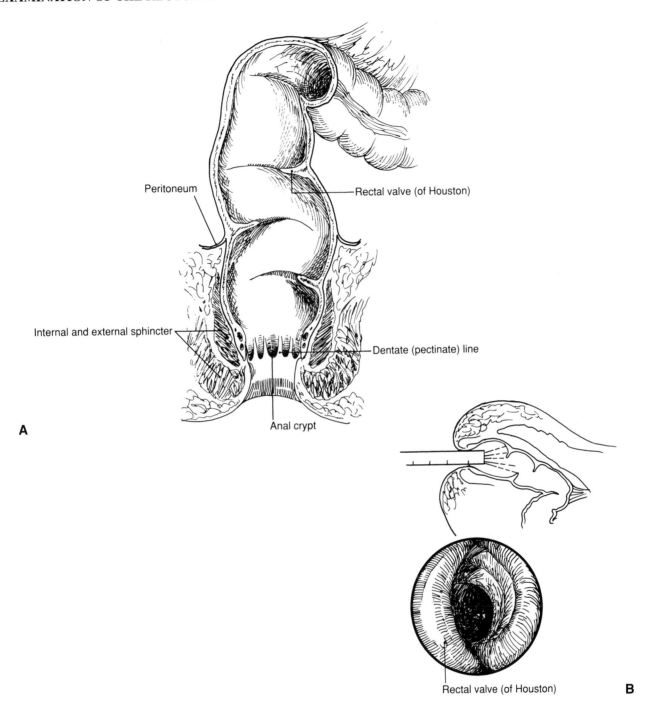

Peritoneum

Rectal valve (of Houston)

Internal and external sphincter

Dentate (pectinate) line

Anal crypt

A

Rectal valve (of Houston)

B

Examination of the Rectosigmoid Colon (Fig. 94.2)

Technical Points

The sigmoid is identifiable by its tendency to collapse, the angulation that occurs at 15 cm, and the concentric appearance of its folds. After passing the scope to its maximum safe extent, gently withdraw it using a turning motion to ensure that the bowel is adequately inspected in each direction. At the rectosigmoid juncture, the rectum, in comparison to the sigmoid, will appear as a larger, more commodious hollow viscus, with less of a tendency to collapse. The rectal valves (of Houston) will appear at intervals. It is necessary to angle the scope carefully to inspect behind the valves, where small lesions may be hidden. Carefully withdraw the scope, allowing the bowel to collapse as you do so. In the lower rectum, take care to inspect the entire rectal ampulla, particularly the area adjacent to the anus. An anoscope may allow improved visualization of the anal area.

Anatomic Points

The junction between the sigmoid colon and the rectum is ill defined at best. This has resulted in the use of a purely arbitrary point—the level of the third sacral element—to delineate between these two portions of the gastrointestinal tract.

Clinically, it is perhaps better to consider the rectosigmoid as a unit. Despite the ambiguities surrounding the terminal colon and beginning rectum, there are several anatomic changes that characterize this boundary. These include a change in peritoneal relationships, the disappearance of haustra, "dispersal" of taeniae coli into a layer of longitudinal muscle completely surrounding the viscus, division of the superior rectal (hemorrhoidal) artery into its left and right branches, and presence of the highest transverse rectal fold (valve of Houston).

FIGURE 94.3
BIOPSY OR POLYPECTOMY

Biopsy or Polypectomy (Fig. 94.3)

Technical and Anatomic Points

Because the biopsy forceps that are used through the rigid sigmoidoscope take a large bite of tissue, they should be used only in the case of obvious polypoid growths protruding into the mucosa or lesions on the valves of Houston. Inadvertent full-thickness biopsy of normal bowel wall can result in bowel perforation. Visualize the lesion from which a biopsy specimen is to be obtained and pass the biopsy forceps through the proctoscope. Take a good bite of the lesion to obtain an adequate sample and then check for bleeding.

Polypectomy can be performed through a rigid proctoscope. To do so, pass a polypectomy snare around the polyp and tighten it around the base of the polyp. Use electrocautery to coagulate the base and then pull the polyp through. Polypectomy is most commonly performed through the flexible colonoscope because examination of the entire colon for other polyps is necessary and visualization is often improved with use of this instrument.

REFERENCES

1. Goligher JC. Diagnosis of diseases of the anus, rectum and colon. In: Goligher JC, ed. *Surgery of the anus, rectum and colon.* 4th ed. London: Bailliere Tindall, 1980:48. (This book is old, but it remains a classic. It contains an excellent description of physical examination and performance of rigid sigmoidoscopy.)

2. Jagelman DG. Anoscopy. In: Sivak MV, ed. *Gastroenterologic endoscopy.* Philadelphia: WB Saunders, 1987:960.
3. Keighley MRB. Injuries to the colon and rectum. In: Keighley MRB, Williams NS, eds. *Surgery of the anus, rectum, and colon.* London: WB Saunders, 1993:1909–1912. (Discusses causes of iatrogenic perforation and management.)

SECTION VI

The Lower Extremity

The final section of the book is devoted to the anatomy of the lower extremity as encountered by the general surgeon. First, a series of chapters on amputations introduce the muscle groups and neurovascular structures. Chapter 95 details techniques for so-called minor amputations of the digits and forefoot. These are often performed by junior residents, yet meticulous attention to patient selection and technique is imperative for proper healing. This is also true for major amputations—the below-knee amputation (Chapter 96) and the above-knee amputation (Chapter 99). Amputation at other levels, such as the Syme amputation, knee or hip disarticulation, and hemipelvectomy, are detailed in the references.

The next few chapters deal with vascular surgery of the lower extremity. Venous anatomy is given first, in two related chapters. Chapter 98 describes the greater saphenous vein through the operations of venous stripping and ligation (and the related topic of harvesting the saphenous vein for vascular conduit). The related minor procedures of saphenous vein cutdown at ankle and groin are presented in Chapter 99.

The femoral artery was first introduced in Chapter 30 and is explored in greater detail in Chapter 100, which is devoted to femoropopliteal bypass grafting.

Finally, Chapter 101 details fasciotomy of the lower extremity and reinforces the anatomy of the section.

CHAPTER 95

Transmetatarsal and Ray Amputations

Transmetatarsal and ray amputations require meticulous patient selection and attention to surgical technique when performed in patients with peripheral vascular disease. Transmetatarsal amputation is performed for gangrene, trauma, or rarely, tumors limited to the distal part of the foot. Part or all of the foot may be resected at the midmetatarsal level. In this chapter, the standard full transmetatarsal amputation is described, followed by a discussion of both partial transmetatarsal and ray amputations.

Skin Incision and Division of Soft Tissues (Fig. 95.1)

Technical Points

Plan a gently curved skin incision that is longer on the plantar surface than on the dorsal surface of the foot. The skin of the plantar surface is stronger and can be pulled up to form a good flap over the tips of the metatarsals. Make the skin incision at about the level of the metatarsal heads (Fig. 95.1A). Divide the soft tissues down to the level of the bone. Secure the digital arteries with suture ligatures (Fig. 95.1B).

Anatomic Points

Division of the skin and superficial fascia of the dorsum of the foot will expose the superficial veins and nerves that occupy the plane between superficial and deep fascia. The anatomy of the superficial venous network varies; however, recall that the greater and lesser saphenous veins begin as continuations of the medial and lateral ends of the dorsal venous arch, respectively. The dorsal venous arch is located roughly over the middle of the second through the fifth metatarsals. The greater saphenous vein begins over the proximal end of the

first metatarsal, and the lesser saphenous vein begins over the cuboid. The branches of two sensory nerves—the superficial peroneal and sural nerves—lie relatively superficial and may be encountered. The superficial peroneal nerve supplies most of the skin of the dorsum of the foot and toes, except for the first interdigital space and apposing sides of digits 1 and 2 (supplied by a branch of the deep peroneal nerve). The sural nerve provides cutaneous innervation to the lateral side of the foot. The nerves are crossed superficially by the superficial veins.

When the deep fascia of the dorsum of the foot is divided, the dorsalis pedis artery, a continuation of the anterior tibial artery, should be identified and ligated (if necessary) before its division. This artery, accompanied by the deep peroneal nerve, lies lateral to the extensor hallucis longus tendon, passes deep to the inferior extensor retinaculum, and is crossed by the extensor hallucis brevis (Fig. 95.1C). At the proximal end of the first intermetatarsal space, it turns plantarward, between the interosseous muscles of this space, to anastomose with the deep branch of the lateral plantar artery, forming the plantar arterial arch. Branches of the dorsalis pedis artery that must be considered in amputations include the first dorsal metatarsal artery. This artery bifurcates, in the cleft between the first two digits at the level of the metatarsophalangeal joint, into two dorsal digital arteries, which supply the contiguous sides of these two digits. The arcuate artery, a lateral branch of the dorsalis pedis artery that lies deep to the intrinsic extensor musculature and that gives rise to the remaining three dorsal metatarsal arteries, crosses the bases of all metatarsals except the first.

In addition to neurovascular structures on the dorsum of the foot, several extensor muscles or tendons have to be

LIST OF STRUCTURES

Metatarsal bones	Superficial peroneal nerve	Digital arteries
Phalanges	Deep peroneal nerve	Extensor hallucis longus muscle
Tarsal bones	Sural nerve	Extensor hallucis brevis muscle
Cuboid	Anterior tibial artery	Inferior extensor retinaculum
Superficial fascia	Dorsalis pedis artery	Extensor digitorum longus muscle
Deep fascia of the foot	First dorsal metatarsal artery	Extensor digitorum brevis muscle
Plantar aponeurosis	Arcuate artery	Peroneus tertius muscle
Dorsal venous arch	Lateral plantar artery	Interosseous muscles (dorsal and
Greater saphenous vein	Plantar arterial arch	plantar)
Lesser saphenous vein	Dorsal arterial arch	Adductor hallucis muscle

FIGURE 95.1
SKIN INCISION AND DIVISION OF SOFT TISSUES

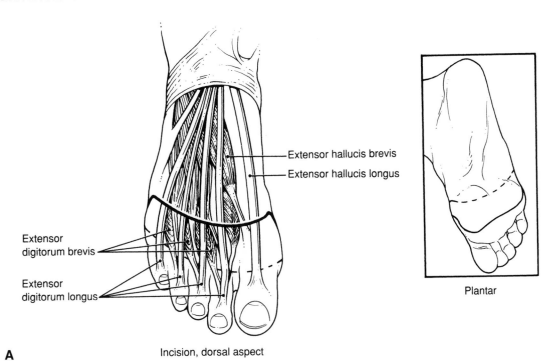

Extensor hallucis brevis

Extensor hallucis longus

Extensor digitorum brevis

Extensor digitorum longus

Plantar

Incision, dorsal aspect

A

Cut tendons

Digital arteries (sutured)

B

Dorsalis pedis artery

Lateral tarsal artery

Dorsal digital arteries

C

FIGURE 95.2
DIVISION OF THE METATARSALS AND COMPLETION OF THE AMPUTATION

A — Periosteal elevator   Metatarsals (divided in their midshaft) **B**

divided to provide unobstructed access to the periosteum. These include the tendons of the extensor hallucis longus and brevis muscles and the multiple tendons of the extensor digitorum longus and brevis muscles. The tendon of the peroneus tertius muscle inserts on the base of the fifth metatarsal and is at that point proximal to the line of resection.

Division of the Metatarsals and Completion of the Amputation (Fig. 95.2)

Technical Points

Use a periosteal elevator to elevate periosteum and soft tissues from the metatarsals at the point of division (Fig. 95.2A). Divide the metatarsals cleanly just behind their heads, using a pneumatic bone saw or bone cutters. A pneumatic saw is preferable because it cuts cleanly without splintering. If you use bone cutters, be careful to smooth the metatarsal shafts after division and remove any splinters of bone. A rongeur is convenient for this.

Be careful not to strip back past the level of amputation because this would separate soft tissue from bone and create dead space.

The amputation may then be rapidly completed by transecting the plantar tendons and remaining soft tissues posteriorly. Divide the tendons flush with the surrounding soft tissues (Fig. 95.2B).

Irrigate the stump and secure meticulous hemostasis.

Anatomic Points

Elevation of the periosteum of the metatarsals will detach the origins and insertions of the muscles that attach to the shafts of these bones. This includes the four dorsal interossei muscles,

which lie in the dorsal aspect of each intermetatarsal space, as well as the three plantar interossei muscles that lie just deep to the former muscles (there is no plantar interosseous muscle in the first intermetatarsal space).

Subsequent division (from dorsal to plantar) of the soft tissues of the plantar aspect of the foot will first divide the dorsal and plantar interosseous muscles, the intrinsic plantar muscles of the little toe (the flexor digiti minimi brevis and abductor digiti minimi), and two of the three intrinsic plantar muscles of the great toe (the flexor hallucis brevis and adductor hallucis). Division of these muscles exposes the fascial plane in which lie the plantar metatarsal arteries

FIGURE 95.3
CLOSURE OF THE AMPUTATION

— Drain

Tailored flap (completed)

FIGURE 95.4
PARTIAL TRANSMETATARSAL AMPUTATION AND RAY AMPUTATION

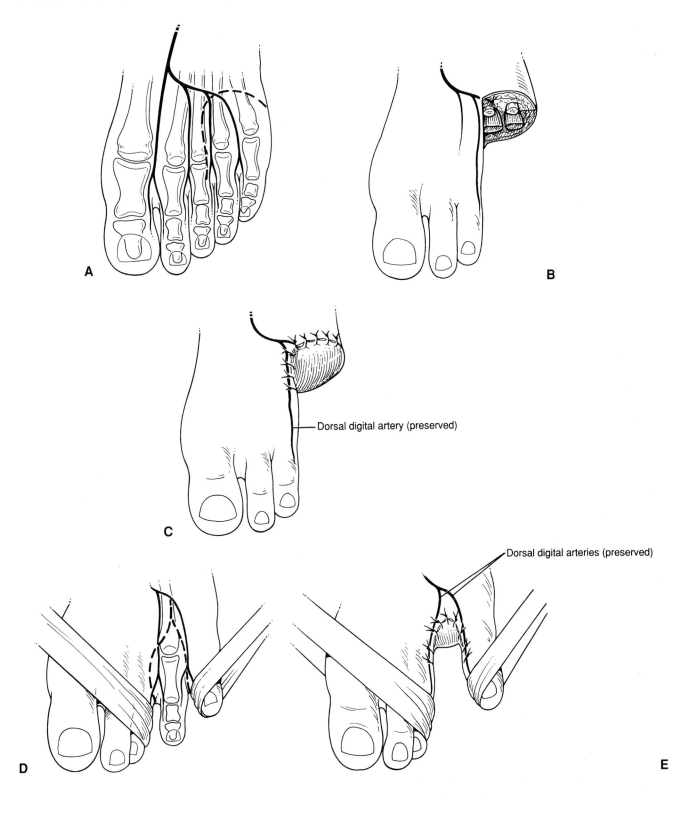

Dorsal digital artery (preserved)

Dorsal digital arteries (preserved)

that arise from the plantar arterial arch (from the most lateral intermetatarsal space to the most medial metatarsal space) and the medial plantar artery. Because of the proximal location of the plantar arch, the metatarsal arteries and the medial plantar artery will be divided; these are large enough to require ligation. The digital nerves (branches of the medial and lateral plantar nerves) that accompany these arteries will also be divided.

After division of the neurovascular structures, the soft tissues of the oblique head of the adductor hallucis and tendons of the flexor digitorum longus and hallucis longus (including the attached lumbrical muscles) are next divided. This exposes the fascial plane that contains branches of the medial plantar and lateral plantar nerves, which are also divided. These are primarily sensory branches. Division of these nerves and the accompanying connective tissue exposes the flexor digitorum brevis, the last muscle that must be divided. When this muscle is divided, the deep surface of the plantar aponeurosis, an expression of deep fascia, is exposed. The plantar aponeurosis, superficial fascia, and plantar skin are firmly attached to each other, and because no major vascular structures are present in these layers, they can be divided with impunity.

Closure of the Amputation (Fig. 95.3)

Technical and Anatomic Points

Close the soft tissues over the metatarsal heads in layers, using interrupted Vicryl sutures. Tailor the flap so that there are no "dog ears" and so that it can be brought together without tension. If the flaps come together under tension, resect additional metatarsal bone to allow comfortable closure.

Approximate the skin carefully. Handle the skin edges with care to avoid traumatizing tissues that are probably ischemic. A drain may be placed under the flap, if desired.

Partial Transmetatarsal Amputation and Ray Amputation (Fig. 95.4)

Technical Points

Partial transmetatarsal amputation is occasionally performed when one or two digits are involved and the rest

of the foot is thought to be salvageable. It can be done as an open or closed procedure but is more commonly done open.

The skin incision in this case passes down between the toes along a line between the two metatarsal shafts and then crosses over the head of the metatarsals. Again, the posterior flap should be made longer than the anterior one.

It is important to spare the digital artery going to the adjacent toe that is to remain. If this artery is ligated or traumatized, the ischemia may progress to involve this digit as well.

Clean the metatarsal heads of the periosteum and divide the bones in their midshaft, as previously described. Closure is similar to that done in complete transmetatarsal amputation.

Alternatively, the flap may be left open to granulate. It may then be closed secondarily, or covered by split-thickness skin grafts. This approach is slow and requires meticulous wound care during the postoperative period; however, it may result in salvage of part of the foot when infection is present, particularly if arterial inflow can be improved after the infection clears.

Ray amputation is performed when only one digit needs to be removed. Outline a tennis racquet–shaped incision around the base of the affected toe. Divide the soft tissues as described earlier, being careful to spare the digital vessels to the neighboring toes. Divide the metatarsal in its midshaft portion. In this case, it is safest to use bone cutters, which can be placed precisely around the bone in a relatively small working space. Smooth the end of the metatarsal with a rongeur. Close the small incision in layers.

Anatomic Points

Remember that there are both dorsal and plantar digital arteries and that of the two, the plantar arteries are larger. Dorsal and plantar digital arteries are branches of dorsal and plantar metatarsal arteries, respectively. Digital arteries actually arise quite distally in the interdigital space, so that it is necessary to preserve the metatarsal artery in its entirety, with ligation and division of only the digital arteries supplying the digits to be removed.

REFERENCES

1. Chang BB, Jacobs RL, Darling RC III, et al. Foot amputations. *Surg Clin North Am* 1995;75:773–782. (Discusses alternatives, emphasizing management of patients with peripheral vascular disease.)
2. Clark N, Sherman R. Soft-tissue reconstruction of the foot and ankle. *Orthop Clin North Am* 1993;24:489–503. (Presents thorough discussion of management options for trauma.)
3. Early JS. Transmetatarsal and midfoot amputations. *Clin Orthop Relat Res* 1999;361:85–90. (Discusses patient selection, technique, alternative approaches.)
4. Effeney DJ, Lim RC, Schecter WP. Transmetatarsal amputation. *Arch Surg* 1977;112:1366.
5. Little JM. Transmetatarsal amputation. In: Malt RA, ed. *Surgical techniques illustrated: a comparative atlas.* Philadelphia: WB Saunders, 1985:578.
6. Sizer JS, Wheelock FC. Digital amputations in diabetic patients. *Surgery* 1972;72:980.
7. Wagner FW. The Syme amputation. In: American Academy of Orthopaedic Surgeons. *Atlas of limb prosthetics: surgical and prosthetic principles.* St. Louis: CV Mosby, 1981:326. (Provides a clear description of an alternative to below-knee amputation in selected patients.)
8. Wheelock FC. Amputation of individual toes. In: Malt RA, ed. *Surgical techniques illustrated: a comparative atlas.* Philadelphia: WB Saunders, 1985:582.
9. Wheelock FC. Transmetatarsal amputation. In: Malt RA, ed. *Surgical techniques illustrated: a comparative atlas.* Philadelphia: WB Saunders, 1985:572.

CHAPTER 96

Below-knee Amputation

Most amputations are performed for ischemia. The choice of the level of amputation requires mature judgment. Although it is important to salvage as much length as possible, a poor initial choice of level may doom the patient to a second amputation, often at a significantly higher level. References at the end discuss factors to consider in selecting an amputation site as well as the utility of several commonly performed tests.

When below-knee amputation is performed for ischemia, the stump should be made long enough to allow fitting of a prosthesis, but not so long that viability is sacrificed. Below-knee amputation that is performed for trauma, in the presence of normal arteries, may be performed at a lower level.

In this chapter, the standard procedure for below-knee amputation, as performed for ischemia, is described. References at the end detail alternative techniques, including amputation for trauma or tumor.

Skin Incision and Development of Flaps (Fig. 96.1)

Technical Points

Plan a skin incision with a long posterior flap. The length of the posterior flap should approximate the transverse diameter of the leg. As extra length of flap can always be trimmed; it is advisable to make the flap too long at the initial incision. Divide the minimal soft tissues anterior to the tibia. Plan to divide the tibia about four fingerbreadths below the tibial tuberosity. If the amputation is being performed for trauma, a longer stump may be tailored. Generally, when amputation is done for ischemia, a shorter stump is desirable.

Identify and ligate the greater saphenous vein in the medial aspect of the anterior incision. Divide all soft tissues down to the tibia anteriorly and through the fascia of the muscles laterally.

To limit blood loss, do not create the posterior skin incision at this point.

Anatomic Points

The division of the tibia about four fingerbreadths inferior to the tibial tuberosity corresponds to approximately the level of the greatest circumference of the leg. At this location, the greater saphenous vein and accompanying saphenous nerve are located in the superficial fascia just posterior to the medial border of the tibia, that is, in the fascia overlying the tibial origin of the soleus muscle. No important structures lie in the superficial fascia anterior to the greater saphenous vein. The anteromedial surface of the tibia lies just deep to the superficial fascia. Hence, the anterior border of the tibia is a useful landmark, and no muscles must be divided to expose it.

Lateral to the anterior border of the tibia, the deep fascia covering the muscles of the anterior compartment of the leg must be divided. At the usual level of amputation, the muscle most closely associated with the tibia is the tibialis anterior; posterior to this is the belly of the extensor digitorum longus muscle. The belly of the extensor hallucis longus may be encountered between the extensor digitorum longus and the tibialis anterior if a low below-knee amputation is performed.

When the fascia is divided still more posterolaterally, the anterior intermuscular septum will be encountered; this forms the anterior wall of the lateral compartment. Division of the deep fascia of the lateral compartment exposes the belly of the peroneus longus muscle. Continued circumferential division of the deep fascia should allow visualization of the posterior intermuscular septum, which separates the lateral compartment muscles from the posterior compartment muscles.

LIST OF STRUCTURES

Tibia	Deep fascia	Tibialis posterior muscle
Tibial tuberosity	Interosseous membrane	Tendon of plantaris muscle
Fibula	Gastrocnemius muscle	Popliteal artery and vein
Greater saphenous vein	Soleus muscle	Anterior tibial artery and vein
Lesser saphenous vein	Tibialis anterior muscle	Posterior tibial artery and vein
Saphenous nerve	Extensor digitorum longus muscle	Peroneal artery and vein
Common peroneal nerve	Extensor hallucis longus muscle	
Superficial fascia	Peroneus longus muscle	

FIGURE 96.1
SKIN INCISION AND DEVELOPMENT OF FLAPS

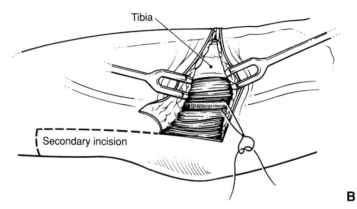

Division of the Tibia and Fibula (Fig. 96.2)

Technical Points

Strip the periosteum from the tibia circumferentially with a periosteal elevator. Divide the tibia with a pneumatic bone saw 1 to 2 cm above the level of the skin incision. If a pneumatic saw is not available, a Gigl wire saw works well.

Angle the cut on the tibia upward as you progress anteriorly so that the anterior edge of the tibia does not form a sharp projection that could traumatize the stump.

Divide the fibula several centimeters higher than the tibia. It is often convenient to do this with bone cutters, so that the bone can be divided high up within the soft tissues of the stump. Carefully smooth the end of the fibula with a rongeur

FIGURE 96.2
DIVISION OF THE TIBIA AND FIBULA

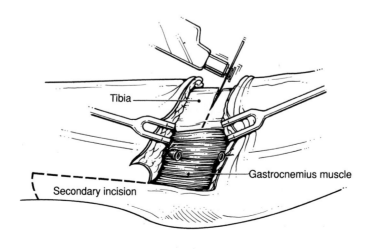

and remove any spicules of bone that are left in the wound after the fibula has been divided.

Anatomic Points

Elevation of the tibial periosteum does not require division of any muscles because the periosteum can be entered on the anteromedial surface of the tibia. Exposure of the fibula, however, demands division or detachment of the origins of the extensor digitorum longus muscle in the anterior compart-

ment, the peroneus longus muscle in the lateral compartment, and the soleus and tibialis posterior muscles in the posterior compartment. As you expose the fibula, be careful to avoid inadvertent injury to the vessels in the region. Anterior to the interosseus membrane, in close proximity to the fibula, are the anterior tibial vessels. The posterior tibial vessels, as well as the peroneal vessels, lie in the plane between the superficial and deep posterior compartments—that is, deep to the soleus and superficial to the tibialis posterior muscles. The peroneal vessels are in close proximity to the fibula.

FIGURE 96.3
COMPLETION OF THE AMPUTATION

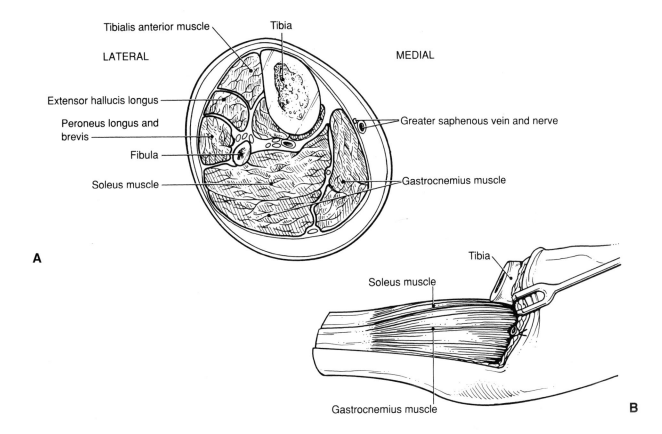

Completion of the Amputation (Fig. 96.3)

Technical Points

Behind the tibia, identify the posterior tibial artery and vein and suture-ligate them. Identify the common peroneal nerve, ligate it, and transect it cleanly under traction, allowing it to retract into the depths of the stump.

Within the deep flexor muscle compartment, identify and suture-ligate the deep vessels. The level of amputation and the variable level of trifurcation of the popliteal artery into anterior tibial, posterior tibial, and peroneal branches influence the number and exact location of these neurovascular bundles. The tibial nerve accompanies the

posterior tibial vessels and must be ligated and divided under tension.

Develop the posterior flap to include the soleus muscle. Enter the plane between the gastrocnemius and soleus muscles by dividing the posterior crural septum laterally. The plane between the gastrocnemius and soleus muscles is generally avascular and can rapidly be developed by blunt dissection. Laterally and medially, it is necessary to incise the fascial attachments that anchor the two muscles together.

Complete the posterior skin incision. Identify and ligate the lesser saphenous vein. Transect the soleus muscle and remaining soft tissues at the level of the skin incision to complete the amputation.

Anatomic Points

The anterior tibial vessels pass into the anterior compartment through a gap in the interosseus membrane just inferior to the proximal tibiofibular joint. To expose these vessels, and as a necessary part of the amputation, the tibialis anterior, extensor digitorum longus, and extensor hallucis longus should be divided. The nerve that accompanies these vessels in the anterior compartment is the deep peroneal nerve, a branch of the common peroneal nerve. It is not necessary to divide the deep peroneal nerve at this level because the common peroneal nerve will be divided next.

The common peroneal nerve, which wraps around the lateral aspect of the fibula just inferior to its head, should be found deep to the peroneus longus. The common peroneal nerve can be located by tracing the deep peroneal nerve proximally to the point where the superficial peroneal nerve is seen to innervate the peroneal muscles. Division of the common peroneal nerve then involves nerve division proximal to this point. The peroneus longus muscle, if not divided earlier, should be divided after division of the common peroneal nerve.

After division of the muscles, nerves, and vessels in the anterior and lateral compartments, it is necessary to identify and divide neurovascular structures in the posterior compartment. At the level of tibial division, the posterior tibial vessels accompanied by the tibial nerve, and possibly the peroneal vessels, should be located after the tibialis posterior is divided. These neurovascular structures should be found on the deep (anterior) side of the deep transverse fascia, a septum separating the superficial and deep posterior compartments.

After division of the posterior compartment's neurovascular structures and the tibialis posterior, all that remains connecting the distal segment from the proximal leg are the muscles associated with the calcaneal tendon, the posterior crural fascia, the superficial fascia, and the skin. The plane between the gastrocnemius and soleus muscles is typically avascular. Frequently, the small saphenous vein, which ascends in the superficial fascia or a deep fascia compartment in the midline of the calf, passes between the two heads of the gastrocnemius muscle to enter the popliteal vein posterior to

FIGURE 96.4
CLOSURE OF THE STUMP

the knee joint. As the plane between the gastrocnemius and soleus muscles is developed, the tendon of the plantaris muscle can be observed passing from lateral to medial on the superficial surface of the soleus muscle.

Closure of the Stump (Fig. 96.4)

Technical and Anatomic Points

Irrigate the stump carefully and secure hemostasis. If bleeding from the marrow cavity of the tibia is a problem, use bone wax to close the cavity. Use only the minimal amount necessary because this acts as a foreign body and may potentiate infection. Pull the posterior flap up and suture it to the anterior flap. Tailor the flap in such a way that there are no "dog ears." Close the fascia securely with interrupted 2-0 Dexon sutures first.

Then close the subcutaneous tissues and skin. Handle the skin carefully and atraumatically. Particularly in the presence of ischemia, rough handling may jeopardize subsequent healing of the flaps. Meticulously approximate the skin edges.

Dress the stump carefully. Consider using a well-padded, posterior splint to prevent flexion contracture at the knee. Do not use tape on the skin of an ischemic extremity.

REFERENCES

1. Allcock PA, Jain AS. Revisiting transtibial amputation with the long posterior flap. *Br J Surg* 2001;88:683–686. (Reaffirms value of technique.)
2. Burgess EM. Disarticulation of the knee: a modified technique. *Arch Surg* 1977;112:1250. (Describes an alternative to below-knee amputation.)
3. Hicks L, McClelland RN. Below-knee amputations for vascular insufficiency. *Am Surg* 1980;46:239.
4. Kaufam JL. Alternative methods for below-knee amputation: reappraisal of the Kendrick procedure. *J Am Coll Surg* 1995;181:511–516.
5. Porter JM, Mayberry JC, Taylor L Jr, et al. Chronic lower-extremity ischemia: part II. *Curr Probl Surg* 1991;28:93–179. (Presents excellent review.)
6. Rush DS, Huston CC, Bivins BA, et al. Operative and late mortality rates of above knee and below-knee amputation. *Am Surg* 1981;47:36.
7. Smith DG, Fergason JR. Transtibial amputations. *Clin Orthop Relat Res* 1999;361:108–115. (Reviews alternative techniques and outcomes.)
8. Song EK, Moon ES, Rowe SM, et al. Below knee stump reconstruction by turn-up technique: report of 2 cases. *Clin Orthop Relat Res* 1994;307:229–134.
9. Wheelock FC, Little JM, Dale WA, et al. Below knee amputation. In: Malt RA, ed. *Surgical techniques illustrated: a comparative atlas.* Philadelphia: WB Saunders, 1985:544.
10. Winburn GB, Wood MC, Hawkins ML, et al. Current role of cryoamputation. *Am J Surg* 1991;162:647–650. (Describes temporizing maneuver in infected cases.)

CHAPTER 97

Above-knee Amputation

Above-knee amputation is performed when it is not possible to save the knee joint because of the extent of injury or ischemic damage. Generally, the longer the stump, the better. The limiting factor is usually the condition of the skin and the soft tissues above the knee. If there is a question about the extent of gangrene or infection in the subcutaneous tissues in the skin, perform a guillotine amputation at the lowest possible level, leaving the stump open. When the infection is controlled, revise the amputation.

Position of the Patient and Development of Flaps (Fig. 97.1)

Technical Points

Position the patient supine with the leg draped free. Plan symmetric fish-mouth skin flaps anteriorly and posteriorly. The flaps should be of approximately the same size and length. Gently curve the fish-mouth to avoid interfering with the blood supply to the tip of the flap.

Make a skin incision and deepen the incision down to the fascia overlying the muscle groups. Identify and ligate the greater saphenous vein in the medial portion of the anterior flap. Incise the fascia sharply.

Anatomic Points

The greater saphenous vein and a variable number of tributaries are the only structures of consequence in the superficial fascia of the thigh. The course of the greater saphenous vein can be approximated by a line running from a point 8 to 10 cm posterior to the medial side of the patella to a second point that is level with, and 4 cm lateral to, the pubic tubercle. Note that, in the thigh, the larger veins of this system are in a plane between two layers of superficial fascia. Frequently, a large communicating branch between the lesser and greater saphenous veins ascends obliquely around the medial side of the thigh; other large tributaries join the greater saphenous vein on its anterolateral side. One fairly common variant of the greater saphenous system that would necessitate additional vein ligations is duplication of the greater saphenous vein in the more distal part of the thigh. When such duplication occurs, one of the vessels is typically deeper than the other, although both are still within the superficial fascia.

The deep fascia of the thigh, or fascia lata, is not of equal thickness throughout. It is thicker proximally and especially laterally, where it is reinforced by the iliotibial tract, which is actually the long, flat tendon of insertion (to the lateral condyle of the tibia) of the tensor fascia lata and most of the gluteus maximus. In addition, the fascia lata is thickened distally about the knee joint, where it is reinforced by fibrous expansions from the biceps femoris muscle laterally, the sartorius muscle medially, and the quadriceps femoris muscle anteriorly.

LIST OF STRUCTURES

Superficial fascia of the thigh	Lesser saphenous vein (small saphenous vein)	Adductor magnus muscle
Fascia lata (deep fascia of the thigh)	Popliteal vein	Gracilis muscle
Iliotibial tract	Femoral artery	Semimembranosus muscle
Lateral intermuscular septum	Superficial femoral artery	Semitendinosus muscle
Anteromedial intermuscular septum	Profunda femoris artery	Gluteus maximus muscle
Posteromedial intermuscular septum	Popliteal artery	Sartorius muscle
Femoral nerve	Inferior gluteal artery	Tensor fascia lata muscle
Obturator nerve	Ischiatic artery	Biceps femoris muscle
Sciatic nerve	Femur	Quadriceps femoris muscle
Saphenous nerve	Adductor (Hunter's) canal	Vastus lateralis muscle
Femoral vein	Adductor longus muscle	Vastus medialis muscle
Greater saphenous vein (great saphenous vein)	Adductor brevis muscle	Vastus intermedius muscle
		Rectus femoris muscle

FIGURE 97.1
POSITION OF THE PATIENT AND DEVELOPMENT OF FLAPS

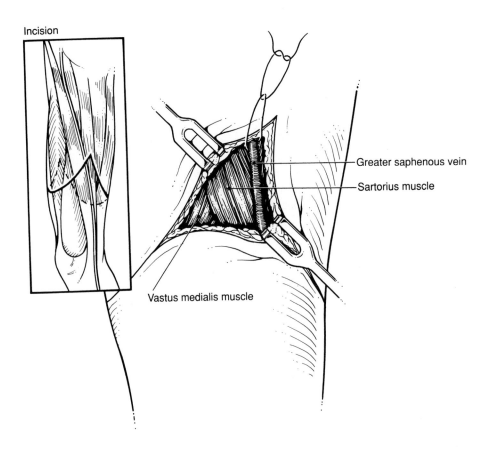

Incision

Greater saphenous vein

Sartorius muscle

Vastus medialis muscle

Division of the Anterior Muscles and Femoral
Vessels (Fig. 97.2)

Technical Points

Divide the sartorius, rectus femoris, and vastus lateralis muscles sharply. The femoral artery and vein lie between the sartorius and vastus medialis muscles and are surrounded by soft tissue. They will be encountered in the medial aspect of the dissection after the muscles have been divided. It is safest to divide first all the muscles lying directly anterior to the femur, then to progress medially, working carefully to identify and protect from harm the femoral artery and vein. Suture-ligate and divide each vessel individually. Continue to divide the medial muscles, working posteriorly until the medial aspect of the femur is accessible.

Laterally, only the vastus lateralis and vastus intermedius muscles need to be divided to expose the femur. No major neurovascular structures should be encountered.

Anatomic Points

A conceptual scheme of the compartmentalization of the thigh is helpful to visualize throughout the procedure. At the levels where most above-knee amputations are made, there are three compartments in the thigh, each separated by intermuscular septa. The anterior compartment is bounded by the lateral intermuscular septum, lying between the vastus lateralis muscle and the short head of the biceps femoris muscle and attached to the fascia lata and linea aspera of the femur, and an anterior medial intermuscular septum, lying between the vastus medialis and adductor muscles and likewise attached to the fascia lata and linea aspera of the femur. Muscles in this compartment are all innervated by the femoral nerve and include both the sartorius and the quadriceps femoris. The *quadriceps femoris muscle* is the collective term for the vastus lateralis, vastus medialis, vastus intermedius, and rectus femoris muscles. The anterior boundary of the medial or adductor compartment is the anteromedial intermuscular septum. The posterior boundary is a posteromedial intermuscular septum, perhaps more theoretical than actual, which lies between the adductor magnus muscle and the hamstring muscles. Muscles in this compartment, innervated by the obturator nerve, include (at amputation levels) the adductor longus, adductor brevis, and adductor magnus muscles as well as the gracilis muscle. The posterior compartment is bounded by the lateral and posteromedial intermuscular septa. The muscles in this compartment include the semimembranosus, semitendinosus, and biceps femoris. These muscles are innervated by the sciatic nerve. A fourth compartment includes muscles (gluteus maximus and tensor fascia lata) innervated by the gluteal nerves; however, neuromuscular structures of this compartment are seldom encountered in a typical amputation.

The sartorius muscle arises from the anterosuperior iliac spine and spirals inferomedially to insert on the medial

FIGURE 97.2
DIVISION OF THE ANTERIOR MUSCLES AND FEMORAL VESSELS

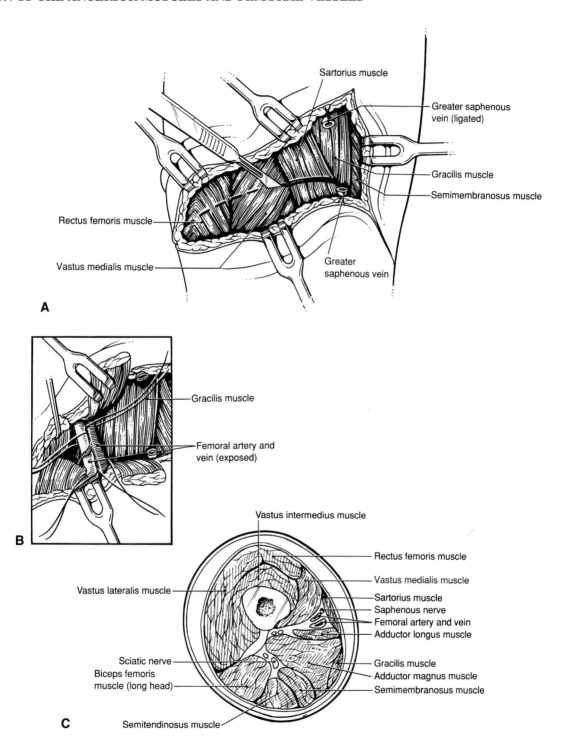

aspect of the tibia. In the proximal third of the thigh, it forms the lateral boundary of the femoral triangle and is thus lateral to the femoral vessels and nerves. In the middle third of the thigh, it forms the roof of the adductor (subsartorial or Hunter's) canal. This triangular intermuscular canal, whose other boundaries are the vastus medialis muscle laterally and the adductor longus and magnus muscles medially, contains

the (superficial) femoral artery and vein, the saphenous nerve, and the nerve to the vastus medialis muscle.

The rectus femoris muscle, the most anterior division of the quadriceps femoris muscle, arises from the anteroinferior iliac spine and from a groove superior to the acetabulum. As its name implies, the muscle then passes straight down the thigh to insert, through the patellar ligament, on the tibial tuberosity. In the upper thigh, it is essentially deep to the sartorius. In the middle third of the thigh, it is primarily lateral to the sartorius, whereas in the distal third of the thigh, it is immediately lateral to the vastus medialis muscle.

Lateral to the rectus femoris muscle is the vastus lateralis muscle, which originates from the intertrochanteric line, greater trochanter, lateral tip of the gluteal tuberosity, and proximal half of the lateral lip of the linea aspera. The largest component of the quadriceps femoris muscle, the vastus lateralis, is superficial to the vastus intermedius muscle. Quite proximally, it is deep to the tensor fascia lata. Its fibers are directed inferomedially, inserting onto a strong aponeurosis and tendon that ultimately contributes to the patellar ligament.

The vastus medialis muscle, which originates primarily from the medial lip of the linea aspera, is covered in the middle third of the thigh by the sartorius muscle. In the distal third of the thigh, it lies between the sartorius and the rectus femoris muscles. Like the vastus lateralis muscle, it is superficial to part of the vastus intermedius muscle. From its long origin, its fibers are directed inferolaterally to insert on the common aponeurosis and tendon that ultimately contributes to the patellar ligament. Remember that this muscle forms the lateral wall of the adductor canal.

The final anterior compartment muscle to be divided is the vastus intermedius. This deep, thin muscle has a fleshy origin from the proximal two thirds of the anterior and lateral shaft of the femur. These muscular fibers run anteroinferiorly to attach to the deep part of the common quadriceps tendon.

Division of the muscles within the medial compartment necessitates identification and protection of the contents of the adductor canal. If the level of amputation is at or above the midthigh, this will include the nerve to the vastus medialis muscle, which lies lateral to the femoral artery.

Regardless of the level of amputation, two medial compartment muscles—the gracilis and adductor magnus—will be divided. The gracilis muscle, the most superficial of the medial compartment muscles, originates from the ischiopubic ramus and inserts on the medial aspect of the tibia posterior to the insertion of the sartorius muscle. The adductor magnus muscle also arises from the ischiopubic ramus and the ischial tuberosity. From this origin, it fans out to insert along the entire medial lip of the linea aspera, medial supracondylar line, and adductor tubercle. This extensive insertion is interrupted by five osseoaponeurotic openings. The most distal of these openings, located approximately at the junction of the middle and distal thirds of the thigh, is the adductor hiatus. The femoral artery and vein pass into the popliteal fossa through this hiatus, becoming the popliteal artery and vein. The more proximal four openings, which are much smaller, transmit the perforating branches of the profunda femoris artery, the last of which is the termination of this artery. The openings, the most distal of which is approximately at the midthigh level, are posterior to the adductor longus muscle.

In amputations involving the proximal third of the femur, the adductor longus muscle must also be divided. This muscle arises from the body of the pubis, and its fibers fan out to its insertion on the linea aspera. It lies anterior to the adductor

brevis and adductor magnus muscles. The anterior branch of the obturator nerve, along with the corresponding branch of the obturator artery and, more inferiorly, the profunda femoris artery, lies in the plane between the adductor longus and the more posterior adductor muscles.

Division of the Femur and Completion of the Amputation (Fig. 97.3)

Technical Points

When a sufficient amount of muscle has been divided, circumferentially strip the periosteum from the femur with a periosteal elevator. Retract the muscles and soft tissues of the stump and divide the femur obliquely with a pneumatic or Gigli saw. Angle the cut so that the anterior surface is slightly shorter than the posterior surface. Use a rasp to smooth the cut surface of the bone. If the cavity of the marrow tends to ooze, apply bone wax to seal the cavity.

The profunda femoris artery and vein lie close on the bone and may be encountered as the bone is divided. Careful stripping of the periosteum should elevate these vessels, which can then be ligated.

The sciatic nerve lies medially and posteriorly, between the biceps femoris and the semitendinosus muscles. Ligate and cleanly divide the sciatic nerve under tension, allowing it to retract. Cut the sciatic nerve and then clamp and tie it with a heavy nonabsorbable suture. Allow it to retract into the stump.

Divide the remaining muscles and soft tissues rapidly, achieving temporary hemostasis by applying pressure. Definitive hemostasis is more easily obtained after the amputation is completed.

Anatomic Points

After division of the femur, the structures in the posterior compartment of the thigh must be divided. If the femur is divided distal to the level of the adductor hiatus, the popliteal artery and vein will be encountered. Posterior to these, but with varying degrees of approximation to vascular structures (depending on the level of amputation), the sciatic nerve will be encountered. This nerve is posteromedial and can present as a medial tibial nerve and a lateral common peroneal nerve. In the more distal part of the thigh, the sciatic nerve is located in the connective tissue posterolateral to the biceps femoris muscle. More superiorly, the long head of the biceps femoris muscle (which arises from the ischial tuberosity) crosses posterior to the sciatic nerve to join the short head of the biceps femoris (which arises from most of the lateral lip of the linea aspera) to insert on the lateral femoral condyle and head of the fibula. It should be noted that the sciatic nerve is accompanied by the slender ischiatic artery, typically a branch of the inferior gluteal artery. This artery represents the proximal part of the original axial artery of the extremity and occasionally can be the primary vascular supply to the lower extremity.

Two other muscles, both of which lie in the posterior compartment, must be divided to complete the amputation.

FIGURE 97.3
DIVISION OF THE FEMUR AND COMPLETION OF THE AMPUTATION

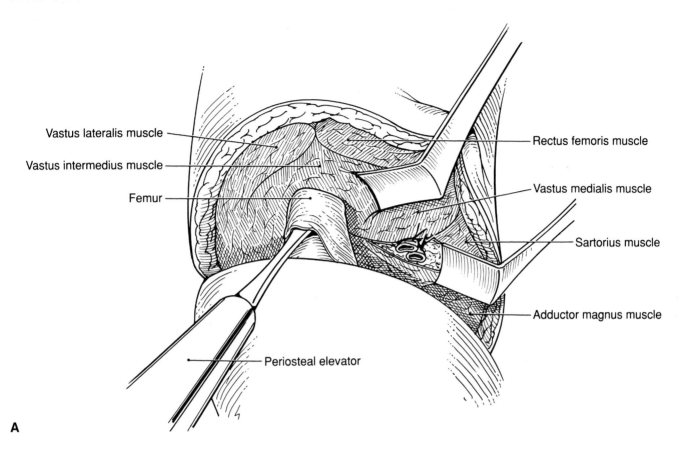

Vastus lateralis muscle

Vastus intermedius muscle

Femur

Periosteal elevator

Rectus femoris muscle

Vastus medialis muscle

Sartorius muscle

Adductor magnus muscle

A

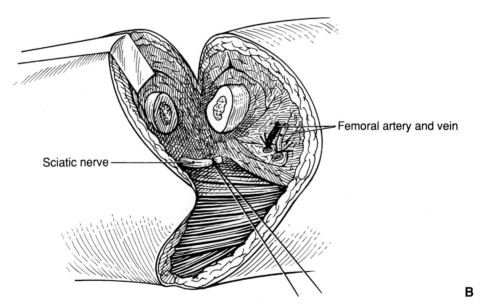

Sciatic nerve

Femoral artery and vein

B

These posteromedial muscles are closely related, spatially and functionally, to each other. Of the two, the semitendinosus muscle is most superficial. It arises from the ischial tuberosity by a tendon in common with the long head of the biceps femoris. It presents as a fleshy, fusiform muscle belly that ends about midthigh in a long, rounded tendon inserting on the medial tibial surface posterior to the insertions of the sartorius and gracilis muscles. The other muscle is the semimembranosus muscle, which arises by a flat tendon from the ischial tuberosity that rapidly develops into an aponeurosis. About midthigh, fleshy fibers arise to constitute the belly of the semimembranosus muscle. These fibers converge on a distal aponeurosis slightly proximal to the knee, and this aponeurosis changes to a complex tendon that basically inserts into the medial tibial condyle.

FIGURE 97.4
CLOSURE OF THE STUMP

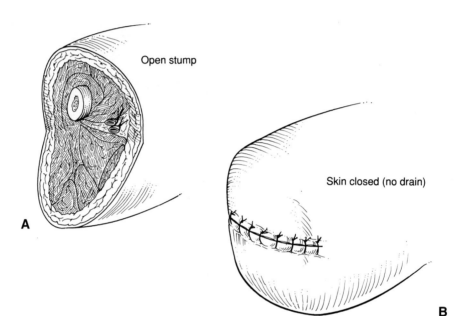

Closure of the Stump (Fig. 97.4)

Technical and Anatomic Points

Check hemostasis in the stump and irrigate it to remove fragments of bone and foreign material. Approximate the muscles over the bone and close the fascia with multiple interrupted 2-0 Vicryl sutures.

Trim the skin flaps so that they oppose each other without "dog ears" and without tension. If the flaps are under tension, revise the stump by shortening the femur. Close the skin with multiple interrupted fine sutures. Place a soft, bulky dressing on the stump.

REFERENCES

1. Berardi RS, Keonin Y. Amputations in peripheral vascular occlusive disease. *Am J Surg* 1978;135:231.
2. Berlemont M, Weber R, Willot JP. Ten years' experience with immediate application of prosthetic devices to amputees of the lower extremity on the operating table. *Prosthet Orthot Int* 1969;3:8.
3. Burgess EM. General principles of amputation surgery. In: American Academy of Orthopaedic Surgeons. *Atlas of limb prosthetics: surgical and prosthetic principles.* St Louis: CV Mosby, 1981:14.
4. Burgess EM, Romano RL, Zettl JH, et al. Amputations of the leg for peripheral vascular insufficiency. *J Bone Joint Surg Am* 1971;53: 874.
5. Couch NP, David JK, Tilney NL, et al. Natural history of the leg amputee. *Am J Surg* 1977;133:469.
6. Gottschalk F. Transfemoral amputation: biomechanics and surgery. *Clin Orthop Relat Res* 1999;361:15–22. (Presents excellent review.)
7. Medhat MA. Rehabilitation of the vascular amputee. *Orthop Rev* 1983; 12:51.
8. Shea JD. Surgical techniques of lower extremity amputation. *Orthop Clin North Am* 1972;3:287.
9. Wheelock FC, Dale WA, Jamieson CW, et al. Above-knee amputation. In: Malt RA, ed. *Surgical techniques illustrated: a comparative atlas.* Philadelphia: WB Saunders, 1985:528.

CHAPTER 98

Ligation, Stripping, and Harvesting of the Saphenous Vein

Jamal J. Hoballah

This chapter covers excision of the greater and lesser saphenous veins first for management of varicosities and second for use as a vascular conduit.

Superficial venous insufficiency and varicose vein formation can develop in the trunk of the greater or lesser saphenous veins and their respective branches. The resulting varicose veins may be asymptomatic or cause a variety of symptoms, including heaviness in the leg, an itching or burning sensation, and venous stasis ulcerations. Compression stockings are often used as the first line of therapy, but symptoms may persist. Difficulty with compliance, particularly during hot weather, and dissatisfaction with the cosmetic appearance of the legs cause many patients to seek other therapy. Surgical removal, described here, has stood the test of time as an effective management. The key principle remains to remove all varicose veins using the smallest skin incisions possible and to minimize complications.

The saphenous vein is usually stripped by inserting a stripper from one end of the vein toward the other. The stripper is usually passed from the distal end toward the groin to avoid catching on valve cusps. The distal end of the vein is then ligated around the stripper, and the vein is pulled out. The branch veins are usually excised using very small incisions through which the branch may be grasped and avulsed—the so-called "stab incision and vein avulsion" technique. Traditionally, the greater saphenous vein was stripped from the ankle to the groin. However, this approach was found to be associated with saphenous nerve injury because of proximity

and adherence of the saphenous nerve to the greater saphenous vein in the lower leg. In addition, the posterior arch vein is usually the main pathway of incompetence in the leg rather than the saphenous vein. Consequently, it is currently recommended to strip the greater saphenous vein from just below the knee level to the groin. The lowest recurrence rates are obtained by combining stripping of the saphenous vein with excision of the associated branches.

Frequently, varicosities are limited to these branches, and the main trunks are relatively normal and of small caliber. Stripping the trunk in this situation may deprive the patient of a vein that could be a useful conduit in the future should the need for lower extremity or coronary revascularization arise. Thus, some surgeons recommend avoiding stripping the saphenous veins when the varicosities are limited to the branches. In this situation, only stab avulsion of the varicosities is performed. This procedure may be complemented by ligation and division of the saphenofemoral junction if this is proved incompetent by duplex ultrasound evaluation.

Stripping the Greater Saphenous Vein: Exposure of the Saphenofemoral Junction (Fig. 98.1)

Technical Points

A 3- to 4-cm transverse incision in the inguinal crease has an excellent cosmetic result. Preoperative duplex ultrasonography allows precise mapping of the veins, including the saphenofemoral junction. It can be especially helpful in

LIST OF STRUCTURES

Femoral artery	Posterior femoral cutaneous nerve	Pubic tubercle
Common femoral vein	Sural nerve	Fascia lata
Greater (great) saphenous vein; saphenofemoral junction	Lateral cutaneous nerve	Saphenous hiatus (fossa ovalis)
	Musculocutaneous nerve	Adductor canal
Lesser saphenous vein	Patella	Sartorius muscle
Femoral nerve	Lateral malleolus	Gastrocnemius muscle
Saphenous nerve	Medial malleolus	
Medial femoral cutaneous nerve	Inguinal crease	

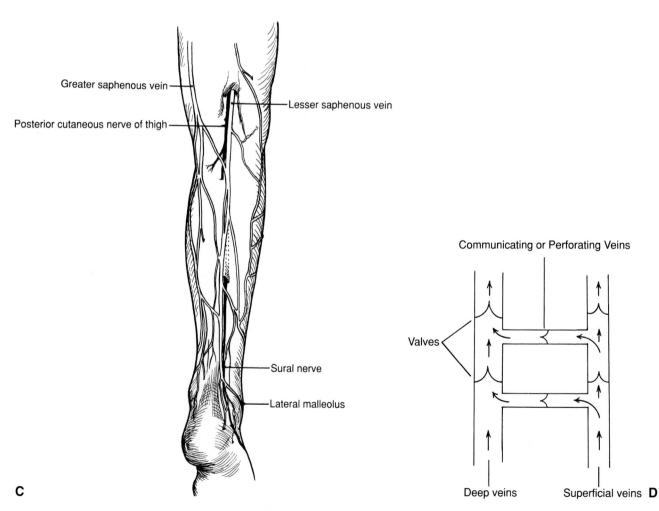

determining the location of the greater saphenous vein just below the knee when the leg is large or the patient obese. If preoperative mapping was performed, center the skin incision over the saphenofemoral junction. Alternatively, use anatomic landmarks and begin the inguinal crease incision 1 cm medial to the femoral pulse and extend it medially for 3 to 4 cm (Fig. 98.1A). If the femoral pulse is not palpable, identify a point midway between the pubic tubercle and anterosuperior iliac spine and begin the skin incision 1 cm medial to this point. Deepen the incision through the subcutaneous tissues and Scarpa's fascia to expose the vein. Often, one of the branches draining into the saphenofemoral junction is encountered first; trace this to the saphenofemoral junction. Skeletonize the saphenofemoral junction, and ligate and divide all the branches draining into it. These branches include the epigastric vein, the circumflex iliac vein, the external pudendal vein, and the anterolateral vein.

Ligate the greater saphenous vein 2 cm distal to the saphenofemoral junction. Apply a clamp to the saphenofemoral junction and divide the saphenous vein, suture-ligating the saphenofemoral junction with 2-0 silk.

Anatomic Points

The greater saphenous vein originates on the medial side of the arch of the dorsum of the foot (Fig. 98.1B). It ascends anterior to the tip of the medial malleolus and then over the subcutaneous surface of the lower end of the tibia. The greater saphenous vein continues up to the knee, where it moves posterior to the back part of the internal condyle of the femur and then follows the course of the sartorius muscle up to the inguinal region. Below the knee, the greater saphenous vein lies in a superficial subcutaneous plane and is accompanied by the great saphenous nerve. The saphenous nerve is a branch of the femoral nerve transmitting sensation from the medial aspect of the leg and foot. Above the knee, the greater saphenous vein gradually moves into a deeper subcutaneous plane and penetrates the fascia lata in the upper thigh through the fossa ovalis to join the common femoral vein. In the thigh, the greater saphenous vein is accompanied by branches of the medial femoral cutaneous nerve. The length of the greater saphenous vein in an adult male is estimated to be 60 cm. Frequently, a duplicate system can be found in the thigh (35%) or in the leg. The vein contains about 8 to 12 valves, with more valves present in the below-knee segment.

The greater saphenous vein has several important branches. The anterolateral and the posteromedial veins represent the main branches in the thigh. The posterior arch vein (vein of Leonardo) is the main branch in the leg and deserves special attention because it has numerous perforators. It runs parallel and posterior to the saphenous vein in the leg and usually joins the saphenous vein just below the knee.

The lesser saphenous vein starts posterior to the lateral malleolus along the lateral border of the Achilles tendon (Fig. 98.1C). It crosses above the Achilles tendon and reaches the midline of the posterior aspect of the leg. The lesser saphenous vein continues upward in the subcutaneous tissues and usually penetrates the muscular fascia at the level where the tendon of the gastrocnemius muscle starts. The vein runs just below the fascia to join the popliteal vein between the heads of the gastrocnemius muscle. The lesser saphenous vein is accompanied by the lesser saphenous nerve and measures about 30 cm.

In addition to draining into the femoral and popliteal veins through the saphenofemoral and saphenopopliteal junctions, the greater and lesser saphenous veins and their branches communicate with the deep veins through communicating veins that perforate the deep fascia to join the deep venous system. These perforating veins are frequently paired, are spread throughout the lower extremity, and may be as numerous as 60 perforators per extremity. Typically, when lying supine, the superficial venous system empties the blood into the deep venous system through the saphenofemoral or saphenopopliteal junctions. During standing or walking, the perforating veins become the major route of blood flow from the superficial to the deep system. Except for those smaller than 2 mm in diameter, perforators tend to have valves that help prevent the blood refluxing from the deep to the superficial venous system during muscle contractions (Fig. 98.1D). In the presence of deep venous obstruction, the perforators become an important collateral route, diverting the flow from the deep to the superficial system. Although most perforators are unnamed, some carry the names of those who described them. May or Kuster perforators connect the greater saphenous vein in the ankle and foot to posterior tibial and plantar veins. Bassi perforators connect the lesser saphenous vein to the posterior tibial and peroneal veins posteriorly in the lower leg. Cockett perforators are three sets of veins connecting the posterior arch vein to the posterior tibial veins and are located proximal to the medial malleolus. It is worth mentioning that in the leg, most of the perforators draining to the gastrocnemius, soleus, and posterior tibial veins originate from the posterior arch vein of Leonardo rather than the greater saphenous vein. Boyd perforators connect the greater saphenous vein to the gastrocnemius vein. Dodd perforators connect the greater saphenous vein to the superficial femoral vein.

Stripping the Greater Saphenous Vein: Distal Dissection and Stripping; Lesser Saphenous Vein (Fig. 98.2)

Technical Points

Below the knee, make a 1-cm transverse or longitudinal incision over the marked greater saphenous vein. The vein is usually identified directly beneath the skin. Ligate the distal end of the vein (Fig. 98.2A) and make a small venotomy proximal to the ligature. Introduce the stripper, guide it up to the groin, and allow it to exit from the ligated inguinal end of the saphenous vein. Apply an olive-shaped head to the distal end of the stripper, securing it with a ligature around the vein. Divide the vein distal to the venotomy. Apply the handle on the inguinal end of the stripper (Fig. 98.2B,C). Steadily and firmly pull the stripper, applying mild pressure on the stripper head and gentle countertraction on the skin, to extract stripper and vein from the inguinal incision (Fig. 98.2D).

FIGURE 98.2
STRIPPING THE GREATER SAPHENOUS VEIN: DISTAL DISSECTION AND STRIPPING; LESSER SAPHENOUS VEIN

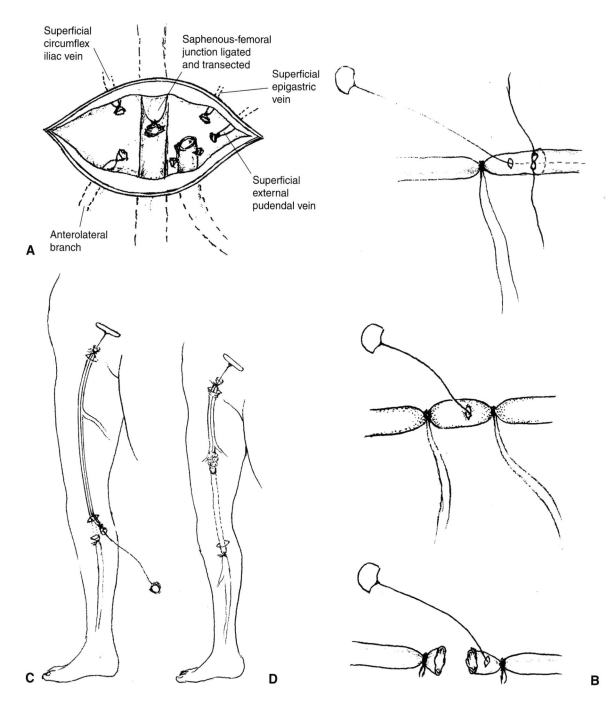

If the vein is to be stripped from the ankle, make a 1-cm transverse or longitudinal incision 1 cm anterior and superior to the medial malleolus. Identify and mobilize the saphenous nerve away from the vein. Pass the stripper and remove the vein as previously described.

After stripping the vein, roll a towel over the medial aspect of the extremity to express any blood collecting in the track of the stripped vein. Irrigate the wound and close it with 3-0 absorbable sutures for the subcutaneous tissue and 4-0 absorbable subcuticular sutures for the skin. Apply elastic bandages from the ankle to the upper thigh.

To strip the lesser saphenous vein, place the patient in the prone position. Make a 2- to 3-cm transverse skin incision behind the knee over the marked vein. Identify the lesser saphenous vein just beneath the skin and trace it to the saphenopopliteal junction. Next, make a 1-cm transverse or

FIGURE 98.3
EXCISION OF BRANCH VARICOSITIES USING STAB AVULSION TECHNIQUE

A
B

longitudinal incision over the lateral aspect of the ankle to identify the distal end of the vein. Identify and separate the sural nerve from the distal vein. Strip the vein as described previously.

Excision of Branch Varicosities Using Stab Avulsion Technique (Fig. 98.3)

Technical Points

It is essential that all the branches be accurately marked with the patient standing upright using marking ink. Make a 1- to 2-mm stab incision along the side of the branch to be removed using a number 11 blade or a 14-gauge needle. Introduce a crochet hook and pass it under the anticipated location of the vein. Withdraw the hook, catching a loop of the vein (Fig. 98.3A). Grasp the loop with a fine hemostat and tease it

out of the incision. Divide the vein loop between two clamps (Fig. 98.3B). Gently pull one end of the transected vein, using a rotating movement. Gently peel away any surrounding soft tissues. Reapply the clamp closer to the skin and again pull the vein until it is avulsed. Repeat the technique with the other end of the transected vein. Make another stab incision 6 to 8 cm from the prior incision along the anticipated course of the vein and repeat. Continue this procedure until all the branches have been excised.

Exposure and Harvesting of the Greater Saphenous Vein for Bypass Procedures (Fig. 98.4)

Technical and Anatomic Points

The greater saphenous vein is considered the gold standard with which all other conduits are compared when performing infrainguinal reconstructions. It is also the most commonly used conduit in coronary revascularization. When used for infrainguinal revascularization, the greater saphenous vein is either harvested or kept in its bed (*in situ* bypass; see Chapter 100), a procedure that requires disruption of its valves to allow for blood flow. When harvested, the vein is either reversed (reversed vein bypass) or used nonreversed, which also necessitates disruption of its valves (nonreversed vein bypass). Valve disruption is usually performed using a valvulotome. Improper valvulotomy may injure the vein or fail to disrupt the valves completely. A good-quality saphenous vein that measures 3 cm or greater in diameter will perform equally well as a reversed, nonreversed, or *in situ* bypass. Small veins (<3 cm in diameter) tend to perform better if used in an *in situ* or nonreversed fashion.

It is essential to use proper technique to avoid injury, which may occur by one of several mechanisms. First, the vein wall can be crushed with the forceps during dissection. Consequently, try to grasp only the adventitia with the forceps. Excessive traction applied to a Silastic loop passed around the vein may injure the conduit. Injury can also occur if small branches are inadvertently avulsed during the dissection or if branches are ligated very close to the body of the graft, thus narrowing the lumen. Overdistention of the vein may result in significant endothelial damage. Avoid this by monitoring intraluminal pressure and keeping it below 300 mm Hg. Chilled whole blood, or a cold solution of Ringer's lactate

(1 L) or dextran 40 (1 L) mixed with 5,000 U of heparin and 60 mg of papaverine, can be used to distend the vein or to run through the conduit while harvesting. This maintains flow and helps avoid the formation of intraluminal thrombi. Finally, it is important to keep the exposed or harvested vein moist and avoid desiccation injury. Avoid this by covering the vein with gauze soaked with warm saline. Adding papaverine (60 mg/500 mL) may help decrease spasm in the conduit.

Preoperative evaluation of the greater saphenous vein with duplex ultrasonography allows the location to be mapped. The skin incision can then be made over the marked skin. Alternatively, use anatomic landmarks. At the ankle level, make a longitudinal incision 1 cm anterior and superior to the medial malleolus. Identify the vein directly beneath the skin. At the inguinal region, begin the incision 1.5 cm medial to the femoral pulse and extend it at a 30-degree angle to the vertical axis of the lower extremity. If the femoral pulse is not palpable, begin the incision 1.5 cm medial to a point midway between the pubic tubercle and the anterosuperior iliac spine. Deepen the incision through the subcutaneous tissues and Scarpa's fascia to expose the vein.

The entire vein can be exposed through a single long incision (Fig. 98.4A) or through multiple 6- to 8-cm incisions separated by 4- to 6-cm skin bridges in an attempt to minimize the morbidity of the single long incision (Fig. 98.4B). Currently, various methods are also available to allow for endoscopic harvesting of the greater saphenous vein through

---

FIGURE 98.4
EXPOSURE AND HARVESTING OF THE GREATER SAPHENOUS VEIN FOR BYPASS PROCEDURES

Greater saphenous vein

A

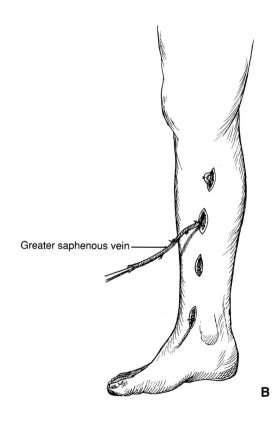

Greater saphenous vein

B

FIGURE 98.4   (Continued)

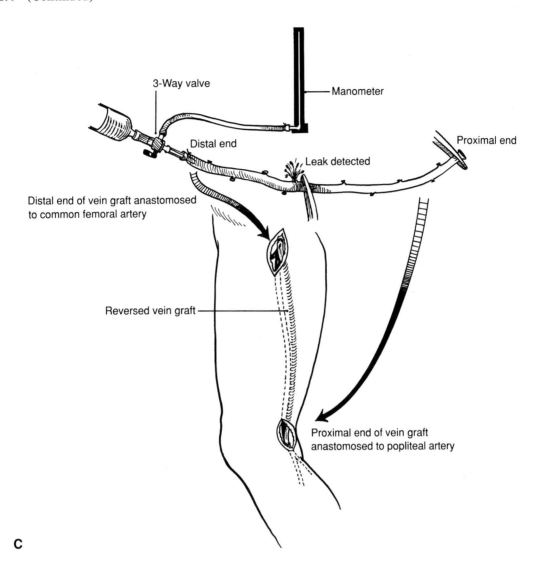

C

a single small inguinal incision and or additional 1- to 2-cm incisions placed at various locations above or below the knee.

Identify a side branch near the most distal part of the vein and introduce a blunt-tipped needle through this site (Fig. 98.4C). Tie the needle in place with a silk ligature and allow the distention solution to drip slowly into the vein lumen. Alternatively, ligate and divide the vein at its most distal end, and use this site to introduce the blunt-tipped needle. Gently encircle the vein with a Silastic loop; lift it and free it of surrounding tissue with sharp dissecting scissors. Identify, ligate, and divide all tributaries.

If the conduit is to be used in the nonreversed fashion, leave long 3-mm stumps on several branches along the body of the vein. Introduce the valvulotome through the distal end of the vein and through these stumps (see Fig. 100.5).

When the greater saphenous vein is not available, the lesser saphenous vein represents a good alternative autogenous conduit. Because of its small length, the lesser saphenous vein is typically used for short bypasses or bypass revisions. When

contemplating using the lesser saphenous vein, preoperative assessment with duplex ultrasonography and mapping of its course is recommended. If vein mapping is not available, begin a longitudinal skin incision in the middle of the posterior aspect of the calf. Deepen this incision through the subcutaneous tissue until the fascia is identified. Incise the fascia, exposing the saphenous vein directly underneath it. The lesser saphenous vein can be harvested with the patient lying prone or supine. Both involve some compromise. The prone position provides the best exposure but will usually require turning the patient back to a supine position and again prepping and draping. When the patient is lying supine, external rotation of the leg and the gastrocnemius muscle will allow access to the lesser saphenous vein. However, the junction to the popliteal vein remains challenging to expose from this approach. The lesser saphenous vein can also be approached through a medial skin incision; however, this requires the creation of large skin flaps and allows access to only a short segment of the vein.

REFERENCES

1. Allen KB, Shaar CJ. Endoscopic saphenous vein harvesting. *Annu Thorac Surg* 1997;64:265–266.
2. Crane C. The surgery of varicose veins. *Surg Clin North Am* 1979;59: 737.
3. Goren G, Yellin AE. Ambulatory stab avulsion phlebectomy for truncal varicose veins. *Am J Surg* 1991;162:166–174.
4. Large J. Surgical treatment of saphenous varices, with preservation of the main great saphenous trunk. *J Vasc Surg* 1985;2:887.
5. Nabatoff RA. The short saphenous vein. *Surg Gynecol Obstet* 1979;149: 49.
6. Samuels PB. Technique of varicose vein surgery. *Am J Surg* 1981;142: 239.
7. Thomson H. The surgical anatomy of the superficial and perforator veins of the lower limb. *Ann R Coll Surg Engl* 1979;61: 198.

CHAPTER 99

Venous Access: Saphenous Vein Cutdown

The greater saphenous vein can be used as an anatomically constant and easily cannulated vein for emergency venous access. The saphenous vein at the ankle is constant, although it may be involved by varicose vein disease in elderly patients. In children, it is a useful route of access, especially because it is somewhat removed from the central area and thus out of the way of resuscitative attempts. Bony landmarks render the vein easy to find.

The greater saphenous vein at the groin is sometimes used for introduction of an extremely large catheter, such as a sterile oxygen flow catheter, through which blood and intravenous fluids can be infused rapidly in a patient with traumatic injuries. The techniques of saphenous vein cutdown at the ankle and the groin are described in this chapter. Alternatives are discussed in the references at the end.

LIST OF STRUCTURES

Common femoral vein
  Greater saphenous vein
  Saphenofemoral junction
  Superficial epigastric vein
  Superficial circumflex iliac vein
  Superficial external pudendal vein

Medial malleolus
Patella
Inguinal ligament
Superficial fascia
Fascia lata
  Saphenous hiatus (fossa ovalis)

Femoral nerve
  Saphenous nerve
  Medial femoral cutaneous nerve
  Anterior femoral cutaneous nerve

FIGURE 99.1
SAPHENOUS VEIN CUTDOWN AT THE ANKLE

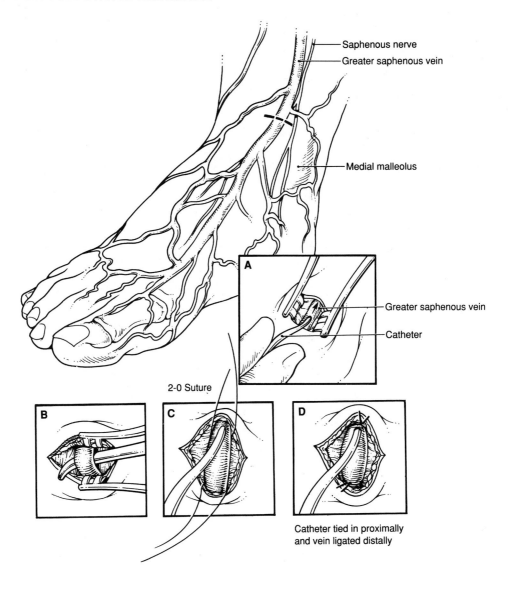

Saphenous nerve
Greater saphenous vein
Medial malleolus

A

Greater saphenous vein
Catheter

2-0 Suture

B

C

D

Catheter tied in proximally
and vein ligated distally

Saphenous Vein Cutdown at the Ankle (Fig. 99.1)

Technical Points

Place the leg in external rotation and prep the medial aspect of the ankle from the medial malleolus around to the anterior aspect of the ankle. Infiltrate the area of the proposed skin incision, which will be two fingerbreadths above and two fingerbreadths medial to the medial malleolus. Make a transverse incision through the skin. The greater saphenous vein will lie immediately under the skin. Take great care not to enter the vein while making the initial skin incision. Spread tissues in a longitudinal fashion as you look for the saphenous vein. The saphenous vein is usually at least 3 to 5 mm in diameter and often is even larger.

Elevate the saphenous vein into the field and clean it by sharp and blunt dissection. Identify and protect the saphenous nerve. Place ligatures proximally and distally and make a venotomy on the anterior surface of the vein. Introduce the catheter and secure it, tying the catheter into place proximally and ligating the vein distally.

Anatomic Points

The greater saphenous vein is typically the largest and, in most cases, anatomically the most consistent of the superficial veins. It starts on the medial side of the dorsal venous arch of the foot, passing from there 2.5 to 3 cm anterior to the medial-most projection of the medial malleolus. From there, it courses up the medial side of the leg, passing posterior to the knee joint, about 8 to 10 cm posterior to the anteromedial border of the patella. It then ascends in the superficial fascia of the thigh to a point about 2.5 cm distal to the inguinal ligament,

FIGURE 99.2
SAPHENOUS VEIN CUTDOWN AT THE GROIN

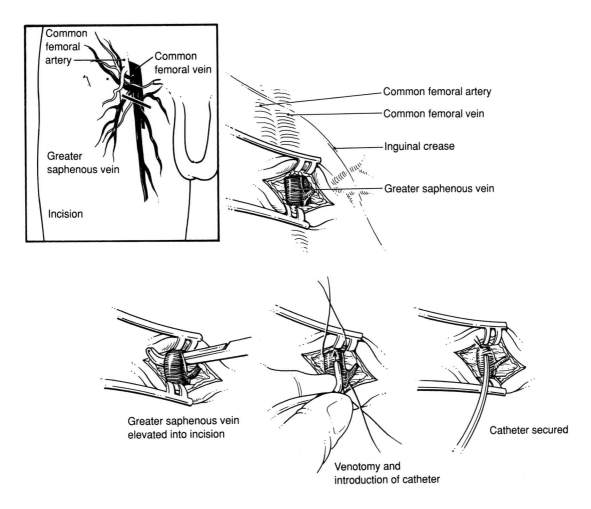

Greater saphenous vein elevated into incision

Venotomy and introduction of catheter

Catheter secured

where it passes through the saphenous hiatus (fossa ovalis) of the fascia lata to terminate in the common femoral vein.

At the ankle, the greater saphenous vein is very superficial and thus can be injured when making the initial skin incision. The saphenous nerve is a sensory branch of the femoral nerve. It typically runs immediately anterior to the greater saphenous vein.

Saphenous Vein Cutdown at the Groin (Fig. 99.2)

Technical Points

Place the extremity in moderate external rotation. The skin incision will be made medial to the femoral pulse, about two fingerbreadths below the inguinal crease. Make a transverse incision about 4 cm in length. The saphenous vein will lie on the subcutaneous fat and will be relatively superficial.

Identify the saphenous vein and elevate it into the incision. Make a venotomy on the anterior surface of the vein and introduce the catheter as previously described. Secure the catheter in place and close the incision with absorbable suture material.

Anatomic Points

The inguinal skin crease does not always directly correspond with the location of the deeper inguinal ligament. In thin people, the skin crease is immediately superficial to the ligament, but in most people, it is 2 to 3 cm distal. Because the saphenous hiatus (fossa ovalis) is located about 2.5 to 3 cm distal to the inguinal ligament, the initial skin incision for exposure of this vein should always be distal to the skin crease (i.e., one should attempt to gain access to the vein while it is in the superficial fascia, not at the hiatus itself).

In its course through the thigh, the saphenous vein lies deeper than it does in the lower leg. Typically, it is located between two layers of superficial fascia, its depth being dependent on the amount of adipose tissue in the thigh. In its upper part, it typically receives large tributaries draining the posteromedial and anterolateral thigh as well as the smaller peri-inguinal veins (superficial epigastric, circumflex iliac, and external pudendal veins). In addition, it frequently is closely related to branches of the medial femoral cutaneous nerve, or to other sensory branches (eg, anterior femoral cutaneous nerve) of the femoral nerve.

REFERENCES

1. American College of Surgeons Committee on Trauma. Shock. In: *Advanced trauma life support manual.* 6th ed. Chicago: American College of Surgeons, 1997:133–146. (Presents excellent discussion of alternatives, including percutaneous femoral line placement and interosseous infusion.)
2. Hansbrough JF, Cain RL, Millikan JS. Placement of 10-gauge catheter by cutdown for rapid fluid replacement. *J Trauma* 1983;23:231. (Provides classic description of rapid infusion line placement.)
3. Redo SF. Venous cutdown procedures. In: *Atlas of surgery in the first six months of life.* Hagerstown, MD: Harper & Row, 1978. (Provides excellent discussion of issues related to infants.)

CHAPTER 100

Femoropopliteal Bypass

Kenneth B. Simon

A variety of conduits have been used to bypass obstructed segments of the femoropopliteal system. Autogenous saphenous vein is the graft preferred by most surgeons. The saphenous vein may be removed completely from the contralateral leg, as described in Chapter 98, and used in a reversed fashion. Alternatively, an *in situ* bypass may be performed. In this chapter, the technique of *in situ* saphenous vein bypass is described.

Sites of Groin Incision (Fig. 100.1)

Technical Points

Place the patient supine on the operating table with the thigh mildly externally rotated, flexed, and elevated at the level of the knee joint. Palpate the inguinal ligament and identify the pubic tubercle and anterosuperior iliac spine. Place a longitudinal skin incision centered over the femoral artery (Fig. 100.1A). This skin incision should extend from 2 to 3 cm above the inguinal ligament to about 10 cm below the inguinal ligament. The profunda femoris artery usually takes off from the common femoral artery at the level of the inguinal ligament or about 1 to 3 cm distal to it. The skin incision must, therefore, extend above the inguinal ligament to expose the common femoral artery adequately. If the incision or dissection is below the usual anatomic bifurcation of the common femoral artery, only the superficial femoral artery will be seen.

Several lymph nodes will be found anterior to the femoral artery in the femoral canal (Fig. 100.1B). Be careful to avoid injury to the lymphatic channels and lymph nodes in this area. Disruption of the lymphatic system can result in lymphorrhea, lymphocele formation, or wound problems. Dissect the common femoral, profunda femoris, and superficial femoral arteries gently. A small venous branch courses over the profunda femoris artery. Ligate and divide this vein to allow access to the profunda femoris distal to its first perforating branch. Obtain proximal control of the common femoral artery and distal control of both the superficial femoral and profunda femoris arteries using Silastic loops.

The greater saphenous vein is superficial and medial to the common femoral artery. The groin incision diagrammed allows for excellent exposure of the saphenous vein. Either continuous or interrupted skin incisions may be used to perform an *in situ* bypass.

LIST OF STRUCTURES

Inguinal ligament
Pubic tubercle
Anterosuperior iliac spine
Femur
   Medial femoral condyle
Superficial circumflex iliac artery and
   vein
Superficial epigastric artery
Superficial external pudendal artery
   and vein
Inguinal lymph nodes
Femoral sheath
Fascia lata
Femoral artery
   Superficial femoral artery
Popliteal artery

Mediosuperior genicular artery
Laterosuperior genicular artery
Middle genicular artery
Anterior tibial artery
Posterior tibial artery
   Peroneal artery
Profunda femoris artery
   Medial femoral circumflex artery
   Lateral femoral circumflex artery
Femoral vein
   Greater saphenous vein
   Lesser saphenous vein
Femoral nerve
Saphenous nerve
Peroneal nerve
Saphenous hiatus (fossa ovalis)

Inguinal lymph nodes
Iliopsoas muscle
Pectineus muscle
Adductor brevis muscle
Adductor longus muscle
Adductor magnus muscle
Adductor tubercle
Adductor canal
Sartorius muscle
Semimembranosus muscle
Semitendinosus muscle
Vastus medialis muscle
Popliteal fossa (space)
Soleus muscle
Calcaneal tendon
Gastrocnemius muscle

FIGURE 100.1
SITES OF GROIN INCISION

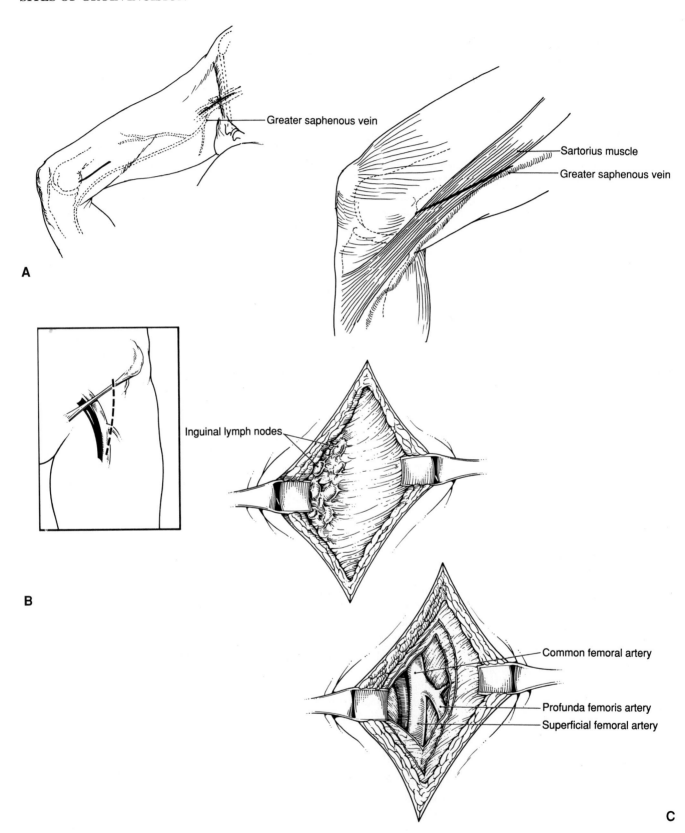

A

B

C

Greater saphenous vein

Sartorius muscle

Greater saphenous vein

Inguinal lymph nodes

Common femoral artery

Profunda femoris artery

Superficial femoral artery

Anatomic Points

The common femoral artery is the most lateral structure in the femoral sheath. It reliably bisects the inguinal ligament. This relationship can be used to locate the femoral artery, even when occlusive disease prevents location of a palpable pulse. The femoral nerve lies immediately lateral to the femoral artery, whereas the femoral vein is immediately medial to the artery.

Exposure of the femoral artery demands dissection through the superficial fascia, fascia lata, and femoral sheath. The superficial fascia in this region contains the superficial circumflex iliac vessels, the superficial epigastric vessels, and the superficial external pudendal vessels. The arteries, which are branches of the (common) femoral artery, all pass through the cribriform fascia of the saphenous hiatus, or penetrate the fascia lata adjacent to the hiatus, to gain access to the superficial fascia. Typically, the veins are tributaries of the greater saphenous vein and either join this vein before its passage through the cribriform fascia or pass through the cribriform fascia independently, draining into the saphenous vein just before it empties into the femoral vein.

The largest vascular structure in the superficial fascia is the greater saphenous vein, which essentially overlies the proximal femoral vein and is thus medial to the femoral artery axis. In its course in the upper thigh, it lies between two layers of superficial fascia and is, therefore, not as obvious as it is in the lower leg. In addition to receiving the small tributaries mentioned earlier, typically, one or more larger tributaries draining the thigh or communicating with the lesser saphenous vein also drain into the greater saphenous vein.

In addition to these arteries and veins, a number of superficial inguinal lymph nodes are found in this area. These constitute two groups: horizontal and vertical nodes. The horizontal nodes (which drain the lower trunk) and their vessels parallel the inguinal ligament and are just inferior to the ligament. The vertical nodes, which drain the inferior extremity, lie in the superficial fascia over the femoral artery. Efferents from these nodes pass through the cribriform fascia and drain into nodes closely associated with the femoral canal, a space in the femoral sheath just medial to the femoral vein through which the lymphatics pass to drain into iliac nodes.

Typically, the so-called common femoral artery passes 4 to 5 cm distally before it bifurcates into the profunda femoris and superficial femoral arteries. The superficial femoral artery is a direct extension of the common femoral artery and generally lies in the same axis. With respect to the axis of the common and superficial femoral arteries, the profunda femoris originates posterolaterally, then curves posteromedially and inferiorly, posterior to the superficial femoral artery. In this part of its course, it crosses the iliopsoas, pectineus, and adductor brevis muscles. It then passes in the plane between the adductor longus and the adductor magnus muscles, where it gives off several branches. Although most of these supply the adductor muscles, typically there are four perforating branches that pass through the insertion of the adductor

magnus muscle to supply the hamstring muscles. The first two perforating arteries usually penetrate both the adductor brevis and adductor magnus muscles, whereas the third and fourth (the termination of the profunda femoris artery) penetrate only the adductor magnus. In addition to supplying the posterior compartment muscles, the penetrating arteries also anastomose with each other and with other arteries, thus providing an important collateral network. Additional branches include the medial and lateral femoral circumflex arteries; these typically arise from the profunda femoris artery, although either or both may arise from the common femoral artery. These arteries, in addition to supplying adjacent muscles, also participate in the arterial anastomosis around the hip joint. Further, the medial femoral circumflex artery provides most of the blood supply to the head of the femur.

Exposure of the profunda femoris artery necessitates skeletonization of the common femoral and proximal part of the superficial femoral arteries. When the profunda femoris artery is exposed and skeletonized, caution should be exercised because the profunda femoris vein and any of its lateral tributaries are anterior to the artery.

Exposure of the Proximal Popliteal Artery (Fig. 100.2)

Technical Points

Flex the knee, externally rotate the knee and thigh, and elevate the leg with rolls placed under the knee joint. Make a 4- to 5-inch long longitudinal incision 1 inch proximal and inferior to the adductor tubercle. The greater saphenous vein is superficial in this location. Be careful not to injure this vein inadvertently.

Use either a long continuous incision or several interrupted incisions along the course of the greater saphenous vein to perform an *in situ* bypass (Fig. 100.2A). Minimize handling of the edges of the skin incision and avoid making the skin flaps too thin. Skin flaps that are thin or traumatized with forceps, especially in patients with ischemia or occlusive vascular disease, usually result in wound problems. Complications, such as wound infections, sloughing of skin flap edges, or sloughing of the skin flap (particularly the posterior flap) often arise in such cases. A gentle, meticulous technique is therefore critical when creating the skin flaps.

Retract the sartorius muscle posteriorly and the tendons of the adductor magnus, semimembranosus, and semitendinosus muscles anteriorly (Fig. 100.2B). Identify the popliteal artery and vein along the posterior medial borders of the femur. Meticulous dissection is required to avoid injuring the venous plexus that surrounds the popliteal artery. Secure the branches of the venous plexus with Silastic loops or fine silk suture.

Anatomic Points

The popliteal artery is exposed through an incision that parallels the anterior border of the sartorius muscle and passes just posterior to the medial condyle. The greater saphenous vein

FIGURE 100.2
EXPOSURE OF THE PROXIMAL POPLITEAL ARTERY

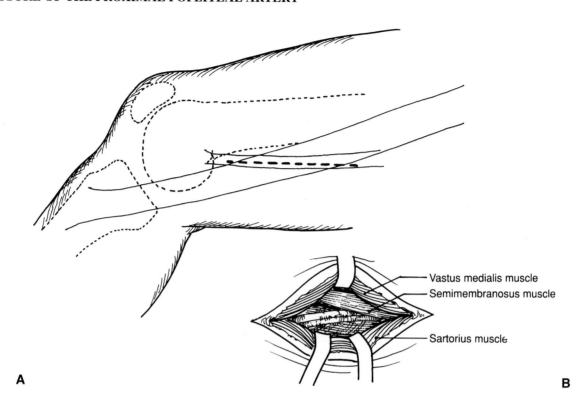

Vastus medialis muscle
Semimembranosus muscle
Sartorius muscle

A

B

and nerve lie posterior to the medial condyle and should not be damaged. The saphenous nerve, a sensory branch of the femoral nerve that provides sensation to the medial leg and foot, passes through the adductor canal along with the femoral vessels. At the level of the adductor hiatus, the saphenous nerve emerges posterior to the sartorius muscle to become superficial.

The popliteal artery is the continuation of the superficial femoral artery after its passage through the adductor canal (adductor hiatus). Exposure of the terminal superficial femoral artery and proximal popliteal artery is accomplished by opening the distal adductor canal, dividing the tendon of the adductor magnus (which forms part of the adductor hiatus), and mobilizing the distal gracilis and medial hamstring muscles. The distal adductor canal is opened by division of the intermuscular fascia between the vastus medialis and sartorius muscles, thereby allowing the sartorius muscle to be retracted posteriorly. Division of the tendon of the adductor magnus opens the adductor hiatus, the anatomic point where the (superficial) femoral artery becomes the popliteal artery. Posterior retraction of the gracilis muscle, as well as of those muscles (semitendinosus and semimembranosus) that form the superomedial boundary of the popliteal fossa, allows visualization of the contents of the popliteal fossa.

Upon exposure of the structures in the popliteal space, one will find the popliteal vein to be superficial to the popliteal artery, and both of these vessels lie deep to the tibial nerve. Note that the popliteal artery is somewhat more medial than

the vein and that the vein is somewhat more medial than the nerve.

In addition to preserving the network of small veins surrounding the popliteal artery, which are almost venular in size, it is important to preserve the genicular arteries, of which there are three in the popliteal fossa. The mediosuperior and laterosuperior genicular arteries arise from the proximal popliteal artery and pass along the floor of the popliteal space to encircle the femur, just above the respective epicondyles. Ultimately, these arteries participate in an arterial plexus around the patella, thus constituting part of the collateral circulation around the knee joint. The small middle genicular artery arises from the deep surface of the popliteal artery, quickly piercing the capsule of the knee joint to supply intrinsic ligaments and the synovial membrane of this joint.

Exposure of the Distal Popliteal Artery (Fig. 100.3)

Technical Points

Flex the knee and externally rotate and elevate the leg using rolls or a pillow. Make an incision, measuring about 7 to 10 cm in length, 1 cm posterior to the tibia and 1 to 2 cm distal to the medial femoral condyle.

An incision to expose the posterior tibial artery for a bypass located even more distally is shown in Fig. 100.6.

Anatomic Points

As on the thigh, the greater saphenous vein and nerve must be identified. The location of the vein can be closely

FIGURE 100.3
EXPOSURE OF THE DISTAL POPLITEAL ARTERY

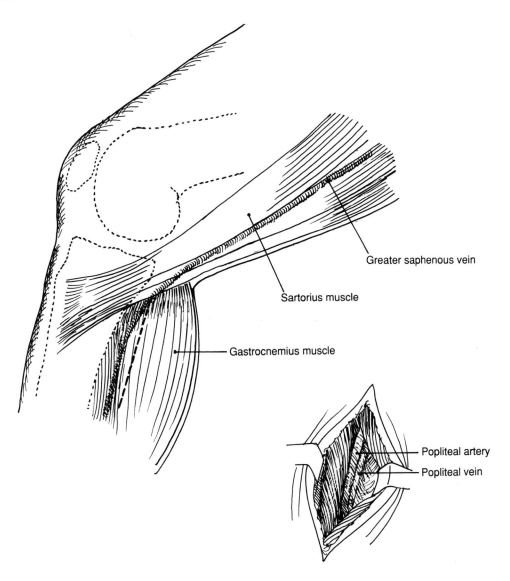

Greater saphenous vein

Sartorius muscle

Gastrocnemius muscle

Popliteal artery
Popliteal vein

approximated by a line connecting the anterior side of the medial malleolus with a point about one handbreadth (8 to 10 cm) posterior to the medial side of the patella. The saphenous nerve accompanies the vein through the superficial fascia.

Exposure of the Distal Popliteal Vessels (Fig. 100.4)

Technical Points

Incise the deep fascia to gain entrance to the popliteal vessels. Retract the soleus and gastrocnemius muscles to expose the distal popliteal artery and vein. Again, be gentle when freeing up the venous tributaries from the popliteal artery. Obtain proximal and distal control of the popliteal artery using vessel loops. If a reversed saphenous vein or prosthetic graft is to be used, create the graft tunnel before heparinization. After securing proximal and distal hemostasis of the

femoral artery and its branches, as well as of the popliteal artery, heparinize the patient with 100 U/kg of heparin. The proximal anastomosis (ie, the anastomosis of the saphenous vein to the common femoral artery) is performed using 6-0 polypropylene suture and a continuous running stitch.

Anatomic Points

To open the lower popliteal space, it is necessary first to open the crural fascia. After this is done, the semimembranosus and semitendinosus tendons must either be divided close to their tibial insertions or mobilized anteriorly. Likewise, the medial head of the gastrocnemius muscle, which originates in the medial femoral condyle and capsule of the knee joint, must be mobilized from these fibrous and bony structures as well as from the popliteus muscle; this may require division of the medial head of the gastrocnemius muscle. The soleus muscle,

FIGURE 100.4
EXPOSURE OF THE DISTAL POPLITEAL VESSELS

Popliteal artery

the deepest of the three muscles whose tendons form the calcaneal tendon, takes part of its origin from the soleal line of the tibia, just distal to the insertion of the popliteus muscle. If necessary, this muscle may be partially reflected from its origin to expose the distal-most part of the popliteal artery and the beginnings of the anterior and posterior tibial arteries.

After these muscles have been mobilized, divided, or both, the distal popliteal vessels should be apparent, wrapped in a common fibrous sheath. Frequently, the distal popliteal vein is represented by anterior and posterior tibial veins that have not yet joined to form a single popliteal vein. Regardless of whether the popliteal vein is single or multiple, the location of the largest vessels is medial to the popliteal artery.

Exposure of the anterior and posterior tibial arteries demands division of the tibial origin of the soleus muscle. If the anterior tibial artery is to be visualized posteriorly, it is also necessary to divide the anterior tibial vein because this lies medial to the artery as these vessels pass through the interosseus membrane. Exposure of the peroneal vessels usually requires complete detachment of the soleus muscle from its tibial origin because the peroneal artery usually arises from the posterior tibial artery some 2.5 to 3 cm distal to the bifurcation of the popliteal artery into anterior and posterior tibial arteries.

Throughout the exposure of the peroneal artery and its branches, care must be taken to avoid the tibial nerve. This nerve accompanies the popliteal vessels and the posterior tibial artery in its course through the leg. Typically, it is more superficial than the artery. Because it is a large nerve, its location is seldom in question.

Passage of a Valvulotome (Fig. 100.5)

Technical Points

Because valves are located anteriorly and posteriorly in the greater saphenous vein, a valvulotome must be passed in a retrograde fashion to destroy them. Use a distal venous tributary of the greater saphenous vein to pass the Mills or Leather valvulotome. Pass a LeMaitre or Hall valvulotome through the distal end of the greater saphenous vein. Allow venous tributaries to remain patent to provide runoff of the arterial inflow until all venous valves have been destroyed. Flow should be evident through the distal end of the greater saphenous vein once the venous valves are incompetent.

Use a bulldog clamp to occlude the greater saphenous vein just distal to the proximal anastomosis. Tailor the distal end of the saphenous vein in a fish-mouth fashion for the distal anastomosis.

Anatomic Points

The number and distribution of valves in the greater saphenous vein are variable, although it can be reliably stated that there are fewer valves in the vein above the knee than below it. Researchers have found that there is usually a valve at the termination of the greater saphenous vein and that there are varying numbers (range of 0 to 11) of variably spaced valves present (averaging one for every 6.6 to 8.8 cm of greater saphenous vein length present). In addition to valves, the surgeon should be aware that there are perforating veins, ranging in number from one to six (but usually two), that provide communication between the greater saphenous and the deep veins of the thigh, with the most constant perforator being located at the midthigh level. Finally, the surgeon should recognize that, with this vein, as with all superficial veins, variation is the rule. Accordingly, the surgeon may find that a variable number of tributaries, some large, drain into the greater saphenous vein, or that the greater saphenous has one or more connections with the lesser (smaller) saphenous vein, or that the greater saphenous vein is doubled in all or part of its course.

FIGURE 100.5
PASSAGE OF A VALVULOTOME

Greater saphenous vein

Valve

FIGURE 100.6
DISTAL ANASTOMOSIS

Greater saphenous vein

Posterior tibial artery

Distal Anastomosis (Fig. 100.6)

Technical and Anatomic Points

Secure proximal and distal control of the popliteal artery and make an arteriotomy 10 to 15 mm in length. Anastomose the greater saphenous vein in an end-to-side fashion using 7-0 polypropylene suture and a continuous running stitch. Upon completion of the anastomosis, ligate all venous tributaries of the saphenous vein close to the main channel to prevent arteriovenous fistula formation.

Obtain an intraoperative angiogram at the completion of the procedure to detect any arteriovenous fistulas. Inject a 50% concentration of contrast media into the saphenous vein just distal to the proximal anastomosis through a 22-gauge needle. All arteriovenous fistulas found on angiography are ligated, but not divided, adjacent to the saphenous vein.

Alternatively, upon completion of the distal anastomosis, check for arteriovenous fistulas using a sterile Doppler flow detector. This modality is an accurate, effective means of locating arteriovenous fistulas, but it often requires more operator experience than does angiography.

Irrigate all wounds with antibiotic-containing solution. Then close the subcutaneous tissue in two layers using absorbable suture. Close the skin using either skin staples or 4-0 absorbable sutures placed with a running subcuticular stitch.

REFERENCES

1. Abbott WM. Prosthetic above-knee femoral-popliteal bypass: indications and choice of graft. *Semin Vasc Surg* 1997;10(1):3–7.
2. Ascer E, Veith JF, Flores SAW. Infrapopliteal bypass to heavily calcified, rock-like arteries: management and results. *Am J Surg* 1986;152:220.
3. Imparato AM, Kim GE, Chu DS. Surgical exposure for reconstruction of the proximal part of the tibial artery. *Surg Gynecol Obstet* 1973;136:453.
4. Karmody AM, Leather RP, Shah DM, et al. Peroneal artery bypass: a reappraisal of its value in limb salvage. *J Vasc Surg* 1984;1:809.
5. Leather RP, Shah DM, Corson JD, et al. Instrumental evolution of the valve incision method of in situ saphenous vein bypass. *J Vasc Surg* 1984;1:113. (Reviews techniques of valve destruction for *in situ* bypass.)
6. Mitchell RA, Bone GE, Bridges R, et al. Patient selection for isolated profundaplasty: arteriographic correlates of operative results. *Am J Surg* 1979;138:912.
7. Pomposelli FB Jr, Jepsen SJ, Gibbons GW, et al. A flexible approach to infrapopliteal vein grafts in patients with diabetes mellitus. *Arch Surg* 1991;126(6):724–727; discussion, 727–729.
8. Schulman ML, Badhey MR, Yatco R. Superficial femoral-popliteal veins and reversed saphenous veins as femoropopliteal bypass grafts: a randomized comparative study. *J Vasc Surg* 1987;6(1):1–10.
9. Skudder PA Jr, Rhodes GA. Hemodynamics of in situ vein bypass: the role of side branch fistulae. *Ann Vasc Surg* 1986;1(3):335–339.
10. Tiefenbrun J, Beckerman M, Singer A. Surgical anatomy in bypass of the distal part of the lower limb. *Surg Gynecol Obstet* 1975;141:528.
11. Tilson MD, Baue AE. Obturator canal bypass graft for infection of the femoral artery. *Surg Rounds* 1981;14.
12. White GH. Angioscopy. *Surg Clin North Am* 1992;72:791. (Presents useful review of a technique in evolution.)

CHAPTER 101

Fasciotomy

Kenneth B. Simon

Strong fascial envelopes surround major muscle groups, dividing them into compartments. Hemorrhage or edema within a compartment causes the pressure within this closed space to rise rapidly. Fasciotomy (incision of the fascia) is indicated when the intracompartmental pressure rises to the point of compromising neuromuscular function. Burns, crush injuries, arterial occlusion or embolism, hypotension, venous occlusion, or trauma may result in compartmental hypertension.

The lower extremity below the knee is most commonly involved. There are four compartments that can be approached either through a single or a double incision. Each approach will be outlined in this section. Fibulectomy fasciotomy, not described in this section, can be found in the references at the end of the section.

Four-Compartment Fasciotomy Through A Single Incision (Fig. 101.1)

Technical Points

Prep the leg circumferentially and drape it in the standard fashion. Make a lateral skin incision overlying the fibula; extend it from the level of the neck of the fibula proximally down to the lateral malleolus. Carry the incision through the skin and subcutaneous tissue down to the fascia encasing the muscles. Identify the lesser saphenous vein and avoid injuring it. The four compartments of the leg will be decompressed through this single incision by the development of skin flaps (Fig. 101.1A).

Incise the skin and subcutaneous tissue on the lateral surface of the leg to expose the fascia encasing the peroneal muscles. Incise the fascia from the head of the fibula down to the lateral malleolus. This decompresses the lateral compartment (Fig. 101.1B).

Undermine the skin flap anteriorly to expose the anterior compartment. Identify the fascia enclosing the anterior compartment. Incise the fascia longitudinally to decompress the compartment. Be careful to avoid damage to the superficial peroneal nerve where it exits between the anterior and lateral compartments in the distal one third of the leg.

Create a posterior skin flap to approach the posterior compartment. Incise the fascia enclosing the posterior compartment to decompress the soleus and gastrocnemius muscles. Take down the attachments of the soleus muscle to the fibula. Retract the soleus and gastrocnemius muscles posteriorly to expose and decompress the deep posterior compartment. Be

LIST OF STRUCTURES

Anterior compartment
Boundaries
  Tibia
  Interosseous membrane
  Fibula
  Anterior intermuscular septum
  Deep fascia
Contents
  Tibialis anterior muscle
  Extensor digitorum longus muscle
  Peroneus tertius muscle
  Extensor hallucis longus muscle
  Deep peroneal nerve
  Anterior tibial artery
Lateral compartment
Boundaries

Anterior intermuscular septum
Fibula
Posterior intermuscular septum
Deep fascia
Contents
  Peroneus longus muscle
  Peroneus brevis muscle
  Common peroneal nerve
  Superficial peroneal nerve
Superficial posterior compartment
Boundaries
  Posterior intermuscular septum
  Transverse crural septum
  Deep fascia
Contents
  Gastrocnemius muscle

Soleus muscle
Plantaris muscle
Deep posterior compartment
Boundaries
  Tibia
  Interosseous membrane
  Fibula
  Transverse crural septum
Contents
  Popliteus muscle
  Flexor hallucis longus muscle
  Flexor digitorum longus muscle
  Tibialis posterior muscle
  Tibial nerve
  Posterior tibial artery
  Peroneal artery

FIGURE 101.1
FOUR-COMPARTMENT FASCIOTOMY THROUGH A SINGLE INCISION

1. Tibialis anterior muscle
2. Extensor hallucis longus muscle
3. Extensor digitorum longus muscle *Anterior tibial artery and deep peroneal nerve

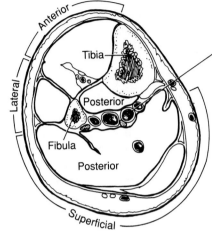

1. Peroneus longus muscle
2. Peroneus brevis muscle
3. Superior peroneal nerve

Popliteus muscle
Tibialis posterior muscle
Flexor hallucis longus muscle
Flexor digitorum longus muscle
Posterior tibial nerve, artery, and vein
Peroneal artery and vein

1. Gastrocnemius muscle
2. Soleus muscle
A 3. Sural nerve

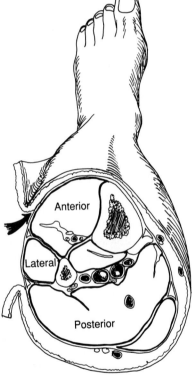

B

careful to avoid injury to the common peroneal and posterior tibial neurovascular trunks when incising the fascia.

The swollen edematous muscles will protrude through the fascial incisions once the compartments are decompressed. Assess the muscles in each compartment for viability. Viable muscle is pink, contracts when stimulated, and bleeds when cut. Cover the exposed muscle fibers with moist gauze to prevent desiccation.

Place loose interrupted nylon sutures through the skin and subcutaneous tissue to approximate the skin edges once the

edema resolves. Sometimes, the muscle will protrude through the incision, preventing secondary approximation of the skin edges. Use a split-thickness skin graft over the muscle when you cannot perform delayed closure of the skin edges.

Anatomic Points

The superficial fascia overlying the lateral aspect of the fibula contains but a few structures of surgical importance. The lesser saphenous vein, which starts on the lateral side of the dorsal venous arch of the foot, passes posterior to the lateral malleolus and peroneal muscle tendons and then ascends for a short distance in the superficial fascia lateral to the calcaneal tendon. It then runs superomedially so that, by mid-calf, it lies in the posterior midline. The point where it pierces the deep fascia can be at the level of the popliteal space or lower. Frequently, comparatively large tributaries connect the lesser and greater saphenous veins, extending diagonally in a superomedial direction from the lesser to the greater saphenous vein. In addition, six or seven perforating veins connect the lesser saphenous vein with the peroneal veins. Typically, the lesser saphenous vein is accompanied by the posterior femoral cutaneous nerve (which provides sensation to the posteromedial thigh, popliteal region, and a variable amount of the posteromedial calf) proximally, and by the sural nerve (which provides sensation to the lower lateral leg and lateral and dorsolateral aspect of the foot) more distally. An incision over the lateral aspect of the leg, extending from the head of the fibula to the lateral malleolus, should avoid these large superficial veins and the major cutaneous nerves.

The four compartments of the leg are formed by the skeletal elements and attached fibrous intermuscular septa. Osteofascial boundaries of the *anterior compartment* include the tibia, interosseous membrane, fibula, anterior intermuscular septum, and deep fascia. Osteofascial boundaries of the *lateral compartment* include the anterior intermuscular septum, fibula, posterior intermuscular septum, and deep fascia. Osteofascial boundaries of the *superficial posterior compartment* are the posterior intermuscular septum, transverse crural septum, and deep fascia. Osteofascial boundaries of the *deep posterior compartment* are the tibia, interosseous membrane, fibula, posterior intermuscular septum, and transverse crural septum.

Although all four compartments of the leg contain muscles, thereby necessitating a neurovascular supply, only three of the four compartments contain major named nerves, and only two of the four contain major named vessels. Contents of the four compartments are described next.

Anterior Compartment. Muscles in the anterior compartment, all of which are involved with dorsiflexion of the foot, include the tibialis anterior, extensor digitorum longus, peroneus tertius, and extensor hallucis longus. They are all innervated by the deep peroneal nerve, a terminal branch of the common peroneal nerve.

The deep peroneal nerve enters the compartment by piercing the anterior intermuscular septum just inferior to the neck of the fibula. It accompanies the anterior tibial vessels, which lie on the interosseous membrane. In addition to supplying all muscles in the anterior compartment and dorsum of the foot, this nerve also provides sensory innervation to the apposing sides of the first and second toes and the first interspace.

The anterior tibial artery, which arises in the lower popliteal region as one of the terminal branches of the popliteal artery, enters the anterior compartment through a gap in the interosseous membrane just inferior to the proximal tibiofibular joint. In its distal course through the anterior compartment, it lies on the interosseous membrane, and through most of its course, it is medial to the deep peroneal nerve. When this artery crosses the ankle joint, it becomes the dorsalis pedis artery.

Lateral Compartment. The only two muscles in the lateral compartment are the peroneus longus and peroneus brevis muscles, both of which are innervated by the superficial peroneal nerve. The superficial peroneal nerve is one of two terminal branches of the common peroneal nerve. This nerve typically arises at the point where the common peroneal nerve pierces the posterior intermuscular septum, at the neck of the fibula, to enter the lateral compartment. The superficial peroneal nerve runs downward, at first lying between the peroneus longus muscle and the fibula, and then passes distally between the two peroneal muscles and the extensor digitorum longus muscle, giving off muscular branches. In the lower third of the leg, it pierces the deep fascia to supply the skin of the lower lateral leg and of the dorsum of the foot, except for the first interspace and adjacent sides of the first two digits.

There are no named arteries in the lateral compartment. The peroneal muscles are supplied by perforating branches of the peroneal artery, which lies in the deep posterior compartment.

Superficial Posterior Compartment. Muscles in the superficial posterior compartment are those plantar flexors that attach to the tuberosity of the calcaneus. These include the gastrocnemius, soleus, and plantaris muscles.

There are no named neurovascular structures in the superficial posterior compartment. The muscles are innervated by branches of the tibial nerve as it passes through the popliteal fossa (although the soleus muscle does receive some innervation from the tibial nerve more distally). Likewise, the primary branches supplying the muscles arise from the popliteal artery, rather than its more distal posterior tibial artery.

Deep Posterior Compartment. Muscles in the deep posterior compartment include the popliteus, flexor hallucis longus, flexor digitorum longus, and tibialis posterior. The latter muscle is basically deep to the two flexors; some clinicians consider it to be a fifth compartment.

The tibial nerve enters this compartment by passing deep to the soleus muscle. Within the posterior compartment, this nerve remains on the deep surface of the transverse crural septum. It is thus superficial to the popliteus muscle, then superficial to the tibialis posterior muscle. Ultimately, it passes posterior to the medial malleolus, between the tendons of the flexor digitorum longus and flexor hallucis longus muscles, to

FIGURE 101.2   (Continued)

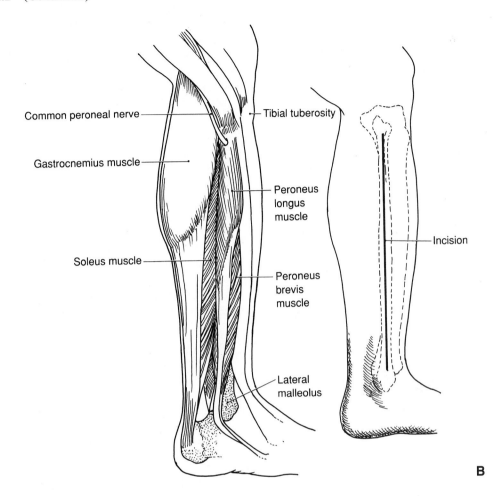

Common peroneal nerve

Gastrocnemius muscle

Soleus muscle

Tibial tuberosity

Peroneus longus muscle

Peroneus brevis muscle

Lateral malleolus

Incision

B

compartment. Decompress the deep posterior compartment by incision of its fascia.

The lateral incision provides access to the lateral and anterior compartments. The incision should extend a distance of 5 to 7 inches along the anterior edge of the fibula. Use Metzenbaum scissors to incise the fascia of the lateral compartment from the knee down to the ankle. Undermine the anterior skin flap to gain exposure to the anterior compartment.

Assess muscle viability in all compartments. Dress the incisions with moistened gauze. Interrupted nylon sutures may be placed through the skin and subcutaneous tissue to approximate the skin edges once the edema resolves.

Anatomic Points

The superficial fascia on the medial side of the leg contains the greater saphenous vein and the accompanying saphenous nerve. The greater saphenous vein starts at the medial end of the dorsal venous arch of the foot and ultimately passes through the saphenous hiatus of the fascia lata to empty into the femoral vein 2 to 3 cm inferior to the inguinal ligament.

In its passage through the superficial fascia of the lower extremity, it passes just anterior to the medial malleolus, then about 8 to 10 cm posterior to the medial side of the patella, and then along the medial side of the thigh to the saphenous hiatus. Its location in the leg can be approximated by a straight line connecting a point on the anterior side of the medial malleolus to a point lying about 10 cm posterior to the medial side of the patella. The saphenous nerve is a branch of the femoral nerve that provides sensation to the medial leg and foot distally to the level of the first metatarsophalangeal joint. As the course of the greater saphenous vein and saphenous nerve lies very close to the medial margin of the tibia, caution should be exercised once the skin has been incised.

Medially, the deep posterior compartment is exposed by splitting fibers of the gastrocnemius and soleus muscles or, alternatively, by detaching soleus muscle fibers from their origin on the middle third of the medial border of the tibia. One should remember that soleus muscle fibers also arise from the soleal line of the tibia, the head and proximal quarter of the fibula, and a fibrous arch superficial to the tibial vessels and nerve.

REFERENCES

1. Finklestein JA, Hunter GA, Hu RW. Lower limb compartment: course after delayed fasciotomy. *J Trauma* 1996;40:342–344.
2. Mabee JR, Bostwick TL. Pathophysiology and mechanisms of compartment syndrome. *Orthop Rev* 1993;22:175–181.
3. Matsen FA, Krugmire RB. Compartmental syndromes. *Surg Gynecol Obstet* 1978;147:943.
4. Mubarak SJ, Owen CA. Double incision fasciotomy of the leg for decompression in compartment syndromes. *J Bone Joint Surg Am* 1977;59:184.
5. Patman RD, Thompson JE. Fasciotomy in peripheral vascular surgery. *Arch Surg* 1970;101:663.
6. Rhodes RS. Compartment syndrome. In: Cameron JL, ed. *Current surgical therapy.* 3rd ed. Philadelphia: BC Decker, 1989:692.
7. Rollins DL, Bernhard VM, Towne JB. Fasciotomy: an appraisal of controversial issues. *Arch Surg* 1981;116:1474. (Presents a clear description of single-incision fasciotomy.)
8. Rorabeck CH. The treatment of compartment syndromes of the leg. *J Bone Joint Surg Br* 1984;66:93.

SUBJECT INDEX